Hand Surgery Update

Hand Surgery Update

Developed by the
American Society for Surgery of the Hand

Published by the
American Academy of Orthopaedic Surgeons
6300 North River Road   Rosemont, IL 60018

Hand Surgery Update

ISBN: 0-89203-150-6
Library of Congress Cataloging-in-Publication Data:
Hand surgery update / American Society for Surgery of the Hand,
    developed by the Hand Surgery Update Committee. — Republished ed.
        p.   cm.
    "A synopsis of important information by established hand surgeons
from recently published articles"—Pref.
    Originally published: Aurora, CO : American Society for Surgery of
the Hand, c1994.
    Includes bibliographical references and index.
    ISBN 0-89203-150-6
    1. Hand—Surgery.   I. American Society for Surgery of the Hand.
Hand Surgery Update Committee.
    [DNLM: 1. Hand—surgery—collected works.   WE 830 H2335 1996a]
RD778.H385   1996
617.5'75059—dc20
DNLM/DLC
for Library of Congress   96-11443
                                                            CIP

Acknowledgments

Hand Surgery Update Committee
Paul R. Manske, MD, Chairman
James R. Doyle, MD
Hill Hastings II, MD
Jesse B. Jupiter, MD
William B. Kleinman, MD
Ralph T. Manktelow, MD
James A. Nunley II, MD
A. Lee Osterman, MD
Clayton A. Peimer, MD
Leonard K. Ruby, MD
Robert C. Russell, MD
Peter J. Stern, MD
Joseph Upton III, MD
Robert L. Wilson, MD
R. Christie Wray, Jr, MD

Contributing Authors and Associate Editors
Richard A. Berger, MD
Allen T. Bishop, MD
Thomas M. Brushart, MD
Glenn A. Buterbaugh, MD
Benjamin E. Cohen, MD
James R. Doyle, MD
Elof Eriksson, MD
Roslyn B. Evans, OTR/L
Paul Feldon, MD
Thomas J. Fischer, MD
Earl J. Fleegler, MD
Louis A. Gilula, MD
Richard D. Goldner, MD
Thomas L. Greene, MD
Douglas P. Hanel, MD
Hill Hastings II, MD
Vincent R. Hentz, MD
Robert N. Hotchkiss, MD
James H. House, MD
Lawrence C. Hurst, MD
Jesse B. Jupiter, MD
Thomas R. Kiefhaber, MD
James M. Kleinert, MD
L. Andrew Koman, MD
John O. Kucan, MD
Terry R. Light, MD
Graham D. Lister, MD
Dean S. Louis, MD
Susan E. Mackinnon, MD
H. Relton McCarroll, Jr, MD
Richard R. McCormack, Jr, MD
James A. Nunley II, MD
A. Lee Osterman, MD
Clayton A. Peimer, MD
Vincent D. Pellegrini, Jr, MD
Leonard K. Ruby, MD
Robert C. Russell, MD
William E. Sanders, MD
Lawrence H. Schneider, MD
Alan E. Seyfer, MD
Peter J. Stern, MD
James W. Strickland, MD
William M. Swartz, MD
Robert M. Szabo, MD
Joseph Upton III, MD
Steven F. Viegas, MD
Andrew J. Weiland, MD
E. F. Shaw Wilgis, MD
Michael B. Wood, MD
R. Christie Wray, Jr, MD
Elvin G. Zook, MD

Credits

We wish to thank the following individuals for contributions to the chapters listed below.

Chapter 7 - Kevin McEnery, MD; Barry Siegel, MD; William Totty, MD; Saara Totterman, MD; Anthony Wilson, MD; Yuming Yin, MD; Mallinckrodt Institute of Radiology and Department of Radiology; Washington University School of Medicine, St. Louis; University of Rochester, New York; Beijing Ji Shu Tan Hospital, Beijing, Peoples Republic of China.

Chapter 11 - Andrew K. Palmer, MD, Professor of Orthopaedic Surgery, State University of New York Health Science Center of Syracuse College of Medicine, Syracuse, New York

Chapter 18 - Michael and Myrtle Baker, Professor and Chairman, Department of Orthopaedics, Pennsylvania State University, Hershey Medical Center

Chapter 19 - Juan Canose, MD

Chapter 27 - Thomas C. Wiener, MD

Chapter 29 - Robert C. Russell, MD, Springfield, IL

Chapter 34 - Owen J. Moy, MD, Buffalo, NY

Chapter 39 - Thomas M. Walsh, MD

Contents

Preface

The field of hand surgery is an ever-changing discipline. In their attempt to maintain an appropriate base of knowledge, students of hand surgery regularly read textbooks and journals, attend CME courses, and listen to colleagues discussing the many aspects of hand surgery. The purpose of the American Society for Surgery of the Hand *1994 Hand Surgery Update* is to present a synopsis of important information by established hand surgeons from recently published articles. The *Hand Surgery Update* text is recommended for residents and fellows, those studying for the CAQ examination in hand surgery, and hand surgeons and physicians as a quick reference to recent information. It is hoped that a new edition of the *Hand Surgery Update* will be published every several years.

I am indebted to Dr. James Urbaniak, former president of the American Society for Surgery of the Hand, whose idea it was to publish such a text, to the hard work of the associate editors whose diligence and prodding kept the project on track to meet the established deadlines, to the numerous hand surgeons who set aside other projects to participate in this one, and to the ASSH Central Office.

The editors dedicate this book to the many hand surgeons who preceded us in establishing a base of information from which we can proceed in furthering the knowledge of hand surgery.

PAUL R. MANSKE, MD
Editor, Hand Surgery Update
June 1994

I

Hand Fractures and Joint Injuries

1

Phalangeal Fractures

Thomas J. Fischer, MD

Introduction

Phalangeal fractures are commonplace and reported incidences have varied. Reports do not include fractures handled before referral to emergency departments, orthopaedic, or hand surgery specialty practices. The quantities of fractures of phalanges are large and present to a variety of practitioners.

This section deals with fracture care of non-articular fractures of the phalanges. Extra-articular fractures of the phalanges can be classified by location in the phalanx; base (proximal metaphysis); shaft (diaphysis); and neck (distal metaphysis). The proximal phalanx (P_1) and the middle phalanx (P_2) share a nearly identical bony shape. The distal phalanx (P_3) has a similar proximal metaphysis (base). P_3 has a unique diaphysis and distal metaphysis (tuft) that anchors a specialized skin structure, the nail plate, and its complex sterile and germinal matrix.

Unique Clinical Issues

Phalangeal fractures are unique in that an isolated fracture can affect the functional unit of the hand and the digit. Digital function can be impaired not only by fracture stability or deformity but equally by concomitant injury to the soft tissues that provide motion, stability, blood flow, and sensation to that digit.

Injury to the soft tissues can be due to direct forces such as crush or sharp laceration, and from indirect forces such as rotation of the digit, terminal impact loading, or various bending forces. Consider the extremes of digital deformity that occur at injuries that tear or crush adjacent structures to the bone. Variations in force magnitude, direction, point of application, and area of contact with the applied force can result in substantially different injury patterns. The fracture pattern, location, and shape only partially determine the treatment. An open, unstable fracture combined with nerve, tendon, and vascular injury must be treated differently than the same fracture pattern in a closed, stable, warm, and sensate digit. Combined soft-tissue injury(ies) may take precedence in deciding the nature of the fracture care. These combined soft-tissue associated lesions influence both the choice of treatment method and the functional outcome. Physical impairment of the functional unit, the digit, easily spills over to adjacent areas and can impair digital performance across the hand, and therefore the functional outcomes of treatment.

Diagnosis

The diagnosis of phalanx fracture is straightforward and is based upon history, physical examination, and radiograph-

ic evaluation. The diagnosis of hidden but significant soft-tissue injuries is more difficult to make and may escape the uninformed or inexperienced practitioner. A history of machine injury, sharp laceration, crush, sport injury, motor-vehicle accident, etc. should be recorded. Knowing the mechanism of injury is important in determining the likelihood of significant associated soft-tissue lesion and in fracture prognosis.

Jupiter and Belsky summarized a fracture classification that allows a basis for the diagnosis of phalangeal fractures.

Table 1-1.

Phalanx	Location	Pattern	Skeleton	Soft Tissue	Reaction to Motion
P (proximal)	Base	Transverse	Simple	Closed	Stable
P_2 (middle)	Shaft	Oblique	Impacted	Open	Unstable
P_3 (distal)	Neck	Spiral	Comminuted		
	Condyle	Avulsion			
	Epiphysis				

With this classification and an accurate inventory of injured soft tissues, fracture management can be discussed and risks and benefits of the treatment plan decided.

Examination

The digit has essential anatomic requirements of length, rotation, and angular alignment that allow for normal functions of pinch, grasp, and hook grasp. Angulation and rotational alignment is determined by comparison of the appearance of the injured digit to the adjacent ones. Assessment of the plane of nailplate alignment is done in digital extension and full flexion. Physical manipulation of the phalanx to assess stability of the fracture and digit deformity may be possible only with digital anesthesia or wrist-block anesthesia to gain sufficient pain control. Anesthesia should be given only after a careful neurologic examination. The ease of closed reduction, the stability of the fracture once reduced, and the "personality" of the fracture are ascertained by manipulation of the digit and its fracture(s).

Inventory of Injured Structures

Thirty percent to 50% of phalangeal fractures are open. The consensus of investigators is that soft-tissue injuries portend a less desirable functional outcome. Unstable open fractures require surgical treatment beyond wound debridement and soft-tissue repair. Significant soft-tissue injury to skin, tendon, nerve, blood vessel, and joint capsule can occur in

50% of open fractures. These have statistically poorer results in total active motion of the digit when compared to open fractures less complicated by soft-tissue injury components. Associated flexor tendon laceration is associated with poor motion outcomes. Nonunion and infection rates are higher in open fractures. Current studies identify the nature of the soft-tissue injury as an indication for clinical outcome, but do not validate the efficacy of treatment methods in preventing poor outcome.

Radiographic Evaluation

Radiographs interpreted without the aid of a clinical examination can give misleading views of the injury. Essential elements of a radiographic evaluation include true AP and true laterals of the affected digit. Splay laterals of the digits in various amounts of flexion to prevent phalangeal override may at best only provide one true lateral of the several digits examined. Care must be taken to ensure that both views are seen on each digit. Radiographic evaluation of the reduced fracture can be done with plain films or video fluoroscopy. Immobilization with synthetic casting tapes or thermoplastic materials for splints facilitates radiographic viewing of the fracture with better clarity than views through plaster. Polytomography is rarely used in diaphyseal injuries to define anatomy and is best used in intra-articular injuries.

Treatment

Treatment plans always must include management of the soft tissues, allowing them to be rehabilitated as fracture stability improves. Implants enhance skeletal stability to withstand the forces of functional aftercare. Indications for operative management include (1) failure of closed reduction to maintain rotation length or angular alignment; (2) intra-articular fracture in which joint congruity is lost, resulting in small joint dysfunction; (3) unstable fractures associated with significant soft-tissue injury in which fracture instability precludes the normal soft-tissue rehabilitation program.

An example of the last indication is an unstable transverse fracture of the proximal phalanx associated with a flexor tendon laceration in zone two. Fractures associated with joint injuries are difficult to rehabilitate when there is soft-tissue injury. Studies by Strickland and Huffaker suggest that less desirable functional outcomes occur when joint or periarticular tissues are injured in the digits. To distinguish periarticular fractures from simpler ones, I will discuss closed and open treatment in the diaphysis separately from similar treatment of the periarticular fracture.

Diaphyseal Injuries

The phalangeal diaphysis is thicker side-to-side than anterior-to-posterior. This increase in radial and ulnar mass is also extended into the soft tissues by the continuation of the osteocutaneous ligaments of Grayson and Cleland. These ligaments anchor onto bone primarily at the mid-portion of the diaphysis, creating a thick band of tissue that creates stability for the fracture when intact. Reduction is difficult when the tip or spike of an oblique or spiral fracture becomes entangled in this stout cord of tissue. Rotational deformity cannot be corrected when this structure is incarcerated in the fracture site. Grossly unstable fractures can result when the osteocutaneous ligaments and flexor and extensor tendon systems are stripped from bone. The balance of forces at the proximal phalanx leads to palmar angulation at the middle phalanx fractures proximal to the FDS insertion and dorsally angulate distal to the FDS insertion. Amounts of comminution vary according to how the magnitude and speed of applied load is absorbed by the cortex. In a closed fracture, the soft-tissue involvement may include the flexor tendon system, as the apex of the fracture angulation may occur at the A_2 or A_4 pulleys. This creates a stenotic deformity of the fibrosseous tunnel that may impede normal flexor tendon excursion. The angulation also creates an effective lengthening of the extensor tendon resulting in an extension lag at the next distal joint, either PIP or DIP.

Unless significantly displaced, long, oblique, and spiral fractures of the diaphysis will prove remarkably stable. When displaced and reduction cannot be readily accomplished, soft-tissue interposition is likely.

Closed Reduction

Closed reduction of phalangeal fractures is readily accomplished with digital nerve block anesthesia. A preferred location for the nerve blockade is infiltration at the level of the metacarpal heads in the palm. This location prevents the further edema and tissue pressures caused by a "ring block" at the level of the web space commissure. Through fracture manipulation the stability can be assessed by the practitioner. Stable, simple gutter splints can protect the fracture from subsequent displacement. Buddy taping to the adjacent digit can provide adequate protection and early assisted motion. Caution must be exercised in the pattern of strapping two digits together; angular forces on the digits may result from the straps that were not present at the time of reduction.

Post-reduction radiographs should be obtained immediately and at three to seven days. Buddy taping or strapping of the digit to the adjacent "well" digit can masquerade as a rotational deformity. Therefore, this method is used to prevent displacement only after adequate reduction is obtained and rotation and angulation are satisfactory. The anesthetized patient can display active composite flexion and extension. Passive flexion can falsely create a "normal" alignment in flexion and should be avoided as it can force the digit to appear of normal rotation. Extending the wrist with the fingers relaxed can create a tenodesis type of finger flexion that can be assessed for rotational malalignment. Immobilization of unstable closed fractures should be continued for three to four weeks.

Strickland and associates showed that digital performance deteriorated when AROM was delayed longer than three weeks. Soft-tissue mobilization can take place with active motion and active motion with blocking techniques. Rapid addition of passive motion and dynamic splinting can take place within four weeks if the fracture is stable. Further delays in mobilizing a stable phalanx because of a tardy radiographic appearance of union have been associated with lowered values for TAM when final results are analyzed. Radiographic appearance of union will lag seven to 10 days behind the clinical appearance of union. Clinical union is manifest by a minimally tender fracture site that is not painful when manipulated and stressed.

Closed Reduction and Percutaneous Fixation

Internal fixation should be considered if the patient's fracture has a loss of reduction; there is comminution; or reduction cannot be held.

Percutaneous fixation can include various implants, from smooth Kirschner wires to absorbable polyglycolic acid pins and percutaneous screw fixation. K-wires can be made to pass across the fracture and affix adjacent cortices or pass intramedullary and act as internal splints that resist bending. In either case, both transverse, short oblique, and spiral fractures are amenable to this treatment if instability persists after closed reduction. Acceptable reduction must be achieved before fixation. Acceptable reduction in the phalanx includes reduction of rotational deformity. Most authors' state that no more than 10° to 15° angular deformity can be accepted. Provisional fixation of the fracture is attained with either traction or a small variety of fracture-reduction clamps. In young, healthy individuals in whom the majority of fractures occur, bone cortex is of sufficient density to require a powered mini-driver. A fresh wire should be used to drill the cortex each time. A drill guide or needle of sufficient inside diameter should be used to guide the pin application. The critical parameters of starting point and pin direction are analyzed and confirmed just as one would line up a billiard shot. Multiple passes perforate and weaken the fracture fragments, embarrass and injure the soft tissue and frustrate the surgeon into accepting a potentially compromised result. Preoperative radiographs and intra-operative fluoroscopy enhance the pin placer's sense of direction as obliquity and dimension of the fracture spikes can be studied.

If a fracture is unstable enough to require an implant, then the minimum requirement for stability is two percutaneous pins unless used as intramedullary devices acting as splints in the isthmus of the phalangeal diaphysis. Once the first pin is in, both cortices engaged, and the fracture clamp still present, a second K-wire is passed across the fracture, usually immediately adjacent to the clamp. Wire should not be placed at the tip of the long oblique or spiral fractures to minimize the risk of iatrogenic comminution. Mid-lateral or mid-axial starting points impale the least amount of mobile flexor and extensor tendons. Distribution of the implants along the fracture site improve overall stability through wider separation of the stability points. Pin placement is a critical step of this technique with regard to starting point, direction, length, and drilling accuracy. Peri-

articular pins usually diminish motion at the DIP and PIP joint levels. The normal, yet minuscule, amount of glide of the collateral ligaments over the condyles and upon their own layered substance is limited. Removal of pins at three to four and one-half weeks allows sufficient time to stretch the scar collagen and maintain good results with maximum joint flexion and extension.

Open Reduction and Internal Fixation

Open reduction of phalangeal fractures may be required to reduce even simple fracture patterns. Hematoma and soft tissue may prevent adequate reduction and are removed by open reduction. Deformity is an indication just as it is for closed reduction. Local exposure may be essential to complete all the steps of reduction. Implants such as plates and screws or intraosseous wire constructs can be applied only with adequate exposure of bone. Plates may provide stability in cases of comminution of fragments or multiple fracture lines that preclude pin fixation. In these instances, plates provide a bridging or spanning function across unstable segments. In other cases multiple fragments may be pulled together by lag-screw fixation through the plate and effect a stable platform to rehabilitate the multiply-injured soft tissues.

Open reduction is considered if closed reduction can be obtained; there may be high-force demands during the soft-tissue rehabilitation; and if there are segmental defects that require bone-graft replacement

Internal fixation that requires an open approach includes (1) multiple intrafragmentary screw fixation; (2) interosseous wire technique (Lister, Ninety-ninety, tension band, sidewinder technique Green/Belsole); (3) plate fixation technique (tension-band plate, lag screw and plate, neutralization plate, buttress plate, spanning plate); and use of (4) intramedullary fixation devices other than K-wires.

Open reduction does not logically proceed to plate fixation. All of the above fixation techniques can be used. In this way difficult clinical problems can be overcome to provide the stability and care needed for the problems identified during examination and diagnosis of the phalanx fracture. Each technique has technical considerations, tricks, traps, and pitfalls that are learned. The surgeon who applies these more complex implants can reach levels of finesse and speed that are enjoyed in most applications of K-wires. The technical ability to apply an implant to bone does not determine the indications for open reduction.

The proximal and middle phalanx can be approached through either a mid-line dorsal skin incision or a mid-axial incision. In the case of the dorsal approach the tendon splitting incision can be central or parasagittal in the interval between central tendon and lateral band. Dorsal skin incisions with tendon approaches that elevate the lateral bands or divide the lateral bands are also possible. Advantages to mid-axial "lateral" approaches and implant placement may include a better gliding surface for the sensitive and low amplitude extensor tendon excursion. Bulky implants placed beneath the extensor tendon may impede normal excursion because of their bulk. Clinical comparisons of the two methods of plate placement, dorsal and lateral, are lacking because implants for lateral placement have only recently been available and widely popularized.

Implants with screw diameter below 2.0mm are acceptable in size and bulk for most phalanx fractures. The middle phalanx sustains implants with l.5mm screw diameter. Wire fixation can be larger for intramedullary devices .054 in or 1.25mm. For interosseous wire techniques, generally .045 in or .035 in wires are used in conjunction with 24-gauge to 28-gauge soft annealed or spooled wire. The type of implant is less important in the fracture care than the indication and the postoperative rehabilitation program. Several studies have demonstrated that adequate strength is obtained with a variety of implants when applied well, as tested in three- and four-point bending. How much fracture stability is needed beyond that provided by the time-tested methods of K-wire fixation is open to question. No good measure has been discovered in biomechanical investigations.

In cases of loss of cortical substance, open reduction can provide length preservation. In addition, grossly comminuted or nonviable shards of dense cortical bone that do not contribute to stability because of size or shape can be excised and replaced by corticocancellous grafts. Grafts and plates can provide immediate stability and rapid reconstitution of bone substance. Functional aftercare for a fracture mechanism that created the substance loss will not be delayed.

External Fixation

External fixation of small bones is achieved by simple constructs of K-wires fixing and reinforcing and methyl methacrylate bars spanning the phalanx. Sophisticated and well-engineered "mini" fixation systems are available. Well-designed external fixation systems for facial fractures have also been added to the devices available.

Indications for external fixation of phalangeal diaphysis fractures include gross comminution with accompanying injury to the soft-tissue envelope extensor, soft-tissue injury in which further open dissection may compromise bone or digit viability, and a segmental defect in which digital length needs to be preserved and formal ORIF delayed. External devices can provide temporary stability until the soft-tissue envelope is restored and other fracture care is possible. Fixators are small enough to allow adjacent digits rather uninhibited AROM/PROM. Apex palmar angulation occurs in fractures of the proximal phalanx treated with external fixation as reported by Parsons.

Periarticular Fractures

The indications for closed reduction of periarticular fractures are similar to those for diaphysis fractures. Special considerations exist because the size of the metaphyseal fragment may preclude manipulative reduction. Risk of adjacent joint stiffness is high.

Subcondylar fractures of the phalanx are a good example. Because a direct hold on the fragment cannot be achieved, manipulation of the joint and the collateral ligaments con-trol the fragment. An adverse position of the joint may be required.

The position needed to reduce and hold the small fragment angle results in excessive flexion of the joint. In the event of a periarticular transmetaphyseal extra-articular fracture of the base of the proximal phalanx, the reduction may not be achieved by closed means. The collateral ligaments are in a palmar position and may not tighten sufficiently in the normal flexion arc of MP flexion during reduction. The digit needs flexion through the fracture to achieve reduction, and if impacted, this may not occur as the joint flexes.

Subcondylar fractures of the phalanx can rotate just as supracondylar fractures of the humerus. The subcondylar volar recess beneath the condyles narrows the anteroposterior diameter of the bone and provides a narrow surface for the fracture to inter-digitate and demonstrate reduction. True lateral and AP radiographs, as well as clinical experience, are necessary to detect malrotation. Little is written about closed treatment of periarticular fractures of the phalanx. The most common pattern is that of the apex palmar proximal P_1 metaphyseal fracture in the child or adolescent. The deformity is easily compensated by growth, and bone remodeling readily occurs in the plane of joint motion. Twenty degrees to 30° of angulation in the base of the growing child under 10 years of age is acceptable. In the adult, that amount of angulation will diminish the P_1 arc of flexion and diminish full fist making.

As the small periarticular fracture fragments are difficult to control in the proximal and distal portions of the phalanx pin, fixation is common. Crossed K-wires from the margins of the condyles and bases provide the control necessary to achieve anatomic reduction. Soft tissues are impaled by these percutaneous pins. Little PIP motion is obtained in the typical P_1 subcondylar fracture fixed with pins while the pins are in place. This problem results in little functional loss in the simple fracture as rehabilitation can start when the fracture is healed. In the injury in which substantial soft-tissue injury occurs, other methods may be necessary to achieve both stability and motion. Eaton/Belsky percutaneous intramedullary wires provide good fixation and are easily applied in the treatment of a proximal metaphyseal fracture. The starting point can be across the metacarpal head and into the base of the reduced phalanx. An alternative is placement of the pin alongside the metacarpal head and into the marginal base of P_1 at a slight centrally converging angle. With this method the MP joint is kept flexed. Pin sites are cleaned and kept immobile while PIP active motion is started. These pins by nature of the starting point provide control of the basilar fracture that otherwise could resume a deformed position due to dorsal cortical comminution or impaction.

Open Reduction and Internal Fixation

Accurate reduction or adequate implant application may be achieved in periarticular fractures only by open reduction. Comminution, impaction, or other displacements may have the same effect on final digit performance. Logically, extra-articular fractures about the joint involve more complex soft-tissue relations. Periarticular fractures are also found to result in final motion with smaller TAM. Studies have yet to conclude whether malunion or iatrogenic influences on periarticular tissues are more important in determining TAM; both are important factors in fracture care.

A unique situation exists when a long spike of phalanx proximal fragment is displaced, shortened, and protrudes into the subcondylar recess of the PIP joint. This mechanical encroachment by a fracture fragment into the periarticular tissues creates a mechanical block to flexion. The alignment and rotation of the phalanx are normal, yet the middle phalanx cannot flex into the palmar subcondylar recess and flexion is permanently restricted.

Minicondylar plates and interosseous wiring techniques provide implants that have low profile, small bulk, and adequate fixation in cancellous bone. These implants extend the abilities of the fracture surgeon to provide a stable platform to rehabilitate the adjacent interphalangeal or metacarpophalangeal joint.

External Fixation

As in the case of the small external fixator applied for diaphyseal fractures, the periarticular fracture that requires external fixation is uncommon. Fixators are usually applied across the joint to provide stable positioning or distraction to these small periarticular metaphyseal fragments.

Complications

Recent reviews indicate that antibiotic use for prophylaxis against subsequent deep infection have not proved efficacious for preventing infection. Studies stressed the importance of removal of nonviable tissues or marginally viable tissues. In open fractures the length of time less than 16 hours from injury to treatment does not alter infection rates. Staphylococcus aureus continues to be the most commonly isolated infecting pathogen; yet wound cultures obtained at the time of injury do not recover this pathogen.

Wounds are characterized by grading systems modified from long-bone open fracture analysis. More "severe" wounds associated with larger wound size, untidy laceration, soft-tissue crush, periosteal stripping, blast injuries, gross wound contamination, and all farm injuries are associated with both higher infection rates and lower values for TAM. Whether the infection or the initial injury is the major determinant of poor outcome has yet to be established. Uninfected cases with the more severe type III wounds have poor results when measured by final TAM.

Annotated Bibliography

Open Fracture Infections

McLain RF, Steyers C, Stoddard M: Infections in open fractures of the hand. *J Hand Surg,* 16A:108-112, 1991.

One hundred forty-six injured hands were classified according to five factors: 1) injury mechanism; 2) injury pattern; 3) fracture type; 4) contamination; and 5) treatment delay. Two hundred sixteen phalangeal fractures were treated. There was an infection rate of 11%. All infections occurred in untidy/crush lacerations. Infections determined poor results as did type of open fracture.

Suprock MD, Hood JM, Lubahn JD: Role of antibiotics in open fractures of the finger. *J Hand Surg,* 15A: 761-64, 1990.

A two-year randomized study of open finger fractures treated prophylactically with antibiotics or not. Digital ischemia was excluded. Antibiotics were of no benefit in reducing the incidence of infection in fractured digits that were viable and surgically debrided.

Biomechanics

Hung LK, So WS, Leung PC: Combined intramedullary Kirschner wire and intra-osseous wire loop for fixation of finger fractures. *J Hand Surg,* 14B:171-176, 1989.

Crossed K-wires failed in flexion with greater deformation than plates, looped wire, or looped wire and K-wire fixed in phalanges. An intramedullary wire combined with loop wire fixation is appropriate for transverse or short oblique fractures.

Nunley JA, Kloen P: Biomechanical and functional testing of plate fixation devices for proximal phalangeal fractures. *J Hand Surg,* 16A:991-998, 1991.

Transverse P_1 fractures were experimentally treated with H plates, straight plates, and mini-condylar plates. Constructs were tested with loads and stress/ strain was measured. Lateral applied mini-condylar plates created less reduction of simulated PIP motion and gave greater strength to simulated loads.

Nonunion

Wray RC, Glunk R: Treatment of delayed union, nonunion and malunion of the phalanges of the hand. *Ann Plast Surg,* 22:14-18, 1989.

Delayed union, nonunion, and malunions were treated with secondary open reduction and internal fixation. Significant gains in TAM and correction of deformity were uniformly seen.

Pediatric

Savage R: Complete detachment of the epiphysis of the distal phalanx. *J Hand Surg,* 15B: 126-128, 1990.

Epiphyseal fractures can be combined with complete soft-tissue detachment from the epiphysis rendering the epiphysis a free fragment.

Surgical Approach

Field LD, Freeland AE, Jabaley ME: Mid-axial approach to the proximal phalanx for fracture fixation. *Contemp Orthop,* 25:133-137, 1992.

A review of the anatomy and technique of phalangeal exposure through a mid-axial approach is presented. Discussion of the technical details of exposure and soft-tissue treatments is excellent.

Soft-tissue Complications

Banerjee A: Irreducible distal phalangeal epiphyseal injuries. *J Hand Surg,* 17B:337-338, 1992.

Soft tissues can create a tongue of tissue that interposes itself into the fracture site. In this case it is a distal phalanx growth-plate separation and a nail fold.

Harryman DT, Jordan TF: Physeal phalangeal fracture with flexor tendon entrapment. *Clin Orthop,* 250:194-196, 1990.

Case report of flexor tendon involvement in fracture site causing irreducible fracture. Review of literature involving growth-plate fractures and soft-tissue complications.

Sanger JR, Buebendorf ND, Matloub HS, Yousif NJ: Proximal phalangeal fracture after tendon pulley reconstruction. *J Hand Surg,* 15A:976-979, 1990.

Case report of bone resorption and pathologic fracture with consideration of cortical circulation. Emphasizes relationship of soft tissues to bone blood supply.

Open Reduction and Internal Fixation

Ford DJ, El-Hadidi S, Lunn PG, Burke FD: Fractures of the phalanges: results of internal fixation using l.5mm and 2mm A.O. screws. *J Hand Surg,* 12B:28-33, 1987.

Screw fixation in 36 patients with unstable articular and extra-articular fracture is 90% satisfactory when measured with TAM.

Freeland AE, Roberts TS: Percutaneous screw treatment of spiral oblique finger proximal phalangeal fractures. *Orthopaedics,* 14:385-386, 1991.

Discussion and description of technique of percutaneous screw application to long spiral fracture of P_1. Limited incisional exposure through a mid-axial incision is described resulting in stable fixation in one case.

Greene TL, Noellert RC, Belsole RJ, Simpson LA: Composite wiring of metacarpal and phalangeal fractures. *J Hand Surg,* 14A:665-669, 1989.

Twenty-one phalangeal fractures in a cohort of 63 hand fractures were treated with composite wiring. Technique and clinical outcomes were detailed for phalanx fractures. Nerve vessel and tendon injury portend a lesser result.

Hastings H: Unstable metacarpal and phalangeal fracture treatment with screws and plates. *Clin Orthop,* 214:37-52, 1987.

Comprehensive review with emphasis on clinical and technical considerations in applying screw and plate implants to bone.

Zimmerman NB, Weiland AJ: Ninety-ninety intraosseous wiring for internal fixation of the digital skeleton. *Orthopaedics,* 12:99-104, 1989.

Excellent description of intraosseous wiring using a bi-plane configuration—"ninety-ninety" wiring technique. One hundred fifty

applications in four years in a variety of transverse bone fixations have resulted in excellent union, low complications, and consistent technical applications.

Intramedullary Nails

Varela CD, Carr JB: Closed intramedullary pinning of metacarpal and phalanx fractures. *Operative Tech,* 13:213-215, 1990.

Description of Hall technique for closed intra-medullary Kirschner wire fixation of proximal phalanx fractures. Technique only; no clinical outcome.

External Fixation

Parsons SW, Fitzgerald JAW, Shearer JR: External fixation of unstable metacarpal and phalangeal fractures. *J Hand Surg,* 17B:151-155, 1992.

Fourteen of 37 fractures treated by external fixation were phalangeal. Early active motion was used with 4.5 weeks of fixation. Two malunions of proximal phalangeal fractures were noted. The difficult and uncommon nature of these fractures was noted. Eighty-five percent had good to excellent results.

Shehadi SI: External fixation of metacarpal and phalangeal fractures. *J Hand Surg,* 16A:544-550, 1991.

Series of metacarpal and phalangeal fractures. Thirty fractures reported; 11 were phalangeal fractures. Methylmethacrylate bars and Kirschner wires were used on middle and proximal phalanges; only four were extra-articular. Eighty-four percent TAM seen postoperatively.

Solinas S, Affanni M: Traitement des fractures des phalanges des doigts avec mini fixateur externe. *Acla Ortho Belgica,* 55:573-580, 1989.

Twenty fractures of phalanges were treated with a specific external fixator. Immediate motion was used when soft-tissue injury allowed. Good results reported in difficult cases without mention of TAM.

Closed Reduction

Maitra A, Burdett-Smith P: The conservative management of proximal phalangeal fractures of the hand in an accident and emergency department. *J Hand Surg,* 17B:332-336, 1992.

Of 2,000 hand fractures, one-fourth were of the phalanx, two-thirds were of the proximal phalanx. Simple fracture care in simple situations can result in good to excellent results in 95.7% of selected fractures.

Open Fractures—Epidemiology

Chow SP, Pun WK, et al: A prospective study of 245 open digital fractures of the hand. *J Hand Surg,* 16B:137-140, 1991.

Prospective study demonstrating that concomitant soft-tissue injuries determine functional outcome (TAM). Flexor tendon injuries in open fractures give significantly poorer results than other associated injuries. Well-controlled indications for treatment and analysis of injuries.

Davis TRC, Stothard J: Why all finger fractures should be referred to a hand surgery service: a prospective study of primary management. *J Hand Surg,* 15B:299-302, 1990.

Six hundred eighty-seven fractures and dislocations were seen in the emergency room. Fifty-four were referred to the hand service primarily. Six hundred twenty-four fractures were treated in the emergency room and referred later. Eighty-two percent had correct diagnosis by radiograph. Twenty-five percent of emergency-room care was deemed unsatisfactory and was altered.

Pun WK, Chow SP, Luk KDK, Chan KC: A prospective study on 284 digital fractures of the hand. *J Hand Surg,* 14A:474-481, 1989.

Displaced fractures are not necessarily unstable and require internal fixation. One in five fractures treated required further

surgical intervention. Skin maceration led to failure of the splint program.

Swanson TV, Szabo RM, Anderson DD: Open hand fractures: prognosis and classification. *J Hand Surg,* 16A:101-107, 1991.

Two hundred open fractures of the metacarpals and phalanges were evaluated for complications. Wound type and general health of the patient has more of a predictive value for complication. Internal fixation demonstrated no increased incidence of wound infection.

2

Metacarpal Fractures

Thomas L. Greene, MD

Introduction

Metacarpal fractures account for as much as 36% of all fractures of the hand. Developments and refinements in both the techniques and devices utilized for the evaluation and treatment of these common injuries continue to help define the specific indications for each method available.

Biomechanics

The point configuration of Kirschner wires and the speed (revolutions per minute) of rotation by the wire driver have demonstrable effects on the load required for insertion and on peak pull out load. Trochar, diamond, and cut-tip wires penetrate cortical bone differently. The trochar point wire produces a hole with the best circumferential fit with bone and the cut-tip wire produces an irregular hole larger than the pin diameter. Insertion at high drill speed (800 rpm) as compared to low drill speed (400 rpm) results in less peak axial loads being reached on cortical entry for diamond and cut-tip wires but not for trochar point wires. Higher drill speeds result in significantly lower pull-out force required for all point types. The trochar point wires inserted at 400 rpm have improved immediate pull-out strength (111.3 N ± 36.9 N) that is significantly different than both the diamond point wires (40.5 N ± 26.7 N) and the cut point wires (7.1 N ± 5.8 N). *In vivo* placement of these wire types in canine metacarpals demonstrates comparable holding ability for the trochar wires (110.4 N ± 30.3 N) and the diamond point wires (117.0 N ± 37.8 N). Both of these point configurations were superior to the cut-tip point wires (55.2 N ± 28.9 N). No noticeable adverse effects associated with thermal necrosis of bone could be ascribed to higher speed insertion or peak load at entry.

Three-point apex dorsal bending and torsional loading of simulated transverse metacarpal fractures have demonstrated the rigidity of fixation to be comparable for dorsal quarter tubular plates applied with 2.7mm screws, with or without an interfragmentary screw. Statistically significant greater values for rigidity in bending and torsion were obtained for the plating techniques as compared to crossed K-wires, intraosseous wire and K-wire combination, or a single intraosseous wire, and were four to six times greater. Maximum bending moments were not improved by the addition of an interfragmentary screw.

Fifth Metacarpal Neck (Boxer's) Fracture

Fractures of the fifth metacarpal neck account for approximately 20% of all fractures in the hand. These fractures are typically seen in young males involved in punching activi-

ties. Treatment recommendations vary from immediate mobilization without splinting to open reduction and internal fixation. The indications for a specific treatment method are not clear-cut. Several large series of Boxer's fractures reviewed retrospectively have addressed the issues of functional outcome and residual deformity and symptoms as they relate to residual angular deformity.

There is universal agreement that rotational deformity is not acceptable and must be corrected initially, as it is directly responsible for residual functional and cosmetic problems. Angular deformity up to 70° has not been associated with functional loss, including residual extensor lag at the metacarpophalangeal joint. There is no demonstrable correlation between the degree of residual angulation and persistent symptoms of pain, disability, grip strength, range of motion, or clinical deformity in patients treated by immediate mobilization without splinting, simple splinting techniques, or more elaborate methods of external immobilization.

Patients treated by immediate motion have had the earliest return to full mobility and functional use of the hand. In a comparison of closed treatment (with or without reduction and splinting) and operative repair (with either closed or open reduction and pinning), all patients had a good functional and cosmetic result without long-term pain or dissatisfaction. Although residual dorsal angulation was less in the operatively treated group, it was at the expense of a longer rehabilitation time and greater cost. A residual extensor lag was more likely in the operative group. It would appear that the only deformity that must be treated is rotational and all other fractures can be treated by immediate active motion without deleterious consequences. Splinting should be used for a brief time, if at all, for pain relief. The cost effectiveness of this nonoperative approach is obvious.

Diaphyseal Fractures: Nonoperative Treatment

Closed treatment of closed diaphyseal metacarpal fractures, particularly of a single metacarpal, is satisfactory for the vast majority of these injuries. Closed reduction followed by external immobilization, in a cast or splint that includes the wrist and one or more digits, is the typical technique employed. The use of a functional cast applied only to the hand, leaving the wrist and digits completely free to allow for active motion, has been demonstrated to maintain reduction, allow earlier return to work and activity, and produce less residual wrist and digital stiffness than fractures treated with more traditional immobilization of the wrist and digits. The patients treated with the functional cast returned to work in one-third the time of the more extensive cast-treated group. Although normal grip strength was achieved by both groups at three months after injury, this goal was achieved faster in the functional cast group. No instances of skin necrosis were encountered in either group.

A functional brace that applies three-point fixation to a fractured metacarpal has been developed that aids both in reduction and immobilization. The brace is adjustable to provide for one pad over the apex of the fracture deformity and two pads, one proximal and one distal, over the bone at the open angle of the fracture. It can be applied to either apex dorsal or apex volar fracture configurations. Although the brace permits motion of the wrist and digits, patients are advised to avoid heavy labor and lifting. The patient can adjust the brace to optimize the fit and comfort as swelling subsides. Very little force is needed to maintain reduction. Residual angular deformity averaged 15° in a group of patients with fractures of the second, third, fourth, or fifth metacarpals treated in the brace as compared to 31° in a group treated with an ulnar gutter splint. The brace-treated patients were generally more pleased with the level of comfort and ability to function during treatment. No comparative evaluation was made of functional outcome. The initial report did not note any skin problems related to the use of this brace. Three cases of skin necrosis encountered in the use of this functional brace led other investigators to evaluate the amount of force developed beneath the dorsal pad. With the brace fitted snugly but comfortably, pressure measurements were an average of 260mm of mercury, an amount well in excess of that required to produce necrosis of skin (100mm Hg for six hours). Subsequent splint modifications may obviate this serious complication.

Diaphyseal Fractures: Operative Treatment

The development of plates and screws and wiring techniques applicable to metacarpal fractures has achieved the goal of open repair of fractures. They provide stable fixation of the fracture, which permits early mobilization of the entire hand and prevents the complications of joint stiffness, tendon adherence, malunion, and nonunion. The indications for open repair are the inability to obtain or maintain a satisfactory closed reduction, open fracture with displacement, displaced intra-articular fracture, replantation, multiple fractures, and severe soft-tissue injury requiring stable fixation to facilitate treatment of the soft tissues. The guiding principle in the management of metacarpal fractures is to use the least invasive method that produces a predictably satisfactory result. The indications for open repair are relative in some circumstances. This is particularly true with regard to the use of closed reduction and percutaneous pinning techniques, which are suitable for isolated displaced fractures.

Percutaneous pin fixation may be achieved directly by pinning at the fracture site or remotely by fixation to an adjacent intact metacarpal or by multiple intramedullary pre-bent blunted 0.045 in diameter K-wires or specially designed curved 0.8mm rods. The latter two methods utilize principles as originally espoused by Rush, Ender, and Pankovich for the treatment of major long-bone fractures.

Metacarpal fractures that are noncomminuted and are either transverse or short oblique are particularly suited to the intramedullary techniques. The insertion site is selected at the farthest distance from the fracture site. If the insertion site needs to be distal, the extensor tendon is split in order to place the insertion site at the metacarpal neck. A small opening in the cortex is made with a drill or bur and a sufficient number of pins are pushed into the canal under image intensification control until it is snugly packed. The pins are then cut short or may be buried within the metaphysis. External support is recommended in the form of a dorsal splint that allows digital motion while maintaining a safe position of posture. The intramedullary technique has been especially useful in the fracture management of the noncompliant patient. A review of 91 displaced hand fractures treated with this technique reported no infections or malunions and only one nonunion.

Many methods of internal fixation of metacarpal fractures have been used, but the underlying objective of providing stable fixation remains the same. Biomechanical studies comparing various fixation devices have shown that simple K-wire fixation and intraosseous wiring with or without additional K-wire fixation do not provide sufficient stability to obviate the need for continued external support. The use of additional external immobilization in these circumstances may contribute to increased stiffness of the hand. Quarter tubular plates and 2.7mm screws have become standard for internal fixation of metacarpal fractures. Occasionally 2.0mm screws and accompanying plates may be necessary if the fracture fragments are small. Interfragmentary screw fixation is suited for long oblique and spiral fractures. Composite wiring techniques, using 0.045 in Kirschner pins and 26-gauge wire loops incorporated about them, compare favorably to plates and screws mechanically; they may be more applicable for treatment of comminuted fractures with small fragments. The effect of any of these techniques at the fracture site is to create interfragmentary compression which enhances stability of the fracture/fixation construct and promotes bone healing. This achieves the goals of open fracture repair of early return of function and primary bone healing.

The results of treating metacarpal fractures with open reduction and stable internal fixation have been uniformly excellent when uncomplicated by extensive soft-tissue injury or loss. Attention to detail and precise operative technique are required, especially when using the small plates and screws. The surgeon is often afforded only one opportunity to correctly drill, tap, and insert the screws; there is little margin for error. Fixation of small fragments with screws may also result in further fracture when the diameter of a tapped hole is more than one-third of the width or diameter of the fragment. Complications related to fracture union are usually the result of inadequate surgical techniques. The fixation may require subsequent removal if an adventitial bursitis develops.

The minicondylar plates have been developed for fixation of periarticular fractures of the metacarpal and phalanges. The 2.0mm blade plate is inserted in the dorsal or lateral aspect of the distal metacarpals. The device has applicability for special situations where stable fixation is needed to allow for early unrestricted motion of intact or partially damaged tendons or joints at risk for stiffness, or for early active or passive motion of divided tendons that are repaired. Contraindications to its use are open epiphysis and a joint fragment narrower than 6mm. As with any metaphyseal blade-plate device, a stable buttress of bone is required opposite the plate and on the compression (palmar) side of the metaphysis. Replacement of lost bone is required when using this device in order to achieve stability. The precise insertion of this device is technically demanding and the surgeon who uses it must carefully practice the technique in a laboratory setting before using it clinically.

An expandable intramedullary device has been applied to transverse and short oblique metacarpal fractures. The device is inserted in a collapsed state and expanded when completely inserted within the canal. Stable fixation has been achieved by contact of the expanded device on the inner cortical surface. Special reamers and templates are used to prepare the intramedullary canal and ensure proper sizing of the device. Rotational stability is difficult to obtain and requires augmentation with a K-wire inserted diagonally across the fracture. Splinting of the hand for six weeks is suggested. The device is inferior to plates and screws on preliminary biomechanical testing.

External Fixation

The use of external fixation for fractures has traditionally been reserved for open injuries with associated soft-tissue or bone loss. Two methods of obtaining external fixation have found clinical applications in the hand. One technique uses commercially manufactured devices (eg., mini-external fixator) consisting of threaded half pins in the bone and connecting rods and clamps. The other uses smooth 0.045 in diameter K-wires, typically in a half-frame configuration, connected with a methylmethacrylate bar. External fixation of both open and closed metacarpal fractures has been shown to be a predictably successful method of treatment. Closed reduction is usually performed after insertion of the pins in locations that avoid interference with tendons

or muscles. An advantage of the commercial devices is the ability to modify fracture alignment during the course of treatment. The average duration of treatment in the external fixator has been one month. Nearly all patients can be expected to recover normal range of joint motion. Mild residual angular deformity occurs among approximately 10% of patients. As anticipated, pin-tract inflammation occurs approximately 10% of the time. A disadvantage of this technique has been the bulk and prominence of the device. Failure of the fixation occurs in up to 10% of cases, usually as a result of a fall onto the hand or inadequate tightening of the clamps.

Fractures in Children

The incidence of fractures of the metacarpal in children under age 12 is 4.7 per 10,000 children. Thirty-six percent of hand fractures involve the metacarpals with the fifth being predominant. A fall on the hand accounts for 37% of fractures and sports and fight injuries account for 45%. Most of the fractures are of the greenstick variety and occur near the epiphysis. Displacement or angulation requiring correction is unusual and is present in only 8.8% of all hand fractures seen, including the phalanges.

Fractures of the epiphysis are uncommon, but when present they occur typically in the second, third, or fourth metacarpals and are the result of a direct axial blow. Growth disturbance may occur in non-displaced Salter II type fractures. Accurate restoration of displaced Salter III and IV type fractures must be achieved. One should be cautious regarding the prognosis for any physeal injury, particularly when the middle three metacarpals are involved.

Delayed union and nonunion of metacarpal fractures in children are rare. The common precursors to the development of these problems has been an associated extensive soft-tissue injury and/or an open fracture. Inadequate early immobilization of the fracture may also contribute to problems with union. Open reduction and bone grafting have been successful for the nonunions with deformity. Observation of a stable nonunion without deformity can result in eventual union after several months.

Annotated Bibliography

Biomechanics

Namba RS, Kabo JM, Meals, RA: Bio-mechanical effects of point configuration in Kirschner-wire fixation. *Clin Orthop Rel Res,* 214:19-22, 1987.

The effects of wire-point configuration and speed of insertion on peak load at cortical entry and force required for pull-out were studied. Lower drill speed (400 rpm) and a trochar point-wire required the greatest pull-out force and created the most uniform hole geometry.

Mann RJ, Black D, Constine R, Daniels AU: A quantitative comparison of metacarpal fracture stability with five different methods of internal fixation. *J Hand Surg,* 10A:1024-1028, 1985.

Apex dorsal three-point bending of transverse metacarpal osteotomies internally fixed by several techniques demonstrated superior rigidity for quarter tubular plates and screws than for Kirschner wires, intraosseous wire with K-wire or a single intraosseous wire. The addition of an interfragmentary screw did not improve the rigidity.

Metacarpal Neck Fractures

Lowdon IMR: Fractures of the neck of the little metacarpal. *Injury,* 17:189-192, 1986.

An evaluation of 57 patients with fifth-metacarpal neck fractures were treated with manipulation and a volar plaster slab. Reduction was not maintained. No definite relationship between the presence of symptoms and residual angulation was demonstrated.

McKerrell J, Bowen V, Johnston G, Zondervan J: Boxer's fracture - conservative or operative management. *J Trauma,* 27:486-490, 1987.

Twenty-five patients treated by a variety of conservative means were compared to 15 patients treated with either closed or open pinning. The conservative group had less extensor lag at follow-up. The residual angulation in the operative group was less but there was a longer rehabilitation time.

Ford DJ, Ali MS, Steel WM: Fractures of the fifth metacarpal neck: is reduction or immobilization necessary? *J Hand Surg,* 14B:165-167, 1989.

Sixty-two patients were treated with immediate mobilization without regard to angular deformity. Recovery was rapid with no long-term functional restriction with residual deformity of up to 70° noted. Fourteen percent of patients were aware of a deformity.

Metacarpal Diaphyseal Fractures

Buchler U, Fischer T: Use of a minicondylar plate for metacarpal and phalangeal periarticular injuries. *Clin Orthop Rel Res,* 214:53-58, 1987.

This specially-designed blade plate has been used for fractures close to the MP joint provided the head fragment is at least 6mm thick. A stable metaphyseal buttress is required. The 2.0mm plate and screws are used for the metacarpal head.

Konradsen L, Nielsen PT, Albrecht-Beste E: Functional treatment of metacarpal fractures: 100 randomized cases with or without fixation. *Acta Orthop Scand,* 61:531-534, 1990.

For the treatment of metaphyseal and diaphyseal fractures of the second through fifth metacarpal, a functional cast applied only to the hand with the wrist and digits free was found to prevent loss of reduction better and allow earlier return to full function than a more extensive cast that included the wrist and digits.

Viegas SF, Tencer A, Woodard P, Williams CR: Functional bracing of fractures of the second through fifth metacarpals. *J Hand Surg,* 12:139-143, 1987.

A three-point fixation brace was used to reduce and immobilize fractures of the second through fifth metacarpals. Less residual angulation was noted than for fractures treated by conventional splints. No complications were noted.

Geiger KR, Karpman RR: Necrosis of the skin over the metacarpal as a result of functional fracture-bracing. *J Bone Joint Surg,* 71A:1199-1202, 1989.

Three patients had skin necrosis beneath the dorsal pad of the Galveston brace. Pressures of an average 260mm Hg were noted beneath the dorsal pad in volunteers with a comfortably fitting brace, far in excess of the amount needed to cause skin necrosis.

Varela CD, Carr JB: Closed intramedullary pinning of metacarpal and phalanx fractures. *Operative Tech,* 13:213-215, 1990.

A technique similar to the Hall technique is described using pre-curved blunted 0.045 in K-wires stacked in the canal of the metacarpals. External splinting was used, maintaining a safe position but allowing digital flexion.

Dabezies EJ, Schutte JP: Fixation of metacarpal and phalangeal fractures with miniature plates and screws. *J Hand Surg,* 11A:283-288, 1986.

Twenty-seven patients in this series had metacarpal fractures treated with plates and screws that allowed early active motion of the hand. They achieved 97% of normal motion at follow-up. Motion was restricted in only one patient and no other complications were noted.

Greene TL, Noellert RC, Belsole RJ, Simpson LA: Composite wiring of metacarpal and phalangeal fractures. *J Hand Surg,* 14A:665-669, 1989.

Thirty-three metacarpal fractures were treated with combinations of 0.045 in Kirschner pins and 26-gauge wire loops tightened about the pins followed by early active motion. All but one patient achieved normal active motion; there were no other complications.

Stern PJ, Wieser MJ, Reilly DG: Complications of plate fixation in the hand skeleton. *Clin Orthop Rel Res,* 214:59-65, 1987.

Twenty-nine plates were applied to the metacarpals for acute fractures and late reconstruction. Complications included angular or rotational deformity, nonunion, and stiffness. Complications occurred in 42% of the reconstructions and 29% of the acute fractures. The small margin for error in the surgical technique is emphasized.

Lewis, RC, Nordyke M, Duncan K: Expandable intramedullary device for treatment of fractures in the hand. *Clin Orthop Rel Res,* 214:85-92, 1987.

A unique device implanted within the canal of the metacarpal for transverse and short oblique fractures has been developed. Problems with rotational control require the use of an additional oblique K-wire. External immobilization is also recommended.

Schuind F, Donkerwolcke, Burny F: External mini-fixation for treatment of closed fractures of the metacarpal bones. *J Orthop Trauma,* 5:146-152, 1991.

Sixty-three closed metacarpal fractures were treated with a half-frame device. Limited open reduction was needed in 26% of cases. Duration of fixation was about one month. Anatomic reduction was maintained 86% of the time. Good or excellent results were achieved in 96.6% of cases.

Royle SG: Rotational deformity following metacarpal fracture. *J Hand Surg,* 15B:124-125, 1990.

Ninety-eight metacarpal fractures treated by closed or open means were found to have a rotational deformity of less than 10° in 25% at final evaluation. In only two cases was there a rotational deformity greater than 10° that required operative repair. Most fractures were of the fifth metacarpal.

Pediatric Metacarpal Fractures

Worlock PH, Stower MJ: The incidence and pattern of hand fractures in children. *J Hand Surg,* 11B:198-200, 1986.

Thirty-six percent of hand fractures in children 12 years of age or younger are of the metacarpal, most often the fifth. Most metacarpal fractures are of the greenstick variety near the epiphyseal head. Less than 10% of all hand pediatric fractures require reduction.

Light TR, Ogden JA: Metacarpal epiphyseal fractures. *J Hand Surg,* 12A:460-464, 1987.

Five cases of metacarpal epiphyseal fractures were reviewed. These occurred in the middle three metacarpals. Two non-displaced Salter II type fractures developed a growth disturbance.

Ireland ML, Taleisnik J: Nonunion of metacarpal extra-articular fractures in children: report of two cases and review of the literature. *J Ped Orthop,* 6:352-355, 1986.

Nonunion of metacarpal fractures in children is predisposed if there is extensive crush or soft-tissue injury or if inadequate immobilization is provided. One patient required open repair and bone graft to obtain union.

3

Intra-articular Fractures in Joint Injuries

Thomas R. Kiefhaber, MD

General Principles

Intra-articular fractures can be classified into four broad categories based upon the mechanism of injury and the resulting fracture pattern: avulsion fractures, shaft fractures that extend into the joint, major articular disruptions, and fracture dislocations. Avulsion fractures result from tension applied through the collateral ligaments or palmar plate, a failure mechanism that creates minimal comminution. Spiral or oblique fractures can extend into the joint producing large noncomminuted fragments. Major articular disruptions and fracture dislocations are caused by longitudinal forces that create comminution and joint surface depression.

A high index of suspicion should be maintained during the examination of injured joints to minimize the chances of overlooking an intra-articular fracture. The involved joint will be swollen and ecchymotic, with tenderness over the damaged structures. Stress testing may reveal instability caused by an underlying fracture or a ligamentous injury. The range of motion will be decreased if the joint is subluxated or a large articular fragment is displaced. A nearly normal range of motion may be found with nondisplaced, stable intra-articular fractures.

Properly positioned and technically perfect radiographs are essential for the accurate evaluation of injuries to the small joints of the hand. A minimum set of radiographs includes an AP, lateral, and oblique. A properly positioned true lateral centered on the injured articulation should always be performed. Both obliques may be useful to delineate the extent of intra-articular involvement. Tomograms are occasionally necessary to obtain an accurate picture of the fracture pattern. The radiograph should include the joints above and below the area of obvious pathology to minimize the chances of overlooking an associated injury.

The technical challenges and possible complications of surgical intervention are high; therefore, the goals and indications for open reduction internal fixation must be clearly defined. Restoration of joint stability is the treatment goal for avulsion fractures. Shaft fractures with joint extensions and major articular disruptions are reduced to correct digital angulation or malrotation and to restore articular surface continuity. The primary indications for treatment of fracture dislocations are to correct subluxation and to restore an acceptable articular surface. Some intra-articular fractures are so extensively comminuted that reconstitution of the joint surface exceeds the surgeon's technical abilities. The older literature recommends primary arthrodesis for these injuries, but more recent studies suggest that a good functional outcome can be attained with traction and immediate range of motion.

Surgery in the small joints of the hand is an extremely demanding technical exercise. Exposure must be wide enough to afford visualization of the articular surfaces without compromising the vascularity of small fragments. Stable fixation that allows immediate postoperative mobilization is preferred. The tendons adjacent to the injured joint are prone to adhesions, a tendency that is increased by surgical manipulation.

The devices available for operative stabilization include Kirschner pins, interosseous wires, pull-out sutures, tension-band wiring, interfragmentary screws, and plates. Kirschner pins have been the mainstay of fixation in the hand because of their versatility and ease of use. Interosseous wires and pull-out sutures are helpful in the treatment of small-avulsion fractures. Interfragmentary screw fixation can be employed in oblique and spiral fractures when the fragment is at least three times larger than the diameter of the screw and preferably large enough to accept two screws. The 1.5mm and 2.0mm A-O condylar plates have proven useful in the management of head fractures of the metacarpal and proximal phalanx.

The outcome of an intra-articular fracture is dependent upon many variables including location, fracture pattern, quality of reduction, and magnitude of associated injuries. Pain and motion may improve up to one year after intra-articular fractures of the hand. In one study, only 27% of the individuals were pain free at early follow-up, but 66% reported no discomfort after 11 years. Aching in cold weather was the most frequent long-term complaint, occurring in one-third of the injured digits. A slow improvement in motion was observed with time but only 60% of the individuals regained a normal arc. Radiographic signs of post-traumatic degenerative arthritis were noted in 17% of individuals. Pain and arthritic changes were not correlated, as several individuals demonstrated erosions and cysts but had no complaints of discomfort. The slow but predictable improvement in motion and pain, and the articular surface remodeling that can be expected, make it advisable to delay reconstructive procedures for at least one year.

Shaft Fractures That Extend into the Joint

Spiral or long oblique shaft fractures can extend into the adjacent joints. Comminution is minimal, but articular surface separation or step-off may be significant. Displaced fractures should be reduced and stabilized. Innovative fixation techniques have been described but most fractures can be treated with Kirschner pins or interfragmentary screws. Lag screw fixation provides compression in addi-

lag screw is

tion to stabilization and is preferred when the length of the fracture line exceeds twice the diameter of the shaft.

Fractures of the Metacarpal Head

Metacarpal head fractures are rare and most frequently affect the immobile index finger. Four basic fracture patterns are observed: avulsions of the collateral ligament, osteochondral injuries, fractures that divide the head into two major parts, and fractures with extensive comminution or loss of bone substance. Radiographic definition of the metacarpal head can be difficult on routine AP, lateral, and oblique views. Brewerton's view profiles the metacarpal heads and tomograms clearly define fracture lines and comminution.

Collateral ligament avulsion fractures are rarely seen at the metacarpophalangeal joint, and are more often seen at the interphalangeal joint. Significant displacement of the fracture fragment is the only indication for operative intervention. Minimally displaced fractures are treated with immediate protected motion. Osteochondral fractures usually present as slices of the articular surface and are associated with open injuries or dislocations. Small osteochondral fragments should be excised to avoid the formation of loose bodies.

Head-splitting fractures bisect the articular surface in an oblique, horizontal, or vertical plane. Articular incongruity interferes with joint motion and increases the risk of posttraumatic degenerative arthritis. Displacement or step-off greater than 1mm should be corrected by ORIF. Extensor tendon adhesions are minimized by utilizing fixation that does not transfix the MP joint. Fracture fragments separated from the shaft in a horizontal plane distal to the collateral ligaments are devoid of all soft-tissue connections and subject to avascular necrosis. Small horizontal fragments should be reduced and fixed with K-wires. Larger fragments can be secured with an AO screw recessed below the cartilage surface or with a Herbert screw.

Unfortunately, the most frequently encountered type of metacarpal head fracture is comminuted with impaction of the articular fragments. Large articular pieces should be reduced, fixed, and supported by bone graft. Highly comminuted fractures should be left *in situ* and treated with an immediate range-of-motion rehabilitation program. The treatment goal is limited to providing a stable, pain-free joint that is devoid of rotational abnormalities. Regardless of the treatment method employed, comminuted metacarpal head fractures rarely regain more than 45° of motion.

Fractures of the Base of the Proximal and Middle Phalanges

Avulsion of the insertion of the collateral ligament at the palmar base of the proximal or middle phalanges rarely occurs in adults. Fragments that involve more than 25% of the articular surface should be anatomically reduced and stabilized to minimize the possibility of posttraumatic degenerative arthritis. Fragments of any size that are dis-

placed greater than 2mm or malrotated compromise joint stability, and ORIF is advised. Large articular pieces are stabilized with an interfragmentary screw, but smaller fragments are more suited to fixation with a pull-out wire or tension-band technique. (Fig. 3-1)

Longitudinal compression produces a spectrum of injuries that range from minimal articular surface depression to fracture dislocations. Symmetrical compression of the joint surface creates stable fracture patterns with frac-

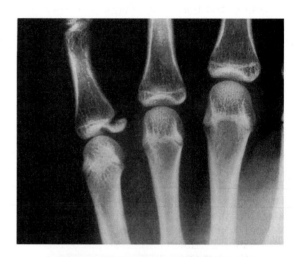

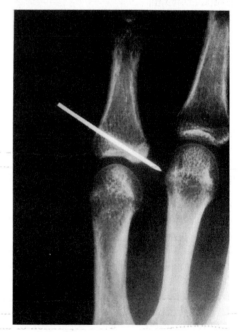

Figure 3-1.   (Top) Pull-off fractures of the base of the proximal and middle phalanx occur at the insertion of the collateral ligament and can result in joint instability. Fracture displacement in excess of 2mm should be corrected by ORIF. Larger fractures should be reduced to restore a smooth articular surface and to restore joint stability. **(Bottom)** Options for internal fixation include Kirschner pin, pull-out wire, tension-band wire, and interfragmentary screw.

ture lines perpendicular to the line of applied force and fragments that have been impacted into soft metaphyseal bone. As the angulatory component of the applied force increases, asymmetric fracture patterns are produced. A large articular fragment can be sheared away from the shaft or a single plateau can be depressed. Both patterns result in significant angulation of the digit. Large fragments with fracture lines parallel to the long axis of the digit are unstable and require ORIF. Articular incongruity of greater than 1mm, or any digital angulation, should be corrected by an anatomic restoration of the articular surface. Depressed articular fragments are elevated and supported with provisional fixation and bone graft. Surgical reconstruction of highly comminuted plateau fractures may be impossible. This type of injury is best treated by limited ORIF to correct asymmetric compression followed by skeletal traction and motion.

Fractures of the Head of the Proximal and Middle Phalanx

The separation of one condyle from the shaft (unicondylar fracture) is the most prevalent fracture pattern in the head of the middle or proximal phalanx. Bicondylar T and Y fractures are less frequently encountered. Displacement of unicondylar fractures causes incongruity of the articular surface and an angulatory deformity of the digit. Reduction can be achieved by traction, but joint compressive forces cause redisplacement that can rarely be prevented by external support. The propensity for loss of reduction justifies stabilization of all unicondylar fractures. Closed reduction and percutaneous pinning is simple and effective, but should only be employed if anatomic reduction of the joint surface can be assured and the pins can be positioned in a plane that does not interfere with the extensor apparatus. If open reduction is necessary, adequate visualization is achieved at the proximal interphalangeal joint by separating one lateral band from the central tendon and at the distal interphalangeal joint by elevating and retracting the terminal tendon. The collateral ligament provides the only blood supply to the condylar fragment and should not be detached. Fixation may be achieved with two Kirschner pins, a single pin coupled with an interosseous compression wire, or interfragmentary screws. (Fig. 3-2) The fixation should be solid enough to allow immediate mobilization. The PIP joint will regain approximately 80° of flexion, but a 20° to 30° flexion contracture is common. The appropriate use of dynamic splints minimizes the extension deficit.

In contrast to unicondylar injuries, nondisplaced bicondylar fractures are stable and can be treated with three weeks of immobilization. Condylar separation or displacement should be corrected to avoid intra-articular incongruity or digital angulation. Closed reduction of bicondylar fractures is impossible since longitudinal traction causes further separation and rotation of the condyles. Through a dorsal approach, the condyles can be reduced and secured to each other using lag screws or Kirschner pins. (Fig. 3-3A and 3-3B) Comminution between the condyles will allow a

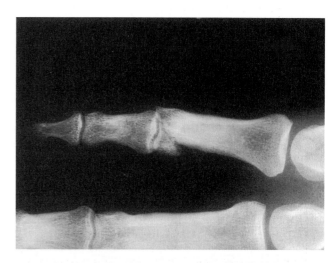

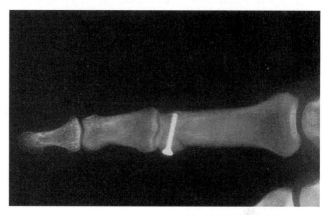

Figure 3-2. **(Top)** Condylar fractures of the head of the proximal or middle phalanges are unstable. **(Bottom)** Once reduced, the condyle can be secured with a percutaneously placed Kirschner pin, or an interfragmentary screw.

compression screw to narrow the width of the head unless the comminuted segment is supported with bone graft. The reconstructed head is fixed to the shaft by Kirschner pins placed to avoid the PIP joint. The large size of the proximal phalanx allows the use of the minicondylar plate for fixation of bicondylar fractures. The distal screw and blade provide excellent compression of the condylar fragments and the side plate secures the head to the shaft. (Fig. 3-3C)

Dislocations and Fracture Dislocations

Carpometacarpal Dislocations

Carpometacarpal (CMC) dislocations and fracture dislocations are infrequently encountered injuries. The majority of CMC dislocations are in a dorsal direction although volar dislocations have been reported. Fifty percent of the isolated CMC dislocations occur at the relatively unstable fifth metacarpal, with its 30° of anterior-posterior motion and

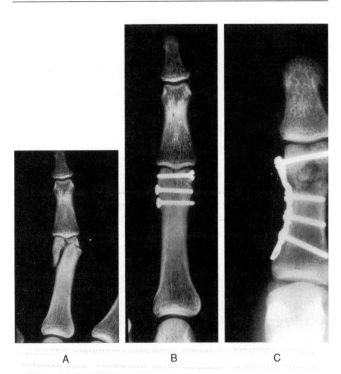

Figure 3-3. **(A)** Bicondylar fractures disrupt the intra-articular surface and the alignment of the head on the shaft. **(B)** The fixation begins by fixing the condyles to each other. The reconstructed head is then secured to the shaft. In this case, one condylar fragment was long enought to allow interfragmentary screw fixation. More commonly, it is necessary to use two Kirschner pins that start at the origin of the collateral ligaments, cross the facture site, and enter the shaft. **(C)** The mini-condylar plate provides secure fixation in larger phalanges.

obliquely-oriented articular surface. Twenty-five percent involve the stable index finger, and 25% the long or ring fingers. Multiple dislocations include the fifth finger 80% of the time, but all combinations have been reported. The usual mechanism of injury for a fourth or fifth CMC dislocation is an indirect force applied through the metacarpal head. Dislocations of the central or radial digits are produced by a direct blow to the base of the metacarpal and are often associated with severe soft-tissue trauma.

The diagnosis of CMC dislocations and fracture dislocations requires a high index of suspicion, a careful physical exam, and a meticulous review of the radiographs. Findings include tenderness at the CMC joint and a volar displacement of the metacarpal head (a sign that may be obscured by swelling). Ulnar deviation and malrotation can be seen in fifth-finger CMC dislocations. The AP radiograph shows disruption of the normal parallel joint lines and superimposition of the base of the dislocated metacarpals on the carpals.

A false impression of metacarpal superimposition will be created if the AP view is obtained with the wrist dorsiflexed. The lateral radiograph is difficult to interpret but most dislocations can be detected by carefully following each metacarpal shaft to its articulation with the carpus. An oblique view in 60° of supination from true lateral profiles the fifth CMC articulation and pronation of 60° allows inspection of the index CMC joint. Chip fractures from the hamate or base of the fifth metacarpal are best visualized by a 15° pronated view, and tomograms are occasionally necessary to clearly delineate carpal fractures. Metacarpal shaft fractures should prompt a search for a dislocation of the adjacent CMC joints, as the two injuries are frequently coexistent.

Longitudinal traction and gentle pressure over the base of the metacarpal usually reduces a CMC dislocation. A capsular flap interposed into the joint, massive edema, or a delay in treatment of more than five days can render closed reduction impossible and necessitate open reduction. Stable, isolated CMC dislocations are treated with three to four weeks of cast immobilization. Percutaneous pin fixation should be performed if postreduction instability is noted. Forces acting on the fifth CMC joint render it particularly unstable; the extensor carpi ulnaris pulls the metacarpal base in a dorsal ulnar direction, the hypothenar musculature angles the head of the metacarpal radially, and the oblique slope of the hamate articulation accentuates the tendency for subluxation. The combination of deforming forces is difficult to counteract with cast immobilization, and a transarticular Kirschner pin is recommended to maintain reduction.

Multiple dislocations are created by high-energy injuries and can be associated with severe soft-tissue damage. Open reduction and Kirschner pin fixation should be performed to assure anatomic apposition of the joint surfaces and maintenance of the reduction until soft-tissue healing restores stability.

Carpometacarpal Fracture Dislocations

Carpometacarpal dislocations can be associated with fracture of the metacarpal or adjacent carpal. Fracture patterns of the metacarpal include small avulsion fragments, fractures with two major components, and comminuted articular surface disruptions. Avulsion fractures, depression of the dorsal articular rim, and coronal split fractures are observed in the carpals. Indications for open reduction include failure of closed reduction secondary to interposition of soft tissue or bone; delayed treatment making closed reduction impossible; compound fracture dislocations that require wound debridement; and multiple fracture dislocations. Chip fractures from either the metacarpal or carpal return to acceptable alignment with joint reduction. Treatment consists of maintaining reduction with a cast or percutaneous pin for three weeks to allow reconstitution of the soft-tissue supports.

The two-part fracture dislocation of the fifth CMC joint has a classic appearance. A small fragment from the radial fourth of the metacarpal base is held reduced by the intermetacarpal ligaments and the remaining articular surface and shaft are pulled dorsally and ulnarly by the extensor

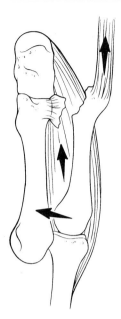

Figure 3-4. The fifth CMC joint is destabilized by the pull of the extensor carpi ulnaris, hypothenar musculature, and slope of the hamate.

carpi ulnaris. (Fig. 3-4) Closed reduction is easily attained with longitudinal traction, but postreduction stability is tenuous; a percutaneous transarticular Kirschner pin eliminates the possibility of re-subluxation and simplifies management. If cast treatment is attempted, the wrist should be held in 45° of dorsiflexion to reduce the pull of the extensor carpi ulnaris, and weekly radiographs obtained to assure maintenance of the reduction.

The treatment of fracture dislocations of the fifth CMC joint still generates debate concerning the need for anatomic correction of joint subluxation and the necessity of restoring a smooth articular surface. An older study reported 14 cases of fifth CMC fracture dislocations that were treated with unrestricted mobilization. At a four-and-one-half year followup, the radiographs demonstrated shortening of the metacarpal, widening of the base, and persistence of articular step-off, but only one patient had significant pain. The authors concluded that anatomic reduction was not necessary. More recent reports suggest that displacement of the fifth CMC joint leads to loss of grip strength, compensatory hyperextension of the MP joint, and an increased chance of developing painful posttraumatic degenerative arthritis. Current recommendations favor complete reduction of CMC subluxation and anatomic alignment of the joint surface.

The principles of anatomic reduction also apply to the carpal articular surface. Open reduction, internal and external fixation, and bone graft are often necessary to accomplish these goals. The comminution can be so extensive that satisfactory reduction is not possible and early range of motion is the best remaining treatment option. Posttraumatic degenerative arthritis of the CMC joint is treated by resection arthroplasty or arthrodesis. Fusion of the normally

mobile fifth CMC joint has theoretical disadvantages, but has proven effective in providing pain relief and increased grip strength.

Metacarpal Phalangeal Dislocations and Fracture Dislocations

Collateral Ligament Injuries

The collateral ligament usually fails at its attachment to the metacarpal head and may include avulsed bone. The radial side of the index finger is most susceptible to injury, but collateral ligament injuries of multiple digits have been reported. Because the cam shape of the metacarpal head makes the collateral ligaments loose in extension and taut in flexion, testing for instability must be done in the flexed posture. The index finger may rotate on the intact ulnar collateral ligament causing palmar subluxation of the radial base of the proximal phalanx, a situation that produces a rotational deformity of the digit.

Conservative treatment of collateral ligament injuries is successful in most cases. Splinting in 50° of MP flexion has been advocated by some authors, but the extended position has also been proposed to allow maximum tightening of the collateral ligaments. Chronic pain and secondary adhesions is a more frequent sequelae than instability, and therefore the maximum period of static splinting should not exceed three weeks. Earlier protected motion, with buddy taping to adjacent digit, is indicated in the ulnar digits and in older individuals. Indications for operative repair of the collateral ligament include avulsion fractures that are displaced more than 2mm or a rotation deformity of the digit.

Metacarpophalangeal Dislocations

Metacarpophalangeal dislocations occur most often in a dorsal direction, and in order of frequency most commonly involve the index, thumb, then small digit. Central, multiple, and volar dislocations are rare. Complex (irreducible) dislocations occur when the palmar plate ruptures proximally and becomes interposed between the dorsally displaced proximal phalanx and the metacarpal head. The trapped palmar plate is the most significant impediment to reduction, but other surrounding soft-tissue structures may also interfere with reduction maneuvers. The lumbrical subluxates to the radial side of the index finger metacarpal head, and the flexor tendons are forced ulnarly. These displaced tendinous structures and palmar plate create a Chinese finger trap that tightens around the metacarpal head when longitudinal traction is applied. (Fig. 3-5) A similar situation occurs in the small finger; the lumbricals and flexor tendons are displaced radially and the abductor digiti minimi wraps around the ulnar side of the metacarpal head.

Simple (reducible) dislocations present clinically with a noticeable deformity, a startling 90° of MP hyperextension. Less deformity is seen in complex dislocations as the proximal phalanx assumes bayonet apposition on top of the metacarpal. A skin dimple in the distal palmar crease, or the

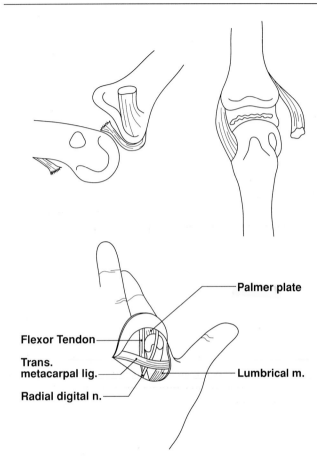

Palmer plate

Flexor Tendon

Trans. metacarpal lig.

Lumbrical m.

Radial digital n.

Figure 3-5. Complex or irreducible MP dislocations are created by interposition of the palmar plate **(Top)** and entrapment of the metacarpal head between the lumbrical and flexor tendons. **(Bottom)**

radiographic presence of a sesamoid within the joint are pathognomonic signs of complex dislocations.

Simple dislocations should be reduced by joint hyperextension and a distally directed pressure applied to the base of the proximal phalanx. Longitudinal traction may convert a dislocation from simple to complex. An attempt may be made to reduce a complex dislocation, but the patient and surgeon should be prepared to perform an open reduction in the event of failure. Open reduction can be achieved through either a volar or dorsal approach. The volar approach is initiated through a transverse incision in the distal palmar crease followed by division of the A₁ pulley to gain exposure of the joint. The index finger radial digital nerve and the ulnar digital nerve to the fifth digit will be tented over the metacarpal head directly beneath the skin and are in danger of division during this approach. Extricating the palmar plate from between the metacarpal head and the base of the proximal phalanx is difficult unless the attachments of the transverse metacarpal ligaments to the palmar plate are divided.

The dorsal approach eliminates the risk of damage to the digital nerves, improves visualization of the dorsally dis-

placed palmar plate, and allows access to metacarpal head fractures. A longitudinal incision is made over the MP joint and the extensor apparatus is displaced distally to allow visualization. The palmar plate can be split in the mid-portion allowing the radial and ulnar halves to fall away from the metacarpal head as the joint is reduced. Approximately 50% of MP dislocations have an associated metacarpal head fracture that can best be treated through the dorsal approach. After reduction of most simple or complex dislocations, the joint is stable and immediate range of motion with protective buddy taping can be initiated.

Proximal Interphalangeal Fractures and Dislocations

Injuries to the Collateral Ligament

Injuries to the proximal interphalangeal joint lateral collateral ligaments occur frequently and can cause extended disability. Ligament failure usually occurs at the attachment to the proximal phalanx or, less frequently, in the midsubstance. The conjoined distal insertion of the collateral ligament and palmar plate can fail through a fracture of the base of the middle phalanx. Asymmetric fusiform swelling and tenderness are observed along the course of the injured ligament. Radiographs may show a chip fracture at the proximal origin of the collateral ligament or a larger fracture from the volar lateral corner of the middle phalanx. Deviation of 20° or more is indicative of a complete collateral ligament rupture. Clinical studies show that all partial collateral ligament tears and most complete disruptions can be effectively treated with seven to 14 days of static splinting followed by protected mobilization. Indications for surgery include radiographic evidence of soft tissues interposed in the joint; a displaced fracture from the middle phalanx or head of proximal phalanx; or continued instability after three weeks of static splinting.

Dorsal Dislocations of the PIP Joint

Dorsal dislocations of the PIP joint are the most frequently encountered articular injury in the hand. Reduction is often accomplished by the patient or a bystander and medical treatment is generally delayed. Biomechanical studies have shown that the palmar plate fails at its distal attachment to the middle phalanx and may pull off a small chip fracture. (Fig. 3-6) The collateral ligaments remain intact in a pure dorsal dislocation. Reduction is easily accomplished under metacarpal block anesthesia with longitudinal traction. Stable reductions may be immediately mobilized in a figure-of-eight or dorsal blocking splint that allows flexion, but prevents the last 20° of extension. Unstable joints must be protected in a position of flexion to prevent redislocation. On rare occasions, the palmar plate fails proximally and can become interposed in the joint, preventing closed reduction. Open reduction is necessary, but the palmar plate does not require repair. Open dislocations should be treated in the operating room with an extension of the skin lacerations and meticulous debridement of the joint. Injuries of this magnitude are associated with failure of one or both of

HYPEREXTENSION

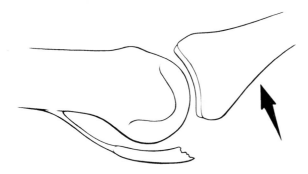

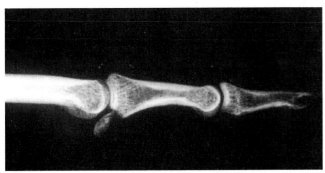

Figure 3-6.   (Top) PIP hyperextension injuries rupture the palmar plate at the distal attachment or through an avulsion fracture. **(Bottom)** Avulsed bone fragments can include up to 30% of the joint surface, but comminution is minimal.

the collateral ligaments. Recommended treatment includes reattachment of the palmar plate, repair of the collateral ligaments, and stabilization of the joint with a temporary transarticular Kirschner pin for three weeks.

Chronic hyperextension of the PIP joint after dorsal dislocation is infrequently encountered if the palmar plate rupture is recognized early and treated appropriately. Hyperextension instability can be treated by tenodesis of one slip of the superficialis, reattachment of the palmar plate, or rerouting of a lateral band palmar to the PIP axis of rotation.

A flexion contracture is the most frequently observed complication following PIP dislocation. Scarring of the palmar plate limits PIP extension and may lead to DIP hyperextension by creating a contracture of the adjacent oblique retinacular ligament. Once established, the resultant pseudoboutonniere deformity is difficult to correct and is best prevented with dynamic extension splints applied as early as six weeks after injury, along with oblique retinacular ligament stretching exercises.

Fracture Dislocations of the PIP Joint

Fracture dislocations of the PIP joint are potentially the most disabling PIP joint injuries and present numerous management difficulties for the treating physician. The mechanism of injury and the resulting fracture pattern are used to define three types of PIP fracture dislocations: hyperextension, impaction shear, and pylon fractures. When the limits of extension are exceeded, the palmar plate avulses at the distal insertion or fails through a fracture of the middle phalanx. The size of the fragment can range from a small fleck to up to 30% of the joint surface, but comminution is minimal. The stability of the reduction should be assessed by testing for redislocation during active range of motion performed under local anesthesia and by carefully scrutinizing the postreduction lateral radiograph for any sign of dorsal subluxation. A carefully applied dorsal blocking splint prevents redislocation of unstable hyperextension injuries and allows immediate active flexion.

An impaction shear injury is produced by a longitudinal load applied to the hyperextended or slightly flexed PIP joint. As the middle phalanx is driven over the head of the proximal phalanx, extensive comminution and impaction of the base of the middle phalanx occurs. The stabilizing effect of the concave base of the middle phalanx and the tether of the palmar plate are lost if more than 50% of the base of the middle phalanx is damaged. The dorsal pull of the extensor mechanism through the central slip, the slope of the remaining dorsal articular surface, and the insertion of the superficialis tendon onto the midshaft of the middle phalanx combine to create a rotational force that causes dorsal subluxation of the middle phalanx base. Successful treatment requires that the deforming forces be counteracted by creating a palmar tether and by reconstructing the palmar buttress of the middle phalangeal articular surface. (Fig. 3–7) Static splints or dorsal blocking splints are inadequate for maintaining the reduction of unstable impaction shear fractures.

Effective treatment modalities include skeletal traction, open reduction internal fixation, and palmar plate arthroplasty. Continuous traction devices have been designed that provide longitudinal traction in combination with a palmarly directed force applied to the base of the middle phalanx. Regardless of the traction method chosen, joint reduction should be monitored by frequent true-lateral radiographs. Recurrent dorsal subluxation should be corrected immediately by adjustments in the device or conversion to an alternative form of treatment. Reconstruction of the middle phalanx base can be achieved by ORIF only if the fragments are large enough to be secured with a Kirschner pin, pull-out wire, or compression screw. Depressed fragments must be elevated, temporarily stabilized, and supported with bone graft. The palmar plate arthroplasty resurfaces the damaged articular surface of the middle phalanx and restores stability by advancing the palmar plate into the fracture defect. The tether of the palmar plate is insufficient to keep the joint reduced if more than 50% of the articular surface has been destroyed. Under these circumstances, it is necessary to restore the convex palmar buttress of the base of the middle phalanx by supporting the palmar plate with bone fragments, bone graft, or one slip of the superficialis tendon.

Patients frequently present with chronic dorsal subluxation of the PIP joint because of a delay in seeking medical

DORSAL DISLOCATION

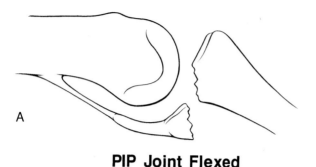

A

PIP Joint Flexed

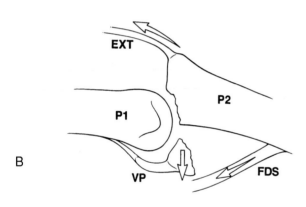

B

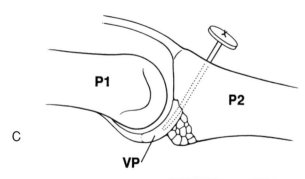

C

Figure 3-7. **(A)** Impaction shear fracture dislocations result from a longitudinal force applied to the slightly flexed or extended PIP joint. **(B)** Loss of the palmar plate tether and the palmar 50% of the middle phalanx base renders the PIP joint unstable. The extensor tendon, superficialis, and slope of the remaining articular surface combine into an unopposed vector that encourages dorsal subluxation. **(C)** When performing a palmar plate arthroplasty, the surgeon must fill any defect behind the palmar plate with chips from the fracture, bone graft, or one slip of the superficialis.

attention or a failed treatment attempt. The motion in a subluxated PIP joint occurs through a hinge action, with the axis of rotation centered at the edge of the fracture. If undamaged articular cartilage remains on the dorsal aspect of the base of the middle phalanx and the palmar aspect of the head of the proximal phalanx, it is possible to re-establish the normal gliding flexion arc by operatively reducing the joint, in combination with extensor tenolysis, PIP capsulotomy, and collateral ligament release. To maintain reduction, it is essential to restore the palmar buttress of the middle phalanx by realigning the palmar articular surface with an opening wedge osteotomy or by resurfacing the fractured surface with a properly supported palmar plate arthroplasty.

A pylon fracture includes a disruption of the dorsal and palmar articular margins and depression of the central articular surface. (Fig. 3-8) Extensive comminution makes anatomic restoration of the articular surface impossible. Longitudinal skeletal traction that allows immediate range of motion provides an acceptable method of treatment. Remodeling of the base of the middle phalanx has been observed and clinical studies have confirmed that most patients obtain an acceptable functional result even though the radiographic appearance of the joint is ominous.

Palmar Dislocations of the Proximal Interphalangeal Joint

Palmar dislocations of the PIP joints are associated with massive soft-tissue damage and can lead to significant long-term joint disability. The collateral ligament ruptures at its proximal attachment and the palmar plate fails distally. The extensor apparatus is split between the central tendon and the lateral band or, more commonly, sustains a complete disruption of the central tendon. An irreducible dislocation can be created if the lateral bands or central tendon become trapped under the head of the proximal phalanx. Reduction may be attempted by simultaneously flexing the MP and PIP joints and gently manipulating the middle phalanx, but open reduction is usually necessary. After open or closed reduction, it is imperative to assess the continuity of the central tendon. An intact central tendon is

AXIAL LOAD

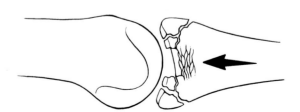

Figure 3-8. A pylon fracture results from a longitudinal force that fractures the dorsal and palmar articular fragments away from the shaft and causes impaction of the central articular surface.

treated with a short period of immobilization followed by a carefully controlled active range-of-motion program. Central tendon disruptions should be treated with six weeks of static splinting or with operative repair. An easily reducible palmar dislocation implies that the collateral ligament, central tendon, and part of the palmar plate have been completely disrupted. Global instability is present and the tendency for redislocation is high. Many surgeons have advocated open reduction, repair of the damaged structures, and fixation of the joint with a transarticular Kirschner pin. Others have reported good results with closed reduction of the joint and temporary percutaneous Kirschner pin fixation.

Avulsion Fractures at the Insertion of the Central Tendon

Proximal interphalangeal hyperflexion or palmar dislocation can create a midsubstance disruption of the central tendon or pull off an avulsion fracture from the insertion to the middle phalanx. If displacement of the fracture fragment is not eliminated by extension of the PIP joint, ORIF should be performed. Fixation is best achieved with a laterally directed pull-out wire, tension-band fixation, or cerclage wire. Postoperatively the PIP joint is held in extension for six weeks, but active and passive flexion of the DIP joint are immediately encouraged.

DIP Dislocations and Fracture Dislocations

The collateral ligaments, palmar plate, flexor digitorum profundus, and extensor tendon combine to provide tremendous inherent stability for the DIP joint. The soft-tissue supports and small moment arm afforded by the short distal phalanx make DIP dislocations rare. Dorsal interphalangeal injuries can be classified by the mechanism of injury: hyperextension, hyperflexion, lateral deviation, and impaction shear. A pure hyperextension force disrupts the palmar plate, but the collateral ligaments and the insertion of the profundus tendon remains intact. The skin and subcutaneous tissue at the DIP joint are firmly bound to the underlying bone and consequently, 64% of DIP dislocations are open. Reduction can be achieved under metacarpal block anesthesia and there is little tendency for redisloca-

tion. Immobilization for pain control can be quickly followed by an active range-of-motion program.

Irreducible dislocations are caused by interposition of the palmar plate, the profundus tendon, or an osteochondral fracture. Open reduction is necessary to extract an interposed palmar plate, but postreduction stability is high and only a short period of immobilization is required. Interposition of the profundus tendon implies rupture of at least one collateral ligament and immobilization should be continued for three weeks.

Isolated collateral ligament injuries are rare and can occur as a midsubstance tear or a bony avulsion of either the proximal or distal end of the collateral ligament. Unless wide displacement of the fracture fragment occurs, ORIF is not necessary. Fractures from the volar base of the distal phalanx can represent an avulsion of the palmar plate or a disruption of the profundus tendon insertion. It is important to distinguish between these two injuries as the treatment and prognosis are very different. Palmar plate avulsion fractures are small, the joint is stable after reduction, and only a short period of immobilization is necessary. Profundus tendon avulsion fractures are larger and not comminuted. It is important to re-establish continuity of the flexor tendon and to reduce the dorsal articular cartilage onto the head of the middle phalanx. A pull-out suture and a transarticular K-wire are frequently necessary to accomplish these tasks.

Impaction shear injuries cause a comminuted fracture of the palmar lip of the distal phalanx that can lead to joint instability. The joint should be reduced and stabilized with a transarticular K-pin. Extensive palmar impaction may require ORIF to restore joint stability. Treatment of pylon fractures is controversial, with some surgeons recommending an attempt at anatomic restoration of the joint surface and others advocating early range of motion. Surgical intervention is difficult, anatomic reduction of the joint is rarely possible, and motion is compromised secondary to tendon adhesions. Some remodeling will occur in this nonweight-bearing joint and a pain-free, functional range of motion can more predictably be obtained with an early range-of-motion program.

Annotated Bibliography

Intra-articular Fractures

Buchler U, Fischer T: Use of a mini-condylar plate for metacarpal and phalangeal periarticular injuries. *Clin Orthop*, 214:53-88, 1987.

The results of 65 fractures treated with the minicondylar plate are presented. The indications for use of the minicondylar plate are clearly defined and the application technique is described in detail.

Hastings H II, Carroll C IV: Treatment of closed articular fractures of the metacarpophalangeal and proximal interphalangeal joints. *Hand Clin*, 4:503-527, 1988.

The authors present a thorough review of the classification and management of intra-articular hand fractures. Techniques of internal fixation are clearly described and well illustrated. The author's own clinical series is used to demonstrate the expected results and possible complications.

Jupiter JB, Sheppard JE: Tension wire fixation of avulsion fractures in the hand. *Clin Orthop*, 214:113-120, 1987.

The technique of tension-wire fixation of avulsion fractures in the hand is described and illustrated with case studies.

McElfresh EC, Dobyns JH: Intra-articular metacarpal head fractures. *J Hand Surg*, 8:383-393, 1983.

The authors present a retrospective review of 103 metacarpal head fractures. An extensive classification system is proposed. Treatment results and management recommendations are presented for each fracture type.

O'Rourke SK, Gaur S, Barton NJ: Long-term outcome of articular fractures of the phalanges: an eleven year follow-up. *J Hand Surg Br*, 14:183-193, 1989.

Fifty-four patients with intra-articular fractures were followed for 11 years. Pain decreased and motion improved with the passage of time. Seventeen percent developed radiographic evidence of posttraumatic arthritis, but only one patient with erosions or cysts complained of persistent pain.

Rayhack JM, Bottke CA: Intraosseous compression wiring of displaced articular condylar fractures. *J Hand Surg*, 15A:370-373, 1990.

The author advocates adding an interosseous wire to a single Kirschner pin for fixation of intra-articular fractures. The interosseous wire is placed in a manner that provides interfragmentary compression and augments rotational control.

Carpometacarpal Dislocations and Fracture Dislocations

Cain JE Jr, Shepler TR, Wilson MR: Hamato-metacarpal fracture-dislocation: Classification and treatment. *J Hand Surg*, 12A:762-767, 1987.

The authors present a classification system and treatment recommendations for CMC dislocations associated with fractures of the hamate.

Clendenin MB, Smith RJ: Fifth metacarpal/hamate arthrodesis for posttraumatic osteoarthritis. *J Hand Surg*, 9A:374-378, 1984.

Seven patients with posttraumatic degenerative arthritis of the fifth CMC joint were treated by arthrodesis supplemented with corticocancellous bone graft. Pain relief was complete and grip strength improved.

Lawlis JF III, Gunther SF: Carpometacarpal dislocations. *J Bone and Joint Surg*, 73A:52-58, 1991.

Fifteen of 20 patients with dislocations or fracture dislocations of the carpometacarpal joints were treated with open reduction internal fixation. Unsatisfactory results were more common in injuries to the second or third CMC joints or in the presence of a concomitant ulnar nerve injury.

Petrie PWR, Lamb DW: Fracture-subluxation of the base of the fifth metacarpal. *Hand*, 6:82-86, 1974.

Fourteen CMC fracture dislocations treated with unrestricted immobilization were followed for four-and-one-half years. Shortening of the metacarpal, widening of the base, and joint line step-off were noted in all cases. Eight patients were pain free, five had minimum pain, and one had significant pain. The authors questioned the need for ORIF.

Rawles JGJ: Dislocations and fracture-dislocations at the carpometacarpal joints of the fingers. *Hand Clin*, 4:103-112, 1988.

This review article includes a description of the pertinent anatomy, a distillation of the literature, and a summary of treatment recommendations.

MP Dislocations and Fracture Dislocations

Bohart PG, Gelberman RH, Vandell RF, Solamon PB: Complex dislocations of metacarpophalangeal joint, operative reduction by Farabeuf's dorsal incision. *Clin Orthop Rel Res*, 164:208-210, 1982.

Bechton's dorsal approach for reduction of complex MP dislocations is described and the advantages of the approach are discussed.

Green DP, Terry GC: Complex dislocation of the metacarpophalangeal joint. Correlative pathological anatomy. *J Bone Joint Surg*, 55A:1480-1486, 1973.

The pathological anatomy of the complex MP dislocation is described in detail and nine cases are reported.

Viegas SF, Heare TC, Calhoun JH: Complex fracture-dislocation of a fifth metacarpophalangeal joint: case report and literature review. *J Trauma*, 29:521-524, 1989.

The pathological anatomy, diagnosis, and treatment of complex CMC dislocations are reviewed.

PIP Dislocations and Fracture Dislocations

Agee JM: Unstable fracture dislocations of the proximal interphalangeal joint. Treatment with the force couple splint. *Clin Orthop*, 101-112, 1987.

The author proposes a force couple constructed of Kirschner wires and rubber bands that maintains joint reduction and allows immediate active range of motion. The results and complications of 16 cases are presented.

Eaton RG, Malerich MM: Volar plate arthroplasty for the proximal interphalangeal joint: A ten year review. *J Hand Surg,* 5:260-268, 1980.

The technical details and potential pitfalls of palmar plate arthroplasty are presented with the results of 24 cases. The range of motion averaged 95° if the procedure was done within six weeks of injury and 78° when the procedure was used to reconstruct a chronic fracture dislocation.

Schenck RR: Dynamic traction and early passive movement for fractures for the proximal interphalangeal joint. *J Hand Surg,* 11A:850-858, 1986.

Ten patients with comminuted fractures of the base of the middle phalanx were treated with a combination of dynamic skeletal traction and passive mobilization. A pain-free arc of motion that averaged 87° was reported.

Stern PJ, Roman RJ, Kiefhaber TR, McDonough JJ: Pilon fractures of the proximal interphalangeal joint. *J Hand Surg,* 16A:844-850, 1991.

The results of three different treatment modalities for PIP pylon fractures are reviewed. The methods utilized included splint, skeletal traction, and ORIF. Skeletal traction produced the best range of motion with the fewest complications.

Vicar AJ: Proximal interphalangeal joint dislocations without fractures. *Hand Clin,* 4:5-13, 1988.

This overview of PIP dislocations presents a detailed description of the pathological anatomy, a review of the literature, and a summary of treatment recommendations.

Zemel NP, Stark HH, Ashworth CR, Boyes JH: Chronic fracture dislocation of the proximal interphalangeal joint—treatment by osteotomy and bone graft. *J Hand Surg,* 6:447-455, 1981.

The authors describe the biomechanics of PIP joint stability as it relates to dorsal fracture dislocations. They propose an osteotomy of the base of the middle phalanx to counteract the deforming forces and restore stability.

DIP Dislocations and Fracture Dislocations

Horiuchi Y, Itoh Y, Sasaki T, Tasaki K, Iijima K, Uchinishi K: Dorsal dislocation of the DIP joint with fracture of the volar base of the distal phalanx. *J Hand Surg Br,* 14:177-182, 1989.

Twelve surgically treated dorsal fracture dislocations of the DIP joint were followed for 6.4 years. Full range of motion was not restored, but all joints were pain free. A classification based upon the mechanism of injury and fracture pattern is proposed.

Simpson MB, Greenfield GQ: Irreducible dorsal dislocation of the small finger distal interphalangeal joint: the importance of roentgenograms–case report. *J Trauma,* 31:1450-1454, 1991.

A case of an irreducible DIP dislocation is summarized. The pathological anatomy and pertinent literature are reviewed.

4

Fractures and Dislocations of the Thumb

Robert N. Hotchkiss, MD

Introduction

The crucial role of the thumb in effective pinch and grasp in opposition with the other digits must be the guiding principle for treatment of injuries to the thumb. In all injuries the ideal of mobility with stability is sought, but in the case of the thumb, motion at the more distal segments (MP and IP joint) should not be coveted at the risk of pain or chronic instability. Contracture of the first web space must also be avoided.

Biomechanical experiments and related calculations have shown that compressive joint reaction forces may be magnified tenfold through the thumb metacarpal and basal joint during pinch.

As with treatment of other fractures in the hand, newer and smaller implants have led to a more facile and flexible approach to internal and external fixation of fractures; however, maintaining length and articular congruity, by whatever technique, remain the task of the surgeon.

Fractures

Phalangeal

Distal phalanx—Mallet thumb injuries occur more rarely than in the digits, but should be treated similarly by splinting for six weeks followed by gentle mobilization. When volar subluxation of the distal phalanx occurs, open reduction with pin fixation reduces the joint and provides articular congruity after healing.

Proximal phalanx—Nonarticular fractures of the proximal phalanx are managed similarly to the other digits. For unstable fractures, K-wire fixation or screw and plate fixation can be used.

Articular fractures involving the IP joint should be restored anatomically to avoid painful deformity. If significant comminution is present, primary arthrodesis can provide a stable and functional thumb with little disability.

Metacarpal

Metacarpal shaft—Unlike metacarpal fractures of the other digits, the thumb metacarpal has little ligamentous support from adjacent soft-tissue structures. Fracture patterns that might be stable in the other digits may not be in the thumb metacarpal, such as oblique fractures of the shaft. Although potentially more unstable, extra-articular deformity of the shaft is also generally better tolerated because of the mobility at the CMC joint.

Fractures of the shaft of the thumb metacarpal have not been reported in the past five years as a separate entity.

Articular Fractures of the CMC Joint

Bennett's

In 1882, Bennett described the fracture pattern which bears his name. His principal recommendations of stable fixation, overcoming the proximal pull of the abductor pollicis longus, have not been changed; only the technology to achieve this goal has changed.

Several studies have documented the importance of restoring the axial length and coaptation of the shaft of the metacarpal to the smaller medial fragment comprising the volar beak ligament. Without bony union of the ulnar-volar fragment and its attachment to the volar ligament to the main portion of the shaft, painful subluxation and decreased pinch strength are more likely.

Most of the controversy surrounds the amount of acceptable intra-articular displacement. Although many authors have recommended an "accurate" reduction of the articular surface, there is evidence that some irregularity (1mm to 3mm of incongruity) is well tolerated and does not lead to progressive disabling arthritis. Two separate retrospective studies of 25 and 41 patients could find no relationship between an imperfect reduction and the development of arthritis at the CMC joint. None of these studies advocated nonoperative treatment of these injuries, but questioned the value of extraordinary effort or measures to alter an imperfect reduction of the articular surface. A stable union of the fracture fragments and volar beak ligament appears to be of greater importance.

Many methods of stabilizing this fracture dislocation have been reported and fall into two categories—direct and indirect stabilization. Direct stabilization of the two fracture fragments requires sufficient size of the usually smaller volar beak portion to accept K-wires or a small lag screw. When the volar ulnar fragment is smaller, most authors have advised using indirect stabilization. Traction techniques, small external fixators, and K-wire fixation to the adjacent index metacarpal have been used with comparable success.

Comminuted Fractures at the Base of the Thumb (Rolando's Fracture)

The principles of deformity and treatment for these fractures are similar to those of the Bennett's fracture. The greater comminution increases the likelihood that indirect methods of reduction and stabilization will be required, but this depends on both the situation and the surgeon.

Interestingly, to date there has been little correlation between the quality of reduction and the occurrence of late symptoms or radiological degenerative arthritis, as with Bennett's fractures.

For fractures with marked bone loss, a technique using external fixation to maximize ligamentotaxis and K-wire fixation of the intra-articular components has been reported with satisfactory outcome. Supplemental bone graft was used as needed to fill voids in the subchondral metaphyseal region of the thumb metacarpal.

Dislocations

Metacarpophalangeal

Dislocations of the thumb MP joint are rare but require the same attention as those of the other digits. Simple dislocation without entrapment of the volar plate can occur, but they may be associated with collateral ligament injuries. Complex dislocations usually require open reduction through a dorsal approach with extrication of the entrapped volar plate. The flexor tendons are often interposed and wrapped around the metacarpal neck.

Carpometacarpal

Acute isolated dislocations of the CMC joint without fracture are rare. Although closed reduction can be accomplished, residual instability and re-dislocation may occur after closed manipulation and pin fixation. Because of the rarity of this injury, there is considerable debate about the pathoanatomy and need for open repair or reconstruction of the volar ligament. The authors of the largest retrospective study advocated prompt closed reduction with careful assessment of stability following reduction. If any instability was noted, pin fixation was recommended.

Ligament Injuries

Ulnar Collateral Ligament Injury (Gamekeeper's Thumb)

The ulnar collateral ligament of the thumb MP joint is commonly injured in skiing and other falls on the outstretched hand. Changes in ski-pole grips have not been shown to reduce the incidence of this injury. A new glove has been designed to protect the MP joint, but studies documenting efficacy have not yet been published or presented.

A mechanically competent ulnar collateral ligament is crucial for effective pinch. Chronic instability can be disabling, reducing the strength of thumb pinch and leading to posttraumatic arthrosis. Since Stener's work demonstrating frequent irreducibility of the ligament, precluding effective apposition and subsequent healing, most authors have advocated immediate open repair for complete disruptions. One recent study has documented a clinically significant loss of pinch strength in those patients treated with repair three weeks after injury. Those treated immediately (within days) demonstrated near-normal pinch strength when compared to the opposite side.

Several techniques and materials have been used for the repair of the ligament. In a recent study, the results of using a prefashioned steel wire was compared with a nonabsorb-

able braided suture. No difference in outcome was noted.

For incomplete tears, functional bracing appears to be as efficacious as casting. In two independent studies, bracing the MP joint alone for six to eight weeks assured the same outcome as plaster casting. Protected motion in flexion and extension was allowed out of the splint on a daily basis in both studies. One study advocated the use of functional bracing after open ligamentous repair.

Radial Collateral Ligament Injury

Injuries to the radial collateral ligament are less common and infrequently studied. These injuries are often unrecognized at the time of injury. There are no recent published series of patients studying the acute injury and its treatment; despite this, some authors advocate immediate open repair for complete tears. Closed treatment with casting for functional bracing has not been compared to open repair.

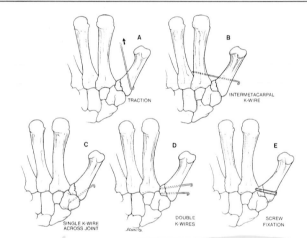

Figure 4-1. Both indirect and direct methods of reduction of the Bennett's fracture can be used. It is important to provide coaptation of the two fragments, irrespective of technique.

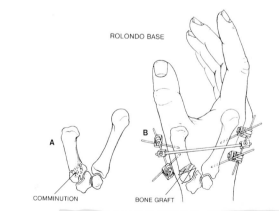

Figure 4-2. A combined technique of external and supplementary internal fixation with bone grafting can be used for complex intra-articular fractures of the basilar joint of the thumb.

Annotated Bibliography

Fractures

Articular Fractures at the CMC Joint

Breen TF, Gelberman RH, Jupiter JB: Intra-articular fractures of the basilar joint of the thumb. *Hand Clin,* 4:491-501, 1988.

The authors describe several techniques for the treatment of intra-articular fractures of the basilar joint of the thumb with detailed explanations of rationale.

Buchler U, McCollam SM, Oppikofer C: Comminuted fractures of the basilar joint of the thumb: combined treatment by external fixation, limited internal fixation, and bone grafting. *J Hand Surg,* 6:556-560, 1991.

Thirteen patients were treated using this combined technique with excellent results.

Foster RJ, Hastings H II: Treatment of Bennett, Rolando and vertical intra-articular trapezial fractures. *Clin Orthop,* 214:121-129, 1987.

The authors review, with helpful diagrams, the methods of direct and indirect treatment for stabilization of fractures at the base of the thumb.

Langhoff O, Andersen K, Kjaer-Petersen K: Rolando's fracture. *J Hand Surg,* (Br) 16:454-459, 1991.

The authors treated 17 patients with Rolando's fracture. Although the authors sought an anatomic reduction of the articular portion of the fracture, radiographic evidence of osteoarthritis or posttraumatic arthritis developed in six of the patients. Interestingly, there was no relationship or correlation between the quality of reduction and the occurrence of late symptoms or osteoarthritis.

Pellegrini VD Jr. Fractures at the base of the thumb. *Hand Clin,* 4:87-102, 1988.

The author carefully reviews the anatomy and kinematics of the basilar joint of the thumb and its importance in treating fractures.

Bennett's Fracture

Cannon SR, Dowd GS, Williams DH, Scott JM. A long-term study following Bennett's fracture. *J Hand Surg Br,* 11:426-431, 1986.

Twenty-five patients with Bennett's fractures were reviewed. Twenty-three of the patients were either minimally symptomatic or asymptomatic. With a follow-up of nearly 10 years, there was no correlation between articular incongruity (offset 1mm to 3mm) and symptomatic arthritis.

Kjaer-Petersen K, Langhoff O, Andersen K: Bennett's fracture. *J Hand Surg Br,* 15:58-61, 1990.

Forty-one patients with Bennett's fractures were followed for an average of seven years. Twenty-one of the 31 patients had no symptoms or disability and the remaining 10 were free of symptoms except for slight pain with weather change. Those with residual deformity of the articular surface had higher rate of

radiologic degeneration, which did not necessarily correlate with clinical outcome.

Dislocations

Miller RJ: Dislocations and fracture dislocations of the metacarpophalangeal joint of the thumb. *Hand Clin,* 4:45-65, 1988.

A comprehensive review of principles of treatment and pitfalls in the treatment of the MP dislocations. A change in ski-pole grips did not appear to influence the incidence of skier's thumb.

Watt N, Hooper G: Dislocation of the trapezial metacarpal joint. *J Hand Surg,* 12B:242-245, 1987.

Twelve patients with acute dislocations of the CMC joint without fracture were treated. Those treated on the day of injury and stabilized were treated only with cast immobilization and did not demonstrate chronic instability. Those treated late or with unrecognized instability with the initial closed reduction developed persistent instability requiring ligamentous reconstruction.

Ligament Injuries

Helm RH: Hand function after injuries to the collateral ligaments of the metacarpophalangeal joint of the thumb. *J Hand Surg,* 12B:252-255, 1987.

Pinch strength was assessed in 34 patients with ligament injuries to the MP joint of the thumb. Ulnar collateral ligament injuries fixed or repaired in a delayed fashion (more than three weeks) demonstrated a 50% decrease in expected pinch strength following repair.

Pichora DR, McMurtry RY. Gamekeeper's thumb: a prospective study of functional bracing. *J Hand Surg,* 14:567-573, 1989.

The authors cautiously recommend functional bracing for all injuries of the ulnar collateral ligament of the thumb; however, instability was greater in those patients with suspected Stener lesions.

Saetta JP, Phair IC, Quinton DN: Ulnar collateral ligament repair of the metacarpophalangeal joint of the thumb: a study comparing two methods of repair. *J Hand Surg Br,* 17:160-163, 1992.

Two materials were used to repair ulnar collateral ligament injuries of the thumb. There was no difference seen between nonabsorbable suture and steel wire.

Sollerman C, Abrahamsson SO, Lundborg G, Adalbert K: Functional splinting vs. plaster cast for ruptures of the ulnar collateral ligament of the thumb: a prospective randomized study. *Acta Orthop Scand,* 62:524-526, 1991.

No difference was seen between patients treated with a functional short thumb spica splint vs. a plaster cast for both operatively and nonoperatively treated tears of the ulnar collateral ligament. In this study, patients with suspected Stener lesions were treated with operative repair.

5

Reconstruction of Finger Deformities

Douglas P. Hanel, MD

Introduction

Finger deformities limit hand function because of pain and malposition. The pain may emanate from either an incongruous arthritic joint or motion at the site of a delayed union. Malposition, especially rotational malalignment, limits motion by interfering with hand closure. Malposition secondary to segmental bone loss leaves the digit worthlessly suspended from surrounding soft tissues. The uniformly dismal long-term results of interphalangeal joint replacement has prompted a closer look at the best methods for small-joint arthrodesis as well as the functional consequences of these fused joints. The best location for osteotomy of phalangeal malunions remains controversial. Osteotomies proximal to the site of malunion have been proposed to prevent tendon adhesion and subsequent loss of motion in the reconstructed digit. Delayed unions are best treated by identifying the physiologic response at the fracture site. Hypertrophic nonunions are managed with reinforced immobilization, whereas atrophic nonunions require bone grafts as well as augmented fixation. Segmental bone loss can be managed with autografts, allografts, or distraction osteogenesis. Autografts remain the mainstay of hand reconstruction with the role of allograft and distraction still being defined. Finally, the best treatment of a hopelessly deformed digit is amputation. When an amputation involves central digits, a unique set of deformities is created that must be corrected to preserve hand function and cosmesis. This chapter reviews recent advances in hand joint arthrodesis, correction of malunion, nonunion and bone loss, and the reconstruction of the hand deformed by central ray resection.

Arthrodesis

Pain, joint destruction, chronic instability, and deformity resulting from trauma or osteoarthritis continue to be indications for small-joint arthrodesis. Joints which must be stable to provide strong lateral pinch, i.e. the index and long finger proximal interphalangeal joint and the thumb metacarpophalangeal joint, are most amenable to fusion. Fusion of the joints whose contribution to hand function requires a larger range of motion results in a significant disability. This is especially true of the ring and small finger proximal interphalangeal joints and to a lesser extent the carpometacarpal joint of the thumb. Although reliable arthroplasties are available for the basal joint of the thumb, the available interphalangeal joint arthroplasties fail to provide sufficient lateral stability after four years. Silastic joint replacements demonstrate severe erosive changes in at least 30% of cases and mechanical failure occurs in all presently utilized hinged prostheses. Until the role of vascularized joint transfer is established or more reliable prosthetic devises are developed, the treatment of choice for interphalangeal joint and thumb metacarpolphalangeal joint destruction is fusion. The question of thumb carpometacarpal arthrodesis vs. arthroplasty is not yet resolved.

The optimal position for the various joint fusions has been reinforced by a number of authors (Table 5-1).

Table 5-1. Position of Small Joint Arthrodesis

	Degrees	
Distal interphalangeal	10-20	Flexion*
Proximal interphalangeal	30-45	Flexion*
Thumb metacarpolphalangeal	15	Flexion
Thumb Carpometacarpal	30-40	Palmar Abduction
	30- 35	Radial Abduction
	≈ 15	Pronation

*progressing from radial to ulnar

In review of 171 interphalangeal joint fusions, flexion of 10° to 20° in the distal interphalangeal joint and 30° to 45° in the proximal interphalangeal joints (progressing from radial to ulnar) was felt to be most appropriate. In another study based on 41 thumb metacarpophalangeal joint fusions, 15° of flexion and 10° of pronation provided optimal pinch position without compromising first web-space breadth. The optimal position for thumb carpometacarpal arthrodesis is 30° to 40° of palmar abduction, 30° to 35° of radial abduction, and enough pronation to accommodate pulp-to-pulp pinch between the thumb, index, and long fingers.

The union rate for all arthrodesis procedures reported in the last 10 years is between 80% to 100%, with the lower fusion rates noted in thumb carpometacarpal joints secured with Kirschner wires. The only distinct advantage of any one fixation method over another is that more rigid fixation allows earlier mobilization. Therefore the procedure chosen should be dependent upon both the familiarity of the surgeon with the procedure and the perceived demands of the patient.

Thumb Carpometacarpal Joint

A greater than 10-year followup of thumb carpometacarpal arthrodesis demonstrated several trends. Normal pinch strength occurred in more than 60% of patients. In one study, 77% of patients were able to contract the thumb to the index, long, and ring pulp and 70% were completely pain-free. In another study there was a 72% decrease in the adduction/abduction arc and a 61% reduction in flexion/extension arc. Despite this loss of motion there were minimal subjective complaints and seldom any demonstrable loss of precision hand function. In both studies, less than 5% of patients developed arthritic changes in the scaphotrapezial articulation, and those who did were successfully managed with silastic or soft-tissue trapezium replacement arthroplasty.

Carroll reported successful arthrodesis using a cup-in-cone technique, in 63 of 64 patients, with three patients requiring secondary grafting to secure union. Other series using Carroll's technique report fusion rates of only 80%. Alternative methods of fixation include bone staples and sliding bone grafts. In a series of eight patients treated with bone staples, five healed within 10 weeks, one healed in 50 weeks, and healing time was not reported in two cases. This compared favorably with the Kirschner-wire fixation used in the 16 other patients. To date, the sliding graft technique is the most successful method described for carpometacarpal joint fusion. Twenty consecutive fusions were successfully performed using a sliding graft (Fig. 5-1).

The consensus of these reports is that carpometacarpal joint arthrodesis is the treatment of choice for patients whose vocations or avocations place high demands for stability and strength upon the thumb. The contraindication to arthrodesis is pantrapezial arthrosis, which occurs in more than two-thirds of patients presenting with thumb pain. Comparing arthrodesis to a variety of arthroplasty procedures in a general population of patients, the overall rate of satisfaction and strength could not be correlated with the type of procedure.

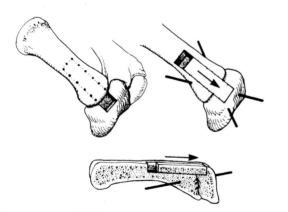

Figure 5-1. Sliding graft method used for 20 consecutive successful trapeziometacarpal arthrodeses. Eight weeks of cast immobilization is necessary with this method. (Reproduced with permission from Doyle JR: Sliding bone graft technique for arthrodesis of the trapezio-metacarpal joint of the thumb; department of Technique. *J Hand Surg,* 16A:363-365, 1991.)

Thumb Metacarpophalangeal Joint

Segmuller has observed that the thumb metacarpophalangeal joint has the least motion of any digital joint and therefore stability of that joint should take precedence over motion. The results of the Segmuller series of 50 fusions using a tension-band technique as well as other studies using a variety of fixation methods portray a high fusion rate and minimal complications. Fusion of the thumb MCP joint leads to a uniformly positive subjective response. Patients report increased strength, thumb ray stability, and the elimination of the painful joint. Objective measurement substantiates this claim. Postoperative thumb pinch strength was always improved when compared to preoperative strength and in a number of cases was even greater than that of the opposite thumb. There is no evidence that fusion of the MCP joint contributes to the acceleration of carpometacarpal or interphalangeal joint dysfunction. Hastings and Hagen did note difficulty with fine pinch in 11 of 18 patients.

Finger Interphalangeal Joints

Biomechanical analysis of crossed Kirschner wires, intraosseus wires, and figure-eight tension bands used for interphalangeal joint fusion fixation suggests that a figure-of-eight tension band is superior in anteroposterior bending and torsion (Figs. 5-2 and 5-3).

Each technique demonstrated the same resistance to lateral bending forces. Placing an interosseous wire dorsal to the axis of flexion is more substantial than placing the wire on or volar to the axis of rotation. Although retrospective studies support these experimental findings with 97% union rates and infrequent postoperative infections, the advantage of this technique over other retrospectively studied fixation techniques is not established. Burton presented 170 successful fusions in 171 attempts using flat osteotomies and cross K-wire technique. The success of this technique demands minimal periosteal dissection, accurate coaptation of medullary bone, circumferential contact of cortical bone, and external immobilization for five weeks to 12 weeks. The technique can be adapted to immature bone by cutting through the secondary ossification centers, preserving the physis, coapting the bone ends, and securing fixation with diverging K-wires. Similar results have been reported using intraosseus wire techniques, cup-in-cone osteotomy with K-wire fixation, dorsal tension band, Herbert screw fixation, an external compression device, power-driven staples, and using a trephine to create a tendon for placement within the medullary canal of the middle phalanx. (Figs. 5-4 and 5-5)

Cast or splint immobilization is recommended with each of these methods. Results are uniformly good for each arthrodesis technique. The development of a fixation method that allows immediate unprotected mobilization and attains a high union rate would be most beneficial.

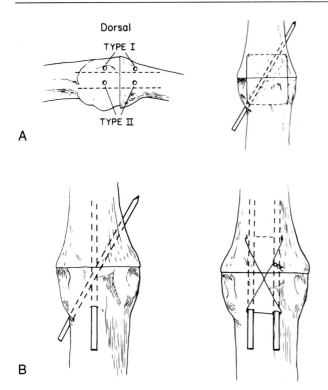

B

Figure 5-2. Four methods of fixation used for arthrodesis of the proximal interphalangeal joint were tested for anteroposterior bending, lateral bending, and torsion. **(A)** Fixation techniques 1 and 2. Technique 1 consists of an oblique Kirschner wire and a tension axis intraosseus loop placed through holes labeled type I. Technique 2 consists of an oblique K-wire and a neutral axis intraosseus loop placed through the holes labeled type II. **(B)** Technique 3 (left) consists of one oblique and one longitudinal K-wire. Technique 4 (right) consists of paired longitudinal K-wires and a dorsal figure-of-eight wire loop. Dorsal figure-of-eight proved to be more resistant to anteroposterior bending. There was no difference in lateral bending. (Reproduced with permission from Kovach JC, Werner WM, Palmer AK, Greenkey S, Murphy DJ: Biomechanical analysis of internal fixation techniques for proximal interphalangeal joint arthrodesis. *J Hand Surg,* 11A:562-566, 1986.)

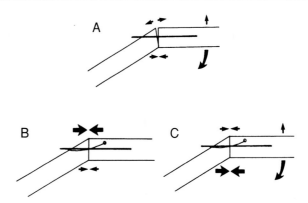

Figure 5-3. Uhl and Schneider illustrate the mechanical advantage of tension-band fixation. **(A)** Arthrodesis with pins alone allows dorsal gapping when the finger is relaxed. **(B)** A dorsal tension band is used to pre-load the dorsal cortex. **(C)** This tension band counteracts the flexors and coverts the forces into palmar compression. If the flexor force exceeds the pre-loaded tension, the system will fail. (Reproduced with permission from Uhl RL, Schneider LH: Tension band arthrodesis of finger joints: a retrospective review of 76 consecutive cases. *J Hand Surg,* 17A:518-522, 1992.)

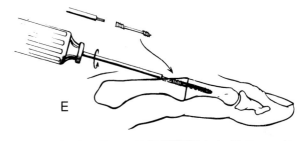

E

Figure 5-4. Herbert screw small joint arthodesis. After preparing the joint surfaces, the Herbert screw is inserted being careful to completely seat the proximal threads. (Reproduced with permission from Ayres JR, Goldstrohm GL, Miller GJ, Dell PC: Proximal interphalangeal joint arthrodesis with the Herbert screw. *J Hand Surg,* 13A:600-603, 1988.)

Malunion

Angular Deformity

Angular malunion of the metacarpal is treated only if there is a painful prominence of the metacarpal head in the palm, usually noted with gripping; if there is tethering of the extensor tendon over the apex of the deformity; or if there is marked clawing of the finger. Angular deformity is poorly tolerated in the second and third metacarpals and even relatively small degrees of angulation (10° to 20°) may create problems. The ulnar two metacarpals, because of the greater mobility of the carpometacarpal joints, are less like-

ly to require correction of deformities. The more proximal sites of malunion within the metacarpal are more likely to create a deformity requiring treatment. The simplest method of correction is a dorsal closing wedge osteotomy. Preoperative planning, with precise drawings of the deformity and the proposed osteotomy, can facilitate the surgery, as there is a tendency for undercorrection of the deformity if one relies on clinical parameters for alignment. Maintaining a partially intact volar cortex or the periosteum greatly enhances stability of the osteotomy and permits fixation with tension-band or intraosseous wiring techniques. Plates and screws may also be used, but are more

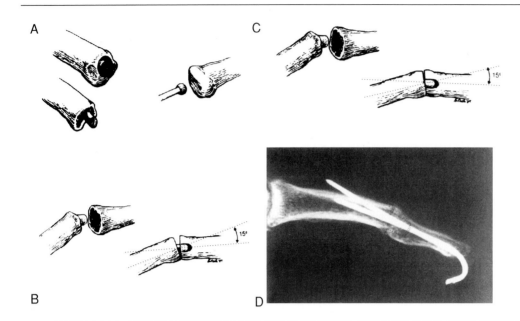

Figure 5-5.   Tenon method of small joint fusion. **(A)** A tenon has been cut in the proximal articular surface with a trephine (left). **(B)** A mortise is fashioned in the opposing articular surface to fit snugly with the previously formed tenon. **(C)** The opposing surfaces are trimmed to fit flush against one another. **(D)** Radiograph showing pinning of the fusion. (Reproduced with permission from Lewis RC, Nordyke MD, Tenny JR: The tenon method of small joint arthrodesis in the hand. *J Hand Surg,* 11A:567-569, 1986.)

limiting if changes in alignment are required after insertion or if there are technical problems with their use.

Rotational Deformity

Two methods for correction of phalangeal malrotation have been advocated: osteotomy at the site of the malunion and osteotomy at the base of the metacarpal. Although osteotomy of the malunion site has the greatest potential for correction of the deformity, this places the adjacent flexor and extensor tendons at risk of injury, adhesions, and subsequent loss of motion. Proximal metacarpal osteotomy avoids these problems.

Proximal metacarpal osteotomy was introduced 30 years ago, and little was written about it until recently. A cadaver study has demonstrated that every 1° of metacarpal rotation corrects approximately 0.7° of phalangeal malrotation. The theoretical amount of phalangeal correction is 18° to 19° in the index, long, and ring and 20° to 30° in the small. The limiting factor to additional rotational correction is the deep transverse metacarpal ligament. Releasing the transverse metacarpal ligament is not recommended because of the resultant loss of the transverse palmar arch and instability of the metacarpophalangeal joint. This procedure has been reported to be "satisfactory" in a number of small series.

In no publication is the amount of deformity (in degrees) or the amount of correction (in degrees) reported. Critics of this procedure point out that although metacarpal rotational osteotomy may correct the apparent finger malrotation, there remains rotational malalignment, albeit to a lesser degree, in complete digital flexion. In addition, the digit assumes an S-shaped appearance in full extension; this is the result of two diametrically opposed angular deformities, the traumatic deformity and the correctional osteotomy, separated by a distance of 3 to 4 cm. If complete correction of a malunion is desired, it can only be done by addressing the malunion site.

A step-cut osteotomy has been used for both metacarpal and proximal phalanx malunions. (Fig. 5-6) The benefits of

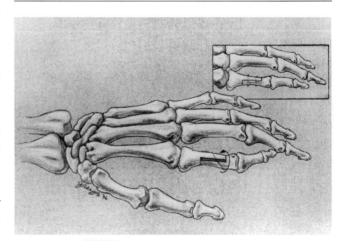

Figure 5-6.   Principle of a step-cut osteotomy. The width of the longitudinal cut (dorsal cortex only) determines the extent of angular correction. The intact palmar cortical hinge combined with internal fixation provides enough stability for early active motion. The direction of the distal transverse limb determines the direction of correction. (Reproduced with permission from Pichora DR, Meyer R, Masear VR: Rotational step-cut osteotomy of metacarpal and phalangeal malunion. *J Hand Surg,* 16A:551-555, 1991.)

this method are that the longitudinal limb of the osteotomy accommodates greater adjustment and presents a larger surface area for healing. Although originally described for metacarpal correction, a recent series presented 16 successfully corrected proximal phalanx malunions. Eleven of the proximal phalanx osteotomies also underwent simultaneous extensor tendon tenolysis and capsulotomies of adjacent joints. Scissoring was corrected in all cases and the osteotomies healed within eight weeks. Increased postoperative motion was reported, although several patients lost up to 15° of motion. The largest series of malunions corrected at the site of deformity comes from the AO center in Switzerland. Thirty-six cases were corrected and maintained with plate and screw fixation. Eighty-six percent of patients had satisfactory digital function. The poor results were related to chronic periarticular injury.

Articular Deformity

A unique malunion problem, which usually presents with limited motion secondary to articular incongruity, is intra-articular malalignment. With time, the incongruity leads to joint destruction manifested as crepitation, pain, increasing angular deformity, and further loss of motion and hand function. This difficult problem has been previously managed with arthroplasty, arthrodesis, or acceptance of deformity. Intra-articular realignment osteotomy has been presented as an alternative treatment. Using direct visualization, the malaligned joint surface is identified and the fracture site taken down. In fractures that are several months old, curretting the maturing callus can reveal the fracture line. If the fracture line is not readily visible then a radiographically assisted osteotomy is recommended. Care is taken to preserve soft-tissue attachments, thereby preserving the vascularity of the bone fragment. The fracture is realigned, secured with rigid fixation, and mobilized early.

The contraindications to this procedure are the presence of severe articular damage in a large portion of the articular surface, and a patient who is unwilling to cooperate with the demanding postoperative therapy. This procedure has been successful in a small number of wrist, thumb, and metacarpal head injuries. The most dramatic results were reported in proximal phalanx condylar malunions when five of six patients demonstrated 50° to 95° of improved motion after the procedure. A poor result occurred in an osteoporotic digit, which required prolonged protection and developed arthrofibrosis. Although the long-term outcome of these osteotomies is not known, the procedure restores alignment, preserves bone stock, and potentially maximizes motion.

Functional limitations may result from inadequately reduced subchondylar or phalangeal neck fractures. A bony block along the volar aspect of the phalanx prevents flexion. This deformity, which represents either apex volar angulation or dorsal translation of the phalangeal head, does not remodel even in children. Three pediatric patients were treated by removal of the bony block, which resulted in gains of 25° to 50° of flexion. The cases were approached through palmar zig-zag incisions that allowed release of the contracted volar capsule and complete visualization of the ostectomy (or bone removal) site.

Nonunion

Metacarpal and phalangeal fractures usually heal within three to six weeks. Open fractures may take more time and are frequently clinically healed long before radiographic consolidation. The diagnosis of delayed union or nonunion is, therefore, vague. Some authors have proposed that at least 12 months must pass before a diagnosis of nonunion in a hand fracture can be made. Others have proposed that a functional approach will provide a better monitor of union, using pain and motion at the fracture site 16 weeks after injury as the criteria for nonunion. This approach is based on the clinical impression that immobilization of a finger beyond four months is associated with seriously compromised digital function and that an aggressive approach is therefore demanded. If one accepts this premise, then delayed union and nonunion of metacarpal and phalangeal hand fractures are the same.

Nonunions occur more frequently in crush-type injuries and involve the proximal phalanx more often than the other phalanges or metacarpals. This is in part due to the increased frequency of proximal phalanx fractures compared to other phalangeal fractures. In addition, the fracture environment of a phalanx is less amenable to healing than the muscular bed that envelops metacarpal fractures. Although in most reported nonunions the initial fracture treatment consisted of either external splints or K-wires, the causal relationship between initial bony treatment and the subsequent failure to heal has not yet been established. It is more likely that the mechanisms of injury, rather than fixation methods, predispose a fracture to nonunion.

In a series of 25 patients with delayed union or nonunion, the recommended treatment varied from the replacement of K-wires to fixation with plates and screws. The need for bone graft was defined by parameters previously used for long bone nonunions. Hypertrophic-reactive nonunions were treated with rigid fixation, such as plate and screws, and were not grafted. (Fig. 5-7)

Non-reactive atrophic nonunions were treated with bone graft in addition to K-wires or plates and screws. (Fig. 5-8)

The 25 nonunions healed within seven to 16 weeks of intervention as confirmed by physical and radiographic findings. In five of 14 patients there was no significant improvement in total digital range of motion after fracture healing. In the remaining patients there was between 5° and 80° of improvement. Despite the discrepancy in range of motion, all patients felt that hand function improved with fracture union. By objective measure, hand strength improved in each case after the fractures united.

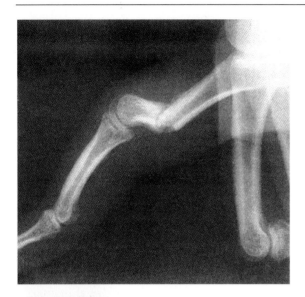

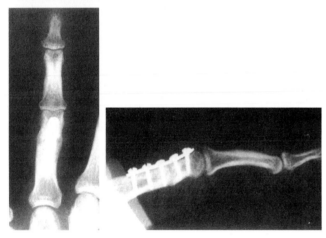

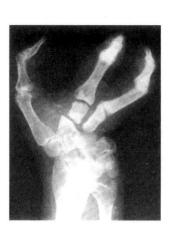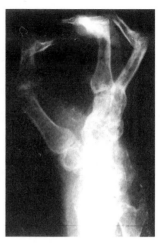

Figure 5-8. **(Left)** An extensive crush injury to the left hand of a 31-year-old cook resulted in a septic nonunion at the base of the second and third metacarpals. Cultures revealed a mixed infection with staphylococcus aureus, enterococci, and Klebsiella. **(Right)** After treatment by debridement, parenteral antibiotics, and a pedicled groin flap, iliac crest graft was used to unite the metacarpals to the distal carpus. (Reproduced with permission from Jupiter JB, Koniuch MP, Smith RJ: The management of delayed union and nonunion of the metacarpals and phalanges. *J Hand Surg,* 10A:457-466, 1985.)

Figure 5-7. A slightly hypertrophic delayed union of the ring finger proximal phalanx **(Top)**. The digital TAM preoperatively was 130°. **(Bottom)** The delayed union was stabilized with a five-hole ASIF plate. An extensor tenolysis and PIP joint capsulotomy were also performed. It is reported that the fracture united, and the fixation plate was removed after seven months; 205° of total active motion was obtained. (Reproduced with permission from Jupiter JB, Koniuch MP, Smith RJ: The management of delayed union and nonunion of the metacarpals and phalanges. *J Hand Surg,* 10A:457-466, 1985.)

Bone Loss

Most traumatic bone defects of the hand are associated with severe soft-tissue injuries. The management of these complex combined injuries requires thorough debridement, skeletal stabilization, and soft-tissue reconstruction. The timing for each of these steps is becoming better defined. Recent protocols for complex injuries to the upper extremity emphasize removal of all potentially nonviable tissue, thereby creating a wound that resembles a defect after the resection of a locally aggressive tumor. These wounds should be made ready for immediate or early closure.

The timing of bone reconstruction is still controversial. Traditionally, soft-tissue coverage and the assurance that the bone graft will be placed in an infection-free environment postponed the process for weeks. In contrast, a recent series of patients with bone defects resulting primarily from gunshot wounds were treated with plate fixation and open cancellous autograft. The 10 hand injuries in this series healed without infection, required 30 weeks to unite, and resulted in satisfactory function in all but one patient. This technique finds its greatest application in the management of metacarpal defects or in those cases where the wound problem is limited to the bone and skin only. When the wound includes exposed vessels and tendons, other methods should be considered.

In one series of 17 patients reported by Freeland, Jabaley, Burkhalter, and Chaves, bone grafting within 10 days of injury effectively stabilized the hands. The authors again emphasized the importance of wound debridement, soft-tissue coverage, and rigid fixation as essential components of management. Büchler and Aiken reported on 18 patients with proximal interphalangeal joint osseous defects, extensor tendon loss, and soft-tissue coverage problems that were treated with proximal interphalangeal joint arthrodesis using a solid block of iliac crest secured by plate and screws. If the distal interphalangeal joint was not

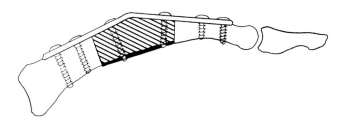

Figure 5-9. Cortical-cancellous composite after fixation with plate and screws. (Reproduced with permission from Buchler U, Aiken AA: Arthrodesis of the proximal interphalangeal joint by solid bone grafting and plate fixation in extensive injuries to the dorsal aspect of the finger. *J Hand Surg*, 13A:589-594, 1988.)

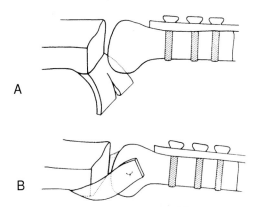

Figure 5-10. After transfer of a composite metacarpal head and shaft allograft, ligamentous stabilization is provided as follows: **(A)** Reconstruction of collateral ligaments can be performed by detaching the volar plate proximally and splitting it longitudinally. **(B)** Each limb of the volar plate is sutured to its side of the allograft metacarpal head. (Reproduced with permission from Trumble TE, Freidlander GE: The use of allogeneic bone in hand injuries. *Techn Orthop*, 1:79-90, 1986.)

destroyed, the extensor mechanism for the distal interphalangeal joint was repaired primarily using tendon grafts when necessary. These procedures require exceptionally good bone carpentry technique. The bone block must be designed to fill the osseous defect, while including the ideal angles for a functional arthrodesis. (Fig. 5-9) The value of careful technique is the restoration of digit length, arthrodesis in a functional position, preservation of distal joint motion (when available), and infection-free healing in all but one case.

In the past, metacarpal defects have been treated with autogenous iliac crest grafts. Alternative autograft sources are presented in a series of 21 patients with hand and wrist defects secondary to either trauma or tumor resection. Metacarpal or phalangeal defects were treated with the diaphyseal-metaphyseal metatarsal segments in 11 cases. Four cases were treated with corticocancellous segments of ulna and three cases were treated with iliac crest. Fixation included "bone impingement" or K-wire fixation followed by prolonged immobilization. Although all the grafts eventually incorporated, no patient gained more than 60% of digit motion and eight had significantly less. Skeletal stabilization has also been obtained with allograft bone. The number of cases using allograft are few. Enthusiastic advocates of allograft reconstruction argue that the architectural similarity of the graft minimizes manipulation, accommodates rigid fixation, and avoids donor-site morbidity as well as the need for general anesthesia. In addition, osteoarticular grafts can be used for reconstruction of joint surfaces. (Fig. 5-10)

Clinical examples of wrist, metacarpal head, proximal phalanx, and middle phalanx replacement have been reported. The allograft-native bone interface seems to heal without problem. The clinical outcome is reported as being good but no parameters for this conclusion are given. Recent investigators, concerned about the potential risk of transmitting fatal diseases from allografts, advocate allograft irradiation and/or treatment with ethylene oxide.

It is hoped that bone donor-site problems will become unimportant as bone transport techniques are developed.

Although lengthening of digits has been practiced for the last 25 years, the recently popularized techniques of Ilizarov have renewed interest in distraction neo-osteogenesis. Unfortunately, we have no additional clinical information to add to the original work of Matev. Reviewing a 20-year experience, Matev points out that although gaps of 3 cm or greater will heal spontaneously in children, the potential for spontaneous osteogenesis in adult digits undergoing distraction is unpredictable. More than one-half of adults will require bone grafts. Similar to long-bone transport, the most common problems arise from pin-tract infections and angulation of the lengthened segment after removal of the distraction device. The first problem can be avoided if fixation pins remain firm; the second problem is avoided by postponing removal of the distractor until there is evidence of consolidation along the full length and width of the bone. A third possible problem, angulation while distracting the digit, can be addressed by passing a K-wire down the axis of the finger being lengthened and simultaneously releasing soft-tissue scars, which may tether the digit as it is mobilized. A clever combination of distraction and vascularized epiphyseal transfer has been presented for the treatment of an intercalary defect in a child. This case report describes using a unilateral frame to distract the digit 2 cm along a longitudinally placed K-wire. After the desired length was achieved, a vascularized metatarsal-phalangeal joint was transferred into the interval created by distraction. (Fig. 5-11) Two and one-half years after transfer, the physes remain open, the digit has grown longitudinally, and a painless mobile joint contributes to a functional tripod grip.

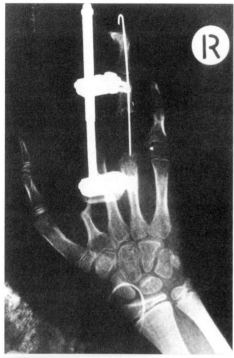

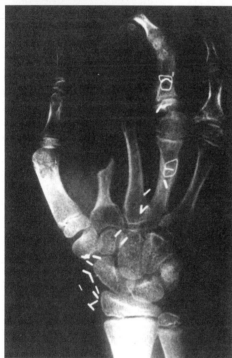

Figure 5-11.   Figures from a case report decribing combined digital lengthening and free vascularized joint transfer. **(Top)** Radiograph of distraction lengthening of 1.9cm. **(Bottom)** Two years postoperatively radiograph demonstrates intact growth plates and articular joint space of transferred metatarsophalangeal joint of a second toe. (Reproduced with permission from Singer DI, O'Brien B.McC, Angel MF, Gumley GJ: Digital distraction lengthening followed by free vascularized epiphyseal joint transfer. *J Hand Surg*, 14A:508-512, 1989.)

Transposition

Severe chronic bony deformities of the finger force the patient and physician to choose between multiple reconstructive procedures or amputation. Single digits with chronic combined injuries, especially if associated with an unreconstructable nerve loss, are best amputated. Border digit amputation is rather straightforward, especially when caution has been taken to minimize neuroma formation, and adequate skin flaps allow tension-free wound closure. Central digit amputations are unique in that the hand is rendered increasingly more unsightly and clumsy as the level of amputation approaches the metacarpal phalangeal joint. The accepted management of this problem is ray resection.

Reconstruction of central ray amputations requires closing the gap created by the amputation while attempting to preserve the web space and maintain rotational and longitudinal alignment of the remaining digits. This assures a cosmetically attractive hand and minimizes hand dysfunction. Web-space preservation is best accomplished by retaining the skin from either the radial or ulnar aspect of the amputated proximal phalanx and insetting the entire web space into the adjacent digit. Because of the mobility

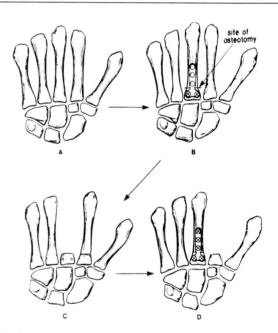

Figure 5-12.   **(A)** Diagram of the native hand prior to procedure. **(B)** T-plate aligned on long finger metacarpal. Transverse limb of T-plate affixed to proximal metaphysis and osteotomy site marked. **(C)** With the plate removed the long ray metacarpal osteotomy is performed and ray resection completed. The index finger is osteotomized and mobilized ulnarly. **(D)** After adjustments for height and repair of the intermetacarpal ligament, osteosynthesis is completed. (Reproduced with permission from Hanel DP, Lederman ES: Index transposition after long finger ray resection. *J Hand Surg*, 18A:271-277, 1993.)

of the ring and small finger carpalmetacarpal joint, it has been recommended that after central ray resection, the gap between metacarpal heads can be closed by imbricating adjacent deep transverse intermetacarpal ligaments. Patients with ring finger amputations are reported to have no problems following web reconstruction, digital rotation, or overall hand appearance after simple approximation and ligament imbrication. However, patients with long finger amputations treated by this method note that the index and ring finger tend to cross as closure of the gap was completed. Although this is a potential cosmetic and functional problem, these patients were reported to be satisfied with the results of their amputation and reconstruction.

The problem of overlapping digits has been recognized since World War II and various osteotomies have been proposed as solutions. The most versatile is transposition of the index finger to the long finger position. This transposition allows complete closure of the gap between the index and ring finger while permitting adjustment of metacarpal height and rotational alignment. Critics have noted that ray transposition is frequently associated with a high incidence of malunion or nonunion and subsequent loss of hand function because of prolonged immobilization. These complications were seen in cases treated with K-wire and cast immobilization and can be avoided with rigid internal fixation using plate and screws for stabilization. (Fig. 5-12)

Patients with chronic problems gained motion after removal of the dysfunctional digit. Eighty percent of pinch and grip strength is retained in acutely injured patients but strength is reduced to 50% in patients with chronic problems.

Alternative methods to simple approximation or digit transposition have been recently described; these include wedge resection of the hamate for closure of the third web space after ring finger amputation and wedge resection of the capitate for closure of the second web space after long finger ray amputation. (Fig. 5-13 and 5-14)

Advocates of wedge osteotomy feel that in the case of ring finger ray resections, simple approximation markedly limits carpometacarpal motion, changes the divergence of the third and fifth digits, and thereby limits the functional outcome. Wedge osteotomy of the capitate is felt to provide better results after long-finger resection because it does not compromise the first web space, does not require prolonged

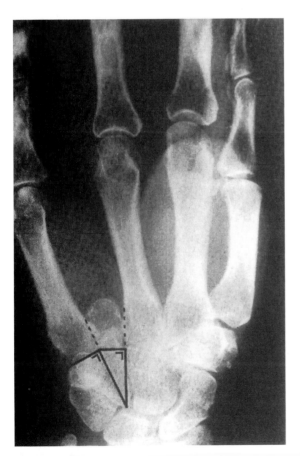 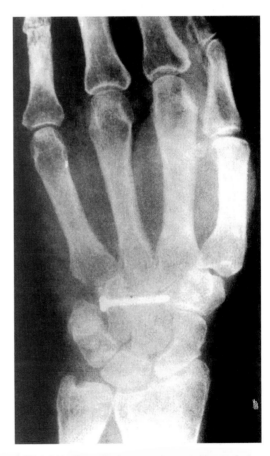

Figure 5-13. **(Left)** Surgical planning for the hamate-capitate wedge osteotomy. **(Right)** Radiograph shows ray transposition and screw fixation. (Reproduced with permission from de Boer A, Robinson PH: Ray transposition by intercarpal osteotomy after loss of the fourth digit. *J Hand Surg,* 14A:379-381, 1989.)

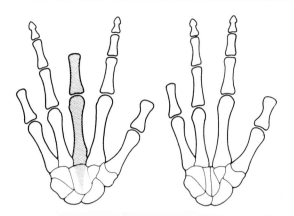

Figure 5-14. Diagrammatic representation of amputation of third ray and V-shaped osteotomy of the capitate **(Left)**. The second and fourth rays have been brought together to close the gap **(Right)**. (Reproduced with permission from Iselin F, Peze W: Ray centralization without bone fixation for amputation of the middle finger. *J Hand Surg,* 13B:97-99, 1988.)

immobilization, or leave a painful index metacarpal stump. However, these theoretical concerns are not manifest in clinical practice. There are no long-term studies that address the affect of carpal osteotomy on intercarpal dynamics or the potential for development of intercarpal arthritis. The functional results of successful wedge osteotomy are reported to be similar to the other reported methods and cosmetically superior according to the authors.

Annotated Bibliography

Arthrodesis

First CMC

Bamberger BH, Stern PJ, Kiefhaber TR, McDonough JJ, Cantor RM: Trapeziometacarpal joint arthrodesis: a functional evaluation. *J Hand Surg,* 17A:605-611, 1992.

This detailed review of 24 patients (16 K-wire, eight bone staples) demonstrates that with thumb CMC joint fusion there is a marked decrease in the flexion/extension arc and abduction/ adduction arc but that there is little functional deficit and minimal subjective complaint.

Carroll RE: Arthrodesis of the carpometacarpal joint of the thumb. A review of patients with a long postoperative period. *Clin Orthop,* 220:106-110, 1987.

Sixty-seven patients, all younger than 50 years of age were followed for three to 25 years after thumb CMC fusion using a cup-and-cone technique. Primary union occurred in 63 with secondary union occurring in three of four initial failures. No patient developed scapho-trapezium-trapezoid arthritis. The author cautions that in older patients, CMC arthrodesis may lead to adjacent joint arthrosis.

Thumb MP Joint

Saldana MJ, Clark EN, Aulicino PL: The optimal position for arthrodesis of the metacarpophalangeal joint of the thumb: a clinical study. *J Hand Surg,* 12B:256-259, 1987.

Fifty females and fifty males were examined while performing 12 common hand functions. Based on these observations the authors recommend fusing the thumb metacarpophalangeal joint in 25° of flexion for men and 20° for women.

Steiger VR, Segmuller G: Arthrodesis of the metacarpophalangeal joint of the thumb. *Handchir Mikrochir Plast Chir,* 21:18-22, 1989.

Forty-one of 50 patients were available for examination after tension-band arthrodesis of the thumb metacarpophalangeal joint. This technique allowed early mobilization and was felt to be uniformly successful. The optimal position of fusion was felt to be 15° of flexion and ten degrees of pronation.

PIP Joint

Burton et al: Small joint arthrodesis in the hand. *J Hand Surg,* 11A:678-682, 1986

A union rate of 99.4% in 171 small joint fusions. Soft-tissue management, metaphyseal abutment, and crossed Kirschner wire fixation is emphasized.

Ijsselstein CB, vanEgmond DG, Hovius SER, van der Meulen JC: Results of small joint arthrodesis. comparison of Kirschner wire fixation with tension band wire technique. *J Hand Surg,* 17A:952-956, 1992.

This retrospective look at 203 PIP and MP joint arthrodeses compares a number of K-wire and interosseus wire fixation techniques to the longitudinal K-wire and dorsal figure-of-eight tension-band technique. Infections, nonunions, and malunions were significantly less for the tension-band technique.

Kovach JC, Werner FW, Palmer AK, Greenkey S, Murphy DJ: Biomechanical analysis of internal fixation techniques for proximal interphalangeal joint arthrodesis. *J Hand Surg,* 11A:562-566, 1986.

Figure of eight tension bands demonstrated superior strength in anteroposterior bending when compared to crossed Kirschner wires and interosseus wires. No differences were seen in lateral bending.

Lewis RC, Nordyke MD, Tenny JR: The tenon method of small joint arthrodesis in the hand. *J Hand Surg,* 11A:567-569, 1986.

A tenon, created by a trephine, is inserted within the medullary canal of the opposite phalanx. Fixation is secured with K-wires. A union rate of 97.7% is reported in 85 joints.

Pellegrini VD Jr, Burton RI: Osteoarthritis of the proximal interphalangeal joint of the hand: Arthroplasty or fusion? *J Hand Surg,* 15A:194-209, 1990.

Fusions provide stable, durable lateral pinch and remain the treatment of choice for the index finger. Preservation of motion in the ulnar digits can be obtained with silicone arthroplasty; however, two- and four-year follow-up reveals progressive periarticular erosion. The question raised in the title remains unanswered.

Uhl, RL Schneider, LH: Tension band arthrodesis of finger joints: a retrospective review of 76 consecutive cases. *J Hand Surg,* 17A:518-522, 1992.

Longitudinal K-wire combined with looped wire tension bands or figure of eight tension bands provided uniformly good results. The most frequent complication was pin penetration of the volar cortex which occurred in 41% of cases. A drill guide is demonstrated which may assist in decreasing the occurrence of this problem.

Malunion

Phalangeal Malalignment Treated With Distant Osteotomy

Gross M and Gelberman R: Metacarpal rotational osteotomy. *J Hand Surg,* 10A:105-108, 1985.

This cadaver study demonstrates that a rotational deformity of up to 18° in the index, long and ring finger and between 20° and 30° in the small finger could potentially be corrected with an osteotomy and rotation of the metacarpal.

Botelheiro JC: Overlapping of fingers due to malunion of a phalanx corrected by a metacarpal rotational osteotomy—report of two cases. *J Hand Surg,* 10B:389-390, 1985.

Two cases, a fourth and fifth digit. This article is followed by an editor's note, which states that "Two of the editors have tried this, once each, without much success. Perhaps this supports the theory that the pen is mightier than the sword."

Phalangeal Malalignment Treated With *in situ* Osteotomy

Lucas GL, Pfeiffer CM: Osteotomy of the metacarpals and phalanges stabilized by AO plates and screws. *Ann-Chir-Main,* 30-38, 1989.

Thirty-six cases of metacarpal/phalangeal malunions were treated with *in situ* osteotomies. Rigid fixation allowed early mobilization. There were no nonunions and no patient lost motion as a result of the osteotomy.

Pichora DR, Meyer R, Masear VR: Rotational step-cut osteotomy for treatment of metacarpal and phalangeal malunion. *J Hand Surg,* 16A:551-555, 1991.

Using a method originally described by O'Donoghue for tibial malunion and later by Manktelow for metacarpal, 23 step-cut

osteotomies successfully realigned seven metacarpal and 16 proximal phalanx malunions. While function was felt to improve in all patients, up to 15° of motion was lost in several cases.

Periarticular Malunion

Light T: Salvage of intraarticular malunions of the hand and wrist. The role of realignment osteotomy. *Clin Orthop,* 214:130-135, 1987.

Hand function and range of motion were improved is six PIP, two CMC, one MP, and one distal radius with intra-articular malalignment treated with intra-articular osteotomy. The time from injury to surgery was six to 52 weeks.

Simmons B, Peters T: Subchondylar fossa reconstruction for malunion of fractures of the proximal phalanx in children. *J Hand Surg,* 12A:1079-1082, 1987.

Three pediatric cases with bony blocks secondary to phalangeal neck fractures were treated with osteotomy and deepening of subchondylar fossa. A volar approach is recommended.

Nonunion

Jupiter JB, Koniuch MP, Smith RJ: The management of delayed union and nonunion of the metacarpals and phalanges. *J Hand Surg,* 10A:457-466, 1985.

Twenty-five delayed unions or nonunions were classified as reactive or nonreactive. Reactive nonunions were treated with modification of fixation whereas nonreactive nonunions required bone graft in addition to the change in fixation.

Bone Loss

Buchler U, Aiken AA: Arthrodesis of the proximal interphalangeal joint by solid bone grafting and plate fixation in extensive injuries to the dorsal aspect of the finger. *J Hand Surg,* 13A:589-594, 1988.

Segmental bone loss involving the PIP joint was bridged with a corticocancellous bone block and rigidly fixed with plates and screws. All 25 digits healed, two with delays. The procedure requires exceptionally good three-dimensional conceptualization and bone carpentry skills.

Calkins MS, Burkhalter WE, Reyes F: Traumatic segmental bone defects in the upper extremity: treatment with exposed grafts of corticocancellous bone. *J Bone Joint Surg,* 9A:1927-1987.

Bone defects in 10 hand injuries were treated with rigid fixation and exposed bone graft. Fixation and critical soft tissue were not exposed. All but one patient healed satisfactorily.

Freeland AE, Jabaley ME, Burkhalter WE, Chaves AMV: Delayed primary bone grafting in the hand and wrist after traumatic bone loss. *J Hand Surg,* 9A:22-27, 1984.

Seventeen patients with 21 bone defects underwent iliac bone grafting within 10 days of injury. Rigid fixation and soft-tissue management were emphasized. There was one fibrous union and one malunion.

Matev IB: The bone-lengthening method in hand reconstruction: twenty years' experience. *J Hand Surg,* 14A:376-378, 1989.

In this invited article the author reviews his method and outcome of digital distraction. His method is not significantly different from other techniques and his experience points out the consistent need for supplemental bone grafts in adult patients.

Rinaldi E: Autografts in the treatment of osseus defects in the forearm and hand. *J Hand Surg,* 12A:282-286, 1987.

Posttraumatic or post-tumor resection bone defects in the forearm, wrist, and hands of 21 patients were treated with various autografts. The 11 traumatic metacarpal or phalangeal defects were reconstructed with metatarsals, partial ulna, or iliac crest. Bony union occurred in all cases; the functional results were mixed.

Trumble TE, Freidlaender GE: Use of allogenic bone in hand injuries. *Techn Orthop,* 1:79-83, 1986.

Among the proposed uses of allografts, a case example and method for metacarpal head replacement is presented.

Transposition

Hanel DP, Lederman ES: Index transposition after long finger ray resection. *J Hand Surg,* 18A:271-277, 1993.

The usual complications of index transposition after long finger ray resection are nonunion and limited function because of prolonged immobilization. These complications were avoided in 10 consecutive cases using rigid internal fixation.

Iselin F, Peze W: Ray centralization without bone fixation for amputation of the middle finger. *J Hand Surg,* 13B:97-99, 1988.

Wedge resection of the capitate was used in 12 patients, yielding cosmetically pleasing results in all patients and an anticipated loss of one-third of grip strength.

Steichen JB, Idler RS: Results of central ray resection without bony transposition. *J Hand Surg,* 11A:466-474, 1986.

Simple approximation, with imbrication of the deep transverse metacarpal ligament was used to reconstruct nine ring finger and four long finger ray resections. Esthetic and functional results were acceptable in all but one case.

II

Carpus and Distal Radius

6

Anatomy and Basic Biomechanics of the Wrist

Richard A. Berger, MD

Introduction

The wrist is a composite articulation interposed between the hand and the forearm. It is responsible for terminal positioning of the hand as a unit, adding to the spatial positioning provided by the axial skeleton, shoulder, elbow, and forearm. Its motions are defined by convention as deviations of the hand, based upon the position of the third metacarpal from a neutral colinear position relative to the forearm bones. The paradoxical demands of extensive mobility and stability make the wrist especially susceptible to mechanical pathologies which are often difficult to treat. Much attention has been directed to understanding the normal pathomechanics of the wrist, and recent basic and clinical research efforts have added substantially to our understanding of this joint. However, many more questions remain before a clear understanding of wrist anatomy and the mechanics will be achieved. This chapter will no doubt change substantially in future editions of this book as a result of research efforts, but stands today as a summary of current concepts of the anatomy and mechanics of the wrist joint.

Development of the Wrist Joint

At approximately the 25th day of gestation, the upper extremity limb buds appear. At day 33, the central carpal flange is seen, and by day 35 mesenchymal condensations are forming the basic structures that ultimately form the carpal bones and associated soft tissues. As in all developing articulating joints, the joints spaces develop by the formation of mesenchymal clefts. At gestational day 37, chondrification of the mesenchymal masses occurs. The carpal bones remain cartilaginous throughout intrauterine life, but maturation of the ligaments and progressive development of surrounding neurovascular structures continues. Ossification of the carpal bones occurs in a relatively consistent fashion. Approximately six months postpartum, the primary ossification centers of the capitate and hamate appear, and at one year the distal radial epiphysis ossifies. The triquetrum begins to ossifiy in the third year, followed by the lunate (fourth year), scaphoid and trapezium (fifth year), and the trapezoid (sixth year). Typically, the distal ulnar epiphysis appears between the fifth through the seventh years. Both the distal radial and ulnar epiphyses close between the 16th and 18th years.

Anatomy of the Wrist—Blood Supply of the Carpus

Extraosseous Blood Supply

The carpus receives its blood supply through branches from three dorsal and palmar arches supplied by the radial, ulnar, anterior interosseous, and posterior interosseous arteries (Fig. 6-1). The three dorsal arches are named (proximal to distal) the radiocarpal, intercarpal, and basal metacarpal transverse arches. Anastomoses are often found between the arches, the radial and ulnar arteries and the interosseous artery system. The palmar arches are named (proximal to distal) the radiocarpal, intercarpal, and deep palmar arches.

Intraosseous Blood Supply

All carpal bones, with the exception of the pisiform, receive their blood supply through dorsal and palmar entry sites, and usually through more than one nutrient artery. Generally, a number of small-caliber penetrating vessels are found in addition to the major nutrient vessels. Intraosseous anastamoses can be found in three basic patterns. First, a direct anastomosis can occur between two large-diameter vessels within the bone. Second, anastomotic arcades may form with similar-sized vessels, often entering the bone from different areas. A final pattern, although rare, has been identified in which a diffuse arterial network virtually fills the bone.

Although the intraosseous vascular patterns of each carpal bone have been defined in detail, studies of the lunate, capitate, and scaphoid are particularly germane due to their predilection to development of clinically important vascular problems. The lunate has only two surfaces available for vascular penetration: dorsal and palmar. From the dorsal and palmar vascular plexuses, between two and four penetrating vessels enter the lunate through each surface. Three consistent patterns of intraosseous vascularization have been identified, based upon the pattern of anastomosis. When viewed in the sagittal plane, the anastomoses form either a Y, X, or an I pattern with arborization of small-caliber vessels stemming from the main branches. The proximal subchondral bone is consistently the least vascularized. The capitate is supplied by both the palmar and dorsal vascular plexuses; however, the palmar supply is more consistent and from larger-caliber vessels. Just distal to the neck of the capitate, vessels largely from the ulnar artery penetrate the palmar-ulnar cortex, while dorsal penetration occurs just distal to the mid-waist level. The intraosseous vascularization pattern consists of proximally-directed retrograde flow, with minimal anastomoses between dorsal and palmar vessels. When present, the dorsal vessels principally supply the head of the capitate, while the palmar vessels supply both the body and the head of the capitate. The scaphoid typically receives its blood supply through three vessels originating from the radial artery: lateral-palmar, dorsal, and distal arterial branches. The lateral-

A
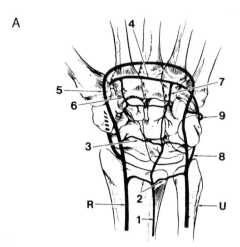

B
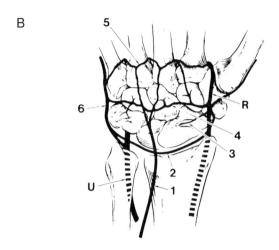

Figure 6-1. **(A)** Anterior blood supply of the carpus. R = radial artery, U = ulnar artery, 1 = anterior interosseous artery, 2 = palmar radiocarpal arch, 3 = palmar intercarpal arch, 4 = deep palmar arch, 5 = superficial palmar arch. **(B)** Posterior blood supply of the carpus. R = radial artery, U = ulnar artery, 1 = posterior interosseous artery, 2 = dorsal radiocarpal arch, 4 = dorsal intercarpal arch, 5 = basal metacarpal arch. (Reproduced with permission from Gelberman RH, Pangais JS, Taleisnik J, et al: The arterial anatomy of the human carpus. Part I: the extra-osseous vascularity. *J Hand Surgery,* 8:367-375, 1983.)

palmar vessel is felt to be the principal blood supply of the scaphoid. All vessels penetrate the cortex of the scaphoid distal to the waist of the scaphoid, coursing in a retrograde fashion to supply the proximal pole. Although there have been reports of minor vascular penetrations directly into the proximal pole from the posterior interosseous artery, substantial risk for avascular necrosis of the proximal pole remains with displaced fractures through the waist of the scaphoid. Overall, it is felt that the remaining carpal bones generally have multiple nutrient vessels penetrating their cortices from more than one side, hence reducing their risk of avascular necrosis by a substantial margin.

Joint Anatomy

Distal Radioulnar Joint

The distal radioulnar joint, although not strictly a part of the wrist, is spatially related to wrist function kinematically and kinetically. The DRUJ is essentially a trochlear joint between the concave sigmoid notch forming the ulnar surface of the distal radius and the convex ulnar head (Fig. 6-2). The radii of curvatures of the articular surfaces forming this joint are dissimilar, with the sigmoid notch possessing a greater radius of curvature than the ulnar head. The ulnar head has approximately 130° of its cylindrical surface covered with articular cartilage. The distal surface of the ulna is composed of the slightly convex head, the styloid process of the ulna, and the fovea at its base. The styloid process is inconsistently variably covered with articular cartilage, varies in length from 3 to 6mm, is on the posterior surface of the ulna, and often exhibits a variable radial curvature.

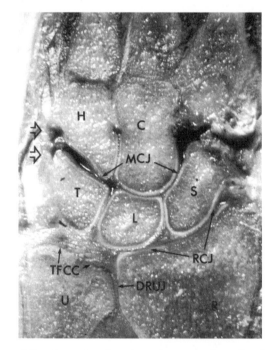

Figure 6-2. Coronal section of a cadaver wrist illustrating the prominent features of the distal radioulnar joint (DRUJ), radiocarpal joint (RCJ) and midcarpal joint (MCJ). Note the triangular fibrocartilage complex articular disc (TFCC) and the distal extent of the TFCC (open arrow heads). R = radius, U = ulna, S = scaphoid, L = lunate, T = triquetrum, C = capitate, H = hamate. (Reproduced with permission from Berger RA: Arthrotomography of the wrist: the triangular fibrocartilage complex. *Clin Orthop,* 172:257-264, 1983.

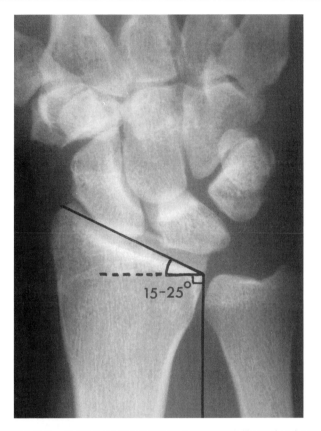

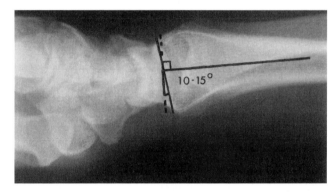

Figure 6-3. **(Left)** Posteroanterior wrist radiograph illustrating the normal range of ulnar inclination of the distal articular surface of the radius. **(Right)** Lateral wrist radiograph illustrating the normal range of palmar inclination of the distal articular surface of the radius.

The foveal region is devoid of articular cartilage and serves as an attachment for the triangular fibrocartilage. Under normal circumstances, the DRUJ is isolated from the radiocarpal joint by a competent triangular fibrocartilage. Degenerative changes and trauma may create perforations in the articular disk region of the triangular fibrocartilage, thus producing a direct communication between the two joints.

Radiocarpal Joint

The radiocarpal joint is formed by the articulation of confluent surfaces of the concave distal articular surface of the radius and the triangular fibrocartilage, with the convex proximal articular surfaces of the proximal carpal row bones. The secant of the concave distal articular surface of the radius is normally inclined palmarly between 10° to 15° and ulnarly 15° to 25° (Fig. 6-3). The distal articular surface of the radius is divided by a fibrocartilaginous ridge, the interfossal ridge, into a triangular-shaped scaphoid fossa and a quadrangular-shaped lunate fossa (Fig. 6-4). The triangular fibrocartilage normally forms a smooth and continuous surface with the distal articular surface of the

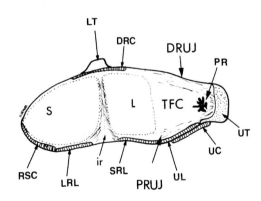

Figure 6-4. Drawing of the proximal surface of the radiocarpal joint from a distal perspective. S = scaphoid fossa, L = lunate fossa, ir = interfossal ridge, LT = Lister's tubercle, TFC = triangular fibrocartilage, PR = prestyloid recess. The capsular ligaments are seen in cross-section: RSC = radioscaphocapitate, LRL = long radiolunate, SRL = short radiolunate, UL = ulnolunate, UC = ulnocapitate, UT = ulnotriquetral, DRC = dorsal radiocarpal DRUJ = dorsal radioulnar, PRUJ = palmar radioulnar.

radius. The pre-styloid recess is located near the ulnar extent of the triangular fibrocartilage, and variably communicates with the ulnar styloid process. The central region of the triangular fibrocartilage is normally quite thin, often appearing translucent, but varies in thickness proportionately with the degree of length discrepency of the distal radius and ulna. The radiocarpal joint is normally isolated from the DRUJ and the midcarpal joint by the triangular fibrocartilage and the proximal row interosseous ligaments, respectively. In approximately 70% of the normal adult population, a direct communication is found between the pisotriquetral joint and the radiocarpal joint. Age-related degenerative defects are commonly found in the central fibrocartilaginous regions of the triangular fibrocartilage and the proximal row interosseous ligaments.

Midcarpal Joint

The midcarpal joint is formed by the mutually articulating surfaces of the proximal and distal carpal rows (Fig. 6-2). Communications are found between the midcarpal joint and the interosseous joint clefts of the proximal and distal row bones, as well as to the second through fifth carpometacarpal joints. Under normal cirumstances, the midcarpal joint is isolated from the pisotriquetral, radiocarpal, and first carpometacarpal joints by intervening membranes and ligaments. The geometry of the midcarpal joint is complex. Radially, the scaphoid-trapezium-trapezoid joint is composed of the slightly convex distal pole of the scaphoid articulating with the reciprocally concave proximal surfaces of the trapezium and trapezoid. Forming an analogue to a "ball-and-socket joint" are the convex head of the capitate and the combined concave contiguous distal articulating surfaces of the scaphoid and the lunate. In 65% of normal adults, it has been found that the hamate articulates with a medial articular facet at the distal-ulnar margin of the lunate, which is associated with a higher rate of cartilage eburnation of the proximal surface of the hamate. The triquetrohamate region of the midcarpal joint is particularly complex, with the mutual articular surfaces having both concave and convex regions forming a helicoid-shaped articulation.

Carpometacarpal Joints

In their most elemental forms, the carpometacarpal joints can be grouped into either fixed or mobile categories. The fixed CMC joints are the second and third, leaving the first, fourth, and fifth as the mobile CMC joints. The functional result of this arrangement allows the second and third metacarpals to form a stable buttress of the palm around which the first, fourth, and fifth metacarpals can rotate. This effectively deepens the palmar cusp and increases the prehensile ability of the fingers.

The first CMC joint is a diarthroidal saddle joint, with concavoconvex surfaces on both the base of the first metacarpal and the distal surface of the trapezium (Fig. 6-5). The axis of orientation of the convex surface of the distal surface of the trapezium is oriented in the anteroposteri-

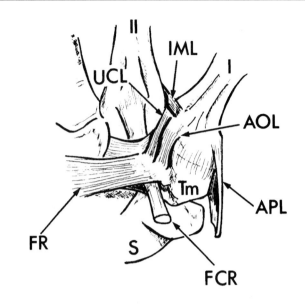

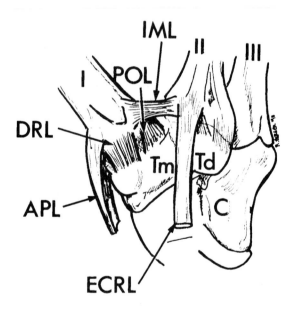

Figure 6-5. **(Top)** Anterior view. I = first metacarpal, II = second metacarpal, Tm = trapezium, S = scaphoid, FR = flexor retinaculum, FCR = flexor carpi radialis tendon, APL = abductor pollicis longus tendon, AOL = anterior oblique ligament, IML = intermetacarpal ligament, UCL = ulnar collateral ligament. **(Bottom)** Posterior view. I = first metacarpal, II = second metacarpal, III = third metacarpal, Tm = trapezium, Td = trapezoid, ECRL = extensor carpi radialis longus tendon, APL = abductor pollicis longus tendon, IML = intermetacarpal ligament, DRL = dorsoradial ligament, POL = posterior oblique ligament. (Reproduced with permission from Imeada T, et al: Anatomy of Trapeziometacarpal Ligament. *J Hand Surgery,* 18A:226-232, 1993.

or plane of the first metacarpal, while the axis of orientation of the convex surface of the base of the first metacarpal is oriented in the medial-lateral plane of the first metacarpal. The first CMC joint is stabilized by a complex network of ligaments recently defined as the anterior and posterior oblique, ulnar collateral, dorsoradial, and intermetacarpal ligaments. The anterior oblique, posterior oblique, and intermetacarpal ligaments attach to the ulnar tubercle of the base of the first metacarpal, forming a "force nucleus" stabilizing the intermetacarpal/carpometacarpal complex through a substantial range of circumduction.

The second and third CMC joints normally have little measureable motion, due to the combination of articular interdigitation through basilar styloid processes on the second and third metacarpals and the extensive ligamentous interconnections between the bases of the metacarpals, the trapezoid and capitate, and between the dorsal and palmar surfaces of the second and third CMC joints. Typically, the third metacarpal styloid process, stemming from the dorso-ulnar surface of the base of the metacarpal, is larger than the second metacarpal styloid process.

The fourth and fifth CMC joints are substantially less constrained than the second and third CMC joints. The geometry of the fourth CMC joint has been described as relatively planar in 86% of adults and somewhat conical in 14%. The base of the fourth metacarpal articulates with the capitate in 82% of the normal adult population. The fifth CMC joint is relatively planar, with only a slight concavity of the distal surface of the hamate matched with a slight convexity of the base of the fifth metacarpal. This results in an increased range of motion of the fourth and fifth CMC joints, averaging 10° to 20° of flexion, respectively, concurrent with a modest range of supination. This motion, however, remains constrained by the strong intermetacarpal and carpometacarpal ligaments, largely limited to the dorsal and palmar surfaces of the respective bones. Additionally, the fifth CMC joint capsule is reinforced by the insertions of the extensor carpi ulnaris tendon and the pisometacarpal ligament.

Interosseous Joints: Proximal Row

The interosseous joints of the proximal row are relatively small and planar, allowing motion primarily in the flexion-extension plane between mutually articulating bones (Fig. 6-2). The scapholunate joint has a smaller surface area than the lunotriquetral joint. Often, a fibrocartilaginous meniscus extending from the membranous region of the scapholunate or lunotriquetral interosseous ligaments are interposed into the respective joint clefts.

Interosseous Joints: Distal Row

The interosseous joints of the distal row are more complex geometrically and allow substantially less interosseous motion than those of the proximal row (Fig. 6-6). The capitohamate joint is relatively planar, but the mutually articulating surfaces are only partially covered by articular cartilage. The distal and palmar region of the joint space is

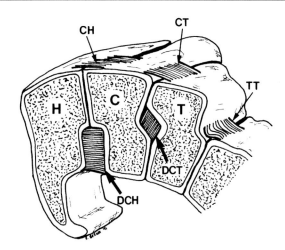

Figure 6-6. Drawing of the cross-section of the distal carpal row from a distal and radial perspective. T = trapezoid, C = capitate, H = hamate, TT = dorsal trapeziotrapezoid ligament, CT = dorsal trapeziocapitate ligament, CH = dorsal capitohamate ligament, DCH = deep capitohamate ligament, DCT = deep trapezocapitate ligament. (Reproduced with permission from An K-N, Berger RA, Cooney WP (Eds): *Biomechanics of the Wrist Joint.* Springer-Verlag, New York, 1991.

devoid of articular cartilage, being occupied by the deep capitohamate interosseous ligament. Similarly, the central region of the trapezocapitate joint surface is interrupted by the deep trapezocapitate interosseous ligament. The trapezium-trapezoid joint presents a small planar surface area with continuous articular surfaces.

Ligamentous Anatomy

Overview

The ligaments of the wrist have been described in a number of ways, leading to substantial confusion in the literature regarding a variety of features of the carpal ligaments. Several general principles have been identified to help simplify the ligamentous architecture of the wrist. No ligaments of the wrist are extracapsular. Most can be anatomically classified as capsular ligaments with collagen fascicles clearly within the lamina of the joint capsule. The ligaments that are not entirely capsular, such as the interosseous ligaments between the bones within the carpal row, are intra-articular. This implies that they are not ensheated in part by a fibrous capsular lamina. The wrist ligaments carry consistent histologic features, which are to a degree ligament specific. The majority of capsular ligaments are composed of longitudinally oriented laminated collagen fascicles surrounded by loosely organized perifasciclar tissue, which are in turn surrounded by the epiligamentous sheath. This sheath is generally composed of the fibrous and synovial capsular lamina. The perifascicular tissue has numerous blood vessels and nerves aligned longitudinally with the collagen fascicles. Currently the function of these nerves is not well understood. It has been hypothesized that these nerves are an integral part of a proprioceptive network, following the principles of Hilton's law of segmental innervation.

The palmar capsular ligaments are more numerous than the dorsal, forming almost the entire palmar joint capsules of the radiocarpal and midcarpal joints. The palmar ligaments tend to converge toward the midline as they travel distally, and have been described as forming an apex-distal "V." The interosseous ligaments between the individual bones within a carpal row are generally short and transversely oriented, and with specific exceptions, cover the dorsal and palmar joint margins. Specific ligament groups are briefly described, and divided into capsular and interosseous groups.

Capsular Ligaments: Distal Radioulnar

The dorsal and palmar distal radioulnar joint ligaments are felt to be major stabilizers of the distal radioulnar joint. These ligaments form the dorsal and palmar margins of the triangular fibrocartilage complex in the region between the sigmoid notch of the radius and the styloid process of the ulna [Figs. 6-2 and 6-4]. Attaching radially at the dorsal and palmar corners of the sigmoid notch, the ligaments converge ulnarly and pass in a cruciate manner such that the dorsal ligament attaches near the tip of the styloid process and the palmar ligament attaches near the base of the styloid process, in the region called the fovea. The palmar ligament has substantial connections to the carpus through the ulnolunate, ulnotriquetral, and ulnocapitate ligaments. The dorsal ligament integrates with the sheath of extensor carpi ulnaris.

Capsular Ligaments: Palmar Radiocarpal

The palmar radiocarpal ligaments arise from the palmar margin of the distal radius and course distally and ulnarly toward the scaphoid, lunate, and capitate (Fig. 6-7). Although the course of the fibers can be defined from an anterior view, the separate divisions of the palmar radiocarpal ligament are best appreciated from a dorsal view through the radiocarpal joint (Fig. 6-8). The palmar radiocarpal ligament can be divided into four distinct regions. Beginning radially, the radioscaphocapitate ligament originates from the radial styloid process, forms the radial wall of the radiocarpal joint, attaches to the scaphoid waist and distal pole, and passes palmar to the head of the capitate to interdigitate with fibers from the ulnocapitate ligament. Few fibers from the RSC ligament attach to the capitate. Just ulnar to the RSC ligament, the long radiolunate ligament arises to pass palmar to the proximal pole of the scaphoid and the scapholunate interosseous ligament to attach to the radial margin of the palmar horn of the lunate. The interligamentous sulcus separates the RSC and LRL ligaments throughout their courses. The LRL ligament has historically been called the radiolunotriquetral ligament, but the paucity of fibers continuing toward the triquetrum across the palmar horn of the lunate renders this name misleading. Ulnar to the origin of the LRL ligament, the

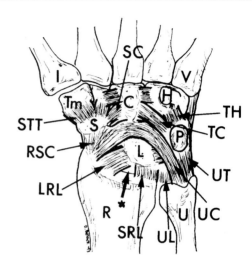

Figure 6-7. Drawing of the palmar capsular ligaments from a palmar perspective. R = radius, U = ulna, S = scaphoid, L = lunate, P = pisiform, Tm = trapezium, C = capitate, H = hamate, I = first metacarpal, V = fifth metacarpal. The ligaments are named as follows: RSC = radioscaphocapitate, LRL = long radiolunate, SRL = short radiolunate, UL = ulnolunate, UC = ulnocapitate, UT = ulnotriquetral, TH = triquetrohamate, TC = triquetrocapitate, SC = scaphocapitate, STT = scaphotrapeziotrapezoid. The asterisk marks the penetration point of the neurovascular source of the radioscapholunate ligament.

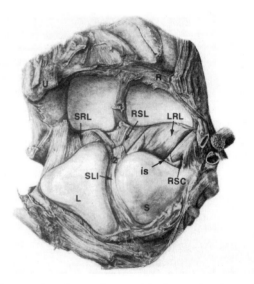

Figure 6-8. Drawing of the radiocarpal joint from a dorsal and distal perspective, with the scaphoid (S) and lunate (L) palmar flexed via a dorsal capsulotomy. RSC = radioscaphocapitate ligament, LRL = long radiolunate ligament, RSL = radioscapholunate ligament, SRL = short radiolunate ligament, SLI = scapholunate interosseous ligament. The RSC and LRL ligaments are separated by the interligamentous sulcus (is). (Reproduced with permission from Berger RA, Landsmeer JMF: The palmar radiocarpal ligaments: a study of adult and fetal human wrist joints. *J Hand Surgery,* 15A:847-854, 1990.)

radioscapholunate ligament emerges into the radiocarpal joint space through the palmar capsule and merges with the scapholunate interossous ligament and the interfossal ridge of the distal radius (Fig. 6-9). This structure resembles more of a "mesocapsule" than a true ligament, as it is composed of small-caliber blood vessels and nerves from the radial artery and anterior interossous neurovascular bundle. Very little organized collagen is identified within this structure. The mechanical stabilizing effects of this structure have recently been shown to be minimal. The final palmar radio-carpal ligament, the short radiolunate ligament, arises as a flat sheet of fibers from the palmar rim of the lunate fossa, just ulnar to the RSL ligament. It courses immediately distally to attach to the proximal and palmar margin of the lunate.

Capsular Ligaments: Dorsal Radiocarpal

The dorsal radiocarpal ligament arises from the dorsal rim of the radius, essentially equally distributed on either side of Lister's tubercle (Fig. 6-10). It courses obliquely distally and ulnarly toward the triquetrum, to which it attaches on the dorsal cortex. There are some deep attachments of the DRC ligament to the dorsal horn of the lunate. Loose connective and synovial tissue forms the capsular margins proximal and distal to the DRC ligament.

Capsular Ligaments: Ulnocarpal

The ulnocarpal ligament arises largely from the palmar margin of the TFCC, the palmar radioulnar ligament, and in a limited fashion from the head of the ulna. It courses obliquely distally toward the lunate, triquetrum, and capitate (Figs. 6-4 and 6-7). There are three divisions of the ulnocarpal ligament, designated by their distal bony insertions. The ulnolunate ligament is essentially continuous with the SRL ligament, forming a continuous palmar capsule between the TFCC and the lunate. Confluent with these fibers is the ulnotriquetral ligament, connecting the TFCC and the palmar rim of the triquetrum. In 60% to 70% of normal adults, a small orifice is found in the distal substance of the UT ligament, which leads to a communication between the radiocarpal and pisotriquetral joints. Just proximal and ulnar to the pisotriquetral orifice is the prestyloid recess, which is generally lined by synovial villi and variably communicates with the underlying ulnar styloid process. The ulnocapitate ligament arises from the foveal and palmar region of the head of the ulna, where it courses distally, palmar to the UL and UT ligaments, and passes palmar to the head of the capitate where it interdigitates with fibers from the RSC ligament to form an arcuate ligament to the head of the capitate. Few fibers from the UC ligament insert to the capitate.

Capsular Ligaments: Midcarpal

The midcarpal ligaments on the palmar surface of the carpus are true capsular ligaments, and as a rule are short and stout, connecting bones across a single joint space (Fig. 6-7). Beginning radially, the scaphoid-trapezium-trapezoid ligament forms the palmar capsule of the STT joint, connecting the distal pole of the scaphoid with the palmar surfaces

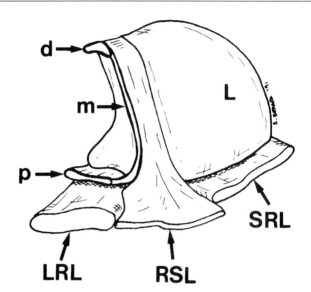

Figure 6-9. Drawing of the scapholunate interosseous ligament, from a radial and proximal perspective, with the scaphoid excised, leaving the lunate (L). The interosseous ligament is divided into dorsal (d), proximal or membranous (m) and palmar (p) region. The radioscapholunate ligament (RSL) merges with the membranous region, after entering the radiocarpal joint between the long radiolunate (LRL) and short radiolunate (SRL) ligaments. (Reproduced with permission from An K-N, Berger RA, Cooney WP (Eds): *Biomechanics of the Wrist Joint,* Springer-Verlag, New York, 1991.)

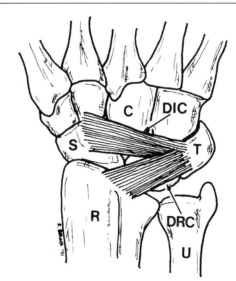

Figure 6-10. Drawing of the dorsal wrist ligaments. R = radius, U = ulna, S = scaphoid, C = capitate. The dorsal radiocarpal ligament (DRC) and the dorsal intercarpal ligament (DIC) share a common attachment on the dorsal surface of the triquetrum (T). (Reproduced with permission from An K-N, Berger RA, Cooney WP (Eds): *Biomechanics of the Wrist Joint.* Springer-Verlag, New York, 1991.)

of the trapezium and trapezoid. Although no clear divisions are noted, it forms an apex-proximal "V" shape. The scaphocapitate ligament is a thick ligament interposed between the STT and RSC ligaments, coursing from the palmar surface of the waist of the scaphoid to the palmar surface of the body of the capitate. There are no formal connections between the lunate and capitate, although the arcuate ligament (formed by the RSC and UC ligaments) has weak attachments to the palmar horn of the lunate. The triquetrocapitate ligament is analogous to the SC ligament. It is a thick ligament, passing from the palmar and distal margin of the triquetrum to the palmar surface of the body of the capitate. Immediately adjacent to the TC ligament, the triquetrohamate ligament forms the ulnar wall of the midcarpal joint and is augmented ulnarly by fibers from the TFCC. The dorsal intercarpal ligament, originating from the dorsal cortex of the triquetrum, crosses the midcarpal joint obliquely to attach to the scaphoid, trapezoid, and capitate (Fig. 6-10). The attachment of the DIC ligament to the triquetrum is confluent with the triquetral attachment of the DRC ligament. Additionally, a proximally thickened region of the joint capsule, roughly parallel to the DRC ligament, extends from the waist of the scaphoid across the distal margin of the dorsal horn of the lunate to the triquetrum. This band, called the dorsal scaphotriquetral ligament, forms a "labrum" which encases the head of the capitate, analogous to the RSC and UC ligaments palmarly.

Interosseous Ligaments: Proximal Row

The scapholunate and lunotriquetral interosseous ligaments form the interconnections between the bones of the proximal carpal row and share several anatomic features. Each forms a barrier between the radiocarpal and midcarpal joints, connecting the dorsal, proximal, and palmar edges of the respective joint surfaces (Fig. 6-9). This leaves the distal edges of the joints without ligamentous coverage. The dorsal and palmar regions of the SL and LT interosseous ligaments are typical of articular ligaments, composed of collagen fascicles with numerous blood vessels and nerves. The proximal regions, however, are composed of fibrocartilage, devoid of vascularization and innervation, and without identifiable collagen fascicles. The RSL ligament merges with the SL interosseous ligament near the junction of the palmar and proximal regions. The UC ligament passes directly palmar to the LT interosseous ligament with minimal interdigitation of fibers.

Interosseous/Intra-articular Ligaments: Distal Row

The bones of the distal carpal row are rigidly connected by a complex system of interosseous ligaments. As discussed below, these ligaments are largely responsible for transforming the four distal row bones into a single kinematic unit. The trapeziotrapezoid, trapezocapitate, and capitohamate joints are each bridged by palmar and dorsal interosseous ligaments (Figs. 6-6 and 6-7). These ligaments are composed of transversely oriented collagen fascicles and are covered superficially by the fibrous capsular lamina, also composed of transversely oriented fibers. This lamina gives the appearance of a continuous sheet of fibers spanning the entire palmar and dorsal surface of the distal row. Unique to the trapezocapitate and capitohamate joints are the "deep" interosseous ligaments (Fig. 6-6). These ligaments are entirely intra-articular, spanning the respective joint spaces between voids in the articular surfaces. Both are true ligaments with dense, colinear collagen fascicles, but are also heavily invested with nerve fibers. The deep trapezocapitate interosseous ligament is located midway between the palmar and dorsal limits of the joint, obliquely oriented from palmar-ulnar to dorsal-radial, and measures approximately 3mm in diameter. The respective attachment sites of the trapezoid and capitate are angulated in the transverse plane to accommodate the orthogonal insertion of the ligament. The deep capitohamate interosseous ligament is found transversely oriented at the palmar and distal corner of the joint. It traverses the joint from quadrangular voids in the articular surfaces and measures approximately 5 x 5mm in cross-sectional area.

Biomechanics of the Wrist

Overview

Within one year after the announcement of the discovery of X-rays, Bryce published a report of a roentgenographic investigation of the motions of the carpal bones. This marked a turning point for basic mechanical investigations of the wrist. The number of published biomechanical investigations of the wrist have increased almost exponentially over the past three decades. As such, a review of all mechanical analyses of the wrist is beyond the scope of this chapter. A general overview of basic biomechanical considerations of the wrist will be presented in the following categories: kinematics, kinetics, and material properties.

Kinematics

The global range of motion of the wrist, measured clinically, is based upon angular displacement of the hand about the "cardinal" axes of motion: palmar flexion-dorsiflexion and radioulnar deviation. The conicoid motion generated by combining displacement involving all four directions of motion is called circumduction. A functional axis of motion has also been described as the "dart-throw" axis, which moves the wrist-hand unit from an extreme of dorsiflexion-radial deviation to an extreme of palmar flexion-ulnar deviation. The magnitude of angular displacement in any direction varies greatly between individuals, but in "normal" individuals generally falls within the ranges described in Table 6-1.

Table 6-1.   Normal Ranges of Motion of the Wrist

Palmar flexion	65-80°
Dorsiflexion	65-80°
Radial deviation	10-20°
Ulnar deviation	20-35°
Pronosupination	5-10°

Several attempts to define the "functional" ranges of wrist motion required for various tasks of daily living as well as vocational and recreational activities have been performed using axially aligned electrogoniometers fixed to the hand and forearm segments of volunteers. Although some variability between results was found, the vast majority of tested tasks could be accomplished with 40° of dorsiflexion, 40° of palmar flexion, and 40° of combined radial and ulnar deviation.

The concept of a "center of rotation" of the wrist has been tested by a number of techniques and widely debated. It is generally agreed, however, that an approximation of an axis of flexion-extension motion of the hand unit on the forearm passes transversely through the head of the capitate, as does a separate orthogonal axis for radioulnar deviation. Remember that the global motion of the wrist is a summation of the motions of the individual carpal bones through the intercarpal joints as well as the radiocarpal and midcarpal joints. Thus, although easier to understand, the concept of a center of rotation of the wrist is at best an approximation and of limited basic and clinical usefulness.

Kinematics: Individual Carpal Bone Motion

As noted previously, the carpal bones are anatomically grouped into two carpal rows: proximal and distal. This concept, however, has been challenged by the introduction of the concept of carpal columns (Table 6-2). The proponents of the columnar theories site longitudinal loading pathways, phylogenetic analogies, and kinematic similarities when justifying the theories. Although these schema should be taken into consideration in any functional description of the wrist, most wrist investigators continue to utilize the conventional terminology of proximal and distal carpal rows. This is largely based upon the observation that the bones within each row display kinematic behaviors that are more similar than those observed between the two rows. Because the kinematic behaviors of the carpal bones are measurably different between palmar flexion-dorsiflexion and radioulnar deviation, these two arcs of motion are considered separately.

Table 6-2. **Carpal Columns as Functional Groupings of Carpal Bones**

Author	Carpal Bone Grouping
MacConaill	scaphoid lunate, triquetrum capitate, hamate, trapezoid
Navarro	lateral (mobile): scaphoid, trapezium, trapezoid central (flexion-extension): capitate, lunate hamate medial (rotation): triquetrum, pisiform
Taleisnik	lateral (mobile): scaphoid central (flexion extension): lunate, trapezium, trapezoid, capitate, hamate medial (rotation): triquetrum

Palmar Flexion-Dorsiflexion

As shown in Figure 6-11, the metacarpals are pulled through the range of palmar flexion and dorsiflexion by the action of the extrinsic wrist motors attaching to their bases. The hand unit, composed of the metacarpals and phalanges, is securely associated with the distal carpal row through the articular interlocking and strong ligamentous connections of the second through fifth carpometacarpal joints. The trapezoid, capitate, and hamate undergo displacement with their respective metacarpals with no significant deviation of direction or magnitude of motion. Due to the strong interosseous ligaments, the trapezium generally tracks with the trapezoid, but remains under the influence of the mobile first metacarpal. The major direction of motion for this entire complex is palmar flexion and dorsiflexion, with little deviation in radioulnar deviation and pronation-supination.

As a generalization, the proximal row bones follow the direction of motion of the distal row bones during palmar flexion-dorsiflexion of the wrist. However, the scaphoid, lunate, and triquetrum are not as tightly secured to the hand unit as are the distal row bones, by virtue of the midcarpal joint. Additionally, the interosseous ligaments between the proximal row bones allow substantial intercarpal motion. Thus, there are measurable differences between the motions of the proximal and distal row bones, as well as between the individual bones of the proximal carpal row. This is most pronounced between the scaphoid and lunate. From the extreme of palmar flexion to the extreme of dorsiflexion, the scaphoid undergoes substantially more angular displacement than the lunate, primarily in the plane of hand motion. There are measurable "out-of-plane" motions between the scaphoid and lunate as well, as the scaphoid progressively supinates relative to the lunate as the wrist dorsiflexes. The effect of the differential direction and magnitude of displacement between the scaphoid and lunate is to create a relative separation between the palmar surfaces of the two bones as dorsiflexion is reached, and a coaptation of the two surfaces as palmar flexion is reached. The extremes of displacement are checked by the "twisting" of the fibers of the interosseous ligaments. Once this limit is reached, the scaphoid and lunate will move as a unit

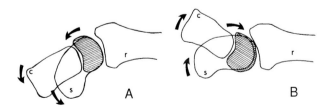

Figure 6-11. Lateral view schematic showing the radius (r), scaphoid (s), capitate (c) and lunate (shaded) during palmar flexion **(A)** and dorsiflexion **(B)** of the wrist. Overall, the proximal row bones move in a similar direction, but with less displacement, compared to the distal row bones.

through the radiocarpal and midcarpal joints. Similar, though of lesser magnitude, behaviors occur through the lunotriquetral joint. In all, the lunate experiences the least magnitude of rotation of all carpal bones during palmar flexion and dorsiflexion. The radiocarpal and midcarpal joints contribute nearly equally to the range of dorsiflexion and palmar flexion of the wrist, when measured through the capitolunate/radiolunate joint column. In contrast, when measured through the radioscaphoid-scaphotrapeziotrapezoid joint column, more than two-thirds of the range of motion occurs through the radioscaphoid joint.

Radioulnar Deviation

As with palmar flexion and dorsiflexion, the bones of the distal row move essentially as a unit with themselves as well as with the second through fifth metacarpals during radial and ulnar deviation of the wrist as shown in Figure 6-12. The proximal row bones, however, display a remarkably different kinematic behavior. As a unit, the proximal carpal row displays a "reciprocating" motion with the distal row, such that the principal motion during wrist radial deviation is palmar flexion. Conversely, during wrist ulnar deviation, the proximal carpal row dorsiflexes. In addition to the palmar flexion-dorsiflexion activity of the proximal carpal row, a less pronounced motion occurs resulting in ulnar displacement during wrist radial deviation and radial displacement during wrist ulnar deviation. Additional longitudinal axial displacements occur between the proximal carpal row bones, as they do during palmar flexion and dorsiflexion. Although of substantially lower magnitude than the principal directions of rotation, these longitudinal axial displacements contribute to a relative separation between the palmar surfaces of the scaphoid and lunate in wrist ulnar deviation and a relative coaptation during wrist radial deviation, limited by the tautness of the scapholunate interosseous ligament. Once maximum tension is achieved, the two bones displace as a single unit. As with palmar flexion and dorsiflexion, the lunate experiences the least magnitude of rotation of all carpal bones during radial and ulnar deviation. The magnitude of rotation through the midcarpal joint is approximately 1.5 times greater than the radiocarpal joint during radial and ulnar deviation.

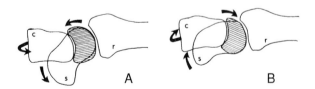

Figure 6-12. Lateral view schematic showing the radius (r), scaphoid (s), capitate (c) and lunate (shaded) during radial deviation **(A)** and ulnar deviation **(B)** of the wrist. The entire proximal row moves in a reciprocating fashion relative to the distal row by palmar flexing during wrist radial deviation and dorsiflexing during wrist ulnar deviation.

Kinematics: Models

Several models have been described to explain the complex interrelated motions of the carpal bones. MacConaill described a progressive congruence in articular contact through the midcarpal joint as ulnar deviation and dorsiflexion are reached, and referred to this mechanism as conjunct rotation. Kauer developed a model of carpal mechanics where the proximal carpal row can assume a finite number of positions relative to the radius. For example, the position of the scaphoid is similar in wrist palmar flexion and radial deviation. This model has been described as a closed kinematic chain. In a similar manner, Lichtman has developed a "closed-ring concept" of carpal mechanics. In this concept, articular contact and ligamentous strain through the radial and ulnar columns of the carpus are responsible for the displacements of the carpal bones. For example, during ulnar deviation, the proximally directed load through the triquetrohamate articulation forces the triquetrum into dorsiflexion. Simultaneously, the scaphotrapeziotrapezoid ligaments pull the distal pole of the scaphoid dorsally resulting in dorsiflexion of the scaphoid. The lunate is rotated dorsally with the scaphoid and triquetrum through the linkage of the interosseous ligament system. Linscheid and associates have described the action of the scaphoid-capitate articulation as a "slider-crank" mechanism, while Gilford felt that a simple three-bar linkage more aptly described the radiocarpal-midcarpal joints, especially when considering their tendencies toward unstable configurations.

Kinematics: Scapholunate Instability

Scapholunate dissociation was the first carpal instability pattern to be studied clinically and in the laboratory. Felt to be the result of traumatic disruption of the scapholunate interosseous ligament, untreated scapholunate dissociation has been associated with the development of "dorsiflexed intercalated segmental instability." Much like a coiled spring, the pre-stressed nature of the scapholunate joint is constrained by the scapholunate interosseous ligament. Division of this structure allows the lunate and triquetrum, the intercalated segments, to dorsiflex relative to the scaphoid, capitate, and radius. This condition has been clinically associated with advanced degenerative disease involving the radiocarpal and midcarpal joints. Radiographic suggestions of scapholunate dissociation include a scapholunate gap greater than 3mm and a foreshortened scaphoid with a cortical ring sign in neutrally deviated posteroanterior radiographs, and measurements of the following angles outside of the accepted normal range: scapholunate (30° to 60°), lunocapitate (+/- 10°), radiolunate (+/-10°). Several investigators have attempted to measure kinematic changes with division of ligaments in cadaver specimens, but reported results have been nonuniform and inconclusive, ranging from only minor rotational changes to immediate dorsal translation of the proximal pole of the scaphoid with concurrent scaphoid palmar flexion and pronation with division of the scapholunate interosseous ligament. Division of the radioscapholunate ligament has not been shown to contribute to scapholunate dissociation. Evidence is mounting that the dorsal region of the scapholunate interosseous ligament and the scaphotriquetral ligaments are the key stabilizers of the scapholunate joint. It is currently felt that clinically evident scapholunate dissociation probably results from initial trauma to the dorsal scaphotriquetral and scapholunate interosseous ligaments with subsequent cyclic loading leading to attenuation of the contiguous ligamentous supports. Once this occurs, progressive carpal collapse patterns become evident.

Kinematics: Lunotriquetral Instability

Just as the scapholunate joint is pre-stressed, dissociation of the triquetrum from the remainder of the proximal carpal row allows the scaphoid and lunate to assume a palmar flexed attitude relative to the capitate and radius. This condition has been called "volar flexed intercalated segmental instability" and again represents a radiographic diagnosis. Division of the lunotriquetral interosseous ligament alone in a cadaveric kinematic study did not produce substantial alterations of lunotriquetral kinematics. However, division of both the lunotriquetral and dorsal scaphotriquetral ligaments produced measureable palmar flexion of the lunate and combined dorsiflexion-supination of the triquetrum.

Kinematics: Limited Arthrodesis

Numerous studies have been completed in the laboratory to evaluate the effect on carpal bone motion effected by limited intercarpal arthrodeses. These studies add substantially to our understanding of the contributions made to global wrist motion by the various intercarpal joints. Overall, arthrodesis of the midcarpal joint has been shown to decrease the range of palmar flexion by approximately 35%, while arthrodesis of the radiocarpal joint results in a loss of palmar flexion of slightly more than 60%. Both arthrodeses limit dorsiflexion, with the greatest effect generated by arthrodesis of the radiocarpal joint. Individual interosseous arthrodeses have been simulated, with resulting measured global ranges of motion of the wrist summarized in Table 6-3. Overall, those arthrodeses crossing the radiocarpal and midcarpal joints are in agreement with the findings noted above. Those arthrodeses between bones within the proximal row reduce wrist range of motion by 10% to 20%, and intercarpal arthrodeses within the distal carpal row have little measurable effect on global wrist motion.

Kinetics

Force Analysis

Force analyses of the wrist have been attempted using a variety of methods, including the analytical methods of free-body diagrams and rigid-body spring models and experimental methods employing force transducers, pressure-sensitive film, pressure transducers, and strain gauges. Due to the intrinsic geometric complexity of the wrist, the large number of carpal elements, the number of tissue inter-

Table 6-3.   Percent of Normal Global Range of Wrist Motion Resulting From Limited Intercarpal Arthrodesis

Study	Arthrodesis Site	RUD	PDM
Rozing and Kauer	RS	61%	40%
	RSL	61%	40%
	SLC	91%	59%
Seradge, et al.	SL	70%	75%
	LT	75%	86%
	SLT	66%	67%
Douglas, et al.	STmTd	73%	83%
	SC	79%	82%
	SL	85%	89%
	LT	97%	95%
	CH	102%	101%
	HT	76%	79%
	CL	71%	64%

RUD = radioulnar deviation
PDM = palmar flexion-dorsiflexion motion
R = radius
S = scaphoid
L = lunate
T = triquetrum
Tm = trapezium
Td = trapezoid
C = capitate
H = hamate

faces to which loads are applied, and the large number of positions that the wrist can assume, these analyses have been difficult and are riddled with assumptions. Thus, relative changes and trends in forces brought about by the introduction of experimental variables are generally more useful than absolute values.

Normal Joint Forces

Experimental and analytical studies of force transmission across the wrist in the neutral position are in general agreement that approximately 80% of the force is transmitted across the radiocarpal joint and 20% across the ulnocarpal joint space. This can be further compartmentalized into forces across the ulnolunate articulation (14%) and the ulnotriquetral articulation (8%). In the neutral position, one investigator reported that 78% of the longitudinal force across the wrist is transmitted through the radiocarpal articulation, with 46% transmitted by the radioscaphoid fossa and 32% by the lunate fossa. Forces across the midcarpal joint in a neutrally positioned joint have been estimated to be 31% through the scaphotrapeziotrapezoid joint, 19% through the scaphocapitate joint, 29% through the lunocapitate joint, and 21% transmitted through the triquetrohamate joint.

In general, it has been shown that forearm pronation increases ulnocarpal force transmission (up to 37% of total forces transmitted) with a corresponding decrease in radiocarpal force transmission. This has been theoretically linked to the relative distal prominence of the ulna that occurs in forearm pronation. The ulnocarpal force transmission increases to 28% of the total in ulnar deviation of the wrist, while radiocarpal forces increase to 87% of the total in radial deviation. Wrist palmar flexion and dorsiflexion have only a modest effect on the relative forces transmitted through the radiocarpal and ulnocarpal joints.

Normal Joint Contact Area and Pressure

Using pressure-sensitive film placed in the radiocarpal joint space, three distinct areas of contact through the radiocarpal joint have been identified: radioscaphoid, radiolunate, and ulnolunate. Overall, it has been determined that the actual area of contact of the scaphoid and lunate against the distal radius and TFCC are quite limited, regardless of joint position, averaging 20% of the entire available articular surface. The scaphoid contact area was greater than that of the lunate by an average factor of 1.5. The centroids of the contact areas shift with varying positions of the wrist, as do the areas of contact. For example, palmar flexion of the scaphoid results in a dorsal and radial shift of the radioscaphoid contact centroid, and a progressive diminution of contact area. With externally applied loads, the peak articular pressures are quite low, ranging from 1.4 N/mm^2 to 31.4 N/mm^2.

The midcarpal joint has been difficult to evaluate using pressure-sensitive film due to its complex shape. It has been estimated that less than 40% of the available articular surface of the midcarpal joint is in actual contact at any one time. The relative contribution to the total contact of the scaphotrapeziotrapezoid, scaphocapitate, lunocapitate, and triquetrohamate joints have been estimated to be 23%, 28%, 29%, and 20%, respectively. Thus, it may be surmised that more than 50% of the midcarpal load is transmitted through the capitate across the scaphocapitate and lunocapitate joints.

Joint Force Alteration With Intercarpal Fusions

Using the rigid body spring model, simulated limited intercarpal arthrodeses invoving the scaphotrapeziotrapezoid, scaphocapitate, and capitohamate joints have shown no more than a 15% reduction of load transmission through the radiolunate joint. However, the combination of capitohamate arthrodesis and capitate shortening has a dramatic effect of radiolunate load reduction and concomitantly increased radioscaphoid, ulnotriquetral, triquetrohamate, and scaphotrapezial joint forces. This effect is probably due primarily to the capitate shortening. Nearly all joint contact shifts to the radioscaphoid joint with STT and SC arthrodeses. Scapholunate, scapholunocapitate, and lunocapitate arthrodeses tend to distibute loads more proportionately through the radioscaphoid and radiolunate joint spaces, but do not duplicate normal joint contact areas.

Joint Force Alteration with Changes in Radius and Ulna Length

Changes in load transmission related to the relative length of the radius and ulna have shown that simulation of a plus-variant ulna of 2.5mm (either by ulnar lengthening or radial shortening) shifts the majority of the transmitted load from the radiocarpal joint (58%) toward the ulnocarpal joint

(42%). The reverse trend occurs with a 2.5mm minus-variant ulna, with a reduction in ulnocarpal load transmission to only 4%. Excision of the TFCC has been shown to reduce ulnocarpal force transmission from 20% to 16%.

Additional studies have been carried out to determine the effect of changing the ulnar inclination of the distal radius, a treatment advocated by some for Kienböck's disease in patients with neutral variance of the ulna. Lateral closing, lateral opening, and medial closing radius osteotomies have been simulated in cadaver wrists and compared to normal values for joint loading characteristics. The lateral opening and medial closing osteotomies increase force transmission to the ulna and nearly eliminate radiolunate forces. In contrast, the lateral closing osteotomy decreases ulnar loading while increasing the loads transmitted through the radiolunate joint. In all three situations, the degree of load shift is proportionately related to the osteotomy angle.

Material Properties of Carpal Ligaments

The material properties of the carpal ligaments have been evaluated to define parameters such as yield strength, stress, strain, and histeresis in isolated bone-ligament-bone cadaveric preparations. Overall, the ligaments of the wrist have not been found to be substantially different in material properties from other mammalian ligament systems. The extrinsic ligaments of the wrist, such as the palmar capsular radiocarpal ligaments, are viscoelastic structures, exhibiting stiffness behavior proportional to strain rate with failure at approximately 100 Newtons. The scapholunate and lunotriquetral interosseous ligaments have been identified as the strongest ligaments in the wrist, requiring force applications greater than 300 Newtons to fail. The strain at deformation for the scapholunate and lunotriquetral interosseous ligaments is substantially greater than the other carpal ligaments, exceeding 50% compared to 10% to 35%. Distraction testing of the radioscapholunate ligament have shown it to be extremely weak, failing at less than 50 Newtons of applied tensile load.

Recently, a series of experiments has been completed that evaluated the material properties of the anatomic subregions of the scapholunate interosseous ligaments. In these experiments the dorsal, palmar, and proximal (membranous) regions were subjected to deformation testing in isolated torsion, translation, and distraction to failure. It was found uniformly that the dorsal region was the strongest of the three, requiring greater than 250 Newtons of applied tensile load. The dorsal region is the principal stabilizer of the scapholunate complex in dorsal and palmar translation, as well as dorsiflexion and palmar flexion. The palmar region also contributes to joint stability, but to a significantly reduced degree. The proximal region, composed of fibrocartilage, has little measurable influence on joint stability. The proximal region is also the weakest in distraction testing, generally failing with application of less than 25 Newtons of tension.

The ligamentous stabilizers of the transverse carpal arch have been recently evaluated, where posteroanterior compressive loads were applied after sectioning the flexor retinaculum and the distal row palmar and dorsal interosseous ligaments. The transversely oriented interosseous ligaments have a significant effect of transverse carpal instability. The flexor retinaculum does not have a significant effect on transverse carpal stability, reducing stiffness to compressive load by less than 8% when divided. However, the width of the carpal tunnel increases significantly (up to 10%) with division of the flexor retinaculum. Division of the flexor retinaculum has not been associated with measurable changes in carpal kinematics.

Pathomechanical Simulations

Simulations of pathologic conditions of the wrist have been attempted in the laboratory to add to our understanding of the pathomechanics and the mechanics of treatment options. The following is a brief selection of laboratory simulations of common clinical situations.

Distal Radius Fracture

As ulnar inclination of the distal radius articular surface decreases, as is often encountered in a malreduced distal radius fracture, ulnar column force increases proportionately. Additionally, changes occur within the radiocarpal joint, with a palmar shift of the radiolunate centroid and a dorsoradial shift of the radioscaphoid centroid. These trends are seen with malposition increments of as little as 10°. Dorsal inclination of the distal radius also affects the load characteristics of the wrist by progressively increasing the radioscaphoid and radiolunate load pressures. These changes are noted consistently with dorsal angulation greater than 30°. Dorsal angulation of the distal radius beyond 20° leads to significant load shifts across the midcarpal joint, due to the relative DISI posture of the proximal carpal row. Shortening of the radius also affects the load patterns, with gross ulnar impingement and disruption of the TFCC noted with radial shortening more than 5mm.

Thus, it has been suggested that relatively normal mechanical loading of the wrist is a reasonable expectation if less than 2mm of radial shortening, less than a 10° loss of ulnar inclination, and less than a 20° loss of palmar inclination can be achieved and maintained.

Scaphoid Nonunion/Malunion

Recent radiographic studies have determined that the normal intraosseous scaphoid angle measures ±32° in the sagittal plane (defined as the angle between tangents drawn on the palmar cortex of the proximal scaphoid and the dorsal cortex of the distal scaphoid) and ±40° in the coronal plane (defined as the angle between tangents drawn on the midcarpal cortex of the proximal half of the scaphoid and the flattened subchondral surface of the distal scaphoid). Just as ligamentous dissociation between the scaphoid and lunate can lead to instability patterns, so can nonunion or malunion of the scaphoid. In an evaluation of carpal kinematics in cadaver specimens with scaphoid osteotomies placed to simulate scaphoid waist fractures, it was found that the proximal and distal fragments move independently, with an increase in net motion of the proximal fragment and a net decrease in net motion of the distal fragment. This uniformly led to a typical "humpback" deformity of the scaphoid as the proximal pole fragment dorsiflexed with the lunate in a DISI pattern. Contact area and pressure studies of simulated scaphoid fractures have revealed that there is no change in the contact area through the scaphoid fossa between intact specimens, specimens with a proximal pole fracture, or specimens following excision of the proximal pole. There is, however, a redistribution of contact tending to increase contact of the scaphoid fossa with the distal fragment, and an increase in the contact pressure in this region. No changes through the radiolunate joint were noted between any of the experimental variables. Keep in mind that these studies do not address loading trends encountered with cyclic loading following scaphoid osteotomy.

Annotated Bibliography

Fetal Development

Landsmeer JMF: *Atlas of Anatomy of the Hand.* Churchill Livingstone, New York, 1976.

Although the information contained in this volume is extensive and detailed, it provides the careful reader with unparalleled information regarding the three-dimensional organization of the wrist in the developing human. Utilizing cross-sectional anatomy eliminates the distortion and bias produced by standard dissection techniques.

Lewis OJ: The development of the human wrist joint during the fetal period. *Anat Rec,* 166:499-516, 1970.

During fetal development, separate radioscaphoid, radiolunate, and ulnotriquetral cavities develop progressively larger communications until a single joint cavity is formed. Initially quite prominent, the distal ulna progressively withdraws from the carpal region.

Vascular Anatomy

Gelberman RH, Panagis JS, Taleisnik J, Baumgaertner M: The arterial anatomy of the human carpus. Part I: the extraosseous vascularity. *J Hand Surg,* 8:367-375, 1983.

The vascular anatomy of the wrist in 25 cadaver specimens was studied by injection and chemical debridement techniques. Three dorsal and palmar arterial arches were consistently identified, contibuted to by the radial and ulnar arteries. Contributions were also noted from the anterior and posterior extensions of the anterior interosseous artery. The major collateral circulation of the wrist is provided by an anastomosis between radial and ulnar recurrent arteries and the anterior division of the anterior interosseous artery.

Panais JS, Gelberman RH, Taleisnik J, Baumgaertner M: The arterial anatomy of the human carpus. Part II: the intraosseous vascularity. *J Hand Surg,* 8:375-382, 1983.

The intraosseous vascular anatomy of all carpal bones except the scaphoid in 25 cadaver wrists was studied by injection and Spalteholz clearing techniques. This manuscript provides the most extensive reference available on intraosseous vascular anatomy of the carpal bones. The carpal bones were classified into three groups based upon common features of vascularity. Group I includes the capitate, scaphoid, and 20% of studied lunates, where large areas of the bones are dependent upon a single vessel. Group II, including the trapezoid and hamate, features multiple areas of vessel entry into the bone without anastomosis. Group III includes the trapezium, triquetrum, pisiform, and 80% of studied lunates, where several penetrating vessels are identified with intraosseous anastomoses, leaving no areas of bone dependent upon a single vessel. Group I bones are at risk for development of avascular necrosis, while AVN rates in groups II and III are low.

Ligament Anatomy

Berger RA, Landsmeer JMF: The palmar radiocarpal ligaments: a study of adult and fetal human wrist joints. *J Hand Surg,* 15A:847-854, 1990.

The palmar radiocarpal ligaments were described as the radioscaphocapitate, long radiolunate, and the short radiolunate ligaments. The radioscaphocapitate ligament was noted to insert primarily into the waist and distal pole of the scaphoid, with extensions into the arcuate ligament supporting the head of the capitate. Few direct insertions into the capitate were noted. The long radiolunate ligament, previously named the radiotriquetral ligament, was noted to terminate at the lunate, and therefore was renamed. The short radiolunate ligament, not previously described, is felt to be a major stabilizer of the lunate.

Berger RA, Kauer JMG, Landsmeer JMF: The radio-scapholunate ligament: a gross and histologic study of fetal and adult wrists. *J Bone Surg,* 16A:350-355, 1991.

The radioscapholunate ligament was found to be a neurovascular extension of the anterior interosseous artery and nerve and the radial artery surrounded by a thick sheath of synovial tissue, which enters the radiocarpal joint space through a defect in the palmar joint capsule between the long and short radiolunate ligaments. It attaches to the scapholunate interosseous ligament distally and the interfossal ridge proximally. This structure may be a vestige of a septum which divides the radiocarpal joint into radiolunate and radioscaphoid clefts that partially regresses during fetal development. It is felt to have minimal direct mechanical effect on the carpus.

Drewniany JJ, Palmer AK, Flatt AE: The scaphotrapezial ligament complex: an anatomic and biomechanical study. *J Hand Surg,* 10A:492-498, 1985.

Twenty-five cadaver specimens were dissected to study the scaphotrapeziotrapezoid and scaphocapitate joints. The scaphotrapezial ligament complex consists of a stout scaphotrapezial ligament on the radial and palmar aspects of the scaphotrapezial joint, weak dorsal and palmar capsules, and a stout scaphocapitate ligament. The ligaments were found to supply resistance to distasis of the scaphotrapeziotrapezoid joint.

Mizuseki T, Ikuta Y: The dorsal carpal ligaments: their anatomy and function. *J Hand Surg,* 14B:91-98, 1989.

The dorsal carpal ligaments were dissected in 50 cadaver specimens. The dorsal radiocarpal ligament was noted to have four basic courses, largely depending upon the degree of insertion into the dorsal surface of the scaphoid. The dorsal intercarpal ligament was found to be quite thin, and coursed from the triquetrum to the dorsal ridge of the scaphoid to the dorsal capsule of the STT joint. The only other connections noted to traverse the midcarpal joint were the dorsal STT and triquetrohamate ligaments.

Palmer AK, Warner FW: The triangular fibrocartilage complex of the wrist—anatomy and function. *J Hand Surg,* 6:153-162, 1981.

Kauer (*Acta Anat Scand,* 93:590, 1975) defined the articular disc as part of an extensive fibrous network attaching to the radius, ulna, triquetrum, lunate, and fifth metacarpal, incorporating the extensor carpi ulnaris tendon sheath. Palmer's study confirmed Kauer's fetal descriptions in adult specimens, and introduced the term triangular fibrocartilage complex, which is the convention most accepted today. Load cell studies revealed that removal of the TFCC redistributed longitudinal loads such that the radius:ulna load-bearing ratio shifted from 60:40 to 95:5. It was also determined that the TFCC is important as a distal radioulnar joint stabilizer.

Taleisnik J: The ligaments of the wrist. *J Hand Surg,* 1:110-118, 1976.

This manuscript provides a comprehensive description of the carpal ligaments, based upon the dissection of 17 wrists. The ligaments were divided into extrinsic (coursing between the carpal bones and either the radius or metacarpals) and intrinsic (coursing entirely between the carpal bones) groups. Additional subclassifications were described, eg, superficial and deep, proximal, and distal.

General Biomechanics

An K-N, Berger RA, Cooney WP, Eds: *Biomechanics of the Wrist Joint.* Springer-Verlag, New York, 1991.

This comprehensive reference of anatomy and current biomechanics of the wrist compiles the research experience of 13 investigators into a single source. Heavily referenced, the topics of discussion include anatomy, individual carpal bone and global wrist motion, force analysis, joint contact area and pressure, osseous strain, material properties, and muscle function.

Youm Y, McMurtry RY, Flatt AE, Gillespie TE: Kinematics of the wrist. I: an experimental study of radialulnar deviation and flexion-extension. *J Bone Joint Surg,* 60A:423-431, 1978.

Radiographic analyses of cadaver and live volunteer wrists suggest that wrist rotation occurs about separate fixed axes for flexion-extension and radioulnar deviation within the head of the capitate. The concepts of carpal height and carpal and ulnar distance ratios were introduced in this manuscript.

Individual Carpal Bone Kinematics

Berger RA, Crowninshield RD, Flatt AE: *Clin Orthop,* 167:303-310, 1982.

Using a three-dimensional sonic digitizer system with miniature triads of spark gaps fixed to each carpal bone and the third metacarpal in cadaver specimens, these investigators describe the motions of each carpal bone as the wrists are passively moved through planar constrained flexion-extension motion and radioulnar deviation. The effects of forearm rotation on carpal bone motion were also tested. The results were reported in terms of screw displacement axes relative to a coordinated system based in the distal radius. Comparisons were made in the magnitude of rotation about the SDAs and the included angles between the SDAs of each carpal bone relative to the third metacarpal. Overall, the bones of the distal row behaved in a similar fashion to the third metacarpal. The bones of the proximal row, however, behaved in a significantly different manner than the third metacarpal during radialulnar deviation, with diminished magnitudes of rotation and increased included angles. No significant differences were noted with changes in forearm rotation.

Lange A de, Kauer JMG, Huiskes R: The kinematical behavior of the human wrist joint: a roentgenstereophotogrammetric analysis. *J Orthop Res,* 3:56-64, 1985.

This manuscript initiated a series of accurate and innovative investigations of carpal kinematics using a technique called roentgenstereophotogrammetric analysis, in which small metal markers are embedded in carpal bones and biplanar radiographs are taken with the wrist in various positions. The results are reported in terms of Euler angle displacements relative to a fixed coordinate system in the radius. Overall, it was found that the proximal and distal rows behave as distinct units, although substantial intercarpal motion is noted between the bones of the proximal carpal row. Forearm rotation produced no overall motion changes; however, the relative contributions of the radiocarpal and midcarpal joints to the arc of flexion did change with forearm rotation.

Ruby LK, Cooney WP, An K-N, Linscheid RL, Chao EYS: Relative motions of selected carpal bones: a kinematic analysis of the normal wrist. *J Hand Surg,* 13A:1-10, 1988.

The authors defined individual carpal bone motion using biplanar radiographic analysis with metal markers implanted in each carpal bone of cadaver specimens. Motions were described by screw displacement axes relative to an anatomic coordinate system in the distal radius. Decreasing magnitudes of rotation during radioulnar deviation of the wrist were noted in the scaphoid, lunate, and triquetrum, respectively. The major direction of rotation of these bones during RUD was palmar flexion-dorsiflexion, but some motion in the radioulnar rotation plane was detected. The magnitude of carpal translation was noted to be minimal in all directions for each bone studied. Intercarpal motion was noted to be much less for the bones of the distal row than for the proximal row bones. The authors concluded that the concept of carpal rows is more kinematically valid than carpal columns.

Kinematics with Intercarpal Arthrodesis

Douglas DP, Peimer CA, Koniuch MP: Motion of the wrist after simulated limited intercarpal arthrodeses. *J Bone Joint Surg,* 69A:1413-1418, 1987.

See Table 6-3.

Masear VR, Zook EG, Pichora DR, Krishnamurthy M, Russell RC, Lemons J, Bidez MW: Strain-gauge evaluation of lunate unloading procedures. *J Hand Surg,* 17A:437-443, 1992.

This study utilized direct surface strain measurements by mounting strain gauge rosettes on the cortical surfaces of cadaveric lunates, followed by simulated STT arthrodesis, capitohamate arthrodesis, and ulnar lengthening osteotomy. Ulnar lengthening of 3mm was consistently associated with reduction of lunate strain. Capitohamate arthrodesis reduced compressive strain but increased shear strain, whereas STT arthrodesis significantly increased both compressive and shear strain in the lunate.

Rozing PM, Kauer JMG: Partial arthrodesis of the wrist: investigation in cadavers. *Acta Othop Scand,* 55:66-68, 1984.

See Table 6-3.

Seradge H, Sterbank PT, Seradge E, Owens W: Segmental motion of the proximal carpal row: their global effect on the wrist motion. *J Hand Surg,* 15A:236-239, 1990.

See Table 6-3.

Viegas SF, Patterson RM, Peterson PD, Roefs J, Tencer A, Choi S: The effects of various load paths and different loads on the load transfer characteristics of the wrist. *J Hand Surg,* 14A:458-465, 1989.

Using pressure-sensitive film in cadaver radiocarpal joints, this paper describes contact areas and pressures within the radiocarpal joint with varying loading pathways (loading proximally through the tendons vs. loading distally through various metacarpal pathways). A consistent finding was the 60:40 scaphoid fossa lunate fossa contact area. Loads greater than 46 pounds do not change the contact areas; however, joint contact pressures correlate positively with load applications. The overall joint contact area does not exceed 40% of the available joint surface area.

Material Properties of Ligaments

Lange A de, Huiskes R, Kauer JMG: Wrist-joint ligament length changes in flexion and deviation of the hand: an experimental study. *J Orthop Res,* 8:722-730, 1990.

Using a roentgenstereophotogrammetric analysis method, the length changes of seven carpal ligaments were measured in cadaver wrists in which metal markers were placed in key ligaments and carpal bones. Short ligaments, such as the short radiolunate ligament, experienced length changes of up to 30%, whereas other longer ligaments did not lengthen more than 20%. The longer ligaments also displayed a greater tendency to curve than did the shorter ligaments. The authors concluded that the radioscaphocapitate ligament plays an important role in stabilizing the capitate in dorsiflexion and deviation, just as the lunate is stabilized by the long radiolunate ligament. The dorsal radiocarpal and palmar triquetrocapitate ligaments stabilize the carpus in the neutral position.

Nowak MD, Logan SE: Strain rate dependent permanent deformation of human wrist ligaments. *Biomed Sci Instrum,* 24:61-65, 1988.

This work represents one of several published manuscripts by the authors reporting on an exhaustive evaluation of the material properties of the major carpal ligaments.

Schuind F, An K-N, Berglund ZL, Rey R, Cooney WP, Linscheid RL, Chao EYS: The distal radioulnar ligament: a biomechanical study. *J Hand Surg,* 16A:1106-1114, 1991.

A stereophotogrammetric analysis of the palmar and dorsal radioulnar ligaments was made as cadaveric forearms were positioned in varying degrees of pronation and supination. Qualitative analysis revealed that the dorsal ligament becomes taut in pronation and the palmar ligament is taut in supination. These impressions were confirmed quantitatively with consistent length changes in the respective ligaments. Mechancial testing applying axial loads to the triangular fibrocartilage revealed significant laxity (mean = 10.4mm), which decreased with forearm pronation. Transverse loading revealed diminished stiffness of the triangular fibrocartilage in neutral forearm rotation.

7

Imaging and Evaluation

Louis A. Gilula, MD

Introduction

A number of imaging techniques are valuable to the surgeon in evaluating and treating patients. Many of these imaging modalities may be expensive and complex to use and interpret. Physical examination is critical. If symptoms are highly supportive of fracture or severe bony abnormality and radiographic examination is normal, additional views to profile the specific site of symptoms may be of value and indeed may be warranted. An additional examination, such as bone scintigraphy or even MRI may detect a fracture or some significant abnormality. A "normal examination" merely states that an abnormality is not demonstrated on that examination. Thus, there is a need to develop a working relationship between the radiologist and primary and secondary care physicians, so that a collaborative team can provide the best patient care. A major problem is that findings of unknown significance may be identified by different imaging techniques. The presence of an anatomic variation or abnormality does not mean that it is symptomatic. Therefore, it is important that the treating surgeon evaluate any reported finding in light of the patient's symptoms to help determine subsequent treatment. Anatomic abnormalities may also be present in the site of symptoms, and some of these findings if treated, may not relieve the patient's symptoms. This chapter presents a brief overview of current uses of the various imaging modalities available for the wrist.

Routine Radiography

Preliminary or Survey Wrist Examination

Routine radiography includes routine survey views, detailed radiographic views, fluoroscopic spot views, and an instability series. The routine radiographic examination can vary, but the minimum must include posteroanterior and lateral views. The posteroanterior (PA) view is obtained with the X-ray beam passing through the posterior aspect of the wrist and the film cassette placed on the palmar aspect of the hand. An anteroposterior (AP) view is obtained with the dorsum of the hand placed on the film cassette and the beam of X-rays passed through the palmar aspect of the hand to exit the dorsum of the hand. The PA view should be obtained with the elbow flexed 90° and abducted 90°, so that the elbow is the same height as the shoulder. This position should be obtained routinely, with the eventuality that ulnar variance determinations sometimes must be made. As the ulna is lowered from this right-angle position and is adducted to the patient's side or when the arm is extended straight in front of the patient, the radius shortens with respect to the ulna. As ulnar variance

may direct a treatment decision, the variation between 1-3mm of ulnar length with respect to the length of the radius may make a significant difference. The PA view of the hand and wrist should be obtained with the palm of the hand flat on the X-ray film cassette to profile the carpometacarpal joints. If the wrist is placed so that the hand is made into a fist or if there is any wrist extension in the PA or AP positions, the carpometacarpal joints may not be in profile.

The PA and AP views provide the best view to survey the carpal bones to look for malalignments and other osseous and joint-space abnormalities. Understanding wrist anatomy on a PA view utilizing concepts of normal parallelism, three smooth carpal arcs (Fig. 7-1) and abnormal overlapping articular surfaces, can enable one to interpret major abnormalities in complex carpal trauma. The concept of parallelism can be helpful if the wrist is seen like a jigsaw puzzle (all bones that normally articulate should fit together like a jigsaw puzzle). This can be observed by looking at

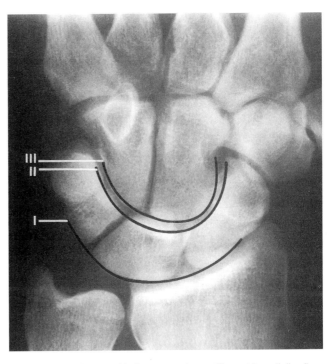

Figure 7-1. PA view with three arcs drawn. Normal "parallelism" can be seen between opposing artiulating cortices of the radius and scaphoid, radius and lunate, lunate and triquetrum, scaphoid and capitate, lunate and capitate, triquetrum and hamate, capitate and hamate, scaphoid and trapezoid and trapezium, and the second through fifth carpometacarpal joints.

normally parallel articular surfaces. In contrast, if there is an articular surface that should normally parallel the articular surface of another bone, but there is overlapping of bones, a dislocation or subluxation at that site should be suspected. This concept of overlapping articular surfaces can be evaluated only when a cortex is in profile and not foreshortened or out of profile.

On the normal PA view of the wrist, three smooth arcs can be drawn (Fig. 7-1). Arc I joins the outer curvatures of the proximal surfaces of the scaphoid, lunate, and triquetrum. Arc II identifies the distal smooth curves of these same three bones. Arc III identifies the proximal surfaces of the capitate and hamate. In the PA neutral position, the arcs should be smooth while changing in radius of curvature from bone to bone. If the arcs are broken, this would be supportive of a fracture, dislocation, or subluxation at the site of the broken arc. In the neutral position (without radial or ulnar deviation), two exceptions to this generality have been recognized: (1) at each joint there will be curvature of the bones; therefore, the arc concept does not apply at each joint margin; and (2) if one bone is narrower in its proximal-distal dimension than the adjacent bone, as sometimes is seen with the triquetrum being narrower than the adjacent portion of the lunate, then the arc at that point would normally not be smooth.

Routinely the lateral view should be obtained with the dorsum of the metacarpals in a straight line with the dorsum of the radius and ulna (Fig. 7-2). Such standardization of wrist positioning makes it easier to recognize alignment abnormalities. Recognition, if the lateral is a fairly true lateral, can be done by identifying the palmar cortex of the pisiform to see if this cortex overlies the midportion of the scaphoid that projects palmar to the palmar surface of the head of the capitate (Fig. 7-2). This method of identifying the correct lateral position uses an ulnar sided structure to overlap on a radial sided structure. Merely using the ulna (with respect to the radius) can present problems, as some people have a prominent ulna dorsally. The lateral view should be obtained at right angles to the PA view, so that a true right angle view of the ulna can be demonstrated.

This can be performed by adducting the wrist to the patient's side while the patient stands erect. Alternatively, two right-angled views can be obtained with the forearm fixed in a holder with the patient's forearm flexed at the elbow, and the arm next to the patient's side. One view is taken with a horizontal beam to get the PA view. A second view is obtained by redirecting the X-ray tube so that the beam is directed from the ceiling toward the floor to get the lateral view.

Two additional views that are recommended as a routine part of the exam are the PA with ulnar deviation and the 45° semisupinated oblique views. The ulnar deviated PA view elongates the scaphoid and provides a good second view of the carpus in the PA position. This view lengthens the scaphoid and provides a second view of the scaphoid waist to exclude scaphoid fractures. As the scaphoid is a commonly injured bone and missed fracture site, it is worthwhile to use this additional view to evaluate the posttraumatic wrist. The semisupinated oblique view is the only

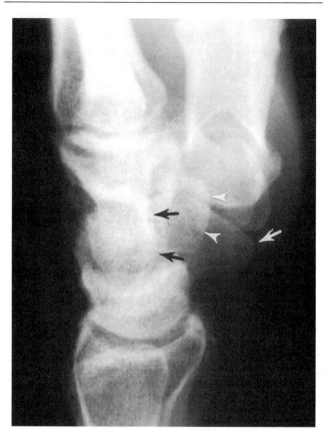

Figure 7-2. A correctly positioned lateral view shows the palmar cortex of the pisiform (arrowheads) projecting over the midpoint between the distal pole of the scaphoid (white arrow) and the palmar cortex of the capitate head (black arrows).

view that profiles the trapeziotrapezoidal joint and commonly shows the scaphotrapeziotrapezoidal joint. In addition to showing this area, an additional view of the remainder of the carpal bones is provided. These four views can be exposed on one X-ray film, limiting the amount of film for the radiographic wrist exam. The soft tissues and underlying bony structures should be observed carefully. When there is focal soft-tissue swelling, the center of this swelling should be scrutinized to see if there is an underlying fracture or other abnormality.

Detailed Radiographic Views

When a patient has point tenderness, specific views may be obtained to profile that site. The carpal tunnel view is helpful to view the palmar tubercle of the trapezium, hook of the hamate, carpal tunnel, pisiform, pisotriquetral, joint and the bony roof of the carpal tunnel. The semisupinated off-lateral view profiles the pisotriquetral joint and is an excellent view to evaluate this articulation. A reverse oblique view (with the palmar aspect of the hand elevated off the table) is a good view to look for a chip fracture off the dorsoradial surface of the scaphoid waist. This view demonstrates the ulnar sided structures and carpal bones in a different plane. The dorsal boss view is an off-lateral view profiling the dorsal boss. Sometimes the dorsal boss may be profiled better when the hand is placed in slight ulnar deviation with the off-lateral view profiling the second and third CMC joint regions. The goal is to profile the dorsal boss to characterize the "boss" to see if it results from osteophyte formation, a separate ossicle, the os styloideum, or a fracture off a normal prominence at the base of the second or third metacarpal. Other detailed specific views are available or can be developed to profile a specific bony prominence. A useful technique to profile a specific tender spot is to obtain multiple exposures on one film at 3° to 5° intervals tangent to the tender site. Such a technique utilizing minimal degrees of obliquity can profile a fracture or an osteotomy site to look for healing.

Fluoroscopic Spots

If overhead views utilizing detailed views are not sufficient to profile a specific structure, obtaining fluoroscopic spots or fluoroscopically directed radiographs can be helpful. Fluoroscopy can allow precise profile of a joint, a cortical surface, and a fracture or osteotomy site. Fluoroscopic evaluation is the easiest and most readily available way to evaluate carpal motion. Usually this examination can be recorded with videotape. Profiling the scapholunate joint precisely while watching its motion under fluoroscopy between radial and ulnar deviation can show if and at what position the scapholunate joint opens maximally. When it is important to identify healing of a fracture or osteotomy site, fluoroscopically controlled spots may be helpful to profile those sites. Alternatively, this fracture or osteotomy site could be evaluated with polytomography or computed tomography to evaluate healing. However, if a fracture or osteotomy site is not profiled, a completely open fracture or osteotomy site may appear healed from overlapping trabeculae (Figs. 7-3). Fluoroscopic spots or detailed views can be utilized to evaluate cortical surfaces for destruction or loss of trabecular structure.

Magnification Views

By utilizing a small focal spot and moving the film away from the part being radiographed, magnification views can be obtained. However, highly detailed views can be obtained with a small focal spot. Such views can be of value when detail of a specific cortical surface or trabecular structure is desired. Ideal machinery for this technique may not be widely available. All of the other techniques within this section of routine radiography should be available at any radiography installation.

Instability Series

A wrist instability series is performed to evaluate carpal bone motion and to see if there is evidence of carpal instability. This examination should include comparison with the opposite side. The static instability series may be performed with or without fluoroscopic control. One advantage of performing an instability series with fluoroscopic control is that motions of the carpal bones can be watched. Utilizing fluoroscopic control, the scapholunate joint can be profiled to look for abnormal diastasis of this joint. A variety of instability views can be obtained. One extensive series is composed of 17 views of each wrist obtained as fluoroscopic spot views. These include PA views with the scapholunate joint in profile with neutral, radial, and ulnar deviation. With the hand prone and without wrist deviation, the hand may be forcefully displaced, alternatively radially and ulnarly, to look for abnormal radiocarpal laxity. The next view obtained is the 30° to 45° semi-supinated oblique view to profile the scaphotrapeziotrapezoidal joint.

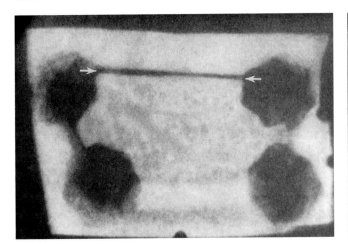 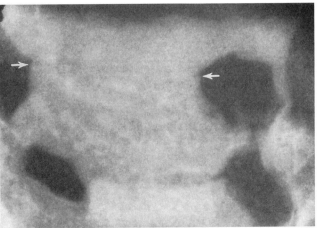

Figure 7-3.   **(Left)** Rat calverial specimen with osteotomy site in profile (between arrows). **(Right)** Same rat calverial specimen with osteotomy site (between arrows) apparently obliterated due to nonprofile of the osteotomy, simulating healing.

Lateral views are then obtained in the neutral, full-flexion, and full-extension positions. These views are obtained to see if there is normal carpal alignment and grossly normal motion. The scapholunate angle is normally between 30° to 60° with 60° to 80° borderline normal, and over 80° generally abnormal. The capitolunate angle is typically less than 30°. Gross motions are easy to remember; bones flex on full flexion and extend on full extension. On flexion the capitate, identifying the distal carpal row, should flex with respect to the midlunate axis. The lunate axis, identifying itself and representing the proximal carpal row, should flex with respect to the midradius axis. On extension, the capitate should extend with respect to the lunate and the lunate should extend with respect to the radius. Next, with the wrist in the neutral lateral position, the wrist is ulnarly deviated and then radially deviated. In these positions, the lunate should tilt dorsally with ulnar deviation and should tilt palmarly with radial deviation. (In other words, the lunate should move in the same direction as the scaphoid.) With the wrist still in the lateral position, the capitolunate instability pattern maneuvers can be performed. These two views are performed with the wrist in slight ulnar deviation, and alternatively palmar and dorsal displacing stresses are performed at the level of the carpometacarpal joints. These two maneuvers are performed to see if the capitate will displace out of the distal lunate concavity, but mainly these maneuvers are performed to see if one or both produce(s) the patient's symptoms. The next view is the off-lateral view profiling the pisotriquetral joint, and finally AP (supinated) views are performed with the fist clenched. These are performed in the neutral, radial deviation, and ulnar deviation positions, with profile of the scapholunate joint. The opposite wrist is also routinely evaluated, as questionable abnormal findings may sometimes be seen bilaterally. This would help raise the question if a finding is a normal variation or the result of bilateral injuries.

The recently proposed tailored instability series is designed to perform a limited instability examination, depending on the abnormality present. This approach suggests that there can be four indications to perform an instability series in some modified manner:

(1) With clinical symptoms of the capitolunate instability pattern, the two CLIP wrist maneuvers should be performed.

(2) If abnormal alignment is present on PA and/or lateral views, a full bilateral instability series is indicated.

(3) With scapholunate symptoms, a minimum examination to identify the widest possible diastasis of the scapholunate joint should be performed. This is accomplished under fluoroscopic control to profile the scapholunate joint in radial, neutral, and ulnar deviations, by also looking at the scapholunate joint in between the extremes of motion, as this joint can widen and narrow at any place during the arcs of motion. These views should be performed in both supine and prone positions. If there is any widening of the scapholunate joint as compared to the normal capitolunate or another normal intercarpal joint, the opposite side should also be evaluated for asymmetry.

(4) With painful popping, clicking, or clunking, the patient may best be evaluated by videotape or cineradi-ography (see following section). This may be combined with a full instability series if this examination demonstrates abnormal bony motion. The full instability series is performed for questionable carpal instability, the most common types of carpal instabilities being VISI, DISI, and rotary subluxation of the scaphoid.

Videotape or Cineradiography

A videotape or cineradiographic examination can be performed to record for later or repeated review of radiocarpal or intercarpal bone motion or motion of an anatomic site. Cineradiography utilizes filming of multiple radiographic exposures at a fast rate and provides more radiation to the patient than the videotape. This technique is available in most cardiology laboratories. Most radiographic departments have videotape capabilities. Videotape can be utilized to record motion, arthrographic examinations, or other types of radiographic procedures performed under fluoroscopy. A videotape examination may include a microphone so that audible sounds are recorded to correlate the popping sound with the movement seen on videotape.

It may be valuable for the examining physician to evaluate the patient with a popping wrist in conjunction with the radiologist. If the patient is to be examined for popping, clunking, or other painful sound in the wrist, it is important that the patient is able to produce this sound repetitively before going to the fluoroscopic suite. When a sound is present only occasionally, it is usually not worthwhile for the patient to show up for a radiographic examination. If it is necessary for the patient to work for a half day or perform some task for a few hours before the popping takes place, then that should be required before the patient comes in for the examination.

Tomography

Tomography is a general term used to describe a wide variety of methods for obtaining a sectional radiographic image. The terms laminography and planigraphy are synonymous with tomography. Conventional (noncomputed) tomography employs conventional radiographic (film/screen) cassettes and uses standard X-ray tubes and generators. The tomographic table and X-ray tube housing are constructed to allow synchronized motion of the tube and film cassette in opposite directions. Both move in an arc or plane and are coupled through a fixed fulcrum. This motion blurs all objects not in the plane of the fulcrum. The level of the plane of imaging can be changed by altering the position of the fulcrum relative to the patient.

Linear tomography, the simplest form of a tomographic X-ray unit, moves the cassette and tube in a linear fashion, usually parallel to the long axis of the table. The main disadvantage of linear tomography is the production of streak-like artifacts from edges parallel to the plane of motion and the resultant inability to effectively blur these edges, even when they are not in the imaging plane. To eliminate these edge artifacts, polydirectional tomography (polytomography) was developed. Polytomography moves the tube and cassette in a complex manner, in opposite directions, maintaining a constant fulcrum. This complex motion is intended to avoid paralleling any anatomic edge, thus producing more complete blurring of structures not in the imaging plane. This complex motion varies with different machines from simple circles and ellipses to complex spirals and hypocycloidals. In general, the more complex the motion, the more complete the blurring.

The aim of polytomography is to produce sharp planar images of the patient's anatomy. The distance through which the tube travels is governed by the angle of the arc through which it swings. The greater this angle, the greater the blurring and the narrower the apparent thickness of the slice. While thin slices improve the separation of structures, they also decrease the apparent image contrast, making certain soft-tissue structures difficult to see. This is less of a problem with bone tomography as the inherent contrast in bone is high. In osteopenic patients, however, this reduction in image contrast may be a problem. The available spatial resolution of polytomography is the same as that of the plain radiograph. The apparent resolution, however, is modified by both the decrease in tissue contrast and the presence of blurring artifact.

Theoretically, polytomography should give us excellent anatomic data. In practice, though, the blurring artifacts and lower image contrast may reduce the diagnostic confidence of the reader. The presence of metallic fixation devices may further reduce this confidence by producing additional dense blurring artifacts across the area of interest. Because the images are planar, it is imperative to obtain two planes at right angles. This eliminates the potential for imaging along the plane of a fracture or other bony defect and rendering it invisible.

In the presence of well calcified bone and in the absence of metallic fixation devices, polytomography provides reliable data about the union of fractures and arthrodeses that may be obscured on the standard radiographs. By eliminating the overlapping structures inherent in three-dimensional data of a conventional radiograph, subtle bony bridging or a clearcut nonunion that could not be seen on the initial radiographs will often become readily visible with polytomography.

In recent years, there has been a tendency for polytomography to be replaced by computed tomography. CT has several advantages over polytomography. In the United States, CT is often more readily available. Polytomography requires well trained and practiced technologists, careful patient positioning, and careful physician supervision. CT, on the other hand, is much less technologist-dependent and can frequently be performed following a simple protocol. In general, the radiation dose is lower with CT, and CT is less time-consuming. The inherent image contrast with CT is much greater than with polytomography and although spatial resolution is much less, the absence of blurring artifact may make structures appear sharper (Fig. 7-4) . The major advantages of polytomography over CT are lower initial cost of equipment and the ability to image in multiple planes. In the hand and wrist this latter advantage is not an issue since the prehensile nature of the distal upper extremity permits direct CT imaging in axial, coronal,

sagittal, and oblique planes. Whichever tomographic method is chosen, careful attention to selection of the appropriate imaging planes is essential.

Bone Scintigraphy (Bone Scan)

Nuclear medicine techniques, especially bone scintigraphy with technetium-99m methylene diphosphonate, are useful to evaluate the wrist. Bone scintigraphy is valuable to identify physiologically active osteochondral abnormalities (i.e., those causing bone repair or remodeling) and provides a sensitive way to look for such abnormalities. In so-called three-phase bone scintigraphy, the first component is an assessment of the local flow (radionuclide angiography) during injection of the radiopharmaceutical. The second phase, the immediate-static or blood-pool phase, shows the distribution of the tracer within the soft tissues after the vascular phase. Two or three hours later, after accumulation of the radiopharmaceutical in bone and the clearance of tracer from the soft tissues, the delayed-phase images depict the local rate of bone turnover. In general, a focal, very intense scintigraphic abnormality will have a good chance to have an imaging explanation, whereas subtle findings may not have an imaging explanation.

Diffusely increased uptake is more suggestive of some type of synovitis or other cause for hyperemia. Any marked focal increased uptake raises the question of some osteochondral problem that should be further evaluated if a plain roentgenographic exam does not show anything. Further evaluation can be done by CT and/or MRI. Generally all fractures should show increased activity by three days (if there is going to be any abnormality at all). Most fractures are apparent within the first 24 hours, but delayed-reaction changes are more likely in elderly patients who form new bone slowly. Bone scintigraphy is a good way to survey for a physiologically active osteochondral problem. If bone scintigraphy is normal in a patient with a painful wrist, then an abnormality, if present, is more likely of soft tissues (especially soft tissues extrinsic to the carpal bones).

Single-photon emission-computed tomography (SPECT) is a type of bone scintigraphy that produces tomographic images in axial, coronal, or sagittal planes. Occasionally SPECT can show abnormalities that were missed by routine bone scintigraphy. However, it may be difficult to perform wrist SPECT in some patients.

Other radiopharmaceuticals, especially gallium-67 citrate, indium-111 labeled leukocytes, and indium-111 labeled polyclonal Ig G, have received attention to evaluate infection. Imaging with these agents is more expensive than routine bone scintigraphy and thus should be utilized only in selected cases. When gallium scintigraphy is performed, the images are compared with routine technetium-99m bone scintigrams. If the uptake of gallium is greater than that of technetium, this supports the presence of an infection or other inflammatory process.

The major value of bone scintigraphy, is to evaluate for possible fracture or underlying physiologically active osteochondral problem to explain a problem for the unexplained painful wrist. For example, bone scintigraphy is helpful when a focal lucent or "cyst-like" defect is seen within a

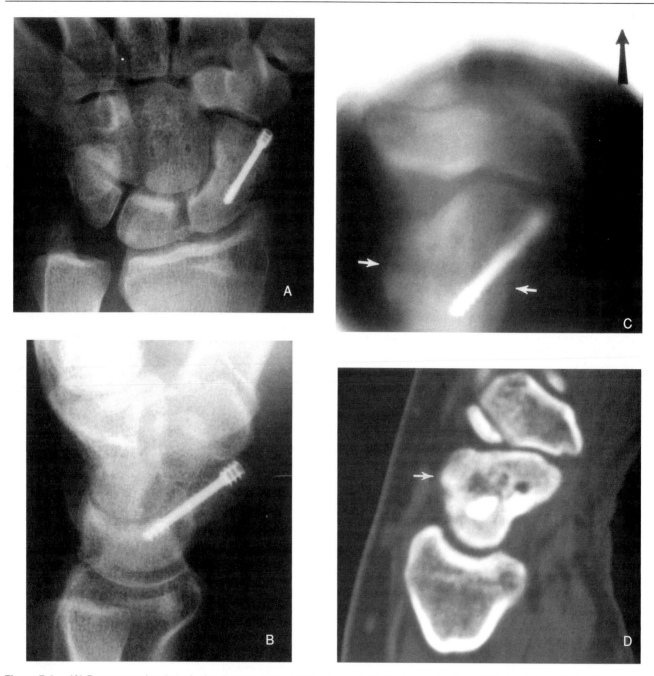

Figure 7-4. **(A)** Posteroanterior view of a healing scaphoid waist fracture with Herbert screw in place. **(B)** Lateral view of a healing scaphoid waist fracture with Herbert screw in place. **(C)** Polytomography of the scaphoid with questionable healing, as there is a lucency in the midportion of the scaphoid (between arrows). **(D)** CT of the scaphoid performed in the long axis of the scaphoid has a waist fracture with Herbert screw in place, with no question that there is solid healing. A hump-back deformity exostosis (arrow) is present, and the metal screw is not causing artifact.

carpal bone. Such lucent defects are commonly seen and are often incorrectly called "cysts." These focal lucent defects may be actually fiber-filled and not cysts; therefore, it is more appropriate to call them "lucent defects." Commonly these defects may be quiescent and have no significance. If there is focal tenderness associated with a lucent defect, bone scintigraphy may be of value to see if the lesion is hot or physiologically active on bone scan.

Such a situation may occur with an active intraosseous ganglia, in which symptoms may be relieved by excision.

Wrist Arthrography

Arthrography is a technique whereby contrast is injected into wrist joints to see if there are abnormal communicating defects between adjacent compartments or if there are abnormal noncommunicating defects. In the wrist there are commonly three separate compartments. The distal radioulnar joint is separate from the radiocarpal compartment. The radiocarpal compartment communicates with the pisotriquetral joint. The midcarpal compartment includes the joints between the scaphoid, lunate, triquetrum, capitate, hamate, trapezoid, and trapezium. The carpometacarpal joints two through five are also filled from the midcarpal compartment. The first carpometacarpal joint does not normally fill from the midcarpal compartment.

Abnormal communication between the midcarpal and radiocarpal compartments occurs through the scapholunate or lunotriquetral ligaments. Less common sites of abnormal communication are through the scaphotrapeziotrapezoidal capsular area (Fig. 7-5), especially radially and palmarly, possibly through the area of the radioscaphocapitate ligament, and through the pisotriquetral joint, probably in the area of the ulnar branch of the palmar extrinsic "v" ligament. Abnormal communication between the radiocarpal and distal radioulnar joints often occurs through the radial aspect of the triangular fibrocartilage. Sometimes communication may occur through the "complex" portion of the triangular fibrocartilage, that is, the soft-tissue attachments along the periphery of the triangular fibrocartilage. Noncommunicating defects may involve the triangular fibrocartilage and especially along the proximal ulnar surface of the triangular fibrocartilage. Contrast collection along the proximal ulnar aspect of the triangular fibrocartilage near the ulnar styloid is consistent with avulsion or perforation into the attachment of the triangular fibrocartilage at this site. Wherever there is abnormal communication, the decision must be made if this is symptomatic or not.

Three-compartment arthrography has been identified to show the maximum number of communicating and noncommunicating defects. It is more correct to call such communication or noncommunicating defects, "defects or perforations" rather than "tears." It is not possible on arthrography to call a communicating or noncommunicating defect or perforation a "tear." Doing so may imply a cause of the defect which is not known. Currently there is no known way to differentiate arthrographically or on MRI between a tear or perforation (communicating defect). A noncommunicating defect is one that does not traverse the entire structure.

Three-compartment wrist arthrography can be performed in a variety of ways. Digital radiography is a technique that allows subtraction of bones and previously injected contrast material (Fig.7-5). The use of digital technique can allow injection of all three joints sequentially by subtracting out the earlier injected joints. However, there is a problem detecting any extravasation of contrast or passage of contrast out of a compartment during motion views after the injecting phase of the procedure, as bones cannot be subtracted if there has been motion of the bones. After the injecting phase, the wrist should be placed through a full range of motion in radial and ulnar deviation, as demonstration of communications may take place only while placing the wrist through the range of radial and ulnar deviation both in prone and supine positions. Contrast flowing from one compartment to the other must be recorded either by

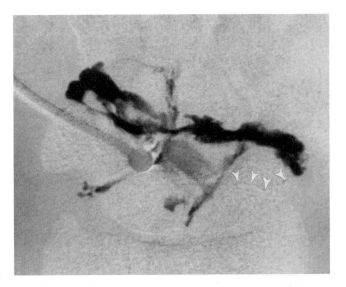

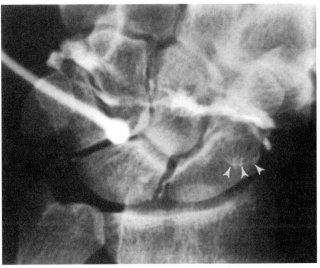

Figure 7-5. Example of digital subtraction **(Top)** showing contrast passing through the scaphotrapezial capsular and radioscaphocapitate ligament area (arrowheads) with the nonsubtrated roentgenogram **(Bottom)** for comparison. The subtraction film is slightly earlier in the injection phase than the nonsubtracted roentgenogram.

videotape or fluoroscopic spots to show the site of communication. When contrast is in the adjacent joint, one may not always be able to detect flow of contrast between compartments without digital subtraction. Therefore, digital subtraction could work with all three compartments injected, but only if all three joints are completely normal, or if all communications took place during the injection phase.

One approach for the three-compartment injection is to inject the midcarpal joint first, which outlines the distal portion of the scapholunate and lunotriquetral ligaments, and then follow this with the distal radioulnar joint injection, if no contrast passed into the radiocarpal joint from the midcarpal compartment. After a short period of time, which may vary between a half-hour to over an hour, utilizing dilute contrast, the radiocarpal joint can be injected. Some authors inject these three joints in different sequences, while other authors wait a longer time between the joint injections. Important features to recognize when evaluating a wrist arthrogram is to see if there has been some method of recording passage of contrast from compartment to compartment, and to see if the wrist has been moved through a range of motion. It is also valuable to use a more dilute type of contrast material or "dye," as this will cause less synovial irritation, less pain, and less post-procedure synovitis. A dilute meglumine salt of approximately 43% concentration can be diluted further with anesthetic to simultaneously provide a test to see if pain is relieved by injecting each joint compartment. One approach is to mix 20cc of this dilute contrast with 10cc of anesthetic. Using a dilute contrast will allow one to more easily see through the contrast and get rid of problems with contrast being too dense to see structures. Anecdotally, many years prior, with use of contrast of 60% to 76%, we encountered an occasional patient with severe post-procedure pain, presumably due to contrast-initiated synovitis. Since use of dilute contrast as above, no such incidences of severe post-procedure pain have been brought to our attention.

The needle can be placed either in the radial or ulnar sides of the midcarpal and radiocarpal joints. The advantage of placing the needle away from the site of symptoms is that if there is extravasation out of the joint compartment away from the needle tip, and in the site of symptoms, it is not necessary to question if the extravasation is needle related. Then the potential pathologic significance of this finding can be evaluated more easily. If the needle is in the site of symptoms, it is difficult to know if the extravasation could be "pathologic" or if it resulted from needle placement.

Capsule defects have been noted by many authors. These may be "communicating" to another compartment or synovial space (as tendon sheath or ganglion) or "noncommunicating" to pass into soft tissues adjacent to the injected joint. It is common for contrast to fill tendon sheaths when the needle passes through a tendon sheath when entering a joint. As abnormal communications from the injected joint may pass into tendon sheaths and adjacent compartments through capsular defects (communicating defects), the needle placement site must be known to evaluate such contrast leakage. The exact significance of capsule defects is uncertain. Perhaps these represent defects in the adjacent extrinsic ligaments. This author is aware of only a few unpublished anecdotal cases in which surgical procedures have been performed for capsular defects, and the results of those procedures are not clear.

Flap-type defects are defects that fill the adjacent compartment from only one compartment. There is some discrepancy in the literature regarding these "one-way" or "flap-type" defects. Some authors feel strongly that all one-way defects through the scapholunate and lunotriquetral ligaments can be filled or shown from the first joint injected as long as that joint is fully distended within the patient's comfort level. However, other authors do not report this same experience. This discrepancy does not exist with respect to one-way defects through the triangular fibrocartilage and through communicating capsule defects. Most literature regarding one-way defects in the triangular fibrocartilage supports the need to inject both the distal radioulnar and the radiocarpal joints to see if there is a one-way defect. Especially if a communicating or noncommunicating defect is not shown from one injected compartment, then the adjacent joint should be injected. Some literature states that if any compartment is not fully distended, then all communicating and noncommunicating defects may not be demonstrated.

Bilateral wrist arthrography is currently being supported. Cadaveric work shows a high incidence of asymptomatic bilateral communicating defects. In many cases these are symmetric. There is a developing belief by some authors that the asymmetric communicating defect may be the one that is more significant and has more likelihood to provide explanation for a patient's pain. Such bilateral symmetric communicating defects seem to be fairly common (Fig. 7-6). Recognition that such defects are bilateral may help eliminate pressure on surgeons to perform some type of procedure for a communicating defect, when the defect is only questionably causing pain. Indeed, when a defect is in the area of pain, finding such a defect on the opposite side will encourage the treating surgeon to be even more cautious about acting on this communication. This knowledge that there are bilateral asymptomatic communicating and noncommunicating defects will have subsequent similar impact on findings detected on MRI, since MRI gradually may replace more routine wrist arthrography, as fine-resolution MRI becomes more developed (see following section on MRI).

The size of ligament defects may vary. Some question has been raised if tiny communicating defects are as significant as large defects. No study has been published correlating the size of defects with pathologic findings. However, if the size and position of defects were routinely recorded on arthrography and/or arthroscopy, this could enable evaluation of the question if there is any correlation between size and location of the defect and potential significance of the defect. The major value of wrist arthrography is to identify sites of communicating and noncommunicating perforations or defects. Other indications for wrist arthrography include demonstration of capsule size, the appearance of possible synovitis or even adhesive capsulitis, capsular outpouchings or ganglia, and a nonunion when contrast passes through a scaphoid waist fracture or possible fibrous or cartilaginous union when contrast does not

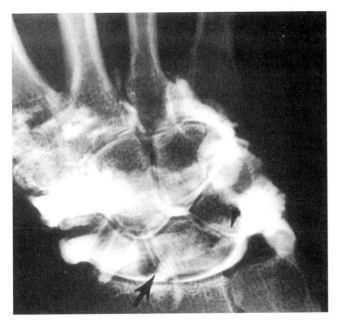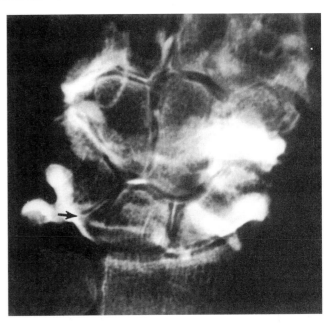

Figure 7-6. **(Left)** Left wrist arthrography in the same patient shows an identical communicating defect of the lunotriquetral ligament (arrowhead) and an intact scapholunate ligament. **(Right)** Right wrist arthrography: bilateral symmetric communicating defects are evident on wrist arthrography. The arrow points to an intact scapholunate ligament, and the arrowhead points to a communicating lunotriquetral defect.

pass through a scaphoid fracture site. Arthrography can also outline some of the cartilage surfaces of the carpal bones, radius, and ulna.

Computed Tomography

Computed tomography is routinely available throughout most of the United States and in many areas of the world. This technique has many applications in the wrist, as it clearly shows fractures, subluxations, intraosseous pathology, and healing or nonhealing of fractures or osteotomies. CT can clearly display joint space widths and demonstrates subtle calcifications and sharp cortical detail. CT has a major advantage over polytomography or tomography in that it does not have the blur associated with polytomography (Fig. 7-4).

Computed tomography should be performed in a tailored manner to give the best possible answer for each presenting clinical problem. This necessitates the presenting problem to be passed from the referring physician to the radiologist. In general, CT sections should be performed at right angles to the surface to be detailed. In other words, to show a fracture line clearly, the wrist should be positioned so that the CT section is passing at right angles to the fracture line. CT sections should be thin enough so that the desired detail is seen. When a thick CT section, as 5-10mm, is obtained, this averages everything within the five to 10mm thick section. If it is desirable to see a 1mm bar or small areas of bony bridging from healing, displaying all information in that 5-10mm thick section as one image could average out that small area of healing so it is not visible. Therefore, it is nec-

essary that thin sections at close intervals be obtained to produce the type of information desired. CT performed in more than one plane may also be necessary to answer specific problems. For instance, if displacement of scaphoid fracture fragments is questioned, at least two CT planes should be obtained for the scaphoid fracture to see if there is palmar or dorsal displacement or rotation of fracture fragments (which can be evaluated easily by sections obtained in the long axis of the scaphoid), and to see if there is radial or ulnar displacement of the scaphoid fragments (which can be evaluated by coronal-plane CT). To evaluate the scaphoid or another carpal bone, 2mm thick sections at 1 or 2mm intervals are usually satisfactory. Sometimes it may be valuable to evaluate a single bone, as the scaphoid, with 2mm thick sections at 1mm intervals in one plane and 2mm thick sections at 2mm intervals in the second plane to decrease the amount of CT time used to image the patient while providing necessary clinical information.

Several different positions are available to position the wrist. The coronal plane can be obtained in two positions, and one such position is obtained with the patient prone on the CT table, with the ulnar side of the hand placed on the tabletop above the head. A second coronal plane can be obtained with the patient prone on the CT table, with the hand extended on a holder and the gantry angled to parallel the carpus. The sagittal plane can be obtained with the patient prone by placing the palm flat on the table with the arm to be examined flexed at the elbow and above the patient's head. Transaxial-plane CTs can be obtained with the arm extended straight over the patient's head in a vari-

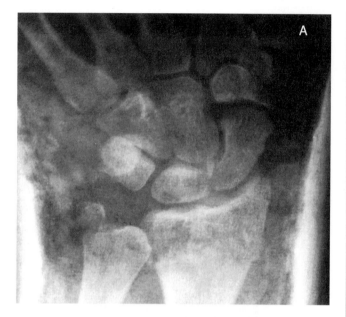

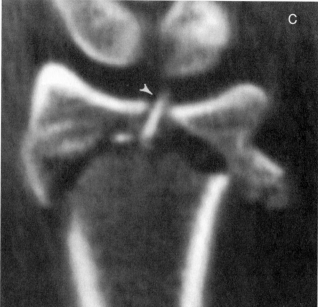

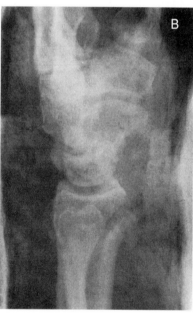

Figure 7-7.   **(A)** PA and **(B)** lateral views of wrist in cast with **(C)** sagittal CT. A fragment (arrowhead) projects in the radiocarpal joint. Even in retrospect this fragment is not seen in A or B.

ety of positions, according to what position the patient can assume comfortably. An oblique sagittal plane or a long axis of the scaphoid plane can be obtained by placing the wrist so that a line between Lister's tubercle and the base of the thumb is placed parallel to the gantry sections. Alternatively, the wrist may be placed so that the gantry is parallel to the axis of a Herbert's screw or K-wire passing through the scaphoid. Placing a metal screw or wire parallel to the gantry sections can make a metallic "streak" artifact much less obvious. To look at the scaphotrapeziotrapezoidal joint, the wrist can be placed in an oblique position so that

the CT sections pass through the STT joint at right angles.

The CT examination can be valuable when the pathology in question has been profiled adequately. A negative CT examination does not mean that the patient is normal; it only means that no abnormality was revealed on that examination. Currently, the major values for CT in the wrist include demonstration of healing of any type of fracture or bone graft procedure and fracture fragment position, especially to identify the presence or absence of pylon fractures or fragments within a joint (Fig. 7-7). Any time fine anatomic bone detail is desired, such as the character of an intracarpal lucency, the CT exam is valuable. CT can show the extent of soft-tissue processes including neoplasia or infection; however, MRI is preferable (when available) to evaluate soft tissues.

Spiral CT, a newer method of computed tomography, obtains planar image data in a continuous acquisition rather than as individual slices. This technique can image an entire wrist in approximately 30 seconds. The resolution in the scanning plane is equal to standard CT. The advantage of this technique is that thin section overlapping images can be acquired efficiently with reduced examination time and radiation exposure for the patient. The reconstructed images allow accurate assessment of acute trauma. Current software provides reconstructed images in an infinite number of anatomic planes, which can greatly aid in the evaluation of complex carpal trauma. Spiral CT also benefits 3-D imaging techniques in providing a complete, registered thin section data set, which is needed for high-quality 3-D reconstructions. Although the resolution of spiral CT reconstructions approaches that of directly acquired images, for the detection of subtle wrist trauma, traditional, nonspiral, directed positioning remains the preferred scanning option.

Three-dimensional CT

Computed tomographic sections can be displayed in a 3-D manner to show carpal bones in entirety or separately. Three-dimensional imaging enables a display of carpal bone(s) from multiple projections. However, to use the advantage of this technique to display carpal surface anatomy, with the closely opposed bones in the carpus, one must usually separate the bones to look at specific anatomic surfaces. Separation of the bones requires an operator's time to identify each bone desired to be saved or removed. Three-dimensional images smooth anatomic surfaces, which make the images more attractive; however, this smoothing effect can eliminate display of hairline fractures and less obvious abnormalities. The ability to rotate the bone in question in "real time" to profile a fracture line is ideal, but is not yet readily available. Utilization of 3-D images allows modeling and preoperative planning, but the cost for this may not yet be reimbursed. At a research level, fracture fragments can be manipulated to plan surgical procedures preoperatively. The major value of 3-D CT is to provide images that more closely approximate what the surgeon will see at operation. This is of most value in cases of complex trauma to enable clear visualization of bone and various fracture fragment displacements.

Magnetic Resonance Imaging

Magnetic resonance imaging has an advantage over radiography, since MRI does not use ionizing radiation. It produces a similar type of cross-sectional anatomy as computed tomography; however, it shows soft-tissue detail and differentiation better than CT and also shows marrow struc-

ture better than CT. MRI is evolving rapidly. Stronger magnets are needed to provide the finer resolution necessary to demonstrate thin structures. Weaker magnets may be adequate to show marrow structure in individual carpal bones and the character of soft-tissue masses. The technical parameters provided by the MRI and its operators vary tremendously, and the technical parameters chosen must be best suited to the individual problem. Surface coils are necessary to improve the quality of the image. The thicknesses of the sections utilized should vary according to the structure desired to be seen. For instance, if a ligament structure of 1 to 2mm thick is in question, 3mm sections are too thick to image the structures clearly and thoroughly. Gadolinium DPA (dyethylenetriamine pentaacetiac acid) is the contrast media commonly utilized with MRI. Some have used gadolinium as an intra-articular contrast agent, but its use is not clearly established. Intravenous injection of gadolinium allows enhancement of more vascular structures as in some soft-tissue tumors and synovial inflammatory processes. MRI is currently the best technique to evaluate neoplasia and infection.

Major uses for MRI include the demonstration of marrow abnormalities, such as avascular necrosis, bone marrow edema, demonstration of the extent of soft-tissue neoplasia, and the detection of occult ganglia or occult glomus tumor. Although some MRI machines are able to image the triangular fibrocartilage (or at least portions of it), the reliable demonstration of intrinsic and extrinsic ligaments has not been widespread (Figure 7-8). With recognition of symmetric bilateral communicating and noncommunicating defects in arthrography, the necessity to demonstrate if a communicating defect is unilateral or bilateral must also be faced with MRI. A major goal for future imaging with MRI is to determine how to differentiate a symptomatic from a nonsymptomatic defect. Finally, an important message for the physician who requests an MRI (or other procedure) is to determine the quality of the exam performed. All equipment and all personnel do not perform equally.

Ultrasonography

Ultrasonography for the hand and wrist is not widely utilized in the United States. In experienced hands, ultrasonography is utilized to evaluate ligaments and tendons, outline known soft-tissue masses, evaluate for fluid collections, and look for and at such other soft-tissue processes as ganglions. This technique can be utilized to identify fluid, especially to see if a mass is cystic or solid. Differentiating an abscess from cellulitis can be accomplished. Sonography can be utilized to identify the location of foreign bodies. A major advantage ultrasound has over CT or MRI is its lower cost. Ultrasonography is not as desirable pictorially, however, due to the difficulty of being readily understood by the clinician. Ultrasonography is highly operator dependent; however, when developed by interested ultrasonographers, it is a good diagnostic technique for specific problems of soft tissues.

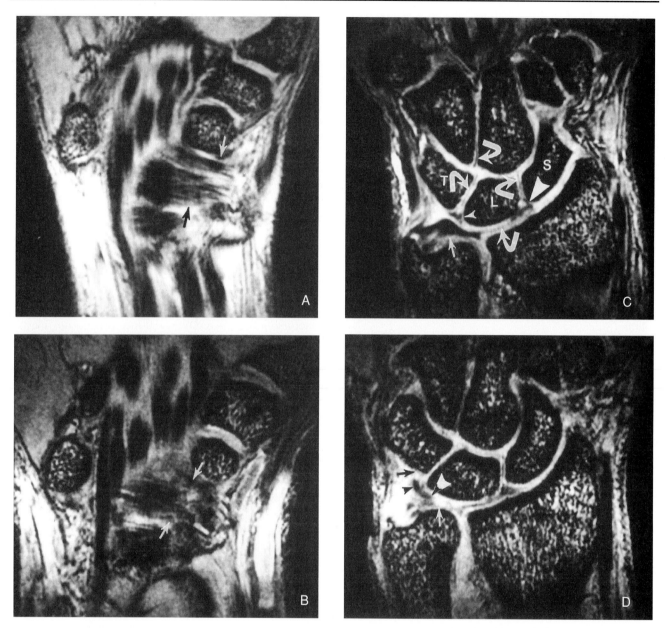

Figure 7-8.   (A) Palmar section shows continuous fascicles of a normal radioscaphocapitate extrinsic ligament (between arrowheads). (MRI is performed with a radiant echo volume acquisition and less than 1mm sections thick). **(B)** In another patient, fascicles in the radio-scaphocapitate ligament are disrupted (between arrows). **(C)** The normal dark triangular fibrocartilage (arrow) extends from the cartilage on the distal radius to insert into the fovea at the base of the ulnar styloid. The normal scapholunate (large arrowhead) and lunotriquetral (small arrowhead) ligaments are structures with mixed signal attaching to cartilage and bone (L = lunate, S = scaphoid and T = triquetrum). The thin black lines represent cartilage surfaces (curved arrows). **(D)** In another patient with perforations of the TFC and lunotriquetral ligament, the normal solid dark structure of the TFC is interrupted (white arrow). The lunotriquetral ligament (arrowhead) is separated from the triquetrum (black arrow) and is still attached to the cartilage on the lunate (large white arrowhead with black tip). Courtesy of Dr. Saara Totterman, radiologist and Dr. Richard Miller, Strong Memorial Hospital of the University of Rochester, Rochester, New York).

Annotated Bibliography

Routine Radiography

Gilula LA: Carpal injuries: analytic approach and case exercise. *AJR,* 133:503-517, 1979.

This article describes an approach to analyze routine radiographs stressing the concepts of parallelism, overlapping articular surfaces, and three normal radiographically identifiable arcs. This article was apparently the first to describe the three carpal arcs and provide an approach to analysis of complex carpal trauma stressing the PA view of the wrist.

Instability Series

Gilula LA, Weeks PM: Post-traumatic ligamentous instabilities of the wrist. *Radiology,* 129:641-651, 1978.

Apparently this is the first summary of basic ligamentous instabilities of the wrist with their radiographic description to appear in radiologic literature.

Louis DS, Hankin FM, Green TL, et al: Central carpal instability-capitate lunate instability pattern. *Orthopedics,* 7:1693-1696, 1984.

This article describes the CLIP wrist and an radiographic approach to its recognition.

Schernberg F: Roentgenographic examination of the wrist: a systematic study of the normal, lax and injured wrist. Part 1: The standard and positional views. *J Hand Surg,* 15B:210-219, 1990.

This article describes appearances and relationship of the carpal bones in 53 normal wrists, 15 lax wrists and 80 injured wrists using frontal and lateral radiographs with the wrist in neutral and other positions.

Schernberg F: Roentgenographic examination of the wrist: a systematic study of the normal, lax and injured wrist. Part 2: Stress views. *J Hand Surg,* 15B:220-228, 1990.

Stress views are described and results of these stress views in injured wrists had pathological radiographic findings confirmed at operation. This article also presents a radiological anatomical classification of wrist instabilities.

Truong NP, Mann FA, Gilula LA, Kang SW: Tailored wrist instability series - Abstract RSNA 1992.

After analysis of 563 instability series, there is presentation of four indications for use of an instability series to decrease the nonindicated wrist instability exams. This presents use of a limited or tailored instability series for most cases where an instability series could be used.

Tomography, Computed Tomography, and Three-Dimensional CT

Belsole RJ, Hilbelink DR, Llewellyn A, Dale M, Ogden JA: Carpal orientation from computed reference axes. *J Hand Surg,* 16A:82-90, 1991.

A CT method to determine mathematical axes of carpal bones is presented. This method decreases the measurement error on plain radiographs.

Biondetti PR, Vannier MW, Gilula LA, Knapp RH: Three-dimensional surface reconstruction of the carpal bones from CT scans: transaxial versus coronal technique. *Comp Med Imag Graph,* 12:67-73, 1988.

The article describes utilization of 3-D in cadaveric and patient wrists and compares two approaches to acquire images for CT scanning and subsequent three-dimensional reconstruction.

Hindman BW, Kulik WJ, Lee G, Avolio RE: Occult fractures of the carpals and metacarpals: demonstration by CT. *AJR,* 153:529-532, 1989.

The use of more than one plane for CT examination of the wrist to demonstrate fractures is emphasized especially to detect occult fractures of the carpals and metacarpals.

Posner MA, Greenspan A: Trispiral tomography for the evaluation of wrist problems. *J Hand Surg,* 13A:175-181, 1988.

This is a good review article for the application of trispiral tomography for the wrist. It shows its use to detect fractures and fracture healing, healing of grafts, and evaluation of intraosseous and subchondral defects.

Stewart NR, Gilula LA: CT of the wrist: a tailored approach. *Radiology,* 183:13-20, 1992.

An approach to tailoring the examination of CT for the wrist is presented. The need to utilize a variety of positions of the wrist to provide answers for each different question presented by the referring physicians is stressed. This article emphasizes that a CT examination may completely miss pathology if not performed in one or more adequate planes.

Bone Scintigraphy

Holder LE: Radionuclide bone imaging in surgical problems of the hand. In Gilula LA, ed.: *The Traumatized Hand and Wrist. Radiographic and anatomic correlation.* WB Saunders, Philadelphia 19-43, 1992.

A wide spectrum of use of bone scintigraphy in the wrist is presented.

Maurer AH: Nuclear medicine evaluation of the hand and wrist. *Hand Clin,* 7:183-200, 1991.

The article reviews the technique of three-phase scintigraphy and its application for study of the hand and wrist.

Arthrography

Hardy DC, Totty WG, Carnes KM, Kyriakos M, Pin PG, Reinus WR, Weeks PM, Gilula LA: Arthrographic surface anatomy of the carpal triangular fibrocartilage complex. *J Hand Surg,* 13A:823-829, 1988.

Noncommunicating defects of the triangular fibrocartilage are described and correlated with histologic sections. Description of normal variations and probable pathologic abnormalities are presented.

Herbert TJ, Faithfull RG, McCann DJ, Ireland J: Bilateral arthrography of the wrist. *J Hand Surg,* 15B:233-235, 1990.

Bilateral wrist arthrography is performed and shows positive arthrograms in the opposite asymptomatic wrist. These authors conclude that unilateral arthrography is of little diagnostic value and recommend the use of the opposite asymptomatic wrist as a control.

Levinsohn EM, Rosen ID, Palmer AK: Wrist arthrography: value of the three-compartment injection method. *Radiology,* 179:231-239, 1991.

The authors of this article popularized triple-joint wrist arthrography. They summarize their results in 300 consecutive patients and conclude that three separate injections into the radiocarpal, midcarpal, and distal radioulnar joints are necessary for a complete wrist arthrographic investigation.

Manaster BJ, Mann RJ, Rubenstein S: Wrist pain: correlation of clinical and plain film findings with arthrographic results. *J Hand Surg,* 14A:466-473, 1989.

The authors find significance between ulnar-sided pain and ulnar arthrographic findings but no correlation between radial pain and scapholunate ligament abnormalities on arthrography. They also find no correlation with scapholunate diastasis and scapholunate ligament abnormalities shown on arthrography.

Wilson AJ, Gilula LA, Mann FA: Unidirectional joint communications in wrist arthrography: an evaluation of 250 cases. *AJR,* 157:105-109, 1991.

The article evaluates unidirectional communications and compares them to those reported by others. The authors suggest that demonstration of communications depends on specific technical factors, such as which joint is injected first, the amount of contrast material used, and the delay between injections. All unidirectional communications through the scapholunate and lunotriquetral ligaments are found from the first compartment injected. Communications through the triangular fibrocartilage are found from either first or second compartments injected.

Magnetic Resonance Imaging

Foo TKF, Shellock FG, Hayes CE, Schenck JF, Slayman BE: High resolution MR imaging of the wrist and eye with short TR, short TE, and partial-echo acquisition. *Radiology,* 183:277-281, 1992.

An approach to obtaining high-resolution images of the wrist is described. Qualities of MRI in this article and the article by Totterman present the basis for high-resolution wrist imaging that should be standard in the future.

Golimbu CN, Firooznia H, Melone CP Jr, Rafii M, Weinreb J, Leber C: Tears of the triangular fibrocartilage of the wrist: MR imaging. *Radiology,* 173:731-733, 1989.

Of 20 patients with surgical correlation, the accuracy of MR imaging to detect TFC tears is 95%. The authors suggest that MRI provides a noninvasive method to study pathologic conditions of the TFC.

Munk PL, Vellet AD, Levin MF, Steinbach LS, Helms CA: Current status of magnetic resonance imaging of the wrist. *Can Assoc Radiol J,* 43:8-18, 1992.

A review of MRI applications of the wrist is provided in this review article.

Totterman SM, Heberger R, Miller R, Rubens DJ, Blebea JS: Two-piece wrist surface coil. *AJR,* 156:343-344, 1991.

A design of a surface coil is described that provides high resolution wrist images.

Totterman SM, Miller R, Wasserman B, Blebea JS, Rubens DJ: Intrinsic and extrinsic carpal ligaments: evaluation by three-dimensional fourier transform MR imaging. *AJR,* 160, 1993, in press.

The ability of MRI to show ligamentous abnormalities with high resolution thin section MRI is stressed in this article. The quality of the work in this paper should set the standard for future work to show thin sections when evaluating anatomy of both extrinsic and intrinsic ligaments.

Trumble TE, Irving J: Histologic and magnetic resonance imaging correlations in Kienböck's disease. *J Hand Surg,* 15A:879-884, 1990.

This is the first article to show correlation between histology using tetracyline labeling to evaluate AVN on MRI. This presents six cases with histologic support for AVN and supports the need to see more than one-half of the lunate involved on MRI to call AVN.

Zlatkin MB, Chao PC, Osterman AL, Schnall MD, Dalinka MK, Kressel HY: Chronic wrist pain: evaluation with high-resolution MR imaging. *Radiology,* 173:723-729, 1989.

MRI is used to evaluate 43 patients having problems of the TFC and intrinsic and extrinsic ligaments of the wrist. The article suggests that MRI is an effective procedure in assessing patients with chronic wrist pain.

Ultrasonography

Hoglund M, Tordai P, Engkvist O: Ultrasonography for the diagnosis of soft-tissue conditions in the hand. *Scand J Plast Reconstr Hand Surg,* 25:225-231, 1991.

On evaluation of more than 100 patients, ultrasound is found to be of value to diagnose ganglions, tendon ruptures, synovitis, tumors, and the presence of foreign bodies. This article discusses the value of ultrasound when the combined expertise of hand surgeons and ultrasonographers is utilized.

8

Scaphoid Fractures

Jesse B. Jupiter, MD

Introduction

The scaphoid, functioning as a mechanical "tie-rod" linking the two carpal rows, will ordinarily concentrate stress in its waist, predisposing this locus to fracture during forced hyperextension.

Weber and Chao, in static loading experiments in fresh cadavers, produced relatively stable waist fractures with bending forces in a dorsal and ulnar direction to the distal pole. Fractures occurred only when the wrist was in 95° to 100° of extension and when the radial portion of the palm received the major load. They observed compressive forces dorsally and tension in the palmar capsule.

Scaphoid fractures secondary to a higher energy of injury may have associated injuries such as "greater arc" injuries within the carpus, including transscaphoid perilunate dislocations or scaphocapitate combined fractures. In addition, more proximal fractures, such as those involving the radial styloid or distal radius, should also alert the surgeon to the likelihood of a greater degree of associated soft-tissue and ligament injury within the carpus. The scaphoid fracture itself may involve the proximal pole, as the disrupted soft-tissue restraints will permit the proximal part of the bone to become wedged against the end of the radius during the forced hyperextension of injury.

In such cases of greater surrounding soft-tissue injury, the scaphoid fracture tends to be displaced into a flexed (humpback) position as a result of the intrinsic oblique loading of the trapezium and trapezoid, which impart both an axial compressive and flexion movement to the distal pole of the scaphoid. This tendency has now been demonstrated in experimental studies by both Smith and associates, and Viegas and associates. In addition, both studies observed that the reproducible scaphoid instability produced increased multiplanar motion at the fracture site with clinical implications both for fracture healing as well as for the later development of arthrosis.

The dorsally angulated or humpback position of the scaphoid was also demonstrated biomechanically to lead to progressive loss of wrist extension. Burgess observed a 24% loss of wrist extension with as little as a 5° increase in flexion of the scaphoid.

Vascular Supply

The unique blood supply of the scaphoid plays an important role in the outcome of injury. Taleisnik and Kelly identified three systems of extraosseous arteries entering the scaphoid from the radial artery. A laterovolar group of vessels was considered the most important source of intraosseous perfusion and was felt responsible for supplying the proximal two-thirds of the bone. Gelberman and Menon identified only two direct vascular leashes entering the scaphoid using indirect dissection techniques with latex injection of the arterial supply followed by debridement with sodium hypochlorite. These investigators suggested that the major blood supply came from branches of the radial artery entering the bone through foramina along the dorsal ridge, which supplied 70% to 80% of the scaphoid including the entire proximal pole. They noted a second group of vessels arising from the palmar and superficial palmar branches of the radial artery to enter the scaphoid in the region of its distal tubercle, perfusing the distal 20% to 30% of the bone. The incidence of observed osteonecrosis with scaphoid fracture being nearly 100% of those involving the proximal one-fifth and 33% of middle thirds is consistent with the nature of the arterial anatomy of the bone.

The location of these vascular leashes will also play a role in consideration of surgical approaches. Botte and associates suggested the palmar approach as least injurious to the important dorsal nutrient branches.

Diagnosis

Following injury, pain localized about the radial side of the wrist, particularly in the anatomic snuff box, must alert the physician to the possibility of a scaphoid fracture. Initial radiographs must have at least four views including a posteroanterior in neutral and ulnar deviation, a lateral, and an oblique view of the wrist. The contralateral wrist should be X-rayed if concern is raised regarding intercarpal alignment. With these radiographs, 98% of scaphoid fractures will be identified by radiologists or orthopaedic surgeons.

Snuff-box tenderness with a negative radiograph is treated by thumb spica splint or cast immobilization for seven to 10 days, followed by repeat examination and radiographs. If tenderness persists despite a negative radiograph, treatment should either be continued (immobilization for seven more days and re-evaluation) or further diagnostic studies should be obtained.

Radionuclide bone scan was shown initially by Ganel and associates in 49 suspected fractures to be accurate in identifying occult fractures with no false negatives. Subsequent studies have identified between a 6% to 16% incidence of false positives with radionuclide scanning. The MRI has perhaps replaced the scan in terms of accuracy, but the expense must be carefully considered.

When assessing a scaphoid fracture, a careful analysis of the lateral radiograph is important to identify the fracture pattern and radiographic signs of instability. Trispiral tomography or lateral axial computed tomography is vital if routine radiographs are difficult to interpret. The computed scans are currently expanding to three-dimensional projections, which may prove valuable for surgical preoperative planning.

Classification

A clear radiographic projection of a scaphoid fracture will allow the injury to be accurately classified. An accurate classification is important not only in management decisions but also in prognosis. Classifications have been developed based upon the intrinsic stability of the fracture as well as on the location and pattern of the injury.

The vast majority of scaphoid fractures (63% to 68%) are located in the scaphoid waist, with 16% to 28% in the proximal third, and 6% to 10% involving the distal third.

Cooney and colleagues have suggested that a stable fracture is one in which the cartilage envelope has not been fully disrupted, and the fracture remains within the bony substance, incompletely separating the two fracture components. In contrast, they note instability to be defined by displacement of the fragments by one millimeter or more as seen on any radiographic projection or angulation demonstrated by a scapholunate angle of greater than 60° and/or a radiolunate angle greater than 15°. In addition, the lateral intrascapular angulation should not exceed 25° ± 5°.

In 1960, Russe defined scaphoid fractures by their orientation as transverse, vertical oblique, or horizontal oblique with transverse fractures being 60% in his series, horizontal oblique 35%, and vertical oblique 5%. His vertical oblique pattern was considered unstable due to shearing forces at the fracture site (Fig. 8-1).

A second and more contemporary classification has been developed by Herbert, who distinguishes four basic types: acute stable, acute unstable, delayed union, and nonunion. Within each type, subdivisions further define the fractures of the tubercle, waist, proximal and distal poles, and fracture-dislocations as well as sclerotic or fibrous nonunions (Fig. 8-2). Herbert considered unstable fractures (Type B) to include distal oblique (B_1); mobile waist (B_2); proximal pole (B_3); fracture-dislocations (B_4); and comminuted and multiple fractures (B_5).

Problems associated with open reduction and internal fixation of unstable scaphoid fractures have included a poor position of the implant, poor alignment of the fracture, subsequent osteonecrosis, and delay in treatment.

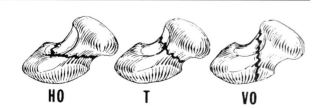

Figure 8-1. The classification system of Russe.

Delayed Union

For stable, aligned fractures seen late (three to six months after injury), some success has been noted with the use of pulsed electromagnetic field stimulation. This combined with a thumb spica cast has been reported to achieve an 80% union rate, although it is less effective for proximal pole fractures and is better used with a long arm thumb spica cast.

Nonunion

As previously noted, recent studies have convincingly demonstrated the association of untreated scaphoid nonunion and the later development of osteoarthritis. Mack and associates observed displacement of the nonunion and instability within the carpus to be major factors in the development of progressive arthritic changes. They also noted an increased incidence of displacement of the nonunion over time, noting the potential for nondisplaced nonunions to angulate and displace over time. Ruby and associates described a definite pattern of arthritic changes beginning at the scaphoid radial styloid joint and progressing to involve the scaphocapitate and capitolunate joints. Vender and associates similarly observed these intercarpal patterns with the end point representing the scapholunate advanced collapse wrist.

Just as with the scaphoid fracture, the scaphoid nonunion can be characterized as aligned, stable vs. displaced or unstable. As noted with delayed unions, there is some enthusiasm for the use of electromagnetic field stimulation; however, to date there has been no controlled patient series comparing immobilization alone with electromagnetic stimulation added to cast immobilization.

The stable aligned nonunion has been effectively treated by a Russe-type inlay corticocancellous bone graft with or without adjuvant internal fixation. Studies from a number of authors suggest union rates of 85% to 97% with this approach. Russe recommends removing of the avascular bone and fibrous tissue at the nonunion site and excavating a trough in the proximal and distal poles. Two corticocancellous struts are placed through a volar approach with the cancellous surfaces facing each other and the remainder of the cavity filled with cancellous bone (Fig. 8-3).

Supplemental fixation with Kirschner wires is recommended and reported by Stark and associates to have a 97% union rate. The K-wires are removed at six weeks and the thumb spica cast continued until union is achieved radiographically.

Avascular Necrosis

Although the presence of diminished vascularity in the proximal pole is not a contraindication to this approach, it does appear to influence outcome. Green reported a union rate with the Russe technique of 92% with good vascularity; 71% when the vascularity was fair; and 0% when bleeding was absent.

TYPE A:
STABLE ACUTE FRACTURES

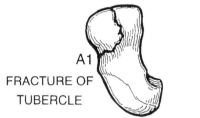

A1
FRACTURE OF
TUBERCLE

A2
INCOMPLETE FRACTURE
THROUGH WAIST

TYPE B:
UNSTABLE ACUTE FRACTURES

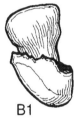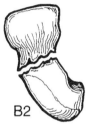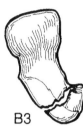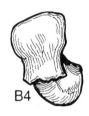

B1
DISTAL OBLIQUE
FRACTURE

B2
COMPLETE FRACTURE
OF WAIST

B3
PROXIMAL POLE
FRACTURE

B4
TRANS-SCAPHOID-
PERILUNATE
FRACTURE DISLOCATION
OF CARPUS

TYPE C:
DELAYED UNION

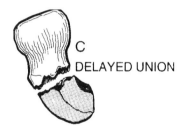

C
DELAYED UNION

TYPE D:
ESTABLISHED NONUNION

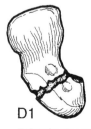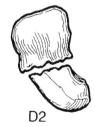

D1
FIBROUS UNION

D2
PSEUDARTHROSIS

Figure 8-2.   The classification system of Herbert.

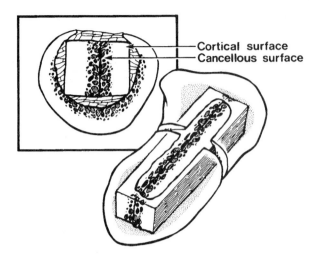

Figure 8-3. The Russe graft performed for a stable nonunion.

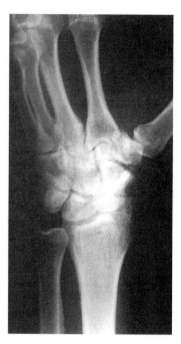

Figure 8-4. An unstable nonunion treated with an intercalated graft and Herbert screw.

It is recommended that the presence of avascular necrosis be confirmed preoperatively. MRI scanning is becoming more widely applied for this purpose and may well prove the most sensitive and specific both for preoperative assessment and postoperative control.

When faced with a completely avascular but stable proximal pole, several vascularized bone grafting procedures have been described. These include the pronator quadratus pedicle graft; a vascularized distal radius graft described by Zaidemberg and associates; or a vascularized bone graft based on the ulnar artery reported by Guimbeteau and Panconi. These vascularized pedicle procedures should be considered in the setting of a stable but longstanding nonunion, cystic degeneration of the scaphoid, or in a recalcitrant nonunion of the proximal pole.

Unstable/Displaced Nonunion

Displaced or unstable scaphoid nonunions are more difficult to treat to gain union. The existence of carpal instability due to an angulated unstable nonunion has become well accepted since the early work of Fisk. Therefore, the goals in treatment should be to restore scaphoid alignment, length, and intercarpal relationship, as well as to gain union.

Fisk designed a wedge-shaped graft to restore the scaphoid alignment. Fernandez modified this technique by resecting the entire nonunion, realigning the scaphoid, and filling the defect with a wedge or truncated wedge graft whose dimensions are based on preoperative plans. Fernandez initially used K-wires for internal fixation but later reported using conventional lag-screw fixation, with union rates of 100% and 95% respectively. A similar approach is reported by a number of authors using the Herbert screw (Fig. 8-4). Cooney and associates noted a lower union rate with a wedge graft and Herbert screw, with complications including incorrect placement of the screw and resorption of the bone graft. They recommend against this approach if there is complete osteonecrosis of the proximal pole.

The contemporary indications for realignment and interposition of an unstable or flexed (humpback) scaphoid nonunion include instability and motion at the nonunion site, cystic resorption at the nonunion, and loss of carpal height.

Malunion

It is becoming apparent that the late consequences identified with malaligned scaphoid nonunions may also be seen with scaphoid fractures that have united but with the flexed "humpback" deformity. Malunion has been identified by Amadio and associates. In a group of 26 patients with intrascaphoid angles greater than 35°, they observed an increased incidence of dorsal intercalary segment instability (DISI) deformity, carpal collapse, weakness of grip, and decreased wrist motion. Loss of carpal height correlated with pain and posttraumatic arthritis.

While the precise indications for corrective osteotomy of a scaphoid nonunion have yet to be established, the symptomatic patient should be counseled regarding the long-term implications of the malpositioned scaphoid and weigh them against possible osteotomy complications, such as nonunion or avascular necrosis.

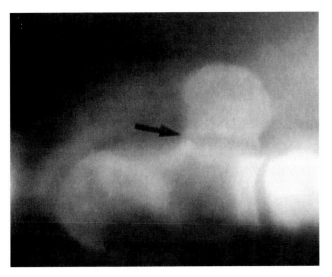

Figure 8-5. A longstanding scaphoid nonunion with scapholunate advanced collapse arthrosis in the wrist.

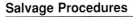

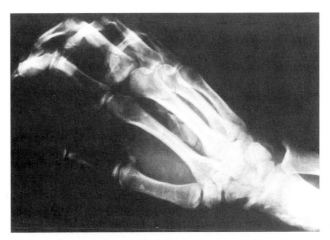

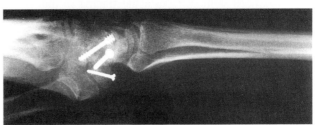

Figure 8-6. **(Top)** A complex fracture-dislocation of the carpus in a young woman with a scaphoid and capitate fracture. **(Bottom)** The scaphoid was fixed with 1.5mm and 2.0mm screws and the capitate with a Herbert screw.

Salvage Procedures

An untreated nonunion that has become associated with intercarpal arthrosis may no longer be suitable for attempts to gain union (Fig. 8-5). While a number of procedures have been reported, there are several that offer the potential for some functional gains.

Radial styloidectomy is technically straightforward and should be considered when arthrosis is localized to this region. This offers the possibility of preserving the existing motion in the wrist. If no intercarpal collapse is present and a small proximal pole nonunion has failed attempts at gaining union, some have recommended excision of the fragment and soft-tissue interposition. Complete scaphoid excision with a silicone replacement has been shown to be effective when combined with fusion of the capitate to the lunate. A proximal-row carpectomy may also preserve motion, although grip strength may be unpredictable. Ultimately, some patients who require a stable and pain-free wrist will be helped by a total wrist arthrodesis.

Capitate Fractures

Isolated fractures are rare. When associated with a scaphoid fracture (naviculocapitate syndrome), the head of the capitate and the proximal scaphoid may rotate together. Careful radiographic evaluation is necessary as the proximal capitate may rotate as much as 180° without a chance of uniting in that position. Avascular necrosis is a risk with these fractures as the blood supply is from an interosseous circulation from distal to proximal (Fig. 8-6).

Fractures of the Trapezium

Two types of fractures have been recognized. These include fractures of the trapezial ridge, which are usually the result of a direct blow, and trapezial body fractures, which are often due to more severe injuries. Ridge fractures, if at the tip (Type II), are generally treated by cast immobilization for three to six weeks. Fractures at the base of the ridge (Type I) may go on to nonunion.

Body fractures are usually intra-articular and require accurate reduction. Either traction alone or traction followed by internal fixation are required.

Pisiform Fractures

These may not be readily apparent and the diagnosis is suggested by local pain and a history of direct trauma. Tomography or CT scans may be required. Treatment is usually a short-arm cast in 30° of wrist flexion and some ulnar deviation. The pitfall in diagnosis is the presence of multiple ossification centers (a normal variant).

Fractures of the Hamate

Hamate body fractures are more likely to be associated with fourth or fifth carpometacarpal fracture-dislocation or with traumatic axial ulnar carpometacarpal dislocations.

Hamate hook fractures are more common but may more difficult to diagnose and are more likely to be seen in athletes. Deep pain with or without ulnar nerve symptoms should suggest the diagnosis. Carpal tunnel radiographic views or 45° supination oblique views demonstrate this area. Tomography more accurately demonstrates the extent of fracture or nonunion.

Excision has been the most recommended treatment, although some have advocated bone grafting with or without internal fixation to retain the pulley effect of the hamate hook on the flexor digitorum profundus with the wrist in ulnar deviation.

Lunate Fractures

Little has been written about acute trauma to the lunate, whereas Kienböck's disease has attracted widespread interest. Fracture has been attributed by some to Kienböck's dis-

ease, although most fractures described in the literature have been small fragments or osteochondral injuries.

Triquetral Fractures

Fractures of the triquetrum are the third most common carpal fracture. Since the triquetrum is encased by strong ligamentous attachments, fractures are often avulsion fragments, most commonly from the dorsal and ulnar aspect.

Compression fractures have been identified and felt secondary to either impaction by the ulnar styloid or with wrist hyperextension and ulnar deviation, forcing the hamate against the posterior projection of the triquetrum. Triquetral fractures may also be seen as part of "greater arc" injuries such as transtriquetral perilunate dislocations.

While isolated avulsion fractures are best treated with cast or splint support, fractures associated with perilunate dislocations are best treated with internal fixation in conjunction with realignment of the carpal architecture.

Annotated Bibliography

Amadio PC, Berquist TH, Smith DK: Scaphoid malunion. *J Hand Surg,* 14A:679-687, 1989.

Forty-five patients with 46 scaphoid fractures were studied more than six months after union using trispiral tomography. Increasing lateral scaphoid angulation, especially with the "humpback" deformity, was associated with progressively poor clinical and radiographic outcomes. The authors concluded that union alone is not a sufficient criterion for success in treating scaphoid fractures.

Beckenbaugh RD, et al: Kienböck's disease. The natural history of Kienböck's disease and consideration of lunate fractures. *Clin Orthop,* 149:98-106, 1980.

Forty-six patients with Kienböck's disease were evaluated over a two- to 27-year period; 72% had a history of wrist injury prior to diagnosis; 67% had evidence of fracture or fragmentation of the lunate. Documented fractures of the lunate were identified followed by both the presence and absence of subsequent Kienböck's disease; which may be explained by the variable bood supply of the lunate. Ten patients were not treated; 36 patients were treated surgically. Patients were relieved of pain and had functional wrists whether they were treated or not and regardless of the type of surgical treatment.

Bishop AT, Beckenbaugh RD: Fracture of the hamate hook. *J Hand Surg,* 13A:135-139, 1988.

Twenty-one cases of hamulus are presented. Diagnosis depends on clinical acuity. The most common symptom is pain in the palm that is aggravated by grasp. Weakness of grasp and dorsal wrist pain are also common. Ulnar nerve paresthesia or weakness and mild carpal tunnel syndrome are frequently present. Tenderness directly over the hamulus is always present, and grip strength typically is diminished. Tenosynovitis, tendon fraying, or tendon rupture may be demonstrated in 25% of the cases and is not related

to the use of steroids. Lateral trispiral tomography is superior to the other diagnostic methods. Excision produced generally excellent results, particularly in patients with an athletic injury or with no associated additional injury. A nonathletic injury or the presence of associated trauma adversely affected results. Immediate immobilization of acute fractures may result in fracture healing and obviate operative intervention. Open reduction and internal fixation is feasible but offers little advantage over excision.

Burgess RC: The effect of a simulated scaphoid malunion on wrist motion. *J Hand Surg,* 12A:774-776, 1987.

The effects of scaphoid malunion on wrist motion were simulated in a cadaveric study. It was found that the loss of wrist extension is proportional to the angular deformity. Loss of radiocarpal extension occurred at 15° of angulation and loss of midcarpal extension occurred at 30° of angulation.

Cooney WP III, Dobyns JH, Linscheid RL: Fractures of the scaphoid: a rational approach to management. *Clin Orthop Rel Res,* 149:90-97, 1980.

Fractures of the scaphoid can be classified into either undisplaced, stable fractures or displaced, unstable fractures by their roentgenographic appearance. When there is greater than 1mm of fracture offset or an instability collapse pattern (dorsal lunate rotation) on the lateral view, an unstable, displaced fracture is present. When doubt exists after reviewing routine films, special views should be obtained, such as radioulnar deviation stress views, traction oblique views, or trispiral tomography. In acute scaphoid fractures in which no displacement of the fracture fragments or lunate dorsal tilting can be seen, a short-arm thumb spica cast provides satisfactory support for fracture union. A wrist position of volar flexion-radial deviation is preferred to the more traditional positions of wrist extension with radial deviation or wrist extension with ulnar deviation with 100% union rate and no malunions. In displaced scaphoid fractures, a long-arm cast is recommended, with reduction of the fracture by wrist flexion and radial deviation. If accurate reduction is not obtained or is lost during the course of treatment, open reduction and internal fixation should be considered.

Fernandez DL: Anterior bone grafting and conventional lag screw fixation to treat scaphoid nonunions. *J Hand Surg,* 15A:140-147, l990.

The results of 20 established nonunions of the scaphoid treated with resection of the pseudarthrosis, anterior corticocancellous iliac bone grafting, and conventional lag screw fixation with the ASIF 2.7mm cortical screw are presented. The union rate was 95% and the average time off work was 8.9 weeks. Review of the relevant literature uniformly shows that the most common reasons for failure are improper internal fixation techniques and/or absence of bone grafting. Successful treatment of scaphoid nonunions with screw fixation and cast-free after-treatment does not depend on the implant used but rather on careful case selection and precise surgical technique.

Fleege MA, Jebson PJ, Renfrew DL: Pisiform fractures. *Skeletal Radiology,* 20:169-172, 1991.

Fractures of the pisiform are often missed due to improper radiographic evaluation and a tendency to focus on other, more obvious injuries. Delayed diagnosis may result in disabling sequelae. A high index of clinical suspicion and appropriate radiographic examination will establish the correct diagnosis. Ten patients with pisiform fracture are presented. The anatomy, mechanism of injury, clinical presentation, radiographic features, and evaluation of this injury are discussed.

Ganel A, Engel J, Oster Z, Farine I: Bone scanning in the assessment of fractures of the scaphoid. *J Hand Surg,* 4:540-543, 1979.

This study demonstrates the reliability of TC-99 bone scans in detecting a fresh scaphoid fracture. No false negative scans were noted. Bone scans may rule out the occult scaphoid fracture, thus limiting the duration of protective splint immobilization.

Gelberman RH, Menon J: The vascularity of the scaphoid bone. *J Hand Surg,* 5:508-513, 1980.

The extraosseous and intraosseous vascularity of the carpal scaphoid was studied in 15 fresh specimens by injection and clearing techniques. The major blood supply to the scaphoid is via the radial artery. Seventy to eighty percent of the intraosseous vascularity and the entire proximal pole are from branches of the radial artery entering through the dorsal ridge. Twenty to thirty percent of the bone in the region of the distal tuberosity receives its blood supply from volar radial artery branches. There is excellent collateral circulation to the scaphoid by way of the dorsal and volar branches of the anterior interosseous artery. An explanation for the cause of scaphoid necrosis on the bases of the vascular anatomy is proposed. The volar operative approach would be least traumatic to the proximal pole's blood supply.

Green DP: The effect of avascular necrosis on Russe bone grating for scaphoid nonunion. *J Hand Surg,* l0A:597-605, 1985.

This article reports a prospective study of 45 patients with nonunion of the scaphoid treated with Russe bone grafting. The operative procedure contains modifications in the technique made by Russe subsequent to his 1960 article. The results support Russe's contention that his operation is not likely to be successful if the proximal pole is avascular. Twenty-four of 26 patients (92%) with good vascularity in the proximal pole achieved solid union. In patients in whom the vascularity of the proximal pole was spotty or diminished, the rate of union dropped to 71% (10 of 14). Most important, none of the five patients in whom the proximal pole was totally avascular achieved successful union. True avascular necrosis is best determined by punctate bleeding points in cancellous bone found at operation, and cannot be accurately predicted by the appearance of preoperative radiographs.

Guimberteau JC, Panconi B: Recalcitrant nonunion of the scaphoid treated with a vascularized bone graft based on the ulnar artery. *J Bone Joint Surg,* 72A:88-94, 1990.

Eight patients with recurrent pseudoarthrosis of the carpal scaphoid were treated by a bone graft from the ulna and vascularized by an ulnar artery pedicle. The graft was taken from the medial aspect of the distal third of the ulna and inserted into the prepared scaphoid. This technique is advocated only for complex recalcitrant nonunion. In all eight patients, primary osseous union occurred in an average of 4.6 months; all were able to resume their previous occupational or athletic actvities.

Herbert TJ, Fischer WE: Management of the fractured scaphoid using a new bone screw. *J Bone Joint Surg,* 66B:114-123, 1984.

A technique has been developed to provide internal fixation for all types of fractures of the scaphoid. This involves the use of a double-headed bone screw. A classification of scaphoid fractures is proposed. The indications for operation include not only acute unstable fractures, but also fractures with delayed healing and those with established nonunion; screw fixation is combined with bone grafting to treat the nonunion. In a prospective trial, 158 operations using this technique were carried out between 1977 and 1981. The rate of union was 100% for acute fractures and 83% overall. This method of treatment appears to offer significant advantages over conventional techniques in the management of the fractured scaphoid.

Mack GR, Bosse MJ, Gelberman RH: The natural history of scaphoid nonunion. *J Bone Joint Surg,* 66A: 504-509, 1984.

Forty-seven nonunions of a fracture of the scaphoid in 46 symptomatic patients are reviewed in order to assess the incidence and severity of degenerative changes of the wrist. The duration of the nonunion ranges from five to 53 years. Three roentgenographic patterns are seen: 23 lesions had sclerosis, cyst formation, or resorptive changes confined to the scaphoid bone (Group I); 14 had radioscaphoid arthritis (Group II); and 10 had generalized arthritis of the wrist (Group III). The duration of Group I nonunions averaged 8.2 years; Group II, 17.0 years; and Group III nonunions, 31.6 years. Fracture displacement and carpal instability correlated with the severity of the degenerative changes. Lunate dorsiflexion of 10° or more was a useful guide to carpal instability. Few of the 47 nonunions were undisplaced, stable, or free of arthritis after 10 years. Based on the high probability of arthritis, it was recommended that all displaced ununited scaphoid fractures be reduced and grafted, regardless of symptoms, before degenerative changes occur. Asymptomatic patients with an undisplaced, stable nonunion should be advised of the possibility of later degenerative changes.

Rand JA, Linscheid RL, Dobyns JH: Capitate fractures. *Clin Orthop Rel Res,* 165:209-216, 1982.

Capitate fractures are serious carpal injuries that should be treated as aggressively as scaphoid fractures, with anatomic reduction obtained by open techniques, if necessary, and by immobilization until the fracture has united. Thus treated, even a capitate proximal pole free of soft-tissue attachments will heal. Anatomic reduction is required for restoration of carpal kinematics. Even with optimal treatment, some posttraumatic carpal arthrosis may be found with long-term follow-up investigations.

Ruby LK, Belsky MR: The natural history of scaphoid nonunion. A review of fifty-five cases. *J Bone Joint Surg,* 67A:428-432, 1985.

The authors reviewed the cases of 56 scaphoid nonunions in 55 patients, none of whom had received treatment of any kind prior to examination. In the 32 patients who had been injured five or more years earlier, arthritis developed in 31 (97%). The one patient in whom osteoarthritis developed less than four years after injury also had avascular necrosis of the scaphoid. The incidence of osteoarthritis increased with time after injury. They concluded that patients with established scaphoid nonunion should be advised that osteoarthritis will most likely develop.

Smith D, Cooney WP III, An K-N: The effects of simulated unstable scaphoid fracture on carpal motion. *J Hand Surg,* 14A:283-290, 1989.

The kinematics of five fresh frozen wrist specimens were studied before and after a simulated scaphoid wrist fracture. To determine change in wrist motion and fracture-site characteristics associated with an unstable wrist, the relative motion of each carpal bone was determined from the movement of implanted carpal markers on biplanar radiographs obtained in neutral and the four extreme wrist positions. The kinematics of the wrist in the specimens, before the osteotomy, were similar to previous studies. After the osteotomy, the proximal and distal segments of the scaphoid moved independently. The distal scaphoid assumed a relatively flexed stance and displayed increased motion. The proximal scaphoid fragment and lunate assumed a relatively extended stance and displayed less motion after the osteotomy. These kinematic abnormalities produced significant interfragmentary motion that would be expected to complicate normal fracture healing. The spontaneous collapse of the two scaphoid fragments produced a dorsal angulation or "humpback" deformity that simulated the clinical situation of displaced scaphoid nonunions. The scaphoid serves an important role in maintaining normal alignment of the carpal bones and producing normal wrist motion.

Stark HH; Richard TA, Zanel NP, Ashworth CR: Treatment of ununited fractures of the scaphoid by iliac bone grafts and Kirschner wire fixation. *J Bone Joint Surg,* 70A:982-991, 1988.

Of 151 ununited fractures of the scaphoid that were treated with iliac bone grafts and Kirschner wire fixation through a volar approach, all but four (97%) healed in an average of 17 weeks. Three of the four failures resulted from obvious technical errors. Neither the preoperative existence of necrosis of the proximal fragment nor the location of the fracture affected the results. When there was mild radiocarpal arthritis preoperatively, it did not pro-gress postoperatively; if there was moderate radiocarpal arthritis preoperatively, progression was seldom seen if a radial styloidectomy was done. Displaced and unstable ununited fractures healed even if the deformity was not corrected completely. The principal benefit of the procedure was relief of pain rather than an increase either in motion of the wrist or in strength of grip.

Teisen H, Hjarback J: Lunate fractures. *J Hand Surg,* 13B:458-462, 1988.

The radiographs of 17 patients with fresh fractures of the lunate bone have been reviewed. The fractures were classified according to their radiological appearances and according to the vascular anatomy of the lunate. A long-term radiographic follow-up examination was performed.

Vender M, Watson HK, Wiener BD: Degenerative change in symptomatic scaphoid nonunion. *J Hand Surg,* 12A:514-519, 1987.

A retrospectve radiographic analysis of 64 patients with symptomatic scaphoid nonunions without previous surgical treatment was accomplished. The results showed a high frequency of degenerative changes occurring in a predictable sequence. For nonunions of four years duration, 75% of patients had radioscaphoid changes, and for those of nine years duration, 60% had midcarpal changes. The pattern of arthritis in scaphoid nonunion is that of the scapholunate advanced collapse wrist resulting from rotary subluxation of the distal scaphoid fragment. The radius-proximal scaphoid fragment joint and the radiolunate joint were consistently spared from degenerative changes, even with severe arthritis. Instability was progressive and associated with an earlier onset of arthritis. Patients with symptomatic scaphoid nonunions appear to have a significant likelihood of arthritis developing.

Viegas SF, Patterson RM, Hillman GR: Simulated scaphoid proximal pole fracture. *J Hand Surg,* 16A:495-500, 1991.

Five fresh cadaver extremities were studied with the use of a static positioning frame, pressure-sensitive film, a microcomputer-based video digitizing system, and a Sun station image analysis system to assess the load-bearing characteristics of the scaphoid in the proximal carpal joint. Specimens were studied in their normal condition after a proximal-pole osteotomy of the scaphoid and after resection of the proximal pole of the scaphoid. The amount of contact area borne through the scaphoid fossa was essentially the same whether the scaphoid was intact, or after a simulated scaphoid fracture of its proximal-pole, or after resection of the proximal pole. The scaphoid contact area and pressure, although overall relatively constant, was redistributed after osteotomy, resulting in an increased contact area under the distal fragment and no change or a slight decrease in the contact area under the proximal fragment of the scaphoid. After resection of the proximal fragment, all scaphoid contact area and pressure was borne by the distal scaphoid fragment. The contact area and pressure characteristics of the lunate remained unchanged in all conditions compared with the normal condition. There were no significant changes in the locations of the centroids of the scaphoid segments and the lunate in any of the conditions tested.

Zaidemberg C, Siebert JW, Angrigani C: A new vascularized bone graft for scaphoid nonunion. *J Hand Surg,* 16A:474-8, 1991.

With the use of standard latex injection techniques with vascular filling of vessels to less than 0.1mm diameter in 10 fresh cadaver dissections, the authors discovered a consistently vascularized bone-graft source from the distal dorsoradial radius. They have used this vascularized bone-graft source with good results in 11 patients with long-standing nonunion of the scaphoid. It is technically easy and seemingly offers the advantages of a decreased period of immobilization and a higher union rate.

9

Avascular Necrosis of the Carpus

Andrew J. Weiland, MD

Introduction

The etiology of avascular necrosis of the carpal bones has yet to be established. Whether in any of the carpal bones, the avascularity is caused by a primarily ischemic event, a traumatic extraosseous vascular interruption, or a microfracture causing an intraosseous vascular interruption is still controversial. There are case reports to support all of these theories. A scaphoid fracture can cause avascular necrosis of the proximal pole of the scaphoid, and a perilunate dislocation can cause avascular necrosis of the lunate, and in these instances the cause of the avascularity is apparent and attributable to a single event. Whether repetitive microtrauma can produce similar results is still under investigation. The knowledge of the etiology of avascularity may lead to earlier diagnosis and treatment of avascular necrosis, and perhaps eventually prevention. Probably, the most recent addition to the understanding of avascular necrosis is magnetic resonance imaging, which can lead to earlier detection of osseous avascularity. Once avascular changes develop, treatment can be instituted to prevent the eventual changes of carpal collapse and arthrosis.

Avascular Necrosis of the Lunate

Etiology

Since the description of lunatomalacia by Kienböck in 1910 much has been written about the cause and treatment of Kienböck's disease. While it has been generally accepted that Kienböck's disease is caused by avascular necrosis of the lunate, whether the microfractures seen in Kienböck's disease are the cause or result of avascular necrosis remains controversial. There is literature to support both a primary ischemic as well as a primary traumatic etiology. Avascular necrosis of the lunate has been reported in diseases known for episodes of ischemia such as sickle-cell anemia. It has also been seen after traumatic disruption of the vascular supply to the lunate such as after scapholunate or intercarpal ligament ruptures, with resultant increased radiodensity of the bone. This situation, however, is usually transient and resolves. Other support for a primary traumatic etiology is that with the use of tomography, transverse fractures of the lunate have been described in 75% of Kienböck's disease. The fracture fragments can be displaced by the capitate, impeding primary healing of the fracture, leading to avascular necrosis.

Hulten demonstrated the association between ulnar negative wrists and Kienböck's disease, and postulated that this predisposed patients and certain individuals to develop avascular necrosis of the lunate. Theoretically, this anatomic variant may selectively overload the lunate at the ulnar border of the distal radius. Whether lack of ulnar support is a cause for traumatic avascular necrosis or a component that leads to collapse in lunates that are avascular has not been shown. Clearly there are patients who are ulnar negative and do not develop Kienböck's disease. Recently, even the presence of ulnar negativity has come into question as being a result of Kienböck's disease rather than a cause. Twenty-year, follow-up studies comparing radiographs at diagnosis to those at re-examination of patients treated conservatively for Kienböck's disease have shown subchondral bone formation in the lunate fossa of the radius. This subchondral bone leads to development of a "pseudo-ulnar negative" wrist, in patients whose wrists were initially ulnar neutral.

Recent studies have shown that the type of vascularity of the carpal bone may influence its susceptibility to avascularity. Twenty percent of lunates receive one nutrient vessel and are thus at higher risk for avascular necrosis from intraosseous disruption (microfracture) or minor extraosseous disruption (ligamentous injury). Eighty percent of lunates receive nutrient arteries from two non-articular surfaces and have intraosseous anastomoses, and are at decreased risk of avascular necrosis due to their rich vascular supply.

Current consensus on the etiology of Kienböck's disease is repetitive microtrauma occurring in a lunate at risk. The ulnar negative position of the wrist increases the selective overloading of the lunate, and lunates with a single nutrient vessel are at increased risk.

Diagnosis

The diagnosis of Kienböck's disease is suspected in the young adult (20 to 40 years of age) with pain and stiffness of the wrist, tenderness over the dorsal lunate, and decreased grip strength, but must be confirmed by radiographic changes. Often patients give a history of a recent hyperextension injury. It is important to obtain standardized posteroanterior radiographs to evaluate the lunate and the ulnar variance of the wrist. For the radiograph, the shoulder is abducted 90°, the elbow flexed 90°, the forearm placed in neutral rotation, and the wrist held in neutral flexion-extension. The classification of Kienböck's disease was described by Stahl and later modified by Lichtman and Weiss, and associates (Fig. 9-1). It is based on the radiographic appearance of the lunate, and dictates treatment. Stage 1 may have no radiographic changes or small fracture lines may be evident. Stage 2 demonstrates sclerosis of the bone, but the size, shape, and relationships of the bone are normal. Stage 3A is characterized by the collapse of the bony structure of the lunate, and 3B combines collapse with associated proximal migration of the capitate and fixed

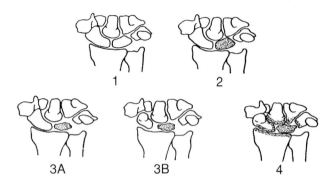

Figure 9-1. Radiographic classification of Kienböck's disease according to the method of Lichtman and associates, modified by Weiss and associates. Stage 1: no change visible in the lunate; Stage 2: sclerosis of the lunate; Stage 3A: sclerosis and fragmentation of the lunate; Stage 3B: Stage 3A with proximal migration of the capitate or fixed rotation of the scaphoid; Stage 4: Stage 3A or B combined with degenerative changes at adjacent intercarpal joints.

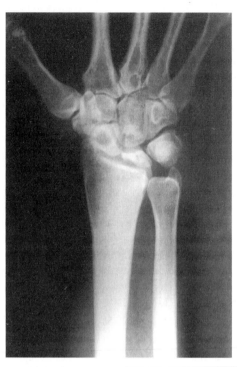

Figure 9-2. Stage 3B Kienböck's disease demonstrating collapse of the bony structure of the lunate with proximal migration of the capitate and fixed rotation of the scaphoid.

rotation of the scaphoid. (Fig. 9-2). Stage 4 demonstrates degenerative changes in the radiolunate and adjacent intercarpal articulations, with joint-space narrowing, osteophyte formation, and even degenerative cysts. Obviously, the prognosis is better for Stage 1 or 2 of the disease, which emphasizes the need for early diagnosis and treatment.

Magnetic resonance imaging has been helpful in the early diagnosis of Stage 1 Kienböck's disease. (Fig. 9-3). A decrease in signal on both T1 and T2 weighted images suggest avascular necrosis even in the setting of normal radiographs. MRI also demonstrates more specificity than radiography or bone scan in diagnosing ischemic necrosis. Loss of signal on T1 weighted images is diagnostic for ischemic necrosis. Normal or increased signal on T2 weighted images implies an earlier stage and a better prognosis. MRI may also be useful to evaluate the lunate for revascularization after operative intervention. (Fig. 9-4). Coronal computed tomography has been advocated for detection of early changes in the avascular lunate. Sclerosis, compression, and fractures of the lunate can be detected earlier by CT scan than by plain radiographs or tomograms.

Treatment

Kienböck's disease can be treated by immobilization, revascularization, ulnar shortening, radial lengthening, limited intercarpal fusion, lunate resection, silicone replacement arthroplasty, limited wrist fusion, and wrist arthrodesis. Initial treatment of Stage 1 Kienböck's disease should consist of immobilization and anti-inflammatory medication. Often, immobilization produces a relative osteopenia of the surrounding carpal bones and makes the sclerosis of the lunate more easily recognizable. If immobilization does not succeed in alleviating symptoms, then surgical intervention should be considered. Long-term results of non-operative treatment for Kienböck's disease have had poor results, with greater than 50% of patients having daily

symptoms because immobilization alone will not prevent the compressive forces across the lunate.

With failure of nonoperative treatment, it is necessary to proceed to surgical intervention. Revascularization with volar radial bone attached to a pronator quadratus flap, the second dorsal metacarpal artery, or a vascularized pisiform transfer have both been advocated. Long-term follow-up is not available, but early results are promising. However, both of these procedures are technically difficult.

Relief of the compressive forces on the lunate can be accomplished either proximally through joint-leveling procedures or distally through limited intercarpal arthrodeses. Capitohamate and scaphoid-trapezium-trapezoid fusions have been described as distally decompressive procedures but significantly reduce wrist range of motion. Joint-leveling procedures are aimed at decreasing the compressive forces on the lunate at the ulnar border of radius by increasing the structural support from the distal ulnar complex. Joint leveling is indicated in patients with ulna minus variant, maintenance of lunate architecture, and lack of arthrosis at the lunate articulations. It is aimed at halting the progession to collapse of the lunate. It can be accomplished by either lengthening the distal ulna or shortening the distal radius. STT fusions and radial and ulnar length-altering procedures of 2mm have been demonstrated to reduce lunate loading by strain gauge measurement. Capitohamate fusions are less effective in reducing lunate load. A two-

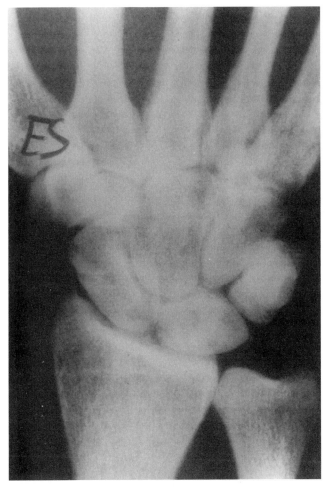

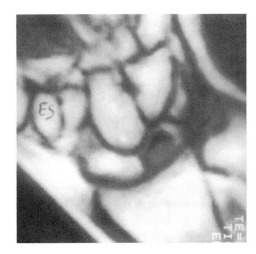

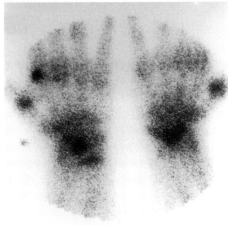

Figure 9-3.   (Left) Stage 1 Kienböck's disease. **(Top Right)** Diagnosed by MRI with decreased signal intensity in the lunate. **(Bottom Right)** Confirmation was made by bone scan. Note the patient has bilateral disease.

dimensional mathematical model of the wrist demonstrates force through the radiolunate articulation to be 30% of the total radioulnar-carpal load. This decreases 45% after a joint-leveling procedure of 4mm. In contrast, limited intercarpal fusions decrease radiolunate force by only 15%. While capitate shortening may decrease the radiolunate load, it significantly increases the load seen by the scapho-trapezial and triquetral-hamate articulations.

Joint-leveling procedures in patients with negative ulnar variance are useful in the early stages of Kienböck's disease including Stage 1-3A and possibly 3B. Shortening of the distal radius provides for pain relief, increased range of motion and grip strength of 30% to 50%, but does not change the radiographic appearance of the lunate. (Fig. 9-5). Continued carpal collapse or disease progression can be expected not to progress. The most important factor affecting outcome after radial shortening may be the age of the patient, as those patients under 30 have significantly improved results. Usually no changes are seen at the distal

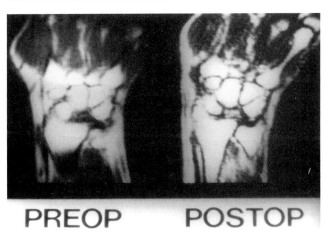

PREOP   POSTOP

Figure 9-4.   MRI demonstrating increased signal intensity in the lunate signifying revascularization after radial shortening.

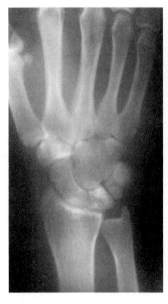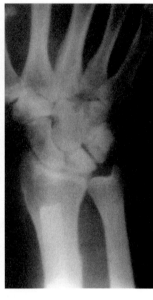

Figure 9-5. **(Left)** Stage 2 Kienböck's disease in a patient with negative ulnar variance. **(Right)** Treated with radial shortening, the patient regained almost full range of motion of her wrist.

radioulnar joint secondary to the 2mm to 3mm of radial shortening, but excessive radial shortening may lead to ulnar-sided wrist pain. Ulnar lengthening produces similar results to radial shortening, but the incidence of nonunion is higher.

By the time patients reach Stage 4, bony changes and disruption of the articular anatomy are present, and revascularization no longer yields a painless radiolunate joint. It is in these patients that a more radical procedure must be performed, including excision of the lunate, proximal-row carpectomy, or wrist arthrodesis. Lunate excision with or without palmaris longus tendon insertion, although initially popular, has been shown to lead to carpal collapse. Rearrangement of the remaining carpal bones may provide a satisfactory result, with ability to perform activities of daily living in 50% of patients. Lunate silicone replacement has yielded poor five-year results. Eighty percent of patients have less than satisfactory results, with dislocation of the prosthesis or silicone synovitis. Limited arthrodeses of the wrist have been described with the stated advantage that some wrist motion can be preserved, but the long-term efficacy of these procedures has yet to be established. With proximal-row carpectomy, some wrist mobility can also be preserved and is indicated in the older patient in whom immobilization is undesirable. It is contraindicated in the

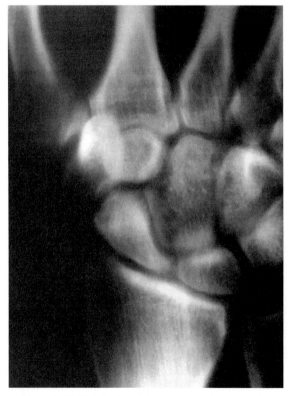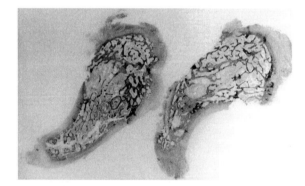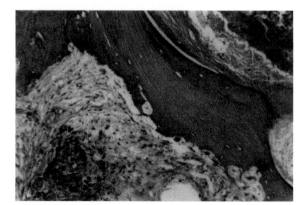

Figure 9-6. **(Left)** Plain radiographs demonstrating avascular necrosis of the scaphoid. **(Top Right)** Histologic section of the excised scaphoid, demonstrating necrosis. **(Bottom Right)** High-power view demonstrating empty lacunae and fibrosis of the marrow.

presence of radiocarpal or proximal capitate arthrosis. The procedure of choice for Stage 4 disease is radiocarpal arthrodesis.

Avascular Necrosis of the Scaphoid and Capitate

Avascular necrosis of the scaphoid occurring in the absence of fracture or trauma is rare. In 1910, Preiser, with whose name this disease has become associated, described five patients with avascular necrosis of the scaphoid without radiographic evidence of scaphoid fracture. The scaphoid is at risk of avascular necrosis because 70% to 80% of the scaphoid, including the proximal pole, is supplied by a single dorsal blood supply without a rich anastomotic system. Whether the ischemic event is intraosseous or extraosseous, the result is the same. The diagnosis is made based on radiographic evidence of sclerosis and fragmentation of the proximal pole of the scaphoid, without evidence of fracture. (Fig. 9-6). Literature on this subject is confusing, as some studies include avascular necrosis following malunion of scaphoid fractures; also most of the literature is based on case reports. The average age of onset of Prieser's disease is 40 years, and most patients have a history of steroid use, remote trauma, or a job requiring repetitive wrist motion.

Patients present with dorsal wrist pain, worsened with activity.

Examination reveals dorsal soft-tissue swelling, tenderness over the scaphoid, and decreased range of motion of the wrist. Radiographs reveal increased density of the scaphoid with possible cystic degeneration and radioscaphoid arthritis. Initial treatment should include immobilization, which is successful in 20% of patients. With failure of immobilization, surgical intervention must be entertained. This can range from arthroscopic drilling of the scaphoid, revascularization procedures, and scaphoid resection with four-quadrant fusion, proximal-row carpectomy, and wrist fusion. Surgery is effective in relieving pain, but does not increase range of motion.

Avascular necrosis of the capitate has been visualized by MRI and documented by case report only. Patients usually complain of pain and stiffness of the wrist, often with crepitation over the capitate. Radiographs usually demonstrate avascular changes of the proximal pole of the capitate. Initial treatment should be conservative with immobilization, which has had some success. If symptoms persist, surgical intervention may be necessary, with partial capitate excision with tendon interpositional arthroplasty having good early results.

Annotated Bibliography

Etiology and Diagnosis

Bourne MH, Linscheid RL, Dobyns JH: Concomitant scapholunate dissociation and Kienböck's disease. *J Hand Surg,* 16A:460-464, 1991.

Six patients had scapholunate dissociation documented radiographically before the onset of Kienböck's disease. Five of the six attributed the wrist pain to a single traumatic event, suggesting a traumatic etiology to lunate avascular necrosis.

Chen WS, Shih CH: Ulnar variance and Kienböck's disease: an investigation in Taiwan. *Clin Orthop,* 255:124-127, 1990.

Corroborates Hulten's hypothesis of the association of negative ulnar variance and Kienböck's disease. One thousand normal Taiwanese subjects had an ulnar variance of 0.313 with only 6% greater than -2.0, compared with 18 patients with Kienböck's disease who had an ulnar variance of -1.22 with 55.6% greater than -2.0.

Friedman L, Yong-Hing K, Johnston, GH: The use of coronal computed tomography in the evaluation of Kienböck's disease. *Clin Radiol,* 44: 56-59, 1991.

Twelve patients with Kienböck's disease were examined with CT scan, plain films, and tomograms. CT scan was more sensitive in demonstrating structural changes including sclerosis, fractures, and compression of the lunate, thus leading to earlier detection.

Gelberman RH, Gross MS: The vascularity of the wrist: identification of arterial patterns at risk. *Clin Orthop,* 202:40-49, 1986.

The carpal vascular anatomy was studied and classified in 75 cadaver limbs. Eight percent of the lunates were noted to have either vessels entering only one surface or large areas of bone dependent on a single vessel, whereas 92% of lunates had a rich intraosseous anastomotic vasculature. A single-vessel vascular pattern is hypothesized to predispose certain lunates to avascular necrosis.

Kristensen SS, Thomassen E, Christensen F: Ulnar variance in Kienböck's disease. *J Hand Surg,* 11B: 258-260, 1986.

Forty-seven wrists with Kienböck's treated with immobilization were re-examined after 20 years. In eight patients, subchondral bone formation in the lunate fossa enhanced the ulnar-negative value of the wrist. Eliminating these patients, no difference in ulnar negativity was found between patients with and without Kienböck's disease.

Lanzer W, Szabo R, Gelberman R: Avascular necrosis of the lunate and sickle cell anemia: a case report. *Clin Orthop,* 187:168-171, 1984.

A case of avascular necrosis of the lunate is reported in a patient with a disease known to cause infarction without a history of trauma. This supports the theory of a primary vascular interruption in the etiology of Kienböck's disease.

Nakamura R, Imaeda T, Suzuki K, Miura T: Sports related Kienböck's disease. *Am J Sports Med,* 19:88-91, 1991.

Ten patients actively involved in sports developed Kienböck's disease after repetitive minimal trauma. This supports the theory of a traumatic etiology to avascular necrosis of the lunate.

Sowa DT, Holder LE, Patt PG, Weiland AJ: Application of magnetic resonance imaging to ischemic necrosis of the lunate. *J Hand Surg,* 14A:1008-1016, 1989.

Twenty-two patients were studied prospectively with radiography, MRI, and bone scan. MRI showed more specificity than radiography or bone scan in diagnosing ischemic necrosis. Focal signal loss on the radial half of the lunate suggested early involvement, and normal or increased signal on the T2 weighted image implied an earlier stage and better prognosis.

Trumble TE, Irving J: Histologic and magnetic resonance imaging correlations in Kienböck's disease. *J Hand Surg,* 15:879-884, 1990.

Six patients with Kienböck's disease diagnosed by MRI, four of whom had radiographic changes, had biopsy specimens demonstrating avascular necrosis of the lunate. This confirms by histopathology the diagnosis of Kienböck's disease in patients with changes seen only on MRI.

White RE Jr, Omer GE Jr: Transient vascular compromise of the lunate after fracture-dislocation or dislocation of the carpus. *J Hand Surg,* 9A:181-184, 1984.

Transient vascular compromise of the lunate is described in three patients with perilunate or lunate dislocations. These cases did not progress to Kienböck's disease, and this argues against a single traumatic etiology for avascular necrosis.

Treatment

Alexander AH, Turner MA, Alexander CE, Lichtman DM: Lunate silicone replacement arthroplasty in Kienböck's disease: a long-term follow-up study.
J Hand Surg, 15A:401-407, 1990.

A five-year follow-up of 10 patients with lunate silicone replacement arthroplasty is discussed. Fifty percent of patients had unsatisfactory results, and the use of lunate silicone replacement arthroplasty is discouraged.

Almquist EE, Burns JF Jr: Radial shortening for the treatment of Kienböck's disease—a 5 to 10 year follow-up. *J Hand Surg,* 4A:348-352, 1982.

Retrospective study of 12 patients with Stage 2 to 3B Kienböck's disease treated with radial shortening. Eleven were satisfied with their treatment at five to 10 years, and returned to their normal activities, though none were relieved of discomfort. No limitations of forearm rotation were noted.

Armistead RB, Linscheid RL, Dobyns JH, Beckenbaugh RD: Ulnar lengthening in the treatment of Kienböck's disease. *J Bone Joint Surg,* 64A:170-178, 1982.

Twenty patients with Stage 2 through 3B Kienböck's disease were followed for 37 months after ulnar lengthening procedures. Ninety percent of patients were satisfied with their result and returned to work; 10% had persistent pain and were unable to return to their previous occupations; 15% percent of patients developed nonunion at the ulnar osteotomy site.

Horii E, Garcia-Elias M, Bishop AT, Cooney WP, Linscheid RL, Chao EY: Effect on force transmission across the carpus in procedures used to treat Kienböck's disease. *J Hand Surg,* 15A:393-400, 1990.

A two-dimensional mathematical model was used to evaluate the effect of force transmission across the carpus in procedures used to treat Kienböck's disease. A 4mm lengthening of the distal ulna was found to reduce radiolunate load by 45%, in contrast to limited intercarpal fusions, which reduced radiolunate load by only 15%. Joint-leveling procedures were shown to almost double the ulno-triquetral joint load, though this is still less than half the value of the normal radiolunate load.

Kato H, Usui M, Minami A: Long-term results of Kienböck's disease treated by excisional arthroplasty with a silicone implant or coiled palmaris longus tendon. *J Hand Surg,* 11A:645-653, 1986.

Thirty-two patients who underwent excisional lunate arthroplasty with silicone implant or coiled palmaris tendon were reviewed at an average of six years. Replacement of the lunate by the palmaris tendon is not recommended because of the progression of carpal collapse. Clinical results were not favorable with silicone replacement arthroplasty in the advanced stages of carpal collapse, although with early collapse results were more favorable.

Kawaii H, Yamamoto K, Yamamoto T, Tada K, Kaga K: Excision of the lunate in Kienböck's disease: results after long-term follow-up. *J Bone Joint Surg,* 70B: 287-292, 1988.

Fourteen patients with Stage 3 Kienböck's disease were followed for 12 years after excision of the lunate. At long-term follow-up, 50% of patients had no pain, with the remainder having mild or severe pain. Carpal collapse developed, but with rearrangement of the carpal bones, range of motion of the wrist was preserved. This offers an alternative treatment for older patients in whom heavy manual work is not necessary. In a younger, more active patient, secondary degenerative changes are more likely to result.

Mikkelsen SS, Gelineck J: Poor function after nonoperative treatment of Kienböck's disease. *Acta Orthop Scand,* 58:241-243, 1987.

Eight year follow-up of 25 wrists with Kienböck's disease treated with immobilization alone revealed that only 20% were pain free, and almost all patients had daily problems.

Nakamura R, Horii E, Iamaeda T: Excessive radial shortening in Kienböck's disease. *J Hand Surg,* 15B:46-48, 1990.

Two patients are presented with the development of ulnar-sided wrist pain after radial shortening of 5mm and 8mm. In both cases ulnar shortening was performed to level the joint and the ulnar-sided wrist pain resolved. Radial shortening of 2mm is recommended and shortening of greater than 4mm is not advised.

Nakamura R, Imaeda T, Miura T: Radial shortening for Kienböck's disease: factors affecting the operative result. *J Hand Surg,* 15B:40-45, 1990.

Factors affecting results after radial shortening for Kienböck's disease in 23 patients over an average of five years were examined. Age was found to be the most important factor, with patients more than 30 years of age obtaining unsatisfactory results. Additionally, radial shortening of greater than 4mm was associated with a poorer outcome. The clinical stage and ulnar variance did not seem to affect the end result.

Trumble T, Glisson RR, Seaber AV, Urbaniak JR: A biomechanical comparison of the methods for treating Kienböck's disease. *J Hand Surg,* 11A:88-93, 1986.

Axially loaded whole-arm specimens fitted with strain gauges were used to evaluate the effect of joint-leveling procedures and intercarpal arthrodeses on lunate compression. Joint-leveling procedures and STT fusions were effective in relieving lunate loads, while capitohamate fusions were ineffective. STT fusions significantly decreased wrist range of motion. With joint-leveling procedures, 90% of the reduction in strain takes place in the first 2mm of length change.

Watson HK, Ryu J, Dibella A: An approach to Kienböck's disease: triscaphe arthrodesis. *J Hand Surg,* 10A:179-187, 1985.

Sixteen patients were followed for an average of 20 months. Eight of the 16 had triscaphe arthrodesis; eight had triscaphe arthrodesis with a lunate silicone arthroplasty. Triscaphe arthrodesis resulted in a 143% increase in extension and a 120% increase in flexion from preoperative value. Ten of the 16 patients had complete pain relief.

Weiss AP, Weiland AJ, Moore JR, Wilgis EF: Radial shortening for Kienböck disease. *J Bone Joint Surg,* 73A:384-391, 1991.

Thirty wrists with Stage 1 to 3B Kienböck's disease were treated with radial shortening and evaluated at an average of 3.8 years. Extension was found to increase 32% and flexion 27% from preoperative values. Seventy percent of wrists had no pain at follow-up, and another 17% of patients had decreased pain.

Avascular Necrosis of the Scaphoid

Ferlic DC, Morin P: Idiopathic avascular necrosis of the scaphoid: Preiser's disease? *J Hand Surg,* 14A: 13-16, 1989.

Attention is brought to Preiser's series of avascular necrosis of the scaphoid in which significant trauma occurred and may have represented scaphoid fractures not detected on the poor quality radiographs of 1910. The distinction is made between avascular necrosis of the scaphoid with and without significant trauma. Five cases of Preiser's disease in four patients are presented, all without significant history of trauma; four of the five cases were associated with carpal tunnel syndrome.

Riley LH, Moore JR, Weiland AJ: Preiser's disease: a report of ten cases. Presented at the 45th Annual Meeting of the American Society for Surgery of the Hand in Toronto, Ontario, Canada. September 24, 1990.

The largest series to date of Preiser's disease in the literature. Eight of 10 patients failed conservative therapy, five patients had proximal row carpectomy and scaphoid excision, four had quadrant fusion, and one patient had failure of capitolunate fusion after scaphoid excision requiring wrist arthrodesis. No significant increase in wrist range of motion occurred following surgical intervention.

Viegas SF: Arthroscopic treatment of osteochondritis dissecans of the scaphoid. *Arthroscopy,* 4:278-281, 1988.

Avascular necrosis of the scaphoid was treated with arthroscopic drilling of the lesion and preliminary results at nine months, demonstrating dramatic relief of symptoms. Long-term results are not available.

Avascular Necrosis of the Capitate

Kimmel RB, O'Brien ET: Surgical treatment of avascular necrosis of the proximal pole of the capitate—a case report. *J Hand Surg,* 7A:284-286, 1982.

One case of avascular necrosis of the proximal pole of the capitate in a patient with a history of repetitive activity was treated surgically with proximal-pole excision and palmaris longus interpositional arthroplasty. Early results are good at 10 months postoperatively.

Rahme H: Idiopathic avascular necrosis of the capitate bone case report. *Hand,* 15:274-275, 1983.

A case of avascular necrosis of the capitate in an ice-hockey player without a history of antecedent trauma was discussed. The patient was treated conservatively and symptoms resolved so that he was able to resume work.

10

Carpal Instabilities

Steven F. Viegas, MD

Introduction

Gilford, Bolton, and Lambrinudi are attributed with the first reference to carpal instability. Fisk used the term in reference to scaphoid fractures during his Hunterian lecture of 1968. He called the zigzag alignment of the radius and carpal bones resulting from fractures of the scaphoid a "concertina" deformity.

In 1972 and 1975, Dobyns, Linscheid, and collaborators published articles on the topic of traumatic instability of the wrist. Their classification is based primarily on the capitolunate angle in the lateral radiograph. This work offered a means to group and identify different categories of carpal instabilities. These included dorsiflexion instability, palmar flexion instability, ulnar translocation, and dorsal subluxation. It is from these papers that the terms "dorsal intercalated segment instability" or DISI, "volar intercalated segment instability" or VISI, ulnar translocation, and dorsal subluxation originated. It is arguably this body of work that has launched an ever-increasing number of presentations and publications on carpal instabilities. In 1980, Taleisnik suggested expanding the classification system to include static and dynamic forms of instability.

In 1987, Dobyns, Linscheid, and colleagues and again in 1990, Cooney, Dobyns, and Linscheid proposed to further expand and adapt their classification to include the terms carpal instability dissociative and carpal instability nondissociative lesions. These classifications, which are based upon whether or not there is a disruption within or between the carpal bones of the proximal and/or distal row, complement their earlier approach which dealt only with the capitate-lunate-radius alignment.

Terms

Several terms will be defined as used in this section and as described in the literature. This discussion will use the term "dynamic" as follows: there is or would be no evidence of abnormal carpal alignment in the standard AP and lateral radiographs; there is evidence of abnormal carpal alignment in standard AP and lateral radiographs with stress exerted by the patient or by someone else; and/or there is evidence of abnormal carpal alignment in positions other than that assumed by the wrist in standard AP and lateral radiographs. The term "static" is used to address what would be an abnormal carpal alignment in the position assumed by the wrist in standard AP and lateral radiographs.

The term "DISI" is used to describe the following carpal alignment on a standard lateral radiograph: the lunate in an abnormally subluxated palmar and extended posture and the capitate in a position in which the proximal pole is sublux-

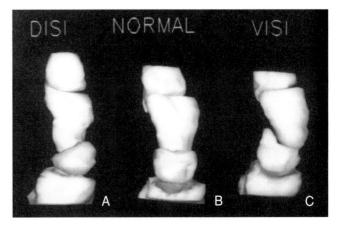

Figure 10-1. A lateral view of a 3-D reconstruction of a CT scan of a wrist with **(A)** a DISI deformity demonstrating the extended posture of the lunate and the flexed posture of the capitate, **(B)** a normal wrist, and **(C)** a wrist with a VISI instability demonstrating the flexed posture of the lunate and the extended posture of the capitate.

ated dorsal to the radiometacarpal axis, with the longitudinal axis of the capitate running from proximal dorsal to palmar distal in the lateral plane (Fig. 10-1).

The term "VISI" will be used to describe the following carpal alignment on a standard lateral radiograph: the lunate in an abnormally subluxated dorsal and flexed posture and the capitate in a position in which the proximal pole is subluxated palmar to the radiometacarpal axis, with the longitudinal axis of the capitate running from proximal palmar to dorsal distal in the lateral plane (Fig. 10-1).

A carpal instability dissociative lesion is caused by the loss of the interosseous ligaments between the individual bones of the carpal rows, resulting in dissociative rather than the normal associative motion between the bones of each row.

A "carpal instability nondissociative lesion" is one in which the normal associative motion between the bones of each carpal row remains intact and the dissociation is between rows, rather than within a row or rows (Fig. 10-2).

An Anatomical Approach Classification

In 1921, Navarro described the carpus as comprised of three vertical columns consisting of the trapezium, trapezoid, and scaphoid in the lateral column, the hamate, capitate, and lunate in the central column, and the triquetrum in the medial column (Fig. 10-3a). Taleisnik modified this

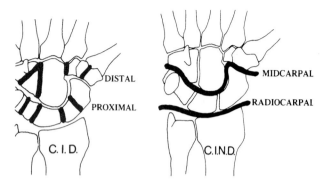

Figure 10-2. Classification of carpal instability. **(Left)** Carpal instability dissociative (CID) is characterized by fractures or ligament tears within the proximal and/or distal carpal row. **(Right)** Carpal instability nondissociative (CIND) is characterized by a ligamentous disruption within the midcarpal joint level and/or within the radial carpal level.

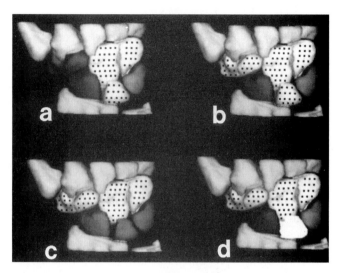

Figure 10-3. The carpus has been explained over the years as being composed of different functional or kinematic units. **(a)** Navarro described the columnar concept of the carpus in 1921. **(b)** Taleisnik modified this concept in 1976. **(c)** Lichtman presented his "ring" model of the carpus. **(d)** More recent kinematic and anatomic studies suggest a model composed of the distal carpal row as one unit and the scaphoid, lunate, and triquetrum of the proximal carpal row acting as separate units.

concept in 1976 to include the trapezium and trapezoid in the central column (Fig. 10-3b). He proposed that both dynamic and static instabilities could be further classified as lateral, medial, or proximal instabilities. Lichtman subsequently proposed "the ring concept," suggesting that the carpus was better represented by a ring model of carpal kinematics in which the distal carpal row and proximal carpal row are connected by a radial link and an ulnar link (Fig. 10-3c). Studies on carpal kinematics and load biomechanics of the carpus suggest that anatomically and functionally, the bones of the distal carpal row are rather tightly bound to each other and act as a single unit, while the bones of the proximal carpal row are much less constrained and act functionally as three individual, although interconnected, units (Fig. 10-3d).

DISI

Scapholunate Dissociation

A number of different lesions have been reported to result in a DISI deformity. The most commonly discussed is that resulting from a ligamentous disruption that includes a disruption between the scaphoid and lunate. This carpal instability pattern has been well described regarding its particular radiologic features (Fig. 10-4), which include the following:

A scapholunate gap: the intercarpal distance between the scaphoid and lunate on the AP radiograph is increased, compared to the other intercarpal spacing. A scapholunate gap greater than 3mm is considered diagnostic of a scapholunate dissociation. This scaphoid gap has been called the "Terry Thomas" sign after the famous English film comedian's dental diastema. This increase in the scapholunate intercarpal distance is noticeable, both in biomechanical and clinical studies in the AP supinated clenched-fist radiographic view.

A shortened scaphoid: the scaphoid assumes a flexed posture as a result of its dissociation from the surrounding

carpus and assumes a shorter appearance on the PA and AP radiographic views.

The cortical ring sign: the flexed posture of the scaphoid results in an end-on view of the scaphoid tubercle/distal scaphoid, which results in this more prominently visualized, circular cortex of the scaphoid.

A DISI pattern of the carpus: the scaphoid assumes a flexed and dorsally subluxated posture, the lunate assumes an extended and volar subluxated posture, and the capitate lies in a flexed posture.

Taleisnik's "V" sign: the intersection of the volar edge of the scaphoid outline when the scaphoid is flexed intersects with the volar margin of the radius at a more acute angle than the normal wrist in which there is a more gentle or wide C-shaped pattern of intersection.

Although ligamentous destabilization of the scaphoid had been discussed previously, Mayfield and associates brought considerable attention and knowledge to the understanding of increasing radial-sided perilunate instability through cadaver studies. In all stages of instability, he found disruption of the scapholunate interosseous ligament.

Perilunate/Lunate Dislocation

Mayfield and associates have demonstrated and described how progressive ligament disruption can result in a dorsal perilunate dislocation and further disruption can result in a volar lunate dislocation. In 1980, Mayfield described the sequential pattern of ligament failure in the wrist. Progressive perilunate instability was classified into four

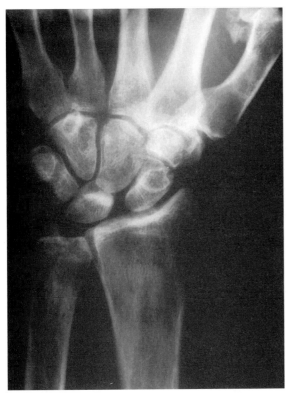

stages. Stage I was scapholunate instability. In Stages II and III, the capitate and triquetrum are progressively peeled away from the lunate. Stage IV is disruption of the dorsal radiocarpal ligament with lunate dislocation. They concluded that the palmar lunate dislocation (Stage IV) represented a more severe stage of disruption than the dorsal perilunate dislocation (Stage II or III) (Fig. 10-5).

Minami, Takahara, and Suzuki compared open scapholunate interosseous ligament repair and reconstruction in patients with lunate and perilunate dislocations in patients with lunate and perilunate dislocations who did not have the SLIL ligament repaired or reconstructed. Their recent clinical and roentgenographic results suggest that repair or reconstruction of the SLIL during open reduction can prevent or reduce the occurrence of carpal instability and improve clinical results.

Recent work by Berger and associates has detailed the differences in the various portions of the SLIO ligament complex, de-emphasizing the importance of the proximal membranous portion of the SLIO ligament as a stabilizing structure on both histologic and mechanical grounds. This membranous portion of the SLIO ligament complex is commonly found to be disrupted in cadaver dissections, while the dorsal segment of the SLIO ligament is not commonly disrupted although it can be found to be attenuated.

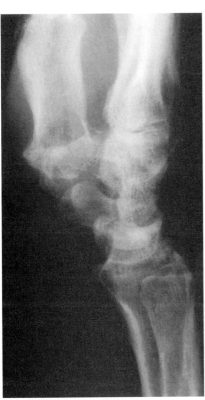

Figure 10-4. **(Top)** An AP and **(Bottom)** lateral radiograph of a scapholunate dissociation with dorsal intercalated segment instability.

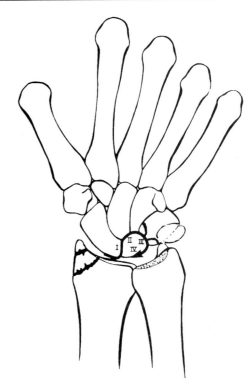

Figure 10-5. A diagram illustrating the four stages of progressive perilunate disruption/instability and the avulsion fractures of the radial styloid and triquetrum that can be associated with these injuries.

In the early stages of Mayfield's classification, the scaphoid is destabilized while the lunate remains, relatively speaking, better supported. In this situation, as Blevens and associates have described, the load mechanics are altered and the lunate load is increased, while the scaphoid load is decreased. With progressive disruption, the lunate also becomes unstable positioning in a palmar-subluxed, extended position with its narrower dorsal lip under the capitate and the load is distributed primarily through the scaphoid, as Viegas and associates reported. Kinematic studies have demonstrated that in a static DISI deformity, the scaphoid essentially maintains a flexed posture, while the lunate remains primarily extended.

SLAC

Watson and associates have described the progressive degenerative changes which they explain as the natural history of chronic scapholunate dissociation and call it scapholunate advanced collapse. These progressive degenerative changes occur first between the radial styloid and the scaphoid, next within the entire radioscaphoid articulation, and then between the lunate and the capitate (Fig. 10-6).

In an attempt to prevent this kind of degenerative arthritis, a number of treatment methods have been described. Dobyns and associates described a method of ligament reconstruction which they later abandoned due to the unpredictability of the procedure. Subsequently, limited fusions became a common method of treatment. Watson popularized the scaphoid-trapezium-trapezoid fusion, the effectiveness of which has been questioned recently, both biomechanically and clinically. Rotman and associates have documented successful treatment of scapholunate dissociation with scapholunate-capitate fusion. Other types of limited carpal fusions have also been utilized to treat scapholunate dissociation. More recently, different types of ligament reconstructions have been reconsidered. Currently there is an increased interest in direct primary repair of the disrupted ligaments. Lavernia and associates reported good results with early and delayed repair of the scapholunate interosseous ligament. Occasionally, they will augment their repair with a capsulodesis as described by Blatt.

Scaphoid Fracture/Malunion/ Nonunion

Other types of pathology that have been demonstrated to result indirectly in a DISI deformity are scaphoid fracture, malunion, or nonunion, and malalignment of the distal radius. These forms of DISI result from bone deformity and/or loss. In scaphoid nonunion, the distal portion of the scaphoid flexes, while the proximal portion of the scaphoid extends, along with the lunate (Fig. 10-7). Nakamura and associates have shown in a series of cases that correction of the nonunion and scaphoid alignment will correct the DISI. The carpal malalignment results from the deformity within the scaphoid, i.e. between its fracture fragments and not from ligament disruption. It remains possible, however, to have a patient with coincidental scaphoid fracture and scapholunate dissocation.

Distal Radius Fracture/Malunion

Malunion of the distal radius can also result in a DISI deformity (Fig. 10-8). Again, the correction of the bone malalignment will correct the carpal instability pattern. Remember that a concomitant distal radius fracture and a ligamentous disruption can occur with either and/or both contributing to the DISI deformity.

Kienböck's

Some cases of Keinböck's disease have been shown to have an associated DISI deformity. In these situations, DISI is usually seen in the more advanced stages of Keinböck's disease and is most likely due to a torsional deformity within the deformed and fragmented lunate.

VISI

There is a relative paucity of cases in the literature of what could be classified as a volar intercalated segment instability. In 1913, Chaput and Vaillant reported on a radiographic study of patients with carpal injuries, one of whom had a typical case of what would now be classified as VISI. Since then, a number of scattered case reports of what we would recognize today as a VISI deformity appeared in the literature.

Despite these isolated reports in the literature, there had not been a consensus of opinion in regard to what pathology was required to result in dynamic and static VISI deformities arising from the area of the lunotriquetral joint. However, clinical cases involving documented disruptions of the lunotriquetral interosseous ligament without any VISI pattern of deformity are not uncommon.

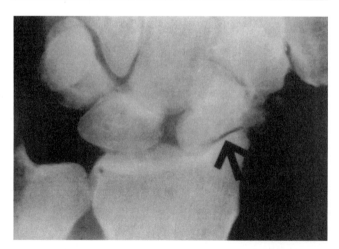

Figure 10-6. An AP radiograph of a wrist with scapholunate advanced collapse illustrating the radioscaphoid joint space narrowing (arrow) and the capitolunate joint space narrowing.

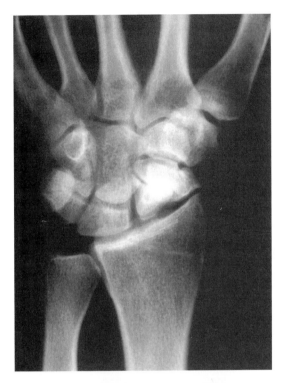

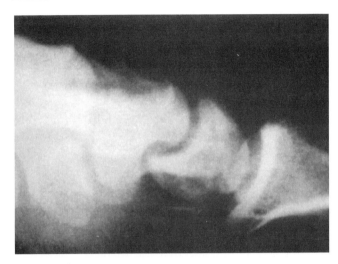

Figure 10-8. A lateral radiograph of a wrist with a distal radius malunion demonstrating a dorsal intercalated segment instability deformity of the carpus.

Lunatotriquetral Dissociation

The etiology most commonly attributed to the development of a VISI deformity was linked to lunatotriquetrum laxity (Fig. 10-9); this would be categorized as a dissociative type of carpal instability. Different authors had speculated that there was a progressive sequence of ligament disruption occurring on the ulnar side of the carpus, similar to what Mayfield, Johnson, and Kilcoyne had described on the radial side of the carpus. Reagan, Linscheid, and Dobyns divided the triquetrolunate instabilities into two groups. Lunotriquetral sprains, which had partial tears in the lunotriquetral interosseous ligament, and lunotriquetral dissociations, which had complete tears of the lunotriquetral interosseous ligament. Others divide triquetrolunate instability into two types, those without radiographic or clinical evidence of VISI and those with an evident VISI deformity.

Cadaver experiments demonstrated increased divergent motion between the lunate and triquetrum following sectioning of the lunotriquetral interosseous and the palmar and dorsal radiotriquetral ligaments. Some studies had also been able to reproduce dynamic VISI patterns with the application of a dorsal force on the capitate and/or hamate. Other cadaver studies which had attempted to reproduce a static VISI deformity had been unsuccessful until Viegas and associates reported on a series of dissections and load studies that presented a staging system of ulnar-sided perilunate instability (Fig. 10-10).

Radiocarpal Dissociation

Viegas and associates demonstrated that the integrity of the dorsal radiocarpal ligaments were critical in preventing a static VISI deformity. In fact, they reported that a static

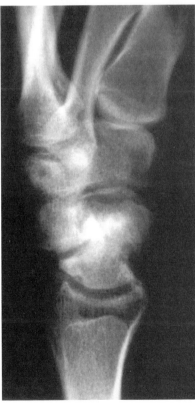

Figure 10-7. **(Top)** An AP and **(Bottom)** lateral radiograph of a wrist with a scaphoid nonunion that has a dorsal intercalated segment instability.

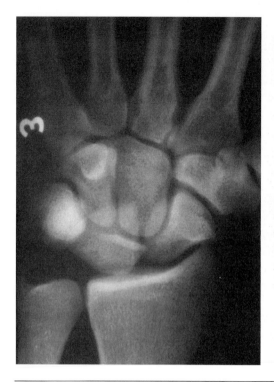 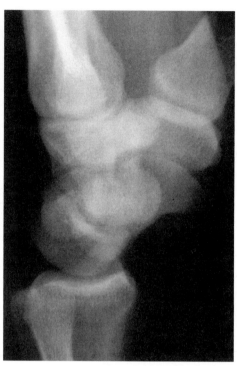

Figure 10-9. (Left) An AP and (Right) lateral radiograph of a patient with a volar intercalated segment instability who had a lunotriquetral dissociation.

VISI deformity can be evident following disruption of the dorsal radiocarpal ligament alone. Horii and associates also found similar results in their kinematic studies and reaffirmed that disruption of the dorsal radiocarpal ligaments is necessary to develop a static VISI deformity.

Several authors have commented on the frequency of a VISI deformity in severe rheumatoid arthritis of the wrist. It is easy to explain the attenuation of the dorsal ligaments by the chronic recurrent inflammation and swelling that

Figure 10-10. Diagrammatic representation of the ligament disruption in the three stages of ulnar-sided perilunate instability. Stage I: the lunotriquetral interosseous ligament is disrupted. Stage II: the palmar radiolunotriquetral ligament is also disrupted. Stage III: the dorsal radioscapholunotriquetral ligament, also called the dorsal radiocarpal ligament, is also disrupted.

often occurs in these patients within the radiocarpal joint. Trumble and associates demonstrated in their clinical series that stabilization of the lunotriquetral joint alone did not prevent the VISI deformity or "clunk." It would seem, in fact, that fusion of the lunate and the triquetrum in a case with a static VISI, as defined by the Stage III instability model, would simply change a CID-VISI into a CIND-VISI.

Triquetrohamate, Capitolunate, Scaphotrapezial Dissociation

A number of other lesions have been reported to result in a VISI deformity. Garth and associates described laxity of the capitotriquetral ligament, which resulted in failure of the triquetralhamate joint, which in turn, they believe, allows a VISI deformity to occur. Trumble and associates also list triquetralhamate disruption as well as capitate-lunate laxity as causes of VISI deformity. Gibson and Hankin and associates have published case reports in which they attribute a VISI deformity to injury of the scaphotrapezial ligament. These kinds of VISI deformities are what Dobyns, Linscheid and associates would classify as carpal instability nondissociative lesions.

Ulnar Translocation

Ulnar translocation or translation is most commonly seen in patients with rheumatoid arthritis of the wrist. Although ulnar translation is one of the types of carpal instability that has been described, there is a paucity of articles in the literature describing specific cases. This type of ulnar translation also has a palmar subluxation component (Fig. 10-11). Posttraumatic ulnar translation is believed to have as a component of its pathology compromise of the volar radial lunate ligament, which subsequently allows the carpus to translate as a unit towards the ulna. Recent studies by Viegas and associates suggest that a much more global ligament disruption is required for ulnar translocation and that there is always a palmar translocation component to the instability. Ulnar translation may also be seen in conjunction with other instabilities such as scapholunate dissociation and triquetral lunate dissociation. Taleisnik categorized ulnar translocation into two types. In Type I, the entire carpus is translated in an ulnar direction, including the scaphoid. In Type II, the scaphoid remains in its normal relation to the radius and the radial styloid-scaphoid distance remains normal, while the remaining carpus translates in an ulnar direction. Volar ligament repair/reconstruction, or alternatively, limited arthrodesis at the radiocarpal joint has been proposed for treatment of ulnar translocation.

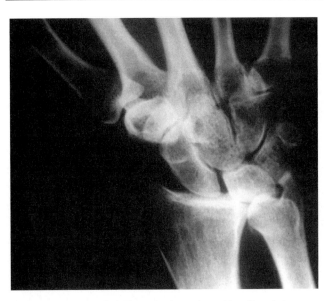

Figure 10-11. An AP radiograph of a patient with a Type I ulnar translocation of the carpus who had rheumatoid arthritis.

Dorsal Subluxation

Dorsal subluxation is the least common of the four types of carpal instabilities originally described by Linscheid and associates. In fact, dorsal subluxation rarely occurs; but, when it does occur, it is usually associated with a Barton's fracture.

Axial Carpal Instability

Axial carpal disruptions have been reported in the literature for decades. Most references are in the form of case reports in which the axial disruption has resulted from a blast or crush injury. It was not until 1989 that Garcia-Elias and associates classified these uncommon injuries into three groups: axial-ulnar disruptions, axial-radial disruptions, and combined axial-radial-ulnar disruptions (Fig. 10-12). Treatment of these injuries consists of open reduction and percutaneous pin fixation in most cases.

Distal Radioulnar/Ulnocarpal Instability

Melone and Nathan have categorized a spectrum of injuries progressing from peripheral ulnar disruption of the triangular fibrocartilage complex into five stages of increasing severity, all of which have as a component distal radioulnar joint instability. Stage I: the common feature of all injuries was peripheral detachment of the TFCC from the ulna styloid. In Stage II, the ECU subsheath was also disrupted. Stage III involves the disruption of the ulnocarpal ligaments, and Stage IV includes disruption of the lunotriquetral interosseous ligaments. Stage V, the final and most severe, involves the disruption of the triquetral capitate and triquetral hamate ligaments. For each stage, the treatment includes operative repair or reconstruction of each of the traumatic injuries.

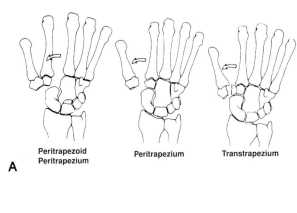

Peritrapezoid
Peritrapezium   Peritrapezium   Transtrapezium

A

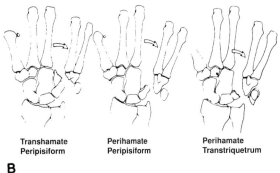

Transhamate   Perihamate   Perihamate
Peripisiform   Peripisiform   Transtriquetrum

B

Figure 10-12. The most common types of axial disruption of the carpus. **(A)** Axial-radial disruptions: peritrapezoid, peritrapezium, and transtrapezium. **(B)** Axial-ulnar disruptions: transhamate, peripisiform, perihamate, peripisiform, and perihamate, transtriquetrum.

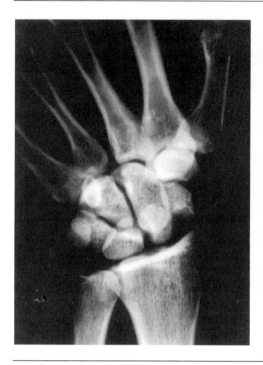
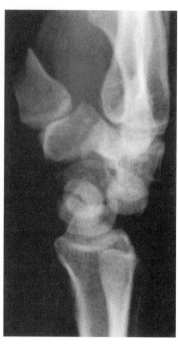

Figure 10-13. Radiographs showing a dorsal transscaphoid perilunate dislocation in both posteroanterior and lateral views.

Carpal Fracture/Dislocations

Carpal fracture/dislocations are less common injuries. Transscaphoid perilunate fracture dislocations are reported to account for approximately 3% of all carpal injuries.

There are two types of transscaphoid perilunate fracture dislocations. The first is the dorsal transscaphoid perilunate fracture dislocation (Fig. 10-13) and the second is the palmar transscaphoid lunate fracture dislocation (Fig. 10-14). Dorsal transscaphoid perilunate fracture dislocation

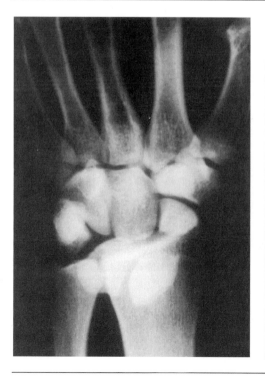
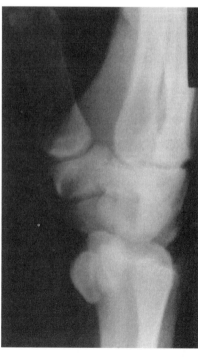

Figure 10-14. Radiographs showing a palmar transscaphoid lunate dislocation in both posteroanterior and lateral views.

is more common than palmar. Treatment in the literature varies from closed reduction and casting to open reduction to primary wrist arthrodesis. Most authors now advocate open reduction and internal fixation. Palmar transscaphoid lunate fracture dislocation is less common; many times it is included as a variant of dorsal transscaphoid perilunate fracture dislocation. Prognosis of this injury is usually poor. Similarly, in comparison to the perilunate/lunate dislocations, it appears that the palmar transscaphoid lunate fracture dislocation is a more severe stage of disruption than the dorsal transscaphoid perilunate fracture dislocation. These injuries represent a sequentially more severe ligamentous disruption.

Viegas and associates have reported good results from treatment of the dorsal transscaphoid fracture/dislocation with open reduction and internal fixation of the scaphoid with a Herbert screw. However, for the palmar transscaphoid fracture/dislocation, additional reduction and repair of the disrupted triquetrolunate and dorsal radiocarpal soft tissues is recommended. A variety of other patterns of carpal fracture/dislocations have been reported and fall into the so-called "greater arc" injuries (Fig. 10-15).

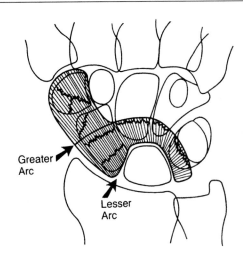

Figure 10-15. A diagram illustrating the area of the "lesser arc" through which the primarily ligamentous perilunate dislocations occur, and the "greater arc" through which carpal fractures are the primary injuries.

Annotated Bibliography

DISI

Almquist EE, Bach AW, Sack JT, Fuhs SE, Newman DM: Four-bone ligament reconstruction for treatment of chronic complete scapholunate separation. *J Hand Surg,* 16A:322-327, 1991.

The authors report on 36 consecutive cases of chronic, complete scapholunate separation treated with a four-bone ligament reconstruction. They used a long, distally based strip of the extensor carpi radialis brevis, which was weaved between the radius, lunate, capitate, and scaphoid using a dorsal and palmar approach. The scapholunate dissociation was additionally reduced by means of a 22-gauge stainless steel wire passed through holes in the scaphoid and lunate. Followup ranged from two to 10 years and averaged 4.8 years. Average postoperative range of motion was 52% of extension and 37° of flexion. Grip strength averaged 73% of the noninvolved side. Preoperative scapholunate gaps seen on radiographs were greater than 4mm, and postoperative gaps radiographically averaged 3.3mm. Eighty-six percent of patients returned to pre-injury activities, including heavy labor. There was no radiographic evidence of advancing arthritic changes at the point of their follow-up review.

Berger RA, Amadio PC, Imadea T, An KN, Cooney WP: The gross and histologic anatomy and material properties of the subregions of the scapholunate ligament. Proceedings, NATO Advanced Research Workshop, Advances in the Biomechanics of the Hand and Wrist, p. 14, Brussels, Belgium, May 22-23, 1992.

The authors reported that the scapholunate interosseous ligament can be divided histologically and biomechanically into three components. The proximal or membranous portion is the weakest ligament. The dorsal component was the strongest both histologically and biomechanically.

Blatt G: Capsulodesis in reconstructive hand surgery. Dorsal capsulodesis for the unstable scaphoid and volar capsulodesis following excision of the distal ulna. *Hand Clin,* 3[1]:81-102, 1987.

Blatt describes the technique he has used successfully to treat scapholunate dissociation with rotatory subluxation of the scaphoid. This treatment consists primarily of a dorsal capsulodesis from the dorsal radius to the dorsal aspect of the scaphoid.

Blevens AD, Light TR, Jablonsky WS, Smith DG, Patwardhan AV, Guay ME, Woo TS: Radiocarpal articular contact characteristics with scaphoid instability. *J Hand Surg,* 14A:781-790, 1989.

Biomechanical study showed division of the scapholunate interosseous ligament produces SL diastasis and dorsoradial translocation of RS contact area. Rotatory subluxation occurred with the addition of sectioning the scaphotrapezium complex or palmar intracapsular radiocarpal ligament (RSL, RC, RLT); periscaphoid ligament disruption tends to shift the lead to the radiolunate joint.

Bourne MH, Linscheid RL, Dobyns JH: Concomitant scapholunate dissociation and Kienböck's disease. *J Hand Surg,* 16:460-464, 1991.

The authors report on six men who had concurrent scapholunate dissociation and Kienböck's disease. Five of the patients attributed the onset of wrist pain to a single traumatic event; three of the patients had radiographic evidence of scapholunate dissociation before the onset of lunate osteonecrosis. The authors suggest that biomechanical factors that may be of significance in the etiology of Kienböck's disease include ulnar minus variance, lesser compliance of the triangular fibrocartilage, ulnar translation of the carpus at impact with shear fracture through the lunate, and disruption of the scapholunate interosseous membrane occurring under similar stress.

Braithwaite IJ, Jones WA: Scapholunate dissociation occurring with scaphoid fracture. *J Hand Surg,* Br, 17B:286-288, 1992.

The authors report on four cases in which scaphoid fracture and scapholunate dissociations appear to have occurred simultaneously in the ipsilateral wrist.

Conyers DJ: Scapholunate interosseous reconstruction and imbrication of palmar ligaments. *J Hand Surg,* 15A:690-700, 1990.

Twenty-eight patients with scapholunate interosseous ligament disruption, carpal instability, and persistent wrist pain were treated by carpal reduction, stabilization, and palmar ligament reconstruction. Twenty-two patients resumed their previous employment, maintained carpal alignment, and had acceptable pain control.

Cooney WP, Linscheid RL, Dobyns JH: Carpal instability: treatment of ligament injuries of the wrist. *Instr Course Lect,* 41:33-44, 1992.

The authors detail a brief review of the anatomy, physiology, and classification of carpal instability and the diagnostic criteria and treatment alternatives. Carpal instability dissociative and carpal instability nondissociative classifications are also explained.

Cooney WP, Dobyns JH, Linscheid RL: Arthroscopy of the wrist: anatomy and classification of carpal instability. *Arthroscopy,* 6:133-140, 1990.

The authors review the arthroscopic anatomy of the wrist and discuss how the arthroscopic examination can be combined with manual manipulation to assess carpal instability. Dissociative and CIND lesions are also reviewed.

Fortin PT, Louis DS: Long-term follow-up of scaphoid-trapezium-trapezoid arthrodesis. Presented at the 59th Annual Meeting of the American Academy of Orthopaedic Surgeons, February 22, 1992.

A series of patients treated with an STT fusion for scapholunate dissociation, Kienböck's, or STT arthritis were followed for an average of 4.8 years. A significant incidence of radioscaphoid and first carpometacarpal joint degenerative changes were identified even when all the recommended criteria for and techniques of STT arthrodesis were followed.

Kleinman WB, Carroll IV C: Scaphotrapeziotrapezoid arthrodesis for treatment of chronic static and dynamic scapholunate instability: a 10-year perspective on pitfalls and complications. *J Hand Surg,* 15A:408-414, 1990.

Retrospective review of 47 wrists in 46 patients who underwent scaphotrapeziotrapezoid fusion for chronic static and dynamic scapholunate instability with follow-up at six months. The complication rate was 52%. Progressive carpal arthrosis was most common in 19% and in each case perfect scaphoid alignment had not been obtained.

Lavernia CJ, Cohen MS, Taleisnik J: Treatment of scapho-lunate dissociation by ligamentous repair and capsulodesis.

J Hand Surg, 17A: 354-359, 1992.

Retrospective review of 21 patients with chronic scapholunate dissociation without degenerative joint disease treated with scapholunate ligament repair. In 14 patients, capsulodesis was added. The average follow-up was three years. Pain was absent or minimal in 19; grip strength and X-ray appearance improved; loss of palmar flexion was 11.5. The scapholunate angle decreased five degrees. The scapholunate gap decreased 0.9mm. Grip strength increased seven pounds.

Linscheid RL, Dobyns JH, Beabout JW, Bryan RS: Traumatic instability of the wrist: diagnosis, classification, and pathomechanics. *J Bone Joint Surg,* 54:1612, 1972.

The classic article describing the four types of posttraumatic instability, dorsiflexion instability, palmar flexion instability, ulnar translocation, and dorsal subluxation. The terms dorsal intercalated segment instability and volar intercalated segment instability were introduced.

Mayfield JK, Johnson RP, Kilcoyne RK: Carpal dislocations: pathomechanics and progressive perilunar instability. *J Hand Surg,* 5:226-241, 1980.

The pathomechanics, ligamentous damage, and degree of carpal instability in perilunate and lunate dislocations were analyzed by experimentally loading 32 cadaver wrists to failure. The mechanism of injury was extension, ulnar deviation, and intercarpal supination. These dislocations occurred in a sequential fashion due to progressive and specific ligamentous disruptions and were classified according to the degree of perilunar instability. Stage I perilunar instability (scapholunate diastasis) had the lowest degree of carpal instability. Lunate dislocations (Stage IV PLI) had the highest degree of carpal instability. Radial styloid fractures were produced in seven as a result of avulsion.

Minami A, Takahara M, Suzuki K: Scapholunate Interosseous Ligament Repair and Reconstruction in Patients with Lunate and Perilunate Dislocations. Presented at the 47th Annual Meeting of the American Society for Surgery of the Hand, November 11-14, 1992.

The authors report the results of 32 patients with lunate and perilunate dislocations treated over a 12-year period. They compared those patients in which the scapholunate interosseous ligament was repaired and/or reconstructed with patients in which the ligament was not repaired or reconstructed. The clinical and roentgenographic results suggest that scapholunate interosseous ligament repair and reconstruction during open reduction can prevent or reduce the recurrence of carpal instability and improve the clinical results.

Mudgal CS, Jones WA: Scapho-lunate diastasis: a component of fractures of the distal radius. *J Hand Surg,* Br, 15B:503-505, 1990.

The authors report on 10 cases of fractures of the distal radius associated with scapholunate dissociation.

Nakamura R, Imaeda T, Tsuge S, Watanabe K: Scaphoid non-union with DISI deformity. *J Hand Surg,* Br, 16B:156-161, 1991.

The authors studied 26 patients with scaphoid nonunions and DISI deformities and 20 additional patients with scaphoid nonunion without DISI deformities. Roentgenographic, arthrographic, and arthroscopic findings were analyzed and used to compare the two groups of scaphoid nonunions. There was no statistically significant difference in the incidence of arthrographically proven scapholunate ligamentous tears between the two groups. The authors believe that ligamentous injury rarely causes DISI deformity in scaphoid nonunion, and anterior wedge grafting alone is sufficient to correct DISI deformity in most cases of scaphoid nonunion.

Pisano SM, Peimer CA, Wheeler DR, Sherwin F: Scaphocapitate intercarpal arthrodesis. *J Hand Surg,* 16A:328-333, 1991.

Review of 17 patients treated with scaphocapitate arthrodesis for rotary scaphoid instability, arthrosis, resistant scaphoid nonunion, and Kienböck's disease. Wrist extension reduced 28°, flexion 40°, radial deviation 14°, and ulnar deviation 14°. Status grip strength averaged 74% of the unoperated side.

Rotman MB, Manske PR, Pruitt DL, Szerzinski J: Scapho-capito-lunate arthrodesis. *J Hand Surg,* 18A:26-33, 1993.

The authors report on 21 patients with an average follow-up of 28 months, treated with scapho-capito-lunate arthrodesis for either chronic incompetence of the scapholunate ligament or a scaphoid nonunion. Eighty-one percent healed after the primary procedure. Range of motion averaged 35° of extension, 30° of flexion, 10° of radial deviation, and 20° of ulnar deviation. Grip strength averaged 70% of the uninvolved side. Pain was significantly reduced in 80% of the patients.

Smith DK, Cooney WP, Linscheid RL et al: Effects of a scaphoid waist osteotomy on carpal kinematics. *J Orthop Res,* 7:590-598, 1989.

Radiographic study of five cadaveric wrists after scaphoid waist osteotomy. There was a tendency for the scaphoid osteotomy to collapse into a dorsally angulated or "hump back" deformity with extremes of wrist position. The scaphoid is important in maintaining the normal alignment of the carpal bones and producing normal wrist motion.

Viegas SF, Patterson RM, Peterson PD, Pogue DJ, Jenkins DK, Sweo TD, Hokanson JA: Evaluation of the biomechanical efficacy of limited intercarpal fusions for the treatment of scapholunate dissociation. *J Hand Surg,* 15:120-128, 1990.

Five fresh-frozen cadaver wrists with Stage III scapholunate dissociation were studied using pressure-sensitive film to compare the differences between various limited carpal fusions used to treat scaphoid instability. Scaphotrapeziotrapezoid and scaphocapitate fusions were found to increase scaphoid fossa load and decrease lunate fossa load even more than in the instability. Scapholunate fusion compared most favorably with the normal load mechanics; however, no fusion was "normal" in all positions tested.

Viegas SF, Tencer AF, Cantrell J, Chang M, Clegg P, Hicks C, O'Meara C, Williamson J: Load transfer characteristics of the wrist; part II, perilunate instability. *J Hand Surgery,* 12A:978-985, 1987.

The authors analyze the load-transfer characteristics of the wrist in increasing stages of perilunate instability as described by Mayfield. Using pressure-sensitive film, they demonstrated that, overall, the scaphoid contact area was found to decrease as the stage of perilunate instability increased, with significant increase in the contact pressures. The location of increased load through the scaphoid fossa coincided with the location where degenerative changes were seen in the proximal wrist joint in clinical cases of scapholunate advanced collapse.

Watson HK, Ballet FL: The SLAC Wrist: Scapholunate advanced collapse pattern of degenerative arthritis. *J Hand Surg,* 9A:358, 1984.

Four thousand wrist radiographic films were reviewed to establish the pattern of sequential changes in degenerative arthritis of the wrist. The most common pattern of degenerative arthritis (57%) was arthritis between the scaphoid, lunate, and radius; 27% of cases occurred between the scaphoid, trapezium, and trapezoid; a combination of these two patterns occurred in 15%.

Watson HK, Hempton RF: Limited wrist arthrodesis. Part I, the triscaphoid joint. *J Hand Surg,* 5:320-327, 1980.

The authors describe their technique of limited wrist arthrodesis of the joints between the scaphoid, trapezium, and trapezoid for localized degenerative arthritis, radial hand dislocations, and certain instability patterns following ligament rupture (rotary subluxation of the scaphoid).

VISI

Alexander CE, Lichtman DM: Ulnar carpal instabilities. *Orthop Clin North Am,* 15:307-320, 1984.

The authors present an explanation of carpal instabilities, including midcarpal and triquetrolunate instability, using the ring concept of carpal kinematics as proposed by Lichtman.

Hankin FM, Amadio PC, Wojtys EM, Braunstein EM: Carpal instability with palmar flexion of the proximal row associated with injury to the scaphotrapezial ligament: report of two cases. *J Hand Surg,* 13B:298-302, 1988.

The authors describe two cases in which the presumed cause of instability was an injury to the extrinsic volar scaphotrapezial ligament complex.

Horii E, Garcia-Elias M, An KN, Bishop AT, Cooney WP, Linscheid RL, Chao EYS: A kinematic study of lunotriquetral dissociations. *J Hand Surg,* 16A:355-362, 1991.

An analysis of carpal motion after sectioning the ligamentous supportive lunotriquetral joints was done using stereoradiographic methods. Two stages of ligament disruption were studied, the first involving complete sectioning of both dorsal and palmar lunotriquetral ligaments and interosseous membrane. Following stage I, altered kinematics of the carpal bones was noted, although it was not until their stage II disruption, which consisted of further sectioning of both the dorsal radiotriquetral and dorsal scaphotriquetral ligaments, that a static volar intercalated segment instability was produced.

Reagan DS, Linscheid RL, Dobyns JH: Lunotriquetral sprains. *J Hand Surg,* 9A:502-514, 1984.

The authors divided the triquetrolunate instabilities into two groups. Lunotriquetral sprains, which had partial tears in the lunotriquetral interosseous ligament, and lunotriquetral dissociations, which had complete tears of the lunotriquetral interosseous ligament. They state that lunotriquetral sprains usually occur from hyperextension and twisting of the wrist. Symptoms include pain, weakness, limitation of motion, and a "click" with lateral motions.

Trumble TE, Bour CJ, Smith RJ, Glisson RR: Kinematics of the ulnar carpus related to the volar intercalated segment instability pattern. *J Hand Surg,* 15A:384-392, 1990.

Dissections were done on cadaver upper extremities to study the carpal kinetics involved in VISI. Disruption of the ulnar half of the volar arcuate ligament and the lunotriquetral ligaments was found to result in lunate rotation, particularly under axial loads.

Trumble TE, Bour CJ, Smith RJ, Edwards GS: Intercarpal arthrodesis for static and dynamic palmar intercalated segment instability. *J Hand Surg,* 13A:396-402, 1988.

Seven patients with VISI deformity were treated with intercarpal arthrodesis. Five of the six patients treated with arthrodesis of the proximal distal rows had pain relief. The patient with arthrodesis limited to the proximal row had a poor result.

Viegas SF, Patterson RM, Peterson PD, Pogue DJ, Jenkins DK, Sweo TD, Hokanson JA: Ulnar sided perilunate instability: an anatomic and biomechanic study. *J Hand Surg,* 15A:268-278, 1990.

Fresh-frozen cadaver dissections and load studies demonstrated a pattern of increasing ulnar-sided instability starting with lunotriquetral interosseous ligament disruption and progressing to a static VISI, CID pattern. The importance of the dorsal ligamentocapsular structures was demonstrated and dorsal radiocarpal instability alone was found to result in static VISI of the CIND type.

Ulnar Translation

Linscheid RL, Dobyns JH: Rheumatoid arthritis of the wrist. *Orthop Clin North Am,* 2:649-665, 1971.

The authors describe the pathoanatomy and pathomechanics which lead to carpal deformities in rheumatoid arthritis of the wrist, including ulnar translation.

Rayhack JM, Linscheid RL, Dobyns JH, Smith JH: Posttraumatic ulnar translation of the carpus. *J Hand Surg,* 12A:180-189, 1987.

The authors describe eight patients with post-traumatic ulnar translation of the carpus. The diagnosis was delayed from two to 23 months in these patients. They report the histories and the variety of treatments used on this group of patients.

Taleisnik J: *The Wrist.* Churchill Livingstone, New York, N.Y., 305-306, 1985.

Taleisnik descibes the Type I and Type II forms of ulnar translation.

Axial Disruption

Garcia-Elias M, Dobyns JH, Cooney WP, Linscheid RL: Traumatic axial dislocations of the carpus. *J Hand Surg,* 14A:446-457, 1989.

Classified as axial ulnar disruptions, axial radial disruptions, and combined axial radial-ulnar disruptions. Prognosis was determined more by the associated soft-tissue injuries than by the carpal derangement itself. Early open reduction and internal fixation and primary repair of damaged structures provide the best opportunity for optimal outcome.

Distal Radioulnar/Ulnocarpal Instability

Melone Jr CP, Nathan R: Traumatic disruption of the triangular fibrocartilage complex, pathoanatomy. *Clin Orthop Re Res,* 275:65-73, 1992.

The authors describe the surgical pathology in 42 cases of traumatic triangular fibrocartilage disruption. From this analysis of the pathoanatomy of these lesions, they develop a spectrum of injury resulting in five basic stages of increasingly ulnar wrist instability. All stages include detachment of the articular disc from its own insertion and are the principal cause of distal radioulnar joint instability. The authors point out that rather than an isolated event, peripheral disruption of the TFC often proved to be the major constituent of more complex lesions that were suitable for surgical repair.

Carpal Fracture/Dislocation

Green DP, O'Brien ET: Open reduction of carpal dislocations: indications and operative techniques. *J Hand Surg,* 3:250-265, 1978.

Forty-nine carpal dislocations in 46 patients are described and the authors suggest an approach for the management of dorsal transscaphoid perilunate dislocation, dorsal perilunate, and volar lunate dislocations. Best results were achieved with open reduction as soon after the injury as possible. Factors in this series that were associated with poorer results were volar dislocation of the proximal pole of the scaphoid with the lunate, severely comminuted radial styloid fractures, extensive osteochondral fractures of the carpal bones, and late open reduction of rotary scaphoid subluxation.

Viegas SF, Bean JW, Schram RA: Transscaphoid fracture/dislocations treated with open reduction and Herbert screw internal fixation. *J Hand Surg,* 12A(6):992-999, 1987.

Eight cases of transscaphoid fracture/dislocations were presented. The authors show the importance of differentiating between a dorsal transscaphoid perilunate fracture/dislocation and a palmar transscaphoid lunate fracture/dislocation. They explain that these are part of a spectrum of injuries with the palmar transscaphoid lunate fracture/dislocation being a more severe injury with less good clinical results following treatment than the less severe dorsal transscaphoid perilunate fracture/dislocation.

11

Triangular Fibrocartilage Complex Injury and Ulnar Wrist Pain

Glenn A. Buterbaugh, MD

Introduction

Ulnar wrist pain is considered by some as the low-back pain of hand surgery. Multiple afflictions occur at this site, and the hand surgeon must keep each in mind in the diagnosis of ulnar wrist pain. The triangular fibrocartilage complex has been extensively studied over the last few years. We have come to better understand the anatomy and biomechanics of the TFCC in the laboratory and have further refined the diagnostic work-up. The disorders have been identified and classified in a pattern of injury.

Alternative lesions, as well, are considered in the diagnosis of ulnar wrist pain, including dislocation, subluxation, and arthritis of the distal radioulnar joint, medial carpal, and lunotriquetral ligament instability, extensor carpi ulnaris subluxation and rupture, calcific extensor and flexor carpi ulnaris tendonitis, hamate hook fractures and pisotriquetral subluxation, and arthritis. The clinical findings for these lesions help define the diagnostic work-up required in the evaluation of ulnar wrist pain.

In the diagnostic work-up, the general principles include a differentiation between acute and chronic injury. Also, the stability of the distal radioulnar joint and medial carpus by palpation as well as the site of localized tenderness are important elements in the initial evaluation. Further examination studies include wrist range of motion and pinch and grip strength. The diagnostic studies include standard PA radiographs of the wrist in neutral forearm rotation to assess ulnar variance specifically as well as the articular surfaces. Other studies helpful in the evaluation of ulnar wrist pain include three-compartment wrist arthrogram and MRI studies for ligamentous and TFCC lesions, as well as CT scan studies to evaluate distal radioulnar joint articulation, the pisotriquetral joint, and the hamate hook.

Anatomy

The term TFCC was introduced to describe the ligamentous and cartilage structure that suspends the distal radius and ulnar carpus from the distal ulna (Fig. 11-1). The TFCC incorporates the poorly identifiable dorsal and volar radioulnar ligaments, the ulnar collateral ligament, the meniscus homologue, as well as the clearly definable articular disk, extensor carpi ulnaris sheath, ulnolunate and lunotriquetral ligaments. The complex arises from the ulnar aspect of the lunate fossa of the radius. It courses toward the ulna where it inserts about the fovea at the base of the ulnar styloid. The fovea is an area rich in vascular foramen, which provides vascularity to the peripheral element of the TFCC, with a more central radial portion being relatively avascular.

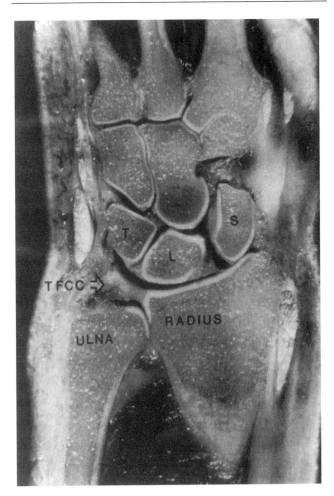

Figure 1. The anatomy of the TFCC is shown providing stability of the distal radioulnar joint. Note the attachments of the TFCC to the fovea of the distal ulna and articular edge of the radius. S, scaphoid; L, lunate; T, triquetrum.

TFCC Lesions: Injury Patterns and Treatment

A classification of TFCC abnormalities has been recently developed based on mechanism and site of injury (Table 11-1).

Traumatic lesions of the TFCC result from a fall on the outstretched upper extremity or hyperrotation injury to the forearm. These traumatic lesions occur from the origin or insertion of the TFCC. Degenerative lesions of the TFCC result from repetitive loading known as ulnar impaction syn-

Table 11-1.   TFCC Abnormalities

Class 1: Traumatic
    A. Central perforation
    B. Ulnar avulsion
        With distal ulnar fracture
        Without distal ulnar fracture
    C. Distal avulsion
    D. Radial avulsion
        With sigmoid notch fracture
        Without sigmoid notch fracture
Class 2: Degenerative (ulnocarpal abutment syndrome)
    Stage:
    A. TFCC wear
    B. TFCC wear
        + lunate and/or ulnar chondromalacia
    C. TFCC perforation
        + lunate and/or ulnar chondromalacia
    D. TFCC perforation
        + lunate and/or ulnar chondromalacia
        + L-T ligament perforation
    E. TFCC perforation
        + lunate and/or ulnar chondromalacia
        + L-T ligament perforation
        + ulnocarpal arthritis

A classification of triangular fibrocartilage complex injuries.

drome. A spectrum of injury results from early TFCC wear to TFCC perforation, lunate chondromalacia, LT ligament tears, and ulnocarpal arthritis.

Traumatic Lesion (Class 1 Lesions—TFCC)

Traumatic lesions are classified as: 1A—a lesion of the horizontal portion of the TFCC (Fig. 11-2), 1B—an avulsion of the complex from the distal ulna either with or without bone (Fig. 11-3), 1C—an avulsion of the complex from its insertion into the lunate or triquetrum (Fig. 11-4), 1D—an avulsion

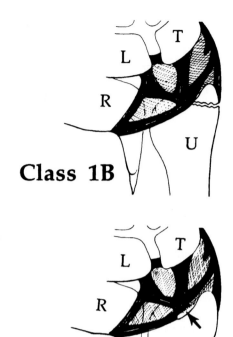

Figure 11-3.   (Top) The ligamentous supports of the ulnar aspect of the wrist (the triangular fibrocartilage complex) illustrating a Class 1B lesion. In this instance, the TFCC is avulsed from the distal ulna with an associated fragment of bone, i.e., the distal ulna. R, radius; U, ulna; L, lunate; T, triquetrum. **(Bottom)** The ligamentous supports of the ulnar aspect of the wrist (the triangular fibrocartilage complex) illustrating a Class 1B lesion. In this case, the triangular fibrocartilage complex is torn free from the base of the ulnar styloid without an associated fracture (arrow). R, radius; U, ulna; L, lunate; T, triquetrum.

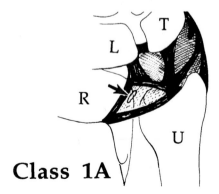

Figure 11-2.   The ligamentous supports of the ulnar aspect of the wrist (the triangular fibrocartilage complex) illustrating a Class 1A perforation. The perforation is a dorsal palmar tear (arrow) just medial to the radial origin of the TFCC. R, radius; U, ulna; L, lunate; T, triquetrum.

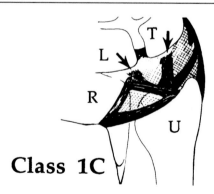

Figure 11-4.   The ligamentous supports of the ulnar aspect of the wrist (the triangular fibrocartilage complex) illustrating a Class 1C lesion. The triangular fibrocartilage complex is avulsed distally from its bony insertion to the lunate by the ulnolunate ligament and/or the triquetrum by the ulnotriquetral ligament (arrows). R, radius; U, ulna; L, lunate, T, triquetrum.

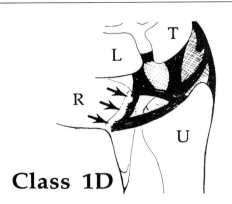

Figure 11-5. The ligamentous supports of the ulnar aspect of the wrist (the triangular fibrocartilage complex) illustrating a Class 1D lesion. Arrows indicate an avulsion of the TFCC from its radial origin. The avulsion can be with or without a fragment of bone. R, radius; U, ulna; L, lunate; T, triquetrum.

of the complex from the attachment to the distal aspect of the sigmoid notch of the radius (Fig. 11-5).

Evaluation and Treatment

Traumatic lesions of the TFCC generally occur secondary to a fall on an outstretched hand or are associated with hyper-rotation injuries to the forearm. Examination of the wrist should include the site of localized tenderness and range of motion of the wrist, including forearm rotation. Pain at the extremes of motion should be noted as well. Evidence of instability by manipulation of the distal ulna with attention to wrist symptoms, clicks, and snaps are noted. Pinch and grip strength as well as routine PA and lateral radiographs complete the exam.

All traumatic lesions of the TFCC should be treated with immobilization when seen acutely, if no instability pattern, subluxation, or fractures are noted. Complete disruption of

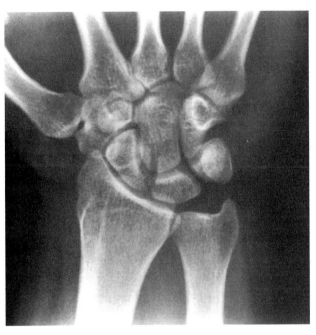

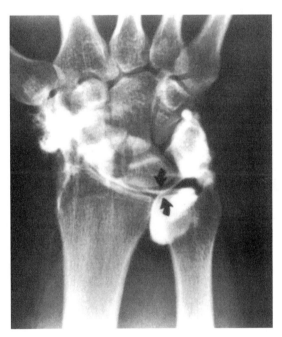

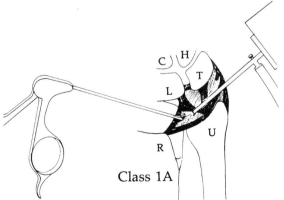

Figure 11-6. **(Top)** Arthrogram identifying a traumatic, horizontal tear in the triangular fibrocartilage (arrows). **(Bottom)** The debridement of the torn portion of the triangular fibrocartilage utilizing a suction punch and the wrist arthroscope. R, radius; U, ulna; L, lunate; T, triquetrum; C, capitate; H, hamate.

the TFCC from the radius, carpus, or ulna is generally associated with a clinical or radiographically detectable instability. In these cases, wrist arthrography and arthroscopy are indicated for evaluation and treatment. With arthroscopy, if the lesion reduces closed, then four weeks of immobilization in ulnar deviation and slight flexion is usually indicated. If positioning does not reduce the torn structures, arthroscopic or open repair is indicated. When the lesion is in the centrum (the avascular portion of the TFCC), arthroscopic debridement has been shown biomechanically and clinically to produce the desired effect. Enlargement of the tear preserving intact the volar and dorsal ligaments frequently relieves the symptomatic clicking and does not disrupt the stability or the load-bearing characteristic of the TFCC. Osterman and associates reported excellent results with arthroscopic limited TFCC debridement for perforations in the avascular region. A relative contraindication to TFCC debridement is an ulnar positive variance.

The technique of wrist arthroscopy is generally performed under regional or general anesthesia with distraction of the wrist in finger traps (Fig. 11-6). The anatomic landmarks on the dorsum of the wrist are identified, including the intervals between the extensor pollicis longus and extensor digitorum communis (three to four portal), extensor digitorum communis and the extensor digiti quinti (four to five portal), and the intervals radial and ulnar to the extensor carpi ulnaris (6R and 6U portals). After the wrist is distended, the arthroscope is carefully introduced by initially using a blunt trochar through the three to four portal. Inspection of the radiocarpal joint begins in sequential fashion with examination of the articular surfaces of the radius, scaphoid, lunate, and triquetrum, as well as the interosseous ligaments, the volar carpal ligament and the TFCC. The TFCC is specifically examined with a probe to "feel" the triangular fibrocartilage perforations if present, as well as to assess the integrity of the TFCC by its "trampolining."

Following careful assessment of all pathology, if partial excision of the TFCC is elected, the perforation should be enlarged to the point where there are no redundant margins. This usually requires removal of the central two-thirds of the triangular fibrocartilage. The instruments generally required are a suction punch, a banana blade or hook knife, and a motorized shaver utilized to "trim up" the margins of the debridement. The wrist is then copiously irrigated with normal saline, and the wounds are closed.

Early motion is encouraged. Patients are allowed to resume activity as symptoms permit. One can expect patients who undergo partial excision of a perforated triangular fibrocartilage to improve markedly within three to six weeks following the procedure for Type 1A and 2C lesions. If the procedure has been done for degenerative lesions with associated chondromalacic changes, particularly in patients with an ulnar positive variance, symptoms may not be completely relieved, but merely improved.

For peripheral tears of the TFCC, arthroscopic or open repair is indicated in lesions that do not reduce closed. Hermansdorfer and Kleinman have identified the trampo-

line test on arthroscopic evaluation in the identification of peripheral tears. Since there is good vascularity of the TFCC in the peripheral regions, suture repair is possible either through an arthroscopic or open technique. They have reported good results in a series of these patients.

Degenerative Lesions (Class 2 Lesions—TFCC)

From Mikic's study in 1978, the TFCC has been shown to undergo changes with age. The term ulnar impaction syndrome has frequently been used to describe the pathologic sequence (Fig. 11-7). Individuals more than 50 years of age have degenerative TFCC changes (many with perforation). Based on this work and the clinical experience of others, degenerative lesions of the TFCC are defined in the following classes: 2A—wear of the TFCC without cartilage abnormality (Fig. 11-8), 2B—wear of the TFCC with either ulnar head or lunate chondromalacia (Fig. 11-9), 2C—degenerative perforation of the TFCC with associated lunate and ulnar head chondromalacia (Fig. 11-10), 2D—the addition of lunotriquetral ligament tear with the findings of 2C (Fig. 11-11), 2E—degenerative arthritis of the

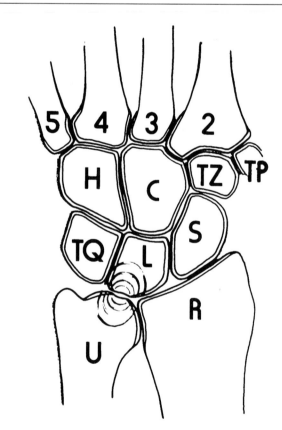

Figure 11-7. The ulnar impaction syndrome with evidence of chondromalacic changes on the ulnar head and lunate. U, ulna; R, radius; TQ, triquetrum; L, lunate; S, scaphoid; H, hamate; C, capitate; TZ, trapezium; TP, trapezoid; 2, 3, 4, 5, metacarpals.

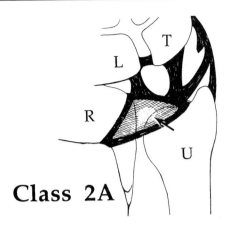

Figure 11-8.   The ligamentous supports of the ulnar aspect of the wrist (the triangular fibrocartilage complex) illustrating a Class 2A lesion. Both the proximal and distal aspects of the TFCC histologically and at times, grossly, evidence degenerative changes as illustrated by the stippling on this illustration (arrow). R, radius; U, ulna; L, lunate; T, triquetrum.

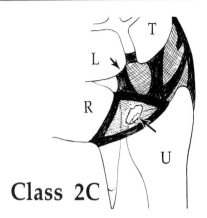

Figure 11-10.   The ligamentous supports of the ulnar aspect of the wrist (the triangular fibrocartilage complex) illustrating a Class 2C lesion. Further progression of the Class 2 degenerative lesions of the TFCC evidences now a large central perforation of the TFC (proximal arrow), as well as the underlying cartilage abnormality of the ulnar head and distally, the medial aspect of the lunate. R, radius; U, ulna; L, lunate; T, triquetrum.

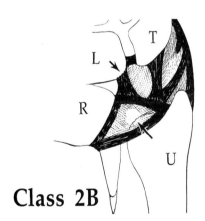

Figure 11-9.   The ligamentous supports of the ulnar aspect of the wrist (the triangular fibrocartilage complex) illustrating a Class 2B lesion. In addition to the degenerative changes of the TFCC seen in a Class 2A lesion (stippling), cartilage erosion of the ulnar head beneath the TFCC is seen (arrow), or of the kissing area of the medial border of the lunate distal to the TFCC (arrow). R, radius; U, ulna; L, lunate; T, triquetrum.

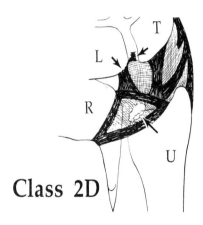

Figure 11-11.   The ligamentous supports of the ulnar aspect of the wrist (the triangular fibrocartilage complex) illustrating a Class 2D lesion. Further progression of the degenerative TFCC abnormalities reveals a through and through perforation of the horizontal portion of the TFC (proximal arrow), cartilage abnormalities of the ulnar head and of an adjacent area of the medial border of the lunate (distal radial arrow), and a disruption of the lunotriquetral ligament (distal ulna arrow). R, radius; U, ulna; L, lunate; T, triquetrum.

sigmoid notch, ulnar head, and ulnar carpus with a large perforation of the TFCC (Fig. 11-12).

Evaluation and Treatment

The evaluation of Class 2 lesions is similar to Class 1 lesions with particular attention to ulnar variance on the neutral PA radiograph. Triple-injection wrist arthrography further defines the pathology and helps determine the lesion class.

The treatment of Class 2 lesions or ulnar impaction syndrome begins with a conservative program of nonsteroidal anti-inflammatory agents, a trial of immobilization until symptoms resolve, and steroid injections into the distal

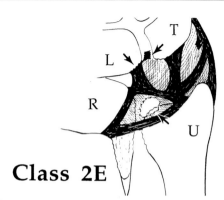

Figure 11-12. The ligamentous supports of the ulnar aspect of the wrist (the triangular fibrocartilage complex) illustrating a Class 2E lesion. The final progression of degenerative TFCC abnormalities reveals the findings of a Class 2D lesion, the additional changes of cartilage abnormalities involving the seat of the ulna, and the sigmoid notch of the radius. R, radius; U, ulna; L, lunate; T, triquetrum.

radioulnar joint and ulnar carpus. If conservative care is unsuccessful after a three-month trial, then treatment to decompress the ulnar impaction is indicated.

Surgical treatment for the ulnar positive patient is a formal ulnar shortening with application of plate fixation (Fig. 11-13) for Class 2A through 2D lesions. Other options include an open-wafer procedure (Fig. 11-14) described by Feldon for Class 2A, 2B, and 2C lesions with the alternative of an arthroscopic wafer procedure for the Class 2C lesions as described by Buterbaugh. In the ulnar neutral patient, Class 2 lesions are treated with arthroscopic limited debridement. Class 2D lesions with TFCC perforation and lunotriquetral ligament tear are treated with an ulnar shortening (with or without lunotriquetral fusion) based on the stability of the lunotriquetral complex after shortening. Alternatives in the treatment of this lesion have included the open-wafer procedure with dorsal capsulorrhaphy of the wrist or combined with lunotriquetral fusion.

Class 2E lesions are best treated with limited ulnar head resection as described by Bowers or Watson, a Suave-Kapandji syndrome, i.e. a distal radioulnar joint arthrodesis with a proximal pseudo-arthrosis popularized by Taleisnik, or a formal Darrach procedure. The choice of the appropriate procedure is based on surgeon preference, the integrity of the complete triangular fibrocartilage complex, and the stability of the distal ulna. The advantages of the limited ulnar-head resection and the Suave-Kapandji procedure are primarily related to maintaining the ligamentous supports of the distal radioulnar joint as well as the biomechanical advantage of maintaining the ulnar column of the wrist. The Darrach procedure, described by Dingman, is a useful salvage procedure, although radioulnar impingement at the resection site and distal tip instability can be problematic. Multiple procedures have been described to reconstruct the unstable distal ulna following a Darrach procedure.

Dislocations of the Distal Radiounlar Joint

Coincident with TFCC injuries, more severe ulnar pathology can occur with major wrist trauma. Isolated dislocations occur involving the distal ulna with the ulna volar or dorsal relative to the distal radius.

Dislocation Distal Radioulnar Joint—Ulna Dorsal

This injury results from hyperpronation with disruption of the dorsal distal radioulnar joint ligaments in partial or complete TFCC injury. Clinically, a dorsal prominence over the wrist is noted with the forearm locked in pronation. Attempts at supination are painful. CT scan of the distal radioulnar joint confirms the diagnosis. Closed reduction with cast immobilization for four weeks in supination is the treatment of choice. Open reduction is required in late cases or when closed reduction is unsuccessful.

Dislocation Distal Radioulnar Joint—Ulna Volar

Volar dislocations of the distal radioulnar joint are associated with forced supination of the forearm or can be secondary to a direct blow. Pathomechanics may require complete disruption of the TFCC. Clinically, the forearm is locked in supination with pain over the distal radioulnar joint. A furrow or indentation is noted on the ulnar side of the distal extensor aspect of the forearm, and there is a prominence on the anterior aspect of the wrist. Evaluation by CT scan will show the volar position of the distal ulna. Treatment, as in dorsal dislocations, consists of a closed reduction with direct pressure over the ulna volarly with gentle forearm pronation. The arm is immobilized in pronation for four weeks. In late cases or in unsuccessful closed reductions, open reduction is required.

Distal Radioulnar Joint Dislocation Associated with Radial Head Fractures (Essex-Lopresti Lesion)

Injuries to the distal radioulnar joint associated with radial head fractures can occur at the time of injury (Type 1) or result from proximal migration following excision of the radial head (Type 2). Migration generally occurs within the first two years following radial head excision.

Treatment recommendations for Type 1 injuries include an open reduction of the radial head or neck fracture with closed reduction and pinning of the distal radioulnar joint. If the radial head is not reconstructable, then a radial head silastic implant with distal radioulnar joint pinning is performed. In Type 2 injuries, a formal ulnar shortening with plate fixation is done to reduce the distal radioulnar joint, and a radial head implant is added to prevent further proximal migration of the radius. Problems associated with silastic radial head implants are recognized, and the implants may require removal at a future time. This area is

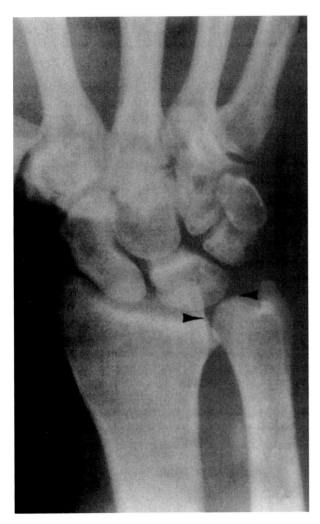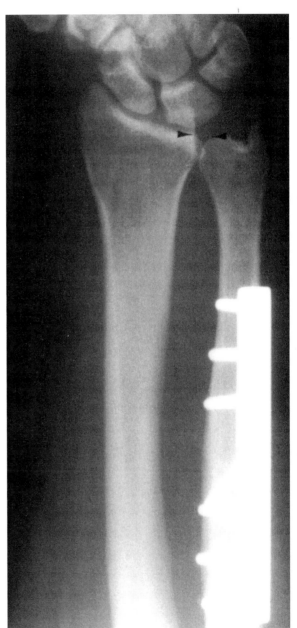

Figure 11-13.   An ulna shortening osteotomy with application of a seven-hole dynamic compression plate is shown. Note the oblique osteotomy and the compression lag screw applied. Note the decompression of the ulnar impaction at the distal radioulnar joint.

being intensely studied for possible attempts at reconstruction of the interosseous membrane. If the distal radioulnar joint shows significant degenerative changes, then reconstructive options including a hemiresection arthroplasty with ulnar shortening, distal radioulnar joint fusion with proximal pseudarthrosis (Suave-Kapandji procedure), or distal ulna excision may be required. A final salvage technique may be conversion to a one-bone forearm.

Subluxation of the Extensor Carpi Ulnaris Tendon

Spinner and Kaplan have described the anatomy of the sixth dorsal compartment and a fiberosseous tunnel overlying 1.5 cm to 2.0 cm of distal ulna. The extensor carpi ulnaris alone occupies this compartment. It is held tight to the ulnar group by the extensor carpi ulnaris tendon sheath. The extensor retinaculum, a separate structure from the ECU

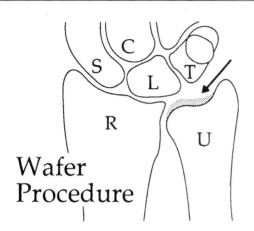

Figure 11-14. Wafer procedure is diagrammed with excision of the distal 2mm of ulnar head. This can be performed as an open technique or arthroscopically.

tendon sheath, passes around the ulna to insert on the palmar aspect of the carpus and soft tissues.

With forced supination, palmar flexion, and ulnar deviation, the ECU tendon can rupture or attenuate the extensor carpi ulnaris tendon sheath to dislocate in a palmar and ulnar direction (Fig. 11-15). The tendon relocates on forearm pronation. This change in position of the extensor carpi ulnaris with forearm rotation produces a clicking or snapping, and in some instances causes pain. Cases have been reported, as well, of partial rupture of the extensor carpi ulnaris associated with subluxation over a prominent portion of the distal ulna causing an abrasion to the undersurface of the extensor carpi ulnaris. Treatment in acute cases should include immobilization in a long-arm plaster splint in pronation with the wrist in slight dorsiflexion and radial deviation. For chronic cases, operative reconstruction usu-

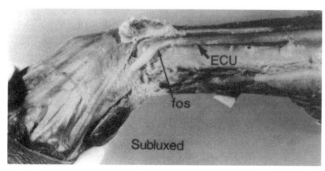

Figure 11-15. Subluxated ECU tendon with extensor retinaculum reflected above shows tendon's fiberosseous sheath attenuated yet intact.

ally is required and involves the medial wall of the extensor carpi ulnaris tendon sheath.

Calcific Tendonitis

The sudden onset of pain without history of trauma to the ulnar aspect of the wrist, particularly associated with repetitive ulnar deviation, can occur. Clinical presentation includes swelling over the extensor carpi ulnaris or flexor carpi ulnaris tendon sheaths with occasional crepitation on range of motion. Radiographs may show calcific deposits within the tendon sheath consistent with calcific tendonitis. Most cases generally respond to oral nonsteroidal anti-inflammatory agents or steroid injection with splinting.

Lunotriquetral Instability

Pain over the ulnar aspect of the wrist distal to the distal radioulnar joint may be associated with disruption of the lunotriquetral ligament. In cases not associated with the ulnar impaction syndrome, well-localized tenderness over this site as well as pain is associated with manipulation of the lunate and triquetrum and/or pain associated with stress at the midcarpal joint. Further progression of these symptoms may lead to a volar carpal instability or VISI pattern or an associated dynamic midcarpal instability. In isolated lunotriquetral instability, with a lunotriquetral ligament tear, ulnar variance is carefully examined for ulnar impaction syndrome (i.e., an ulnar positive variance). In cases of ulnar negative variance, multiple procedures for lunotriquetral instability have been attempted. Wrist dorsal capsulorrhaphy, ligament reconstruction, and lunotriquetral fusion have been tried with mixed results.

Pisotriquetral Subluxation, Dislocation, and Osteoarthritis

Subluxation and dislocation of the pisotriquetral joint have been studied by Vasilas and associates on the radiographic aspects of the pisotriquetral joint. A pisotriquetral view of the joint is required with the forearm positioned 30° supinated off the neutral position. Loss of symmetry between the pisiform and triquetrum is examined and required for the diagnosis. A carpal tunnel view may be helpful in further assessment of this joint.

Pisotriquetral osteoarthritis is more a common problem associated with localized tenderness over the pisotriquetral joint. Frequently on clinical exam, manipulation of the pisiform over the triquetrum causes intense pain. Local anesthetic injection into the pisotriquetral joint confirms the diagnosis. The radiographic views as described above, the 30° supinated view, as well as carpal tunnel views, will frequently show loss of joint space and osteophyte formation (Fig. 11-16).

Initial treatment of pisotriquetral pathology involves rest, nonsteroidal anti-inflammatory agents, and steroid injec-

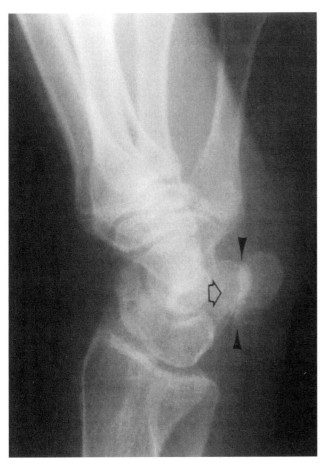

Figure 11-16. Thirty-degree supinated view identifying the pisotriquetral joint. Note the degenerative changes present.

tions into the pisotriquetral joint. If conservative therapy fails, then operative treatment is required with pisiform excision from the flexor carpi ulnaris tendon sheath.

Other Causes of Ulnar Wrist Pain

The complete evaluation of the ulnar aspect of the wrist must include a careful neurologic and vascular exam of the hand. A careful sensory exam as well as motor exam is required for all patients with ulnar wrist pain. Specific attention to the evaluation of the ulnar nerve in Guyon's canal as well as the dorsal cutaneous branch of the ulnar nerve and its anatomic variations are important in this analysis. The vascular status, as well, must be carefully evaluated with an Allen's test to evaluate the patency of the ulnar artery. Other conditions can be referred to the ulnar aspect of the wrist, such as hamate hook fractures, Kienböck's disease, intraosseous and extraosseous ganglions, tumors of the carpal bones, distal ulna and radius, and medial facet arthritis of the lunate.

Conclusion

In the evaluation of the patient with a TFCC injury or ulnar wrist pain secondary to other causes, the clinician must be complete in the evaluation process to confirm the diagnosis. As a general rule, conservative options should be tried in most instances of TFCC injury with operative treatment preserved for patients unresponsive to conservative care or when instability is present. One will frequently see the patient who has undergone multiple procedures for ulnar wrist pain with continued disability. Care must be taken to identify the cause of the problem as well as the subsequent goals of the patient in the rehabilitation of this wrist injury.

Annotated Bibliography

TFCC Lesion: Injury Patterns and Treatment

Bieber W, Linscheid RL, Dobyns JH, Beckenbaugh RD: Failed distal ulna resections. *J Hand Surg,* 113A:191-200, 1988.

Study of 20 patients with failed distal ulna resections suggested that the procedure should be avoided in young patients and those with ligamentous laxity.

Bilos ZJ, Chamberland D: Distal ulnar head shortening for treatment of triangular fibrocartilage complex tears with ulna positive variance. *J Hand Surg,* 16A:1115-9, 1991.

Two to 4mm of cartilage and subchondral bone was excised from the ulnar head in seven patients with a TFCC tear and ulna positive variance. Six patients had either complete or marked improvement in symptoms.

Boulas HJ, Milek MA: Ulnar shortening for tears of the triangular fibrocartilaginous complex. *J Hand Surg,* 15A:415-420, 1990.

The ulna was shortened an average of 2mm in 10 consecutive patients with ulnar wrist pain associated with TFCC tears. Six patients had ulnolunate abutment and/or cartilage degeneration. Pain relief and grip strength were excellent, but flexion decreased an average of 25.8° postoperatively.

Buck-Gramcko D: On the priorities of publication of some operative procedures on the distal end of the ulna. *J Hand Surg,* 15B:416-420, 1990.

A literature review of distal ulna procedures for the treatment of posttraumatic conditions of the distal radioulnar joint. Options are outlined, and included in the discussion are the origins of the names of the procedures attributed to certain authors.

Darrow JC, Linscheid RL, Dobyns JH, Mann JM, Wood MB, Beckenbaugh RD: Distal ulnar recession for disorders of the distal radioulnar joint. *J Hand Surg,* 10A:482-491, 1985.

Thirty-six wrists in 35 patients were treated with an ulnar shortening osteotomy to stabilize or decompress the distal radioulnar joints. Twenty-eight of the 36 wrists had good to excellent results at a 24.5-month follow-up.

Hermansdorfer JD, Kleinman WB: Management of chronic peripheral tears of the triangular fibrocartilage complex. *J Hand Surg,* 16A:340-6, 1991.

In 13 patients with traumatic peripheral separation of the TFCC, reattachment was done with nonabsorbable sutures passed through drill holes at the medial base of the ulnar styloid. Eight of the 11 patients returned to painless activities. Two of the three other patients did well after additional surgery (distal ulna resection in one and ulnar shortening osteotomy in the other).

Minami A, Kaneda K, Itoga H: Hemiresection-interposition arthroplasty of the distal radioulnar joint associated with repair of triangular fibrocartilage complex lesions. *J Hand Surg,* 16A:1120-5, 1991.

Hemiresection-interposition arthroplasty with repair of the torn TFCC was performed in 16 wrists to prevent ulnar head impingement on the TFCC. There was complete pain relief in 10 wrists. Grip strength and range of motion improved in all wrists.

Osterman AL: Arthroscopic debridement of triangular fibrocartilage complex tears. *Arthroscopy,* 6(2);120-4, 1990.

A prospective study of 52 consecutive patients showed that 86% had a positive initial arthrogram and 66% had a positive bone scan at the time of diagnostic arthroscopy; 34% of the tears were linear, 46% central perforation, and 20% ulnar or peripheral perforation. Eleven patients had no visible tear. The author concluded that arthroscopic debridement reduced symptoms without increasing clinical ulnar instability.

Palmer AK: Triangular fibrocartilage complex lesion: a classification. *J Hand Surg,* 14A:594-606, 1989.

TFCC injuries were classified into traumatic and degenerative lesions after analysis of anatomic, biomechanical, and clinical studies.

Palmer AK, Werner FW: The triangular fibrocartilage complex of the wrist anatomy and function. *J Hand Surg,* 6A:l53-162, 1981.

The TFCC is anatomically described as the homogeneous structure composed of the articular disk, the dorsal and volar radioulnar ligaments, the meniscus homologue, the ulnar collateral ligament, and the sheath of the extensor carpi ulnaris. Biomechanical studies suggested that the TFCC functions as a cushion and a major stabilizer of the distal radioulnar joint.

Palmer AK, Glisson RR, Werner FW: Ulnar variance determination. *J Hand Surg,* 7A:376-379, 1982.

The technique of ulnar variance determination is described placing the forearm in a neutral forearm rotation position with the elbow flexed and obtaining a PA radiograph of the wrist. A template is utilized to measure accurately the variance between the length of the radius and ulna.

Palmer AK, Glisson RR, Werner FW: Relationship between ulnar variance and triangular fibrocartilage complex thickness. *J Hand Surg,* 9A:681-683, 1984.

Anatomic data is presented showing an inverse relationship between positive ulnar variance and TFCC thickness.

Palmer AK, Werner FW, Glisson RR, Murphy DJ: Partial excision of the triangular fibrocartilage complex. *J Hand Surg,* 13A;403-406, 1988.

Excision of less than two thirds of the horizontal part of the TFCC cadavers did not alter axial load transmission.

Shaw JA, Bruno A, Paul EM: Ulnar styloid fixation in the treatment of posttraumatic instability of the radioulnar joint; A biomechanical study with clinical correlation. *J Hand Surg,* 15A:712-720, 1990.

Biomechanical testing of nine cadaver specimens showed that the TFCC was the main stabilizer of the radioulnar joint. Internal fixation of the ulnar styloid avulsion fractures restores stability in all forearm rotation positions.

Viegas SF, Pogue DJ, Patterson RN, Peterson PD: Effects of radioulnar instability on the radiocarpal joint: A biomechanical study. *J Hand Surg,* 15A:728-32, 1990.

Computerized analysis of pressure-sensitive film measurement of five cadaver specimens was used to analyze three stages of radioulnar instability. In forearm supination, all stages of radioulnar instability resulted in decreased lunate contact area. In neutral forearm rotation, stage 3 instability demonstrated decreased lunate contact area. In stage 3 instability the lunate high pressure was shifted volar.

Dislocations of the Distal Radioulnar Joint

Buterbaugh GA, Palmer AK: Fractures and dislocations of the distal radioulnar joint. *Hand Clin,* 4(3):361-75, 1988.

A systemic review is presented of the mechanism, presentation, and treatment of fractures and dislocations of the distal radioulnar joint. These injuries included ulna dorsal and ulna volar dislocations as well as lesions associated with fractures of the radial head (Essex-Lopresti lesion) and dislocations of the distal radioulnar joint associated with radial shaft fractures (Galleazzi fractures).

Extensor Carpi Ulnaris Subluxation

Eckhardt WA, Palmer AK: Recurrent dislocation of extensor carpal ulnaris tendon. *J Hand Surg,* 6A:629-631, 1981

Four cases of extensor carpal ulnaris subluxation secondary to sheath attenuation are presented. Sheath reconstruction was successful in relieving symptoms.

Lunotriquetral Instability

Horii E, Garcia-Elias M, An KN, *et al:* A Kinematic study of lunotriquetral dissociations. *J Hand Surg,* 16A:355-62, 1991.

Stereoradiographic analysis of five cadaver specimens showed that the essential lesion to produce a static palmar flexed intercalated segmented instability was transection of the dorsal radiotriquetral and dorsal scaphotriquetral ligaments in addition to the division of the lunotriquetral ligament and interosseous membrane.

Pin PG, Young VL, Gilula LA, Weeks PM: Management of chronic lunotriquetral ligament tears. *J Hand Surg,* 14A:77-83, 1989.

Eleven patients with chronic lunotriquetral ligament tears were treated with lunotriquetral fusion using a compression screw. All patients had fusion achieved at two to five months. Only three patients had persistent pain postoperatively.

Viegas SF, Patterson RM, Peterson PD, *et al:* Ulnar-sided perilunate instability; an anatomic and biomechanic study. *J Hand Surg,* 15A;268-78, 1990.

The spectrum of ulnar-sided perilunate instability is described in three stages based on anatomic disruption and instability. Stage I: lunotriquetral ligament tearing without instability. Stage II: lunotriquetral ligament tear and palmar ligamentous tears with dynamic VISI deformity. Stage III: Complete lunotriquetral disruptions with palmar and dorsal disruption with static VISI deformity.

Pisotriquetral Joint Disorders

Paley D, McMurtry RY, Cruickshank B: Pathologic conditions of the pisiform and pisotriquetral joint. *J Hand Surg,* 12A:110-119, 1987.

This paper reviewed 216 reported cases of pisotriquetral disease in the last 65 years. The authors' experience with 16 cases of pisotriquetral joint disease is described. Pathologic study suggests repetitive trauma leads to dysfunction of the pisotriquetral joint, then to instability, followed by degenerative changes.

Seradge H, Seradge E: Pisotriquetral pain syndrome after carpal tunnel release. *J Hand Surg,* 14A;858-862, 1989.

Pain from the pisotriquetral joint was present in 1.1% of 500 patients six months postoperatively following carpal tunnel release. Pisiform excision was curative.

12

Distal Radius Fractures

William E. Sanders, MD

Introduction

Fractures of the distal radius are very common, usually resulting from falls onto the outstretched extremity. The incidence is as high as 15% of all fractures. Peak occurrence is in the 60 to 70 age group and is higher in women; postural instability and osteoporosis may be contributing factors. Older patients usually sustain fractures with low-energy trauma; young patients sustain fractures with high-energy trauma and the incidence of associated injuries is greater. Despite their frequency, the extent of anatomic disruption, the best treatment options, and the outcome of these fractures are difficult to assess.

Classification

Multiple, sometimes complex classification systems have utilized long-standing eponyms. A classification system should allow outcome studies that evaluate treatment methods and identify the most common fracture patterns to decrease the cost of pretreatment evaluation. A summary of classification systems in current use is shown in Table 12-1.

Table 12-1.

Classification	# Types	Comments
Frykman	8	Widely used for description. Associated ulnar styloid fracture influences classification.
Melone	5	Good for surgical planning (see Figure 12-1).
A O	3 major (over 25 subtypes)	Best for research but too complex for routine use.
Rayhack	4 (3 subgroups)	
Mayo	4	

Unfortunately, many of these classifications are based on plain radiographs. Often only more expensive studies such as polytomes, CT scans, and 3D CT scans allow the surgeon to understand the fracture anatomy, particularly in displaced intra-articular fractures. This author finds polytomes offer the most "bang for the buck." Once the position and/or number of fragments are identified, treatment can be selected.

Associated Injuries

Acute (and delayed) carpal tunnel syndrome can occur from swelling and/or displaced bony fragments.

Intracarpal, radiocarpal, and ulnocarpal ligament injuries are more commonly associated with distal radius fractures in young patients. Triple-injection wrist arthrography and distraction radiographs under anesthesia are most helpful to identify these injuries. There is no consensus regarding concomitant surgical repairs of these associated injuries.

Contusion or separation of the articular cartilage of the radius or carpus may occur. Soft-tissue injuries to surrounding structures (such as stripping of the dorsal retinaculum) are also common.

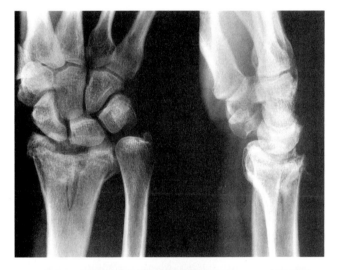

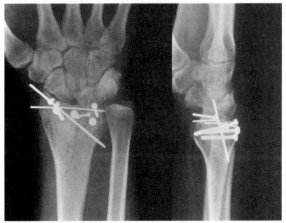

Figure 12-1. A comminuted intra-articular fracture with severe joint depression in a 57-year-old man **(Top)** that was treated by open reduction, autogenous iliac bone graft, and multiple screw and pin fixation **(Bottom)**. No external fixation or protection other than a cast was utilized.

Adequacy of Reduction

Several factors have been identified as prognostic indicators and are used as criteria for an adequate reduction. The relative importance of these is much different in younger than in older patients. These factors and their sequels include the following:

Table 12-2.

Factor	Sequel
Articular stepoff	Arthritis of the affected joint (radioscaphoid, radiolunate, radioulnar). Knirk and Jupiter found that articular depression of >1mm resulted in symptomatic posttraumatic arthritis in 90% of patients they reviewed.
Shortening	Radioulnar joint problems and change in load transmission.
Angulation	Altered wrist mechanics (midcarpal instability) and change in load transmission.

Unfortunately, associated nonosseous injuries are rarely considered. It is difficult to assess the articular cartilage damage. It is not known to what extent associated soft-tissue injuries are responsible for subsequent problems such as pain, limited wrist motion, limited forearm rotation, decreased grip strength, and reflex sympathetic dystrophy. Experience suggests that

- Elderly patients tolerate all types of deformity better than younger ones, and secondary procedures (such as the Darrach resection) are more successful in this group.
- In young patients, restoration of the articular surface is most important. Shortening and angulation can be corrected later if necessary by osteotomy (with good success). However, a malunion of the articular surface is very difficult to address. Many ingenious methods of realigning the articular surface have been reported, such as arthroscopically guided reduction and pinning. Protection of articular cartilage metabolism by drugs or early motion may be helpful.
- Ultimately, treatment of associated (but often unrecognized) soft-tissue injuries may be shown to be of importance.

Concepts of Treatment

It is not sufficient merely to obtain reduction; it must be maintained until healing occurs. The surgeon has only three categorical ways to obtain and maintain reduction: (1) Ligamentotaxis (closed reduction and casting, closed reduction and external fixation). Ligamentotaxis uses traction on the distal osseous structures to reduce the fracture fragments via any intact periarticular ligaments and other soft-tissue structures. (2) Open reduction and/or internal fixation pins, plates, screws. Includes limited open reduction techniques and percutaneous pinning. (3) Obliteration of the defect (bone grafting). The importance of this is proba-

bly underrated. Grafting fills the defect and prevents collapse. It also may aid internal fixation and speed healing so that less deformity occurs before the chosen fixation fails. Autogenous cancellous or corticocancellous grafts are preferable to bank bone because of their osteogenic potential and the current risk of AIDS from bone bank.

Selected combinations of these three are usually applied to a given fracture. Palmer has published an excellent algorithm for treatment selection based on the concepts discussed (Fig. 12-2).

Complications

Malunion may cause pain, decreased motion, distal radioulnar joint problems, secondary arthritis and midcarpal instability. As discussed, changes in radial length and angulation affect load transmission through the TFCC and distal ulna. Palmer and Short have shown that dorsal angular malunion also shifts the areas of maximum transarticular pressure dorsally at the radiocarpal joint.

Distal radioulnar (DRU) joint arthritis can occur following fracture of the distal radius if the fracture is intra-articular into the DRU joint and heals with stepoff or callus. Radial shortening or malunion may also cause radioulnar joint incongruity leading to DRU joint arthritis.

EPL (extensor pollicis longus) rupture is usually seen following nondisplaced distal radius fractures. In these fractures the dorsal retinaculum is not "stripped off" the radius as it is in displaced fractures. The extensor compartments remain intact, and healing callus may narrow the third compartment, resulting in attritional rupture of the EPL. Pain and crepitus at Lister's tubercle with thumb range of motion is an indication for EPL transposition. When rupture occurs, repair is not possible and tendon transfer is required (usually the EIP is used for transfer).

Reflex sympathetic dystrophy (RSD) can occur following any painful injury to the extremity, but is relatively common after distal radius fractures. Mild cases often go unrecognized. Any patient having problems with disproportionate pain or difficulty in regaining finger motion should be examined for RSD and a bone scan obtained for diagnosis (Fig. 12-3). Subclinical carpal tunnel syndrome is a common cause, and may respond to carpal tunnel injection or release. The treatment of RSD is beyond the scope of this section.

Summary of Approach to Treatment

- Study the fracture anatomically (usually by polytomes)
- Select treatment for associated injury(ies)
- Obtain and maintain articular congruity
- Regain length
- Correct angulation
- Consider filling the defect with bone graft
- Remember, the elements of reduction (in order of importance) are articular surface reconstruction, length restoration, and correction of angulation.

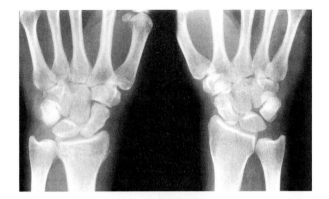

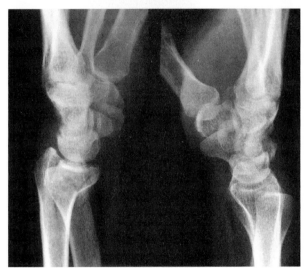

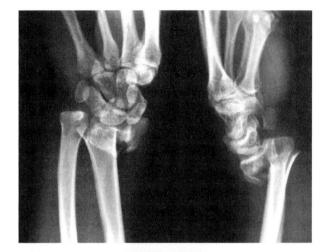

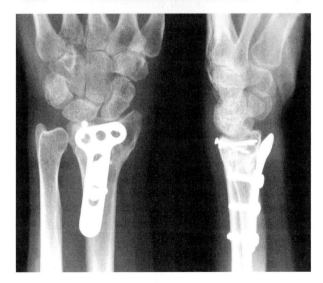

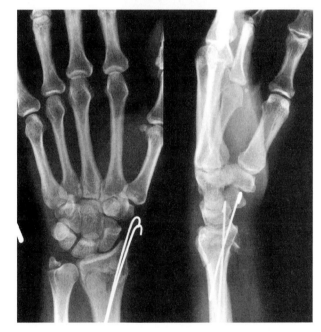

Figure 12-3. A severely displaced distal radius fracture in a 40-year-old woman **(Top)**, treated by closed traction reduction. The two large fracture fragments were anatomically reduced and maintained by percutaneous pinning of the radial styloid **(Bottom)**. The pins were removed at eight weeks.

Figure 12-2. A 35-year-old woman three weeks after a fall resulting in a volar Barton's fracture **(Top)**. There is significant shortening and intra-articular stepoff **(Middle)**. This was treated by open reduction and internal fixation using a combined volar and dorsal approach **(Bottom)**. Satisfactory restoration of the articular surface and improvement in length was obtained. There is mild loss of radial inclination. The normal side is shown for comparison.

A perfect reduction is useless unless it is maintained until healing occurs. Technical perfection and attention to detail are required.

Distal Ulnar Fractures

Fractures involving the distal radioulnar joint include sigmoid notch fractures of the radius and articular fractures (bone and/or cartilage) of the ulnar head. Ulnar styloid frac-

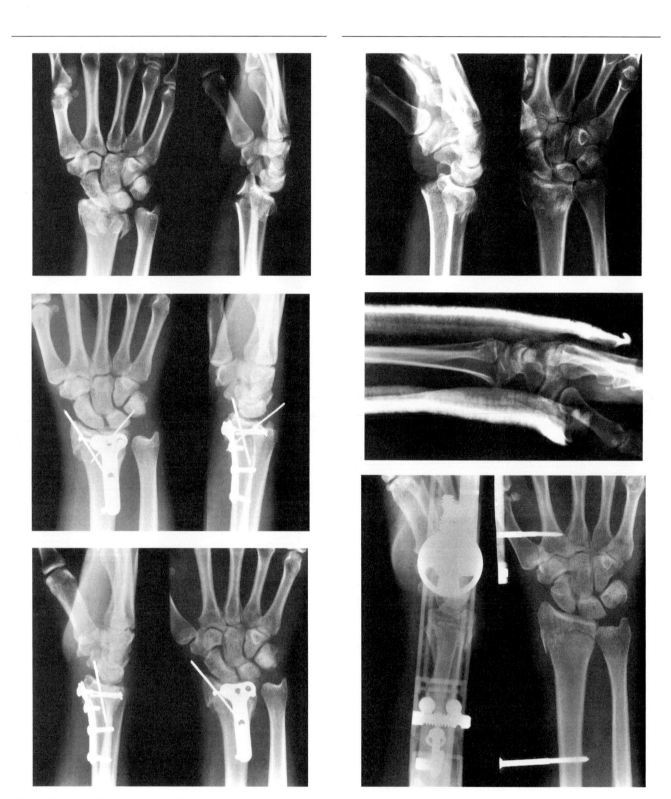

Figure 12-4. A 30-year-old male with a severely comminuted intra-articular fracture of the distal radius **(Top)**. This was aligned with great difficulty by a combination of volar and dorsal approaches. A variety of internal fixation techniques were utilized **(Middle)**. The immediate postoperative results shown were maintained with only slight shortening until healing occurred **(Bottom)**.

Figure 12-5. A significantly displaced distal radius fracture, extra-articular at the radiocarpal joint, intra-articular at the radioulnar joint **(Top)**, that was treated by closed reduction and casting. Radiographs at two weeks showed loss of volar tilt and shortening **(Middle)**. An external fixator was applied with excellent reduction and restoration of a neutral articular tilt **(Bottom)**. Healing was uneventful.

tures may occur alone or in association with a distal radius fracture. Fractures of the radius involving the sigmoid notch are optimally managed by anatomic reduction and internal and external fixation as discussed above. Displaced articular fractures of the ulna should be treated by open reduction. Comminuted ulnar head fractures usually require excision. The TFCC attachment and ulnar shaft length should be preserved if possible. Persistent ulnar wrist pain after injury may be secondary to chondral fractures. These may be identified by arthrotomography.

Isolated ulnar styloid fractures indicate an avulsion of the ulnocarpal ligament complex. These injuries are usually treated by casting in neutral rotation unless the displacement is significant. If the distal radioulnar point is unstable (from an isolated injury, or after stable reduction and fixation of an associated distal radius fracture), ORIF of the styloid fracture and TFCC repair are advocated. Painful styloid nonunions are treated by careful excision of the fragment, leaving intact the ulnar ligaments.

Galeazzi Fractures

This injury is a combination of a distal third radius fracture and subluxation or dislocation of the distal radioulnar joint. Anatomic ORIF of the radius fracture is first performed. If the DRU joint is stable, only casting is needed. If the DRU joint is unstable, repair of the radioulnar ligament(s) and casting are recommended.

Annotated Bibliography

af Ekenstam F, Hagert CG: Anatomical studies on the geometry and stability of the distal radioulnar joint. *Scand J Plast Reconstr Surg,* 19:17-25, 1985.

The distal radioulnar joint is of great importance for normal forearm and hand function. The article presents studies of fresh-frozen and cadaver arm specimens focusing on the articulation surfaces and the ligament structures of the radioulnar joint.

Altissimi M, Antenucci R, Fiacca C, Mancini GB: Long-term result of conservative treatment of fractures of the distal radius. *Clin Orthop,* 206:202-210, 1986.

Two hundred ninety-seven cases involving conservative treatment of wrist fractures are reviewed based on subjective and objective clinical parameters and radiologic features. Radial deviation, volar tilt, and radioulnar index were often out of normal range. Postreduction problems with grip strength, clinical deformity, pain, and numerous compressive neuropathies were noted. Fractures of the distal radius should not be underestimated and conservative management may not produce acceptable results.

Aro HT, Koivunen T: Minor axial shortening of the radius affects outcome of Colles' fracture treatment. *J Hand Surg,* 16A:392-398, 1991.

Shortening of the radius is common after a Colles' fracture. This can significantly alter the transmission of axial forces across the wrist joint, which can result in a permanent disability.

Axelrod TS, McMurtry RY: Open reduction and internal fixation of comminuted, intra-articular fractures of the distal radius. *J Hand Surg,* 15A:1-11, 1990.

A review of 17 patients from 1981-86 with comminuted intra-articular fractures of the distal radius treated by open reduction after failure of closed means. The technical demands of, and the results to be expected from, formal open reduction internal fixation are addressed and discussion concerning the high complication rate often following ORIF is also addressed.

Axelrod TS, Paley D, Green J, McMurtry RY: Limited open reduction of the lunate facet in comminuted intra-articular fractures of the distal radius. *J Hand Surg,* 13A:372-377, 1988.

A technique for lunate facet reduction associated with a distal radius fracture is introduced. This procedure, done under radiographic control involves limited operative exposure and tissue trauma. This method of restoration under fluoroscopy involves both external fixation and percutaneous pinning. The technique and two case reports are presented.

Bartosh RA, Saldana MJ: Intra-articular fractures of the distal radius: a cadaveric study to determine if ligamentotaxis restores radiopalmar tilt. *J Hand Surg,* 15A:18-21, 1990.

Nineteen fresh cadaver wrists were divested of all dorsal and palmar tissues and intrinsic and extrinsic ligaments. A Frykmann VII type fracture was introduced across radiocarpal and radioulnar joints. Attempts were made to reestablish radiopalmar tilt by ligamentotaxis. It was concluded that this method is limited as the sole method for restoring radiopalmar tilt.

Bradway JK, Amadio PC, Cooney WP: Open reduction and internal fixation of displaced, comminuted intra-articular fractures of the distal end of the radius. *J Bone Joint Surg,* 71A:839-847, 1989.

A retrospective study of 16 patients with displaced, comminuted intra-articular fractures of the distal end of the radius treated by open reduction and internal fixation were reviewed. A stepoff of 2mm or more in the distal radius articular surface was associated with an increase in the incidence of posttraumatic arthritis.

Dias JJ, Wray CC, Jones JM: Osteoporosis and Colles' fractures in the elderly. *J Hand Surg,* 12B:57-59, 1987.

A prospective study of 127 patients older than 50 years of age with unilateral Colles' fractures to determine the incidence of osteoporosis and to investigate its influence on bony deformity. Seventy-eight percent were found to be osteoporotic. The final deformity was significantly greater in patients with osteoporosis.

Fernandez DL: Correction of posttraumatic wrist deformity in adults by osteotomy, bone grafting and internal fixation. *J Bone Joint Surg,* 64A:1164-1178, 1982.

A corrective osteotomy for posttraumatic malalignment of the distal radius is reviewed. This reconstructive procedure uses an opening wedge metaphyseal osteotomy combined with insertion of a graft and rigid internal fixation with a plate and screws permitting early motion. This procedure is recommended for young, manually active patients with significant deformity and functional impairment due to malalignment.

Fernandez DL, Geissler WB: Treatment of displaced articular fractures of the radius. *J Hand Surg,* 16A:375-384, 1991.

A presentation of the indications and techniques of surgical restoration of the articular surface of the distal radius and a retrospective radiographic analysis of the results from 40 patients.

Heim U, Pfeiffer KM: *Small Fragment Set Manual.* 2nd Ed;119-161. Springer-Verlag, New York, 1982.

Hirasawa Y, Katsumi Y, Akiyoshi T, Tamai K, Tokioka T: Clinical and microangiographic studies on rupture of the EPL tendon after distal radial fractures. *J Hand Surg,* 15B:51-57, 1990.

A study on the mechanics of ruptured extensor pollicis longus tendons as a complication of fractures in the distal radius is done. A microvascular study on five cadavers revealed that the EPU tendon is subject to mechanical bending and attrition, has no mesotendineum, and has a poorly vascularized portion about 5mm in length, which may be a cause of spontaneous rupture of the tendon.

Knirk JL, Jupiter JB: Intra-articular fractures of the distal end of the radius in young adults. *J Bone Joint Surg,* 68A:647-659, 1986.

A retrospective study of 43 intra-articular distal radius fractures in 40 young adults was conducted. Emphasis was placed on evaluating the critical factors in the assessment and management of the fracture and the development of posttraumatic arthritis with this complex injury.

Leung KS, Shen WY, Leung PC, Kinninmonth AWG, Change JCW, Chan GPY: Ligamentotaxis and bone grafting for comminuted fractures of the distal radius. *J Bone Joint Surg,* 71B:838-842, 1989.

A review of 72 distal radial fractures treated with ligamentotaxis by means of an external fixator for three weeks and bone grafting followed by a carefully monitored program of rehabilitation. Reduction was maintained during healing and more than 80% regained full range of motion in hands, wrists, and forearms with pain-free wrist function. Complications were infrequent and not serious.

Melone CP Jr: Articular fractures of the distal radius. *Orthop Clin North Am,* 15:217-236, 1984.

Based on the experiences of 330 articular fractures of the distal radius, this article defines the patterns of injury and proposes a classification to guide optimal treatment. It also describes techniques that have proved consistently successful for the more complex injuries.

Melone CP Jr: Open treatment for displaced articular fractures of the distal radius. *Clin Orthop,* 202:103-111, 1986.

Maximum recovery of wrist function following articular distal radius fractures depends on acceptable and stable reduction of the radial articular surfaces. In injuries with major disruption, the fracture site may need to be opened in order to preserve the distal radial articulation. This article describes open treatment techniques and analyzes the results of such treatment in cases of complex articular fractures.

Nakata RY, Chand Y, Matiko JD, Frykman GK, Wood VE: External fixators for wrist fractures: a biomechanical and clinical study. *J Hand Surg,* 10A:845-851, 1985.

This article compares *in vitro* the rigidity of four available designs of external fixators and presents the clinical results of one of the fixators.

Palmer AK: Fractures of the distal radius. In Green DP (ed) *Operative Hand Surgery,* 3rd Ed: 929-971. Churchill Livingstone, New York, 1993.

This chapter reviews the anatomy of distal radial fractures along with an in-depth review of the traditional concept of classification and treatment and newer classification and treatment schemes. A preferred method for treating these fractures and their complications, both acute and late in the adult and pediatric amputation is outlined.

Peltier LF: Fractures of the distal end of the radius: a historical account. *Clin Orthop,* 187:18-22, 1984.

Historically, fractures of the distal radius were thought to be dislocations of the wrist. This account reviews the treatment of these fractures along with identification, including three distinct varieties to which the eponyms of Colles, Smith, and Baron have been applied.

Pogue DJ, Viegas SF, Patterson RM, Peterson PD, Jenkins DK, Sweo TD, Hokanson JA: Effects of distal radius fracture malunion on wrist joint mechanics. *J Hand Surg,* 15A:721-727, 1990.

This study investigates the effects that various components of distal radius fracture malunion have on pressure distributions second contact areas in the wrist.

Rayhack JM, Langworthy JN, Belsole RJ: Transulnar percutaneous pinning of displaced distal radial fractures: a preliminary report. *J Orthop Trauma,* 3(2):107-114, 1989.

Maintaining reduction in distal radial fractures can be a major problem. Four to five Kirschner pins are placed percutaneously through the ulna into the radius in an attempt to maintain reduction. The methods and advantages are reviewed and discussed.

Sanders RA, Keppel FL, Waldrop JI: External fixation of distal radial fractures: results and complications. *J Hand Surg,* 16A:385-391, 1991.

Thirty-five distal radial fractures are reviewed in 34 patients (all healed with external fixation) to see if the results warrant the use of external fixation. Frequency of complications and limitations associated with this method require extra care on the part of the surgeon to prevent iatrogenic morbidity that can limit the benefit of external fixation.

Seitz WH Jr, Putnam MD, Dick HM: Limited open surgical approach for external fixation of distal radius fractures. *J Hand Surg,* 15A:288-293, 1990.

Pin placement is frequently associated with complications in use of external fixation. This article presents a technique and the clinical results of a method allowing the visualization of the bony target by using a limited open surgical approach.

Short WH, Palmer AK, Werner FW, Murphy DJ: A biomechanical study of distal radial fractures. *J Hand Surg,* 12A:529-534, 1987.

An experiment using fresh cadaver arms was designed to study the distribution of forces and change in the pressure across the distal radial and ulnocarpal joints after introducing a distal radial fracture. As dorsal angulation increases the changes in the pressure distribution of the ulnar and radial articular surfaces become more concentrated.

Watson HK, Castle TH Jr: Trapezoidal osteotomy of the distal radius for unacceptable articular angulation after Colles' fracture. *J Hand Surg,* 13A:837-843, 1988.

A techinque using trapezoidal corticocancellous bone grafts is used to maintain radiopalmar tilt in Colles' fracture malunions. Functional results in 15 patients were compared with a series using ICBG, plate and screws. The simple technique has the advantage of avoiding disruption of the extensor retinaculum and the need for the reoperation for hardware removal.

III

Tendons

13

Experimental Studies of the Structure and Function of Tendon

James W. Strickland, MD

Introduction

Considerable research has been expended in recent years in an effort to better understand the structure of tendons, their method of function, the biomechanics of their action at the joints they move, and their biologic response to injury and repair. These investigative efforts have given rise to improved methods of tendon repair, a greater emphasis on flexor sheath preservation and restoration, and the early application of stress in an effort to more rapidly increase the strength and gliding of repaired tendons. Although fairly voluminous, tendon research is often contradictory and confusing and the clinical application of some studies is questionable. This chapter reviews some of the most significant recent research in this area and emphasis is placed on the flexor tendons, where most studies have concentrated.

Structure and Anatomy

Tendons are composed of fascicles of long, narrow spiraling bundles of tendon cells (tenocytes) and primarily type I collagen fibers. Both synovial cells and fibroblasts have been identified in the tendon-cell population. The fascicle surface usually has a layer of uniform collagen fibers and elastin. Individual fascicles are capable of sliding past each other with no apparent direct attachments or cellular communications. The surface of the individual bundles of collagen is covered by the endotenon, which surrounds the fascicles, blood vessels, and nerves. A fine fibrous outer layer, the epitenon, is highly cellular and is continuous with the endotenon. Most of the blood vessels and capillaries are contained in this layer. In the palm of the hand, flexor tendon fascicles are covered by a thin visceral and parietal adventitia called paratenon, which is comprised of collagen fibrils that are parallel to the long axis of the tendon. The paratenon is continuous with the synovial mesotenon and provides nutrients to the tendon while allowing tendon gliding.

In the distal palm and digits, the flexor tendons are enclosed in synovial sheaths lined by both a visceral synovial layer that covers the flexor digitorum superficialis and profundus tendons, and a parietal layer that is continuous with the annular and cruciate sections of the sheath and with a proximal mesotenon (Fig. 13-1). The tendons are attached to the sheath only by the filmy vinculae, and the sheaths have predictable segmental thickenings which form strong annular pulleys interposed with thin synovial sections that collapse to allow the pulleys to approximate to each other during digital flexion. The A-2 and A-4 are fibro-osseous annular pulleys arising from the periosteum of the proximal half of the proximal phalanx and the middle third

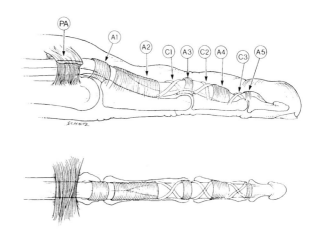

Figure 13-1. The components of the digital flexor sheath are depicted in this drawing. The sturdy annular pulleys (A-1 through A-5) are important biomechanically in keeping the tendons closely applied to the phalanges. The thin, pliable cruciate pulleys collapse to allow full digital flexion. A recent addition has been the palmar aponeurosis pulley which adds to the biomechanical efficiency of the sheath system. Figure 13-1 modified and reproduced with permission from Idler RS: Anatomy and biomechanics of the digital flexor tendons. *Hand Clin,* 1:1:12-13, 1985.

of the middle phalanx, respectively. The A-1, A-3, and A-5 are joint pulleys arising successively from the palmar plates of the metacarpophalangeal, proximal interphalangeal, and distal interphalangeal joints. An important additional annular pulley, the palmar aponeurosis pulley, is composed of the transverse and vertical fibers of the palmar fascia; it is located 1 to 3mm distal to the cul-de-sac of the synovial sheath with an average width of 9mm. It plays an important role in preventing the loss of digital flexion when other proximal components of the sheath have been lost. The condensable cruciate portions of the sheath are the C-1 between the A-2 and A-3 pulleys, C-2 between A-3 and A-4, and C-3 between A-4 and A-5. In the area of the pulleys, flexor tendons have segments that are avascular and have been shown in certain experimental animals to contain tissue that resembles fibrocartilage.

Flexor tendons are usually oval in configuration, compared to extensor tendons in the hand, which are flatter. Tendons such as the flexor digitorum superficialis may arise from a single muscle bundle and act independently, while others such as the flexor digitorum profundus have a common muscle origin for several tendons, resulting in simultaneous function of several digits. Long, extrinsic digital flexor tendon excursion may exceed 8cm in order to produce composite wrist and digital joint flexion, while extensor tendons and the wrist flexors and extensors require considerably less movement. The flexor digitorum profundus acts as the primary digital flexor while the superficialis and the interossei combine for forceful flexion. Digital balance and equilibrium during flexion and extension requires a complex integration of extrinsic and intrinsic activity, and strong forces in the neighborhood of 200 N can be achieved during power grip.

Nutrition

The vascular perfusion of human flexor tendons has been shown to have several sources. Longitudinal vessels enter the tendons in the palm and extend down intratendinous channels; vessels also enter the tendon at the level of the proximal synovial fold or reflection in the distal palm; segmental branches from the paired digital arteries enter the tendons in the flexor sheath through the long and short vincula; and vessels enter the superficialis and profundus tendons at their osseous insertions (Fig. 13-2). The vascularity of digital flexor tendons is richer dorsally and injection studies have identified consistent areas of avascularity. Both the profundus and the superficialis have avascular segments over the proximal phalanx between the synovial reflection and their first vinculum, and the profundus has a second avascular zone over the middle phalanx between its long and short vincula.

Synovial fluid diffusion has been shown to be an alternative nutritional pathway for flexor tendons and may actually function more rapidly and completely than vascular perfusion. Tendon sheath fluid contains concentrations of hyaluronate and several proteins similar to the composition of normal joint fluid. It may provide a significant contribution to the lubrication and nutrition of gliding flexor tendons. The delivery of nutrients from the synovial fluid is apparently accomplished by a pumping mechanism known as imbibition in which fluid is forced into the interstices of the tendon through small ridges or conduits in the tendon surface which are oriented at 90° to each other. This pumping process is enhanced by finger flexion as the tendon glides across the fibro-osseous pulleys.

Biochemical Composition

Normal adult flexor tendons are composed of greater than 95% Type I collagen with the remaining 5% consisting of Type III and Type V collagens. The collagen is arranged in a triple helix of tropocollagen molecules with a three-fold helix around a single protein molecule. While the collagen content of tendons increases with age, the rate of synthesis remains relatively constant.

Biomechanical Properties

Tendons are composed of dense collagen fibers arranged parallel to each other in the direction of the force of the muscle. They possess one of the highest tensile strengths of

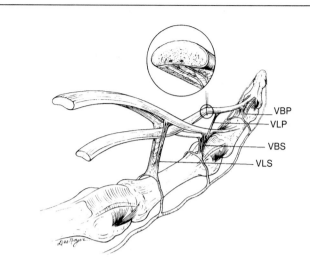

Figure 13-2.   The blood supply to the flexor tendons within the digital sheath is illustrated. The segmental vascular supply to the flexor tendons by means of long and short vincular connections is shown, with the vinculum brevis consisting of small triangular mesentaries located near the insertion of the superficialis and profundus tendons. The vinculum longum to the superficialis tendon arises from the floor of the digital sheath and the proximal aspect of the proximal phalanx and the vinculum longum to the profundus tendon arises from the superficialis at the level of the proximal interphalangeal joint. The cut-away view depicts the relative avascularity of the palmar side of the flexor tendons in Zone 1 and 2 when compared with the richer blood supply on the dorsal side which connects with the vincula. (VBS=vinculum brevis superficialis; VBP=vinculum brevis profundus; VLS=vinculum longus superficialis; VLP=vinculum longus profundus). Figures 13-2 and 13-3 modified and reproduced with permission from Strickland JW: the management of acute flexor tendon injuries. *Orthop Clin of N Am*, 14-4:831-832, 1983.

all soft tissues, which permits the transmission of muscle forces to the skeleton with minimal stretching. Because collagen in different parts of the tendons have different crimp lengths and angles, tendons have great extensibility at low tensile loads and less extensibility at higher loads. The viscoelastic properties of tendons also depends on the architectural interaction of the collagen and elastin fibers. The ultimate strain value for flexor tendons ranges from 9% to 30% with variations resulting from differences in the species, type, and age of the tendons studied and the use of different methods of testing and measurement.

The stress-strain curve for tendons is similar to other collagenous soft tissues such as ligaments. Initially the tendon deforms easily with little tensile force followed by a linear area thought to represent the elastic stiffness of tendon. Microfailure of some fiber bundles may produce small dips and, finally, with additional loading, the tendon ruptures. The rate of loading has little effect on this relationship, although the viscoelastic and viscoplastic characteristics of tendons tend to shift the curve to the right. Immobilization of tendons results in a loss of water content, glycosaminoglycan concentration, and strength, whereas exercise training results in increased collagen fibril size, and increased strength and stiffness. The alteration of mechanical properties is greater in extensor than in flexor tendons, with the difference attributed to anatomic and biochemical differences and the varying loads that the two tendons experience.

Wrist and digital joint movement results either from passive externally applied forces or muscle-tendon forces applied during active movement. While there are modest differences between the calculated flexor tendon excursions required to produce full flexion at all joints distal to the point of measurement, an adjustment between the differing reports would suggest that the superficialis moves about 26mm and the profundus 23mm at midpalm, the superficialis 16mm and the profundus 17mm over the proximal phalanx, and the profundus 5mm over the middle phalanx (Fig. 13-3). The greater the distance a tendon is from the axis of joint rotation, the greater the moment arm and the less motion a given muscle contracture will generate at that joint. Conversely, a shorter moment arm results in more joint rotation from the same tendon excursion.

The moment arm, excursion, and joint rotation produced by the flexor tendons are governed by the constraint of the pulley system. Loss of portions of the digital pulleys may significantly alter the normal integrated balance between the flexor, intrinsic, and extensor tendons. In particular, the A-2 and A-4 pulleys are the most biomechanically impor-

tant and destruction of all or a substantial portion of either pulley may lead to a loss of digital motion and power and produce flexion contractures of the overlying joints (Fig. 13-4). Recent studies using a custom-made loading device determined that the A-2 was the longest and strongest pulley; the A-1 and A-4 the next strongest, and the A-3 the weakest in terms of absolute breaking load because of its shortness. The A-2 and A-4 were found to be mechanically stronger and stiffer than the palmar plate pulleys: A-1, A-3, and A-5.

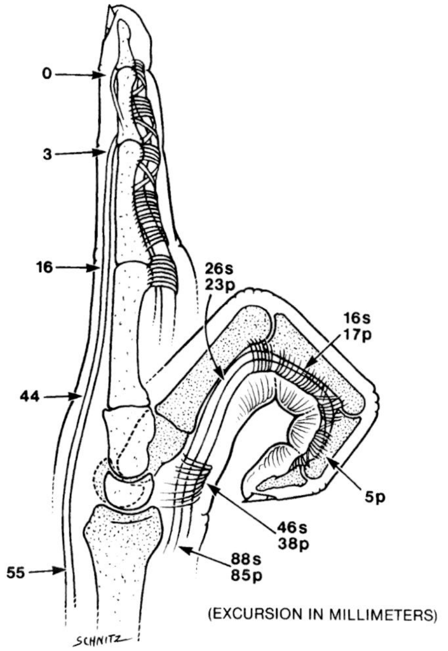

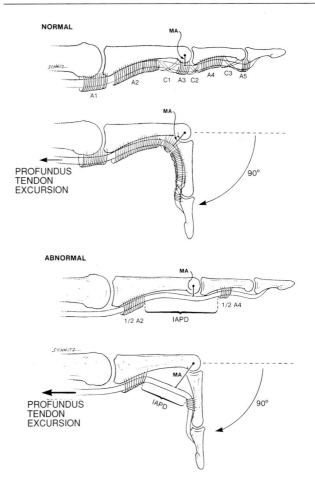

Figure 13-4. The function of the finger flexor tendon pulley system is illustrated. **(Normal)** The arrangement of the annular and cruciate synovial pulleys of the finger flexor tendon sheath. Depiction of the normal moment arm, and profundus tendon excursion, which occurs with the intact fibro-osseous canal as the proximal interphalangeal joint is flexed to 90°. Annular pulleys: A-1, A-2, A-3, A-4, A-5; cruciate pulleys: C-1, C-2, C-3. **(Abnormal)** The biomechanical alteration resulting from the excision of the distal one-half of the A-2 pulley together with the C-1, A-3, C-2, and proximal portion of the A-4 pulley are shown. The distance between the distal edge of the A-2 and the proximal edge of the A-4 pulley is shown as the intra-annular pulley distance. The moment arm is increased and a greater profundus tendon excursion will be required to produce 90° of flexion because of the bowstringing that results from the loss of pulley support.

Figure 13-3. The approximate flexor tendon motion necessary to produce full flexion of digital joints at the forearm, wrist, hand, and digital levels are illustrated. Figures 13-2 and 13-3 modified and reproduced with permission from Strickland JW: the management of acute flexor tendon injuries. *Orthop Clin of N Am,* 14-4:831-832, 1983. Figure 13-3 modified and reproduced with permission from Verdan C: Primary repair of flexor tendons. *J Bone Joint Surg,* 42A:647-657, 1960.

Mathematical equations have been developed to identify the factors influencing digital motion and the moment arm of tendons at a joint. These factors are the distance of the pulley from the joint axis, the perpendicular distance from the edge of the pulley to the longitudinal axis of the bone, and the angle of joint motion.

Any alteration that increases either the distance of the pulley from the axis of the joint or the pulley edge from the longitudinal axis of the bone increases both the moment arm and the tendon excursion necessary to produce flexion of the joint. The average moment arms of the flexor profundus and superficialis at the metacarpophalangeal, proximal and distal interphalangeal joints has been calculated, and, because the profundus has been shown to have a larger moment arm than the superficialis at both the distal and proximal interphalangeal joints, motion at these joints produces differential gliding between the two flexor tendons. The greater the motion at the interdigital joints, the greater the gliding between the two tendons; the hook and the fist position has been demonstrated to produce the most differential motion.

There have been several studies designed to determine the forces generated by various passive and active functions. Mathematical models have been largely unsuccessful because they require kinematic measurements based on the line of action and moment arms of muscles and tendons passing a joint, and must also consider the physiologic constraints of muscles (length-tension and force velocity relationships). Tendon-tension transducers and electromyographic signals have provided measurements that allow the calculation of muscle and tendon forces during isometric activities; strain-gauge transducers have been used to measure the forces in the digital and thumb flexors during operative procedures such as carpal tunnel release. While the methodology used and the results reported from these studies vary, it appears that during passive extension and flexion without resistance, flexor tendons have 2 to 4N of force respectively. Active flexion with "mild" resistance may produce up to 10 N of force, "moderate" resisted flexion up to 17 N, and strong composite grasp as much as 70 N. Firm tip pinch can apparently generate as much as 120 N of tensile load for the index flexor profundus. Forces produced by the flexor superficialis tendon have been shown to be two to seven times less than those produced by the flexor profundus during grasp and pinch. From a clinical point of view, it should be remembered that these loads are substantially increased by the resistance created by a swollen, stiffened finger. Pressure between the pulleys and the flexor tendons may reach as much as 700 mg Hg during active flexion, perhaps explaining the histologic alterations to a cartilage-like material seen in flexor tendons beneath annular digital pulleys.

Tendon Healing

Cellular

After much debate, most investigators now believe that tendons have both an intrinsic and an extrinsic capability to heal and that the relative contribution of each will depend on the type of injury and the method of repair. In the clinical setting, it is probably impossible to isolate the two types of healing. While an overview of current concepts of flexor tendon healing is presented here, the cellular events are similar for all tendons. As with other tissues, tendon healing involves three phases: an inflammatory phase, a fibroblastic or collagen-producing phase, and a remodeling phase. The biologic events that comprise each of these phases are summarized (Fig. 13-5).

Inflammatory Phase

Immediately after tendon injury and repair, the defect is filled with clotted blood, tissue debris, and fluid. Three days after injury, an inflammatory response predominates and is characterized by the presence of cells that originate from the extrinsic peritendinous tissues and intrinsic cells arising from the epitenon and endotenon. The epitenon cells proliferate, migrate into the laceration site, and subsequently bridge the defect. Peritendinous structures also appear to make a fibroblastic and vascular contribution to this initial healing including the synovial sheath, periosteum, subcutaneous tissues, and fascia. These cells appear during the first 48 to 72 hours and proliferate and migrate into the laceration site, where their function is phagocytic involving the removal of cellular debris and collagen remnants, in addition to synthesizing new collagen fibers. The extent to which intrinsic vs. extrinsic fibroblasts contribute to the repair process at the laceration site is not known but may depend on factors unique to a particular injury and the surgical repair.

Fibroblastic/Collagen-Producing Phase

Collagen secretion begins by the fifth day and collagen fibers are formed in a random, disorganized fashion. Fibroblasts become the predominate cell type and collagen content increases for the first four weeks. There is a marked fibroblastic proliferation from the endotenon by the 21st day of the repair process and these fibroblasts participate actively in both the synthesis and resorption of collagen. The fibroblasts and collagen fibrils are initially oriented in a plane perpendicular to the long axis of the tendon, and collagen reorientation is complete by 28 days after injury. The synovium of the sheath has been reconstituted by the 21st day and, as the wound matures, a smooth gliding surface redevelops. At the same time, vascularization increases at the repair site, including penetration of the former "avascular zones" by new vessels extending from the surface epitenon vessels; this occurs in the absence of tendon adhesions. There is increased strength at the repair site beginning at two to three weeks after laceration and repair.

Fibronectin, a glycoprotein found in plasma and on cell surfaces, has been shown to promote fibroblast adhesion to denatured collagen and fibrin and serves as a chemotactic agent for fibroblasts, promoting fibroblast migration into wound beds. As such, fibronectin appears to be an important component of the early tendon healing process. Recent studies have shown that fibroblast chemotaxis and adherence to the substratum in the early days after tendon injury

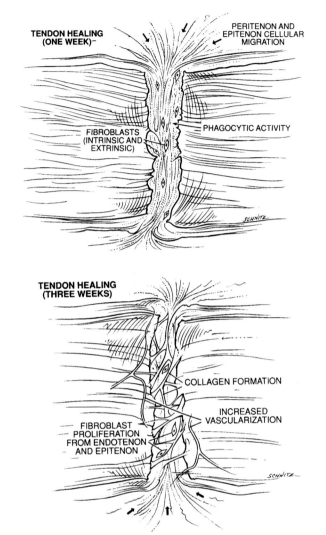

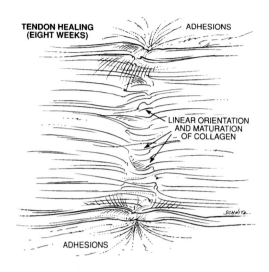

Figure 13-5. Tendon healing. Artist's representation of the biologic sequence. **(Top Left)** At one week an inflammatory response predominates and the laceration site is filled with cells which originate from the extrinsic peritendinous tissues and from the epitenon and endotenon. The cells proliferate and their function is largely phagocytic together with the synthesis of new collagen. **(Bottom Left)** At three weeks there is marked fibroblastic proliferation from the endotenon and epitenon and these fibroblasts participate in both the synthesis and resorption of collagen. The fibroblasts and collagen are in a plane perpendicular to the long axis of the tendon and revascularization increases at the repair site, including penetration of the former "avascular zones" by new vessels. **(Top Right)** At eight weeks, the collagen is mature and realigned in linear fashion. Adhesions are stimulated both by the initial trauma to the tendon and sheath and by immobilization.

and repair appear to be directly related to fibronectin secretion. It increases dramatically in the epitenon adjacent to the repair site seven days after repair and, by 17 days, the fibronectin content has decreased appreciably at the repair site and in the tendon stumps.

Remodeling Phase

By 28 days, the fibroblasts have become more longitudinally oriented and a progressive remodeling and realignment of collagen fibrils occurs. By 42 days, fibroblasts originating from the endotenon play the most active part in the healing process. It appears that the formation of dense collagen tissue leading to tendon adhesions is stimulated both by the trauma to the tendon sheath and immobilization. By six weeks after injury, the repair site gap is completely filled with collagen. At eight weeks, the collagen is mature and realigned in a linear fashion. The ultimate tensile load of

repaired tendons is achieved only after they are subjected to physiologic loading. By 112 days after the injury, there appears to be a complete maturation of the repair site and fibroblasts have reverted to quiescent tenocytes.

Healing flexor tendons are frequently characterized by the ingrowth of fibroblasts from the digital sheath and cellular proliferation of the epitenon, often resulting in dense scar that restricts tendon gliding. These restrictive adhesions are more significant in tendons that have been immobilized. When the synovial sheath has been extensively injured, the extrinsic healing mechanism predominates and adhesions are inevitable. When there is little damage to the flexor sheath from either injury or repair, there is a more favorable balance between the contributions of the epitenon and the endotenon tenocytes and restricting adhesions are not as intense. Gapping or elongation at the repair site may be secondary to strangulation of the microcirculation at the tendon ends, and it has been demonstrated that collagen fills the gap and stretches with cyclic stress. The elongated area becomes the weakest link in the repair chain and the first area to yield. Gaps of 3mm or greater have been associated with increased adhesions and worse results following flexor tendon repair.

Biomechanical

During the inflammatory phase of tendon healing, the strength of the repair is almost entirely that imparted by the suture itself with a modest contribution from the fibrin in the clot between the tendon ends. The strength increases rapidly during the fibroblastic collagen-producing phase when granulation tissue is formed in the defect. When extrinsic healing mechanisms predominate, adhesions between the tendon and its surrounding tissues are inevitable. Conversely, intrinsic healing by the tenocytes usually results in fewer, less dense adhesions. During this phase, collagen fibrils are laid down in a random fashion and have minimal strength. As the collagen is stabilized by cross-linking and realigns itself longitudinally, the strength of the repair increases. In the remodeling or maturation phase, reorganization of the fiber architecture along the direction of muscle force results in a dramatic increase in the mechanical strength of the healing tendon.

It has been established that a healing tendon can be strengthened by the application of tension forces, which may cause a more rapid realignment of the molecules in collagen fibers. In a series of outstanding laboratory investigations, Gelberman and his coworkers demonstrated that passive mobilization led to a more rapid recovery of tensile strength, fewer adhesions, improved excursion, better nutrition, and minimal repair-site deformation of repaired canine flexor tendons when compared to immobilized repairs. They concluded that passive mobilization enhances healing by stimulating maturation of the tendon wound simultaneously with the remodeling of tendon scar. While many questions remain to be answered, it would appear that the most effective current method of returning strength and excursion to repaired tendons would involve the use of a strong gap-reducing suture technique followed by the application of controlled stress on the repaired tendon.

Soluble Factors Influencing Tendon Healing

Considerable research is being conducted in an effort to understand the influence that soluble polypeptides including mitogens (growth factors and hormones), as well as chemotactic and differentiating factors exert on the cellular sequence of tendon repair. These factors have been demonstrated to play a role in both normal physiologic and pathologic processes. They stimulate cell proliferation, matrix synthesis, and cell differentiation; their specific activity varies with the concentration. They may act alone or in synergy with other factors, and a better understanding of their mechanism of action may lead to improved methods of controlling the biologic events associated with tendon healing. One such factor, platelet-derived growth factor, stimulates DNA synthesis and cell division. Its interaction with the cell may provide important information about the regu-

latory mechanisms that control fibroblastic growth during tendon repair.

Another factor, TGF-ß, is a soluble polypeptide that is present in a variety of cells and stimulates the production of fibronectin and collagen by dermal fibroblasts *in vitro.* TGF-ß has been shown to induce fibroblast chemotaxis and its release from platelets, lymphocytes, monocytes, and macrophages may be important for the migration of cells into the tendon repair site. In addition, TGF-ß can induce further differentiation of fibroblastic cells for enhanced synthesis of collagen and this stimulatory activity can be blocked by specific antibodies to TGF-ß. TGF-ß can also cause a strong angiogenic response, which is important in tendon healing. Although it may function by itself, *in vivo,* it also appears to act in concert with other polypeptide growth factors, such as epidermal growth factor, platelet-derived growth factor, and basic fibroblastic growth factor. Important investigation of the cellular role of these factors on the healing response of tendons is ongoing.

Adhesion Formation and Control

Factors that influence the formation of excursion-restricting adhesions around repaired tendons include trauma to the tendon and sheath from the initial injury or from the reparative surgery, tendon ischemia, immobilization, gapping at the repair site, and sheath excision. Adhesions have been shown to form quantitatively in proportion to the extent of tissue crushing and the number of surface injuries to the tendon. Disruption of the vincular system has also been associated with a decrease in tendon excursion. There is considerable debate as to whether sheath repair is favorable for adhesion reduction.

Various biochemical agents have been studied in an attempt to modify adhesion formation around tendon repairs. These agents include steroids, antihistamines, and anti-inflammatory drugs. Anabolic steroids (dexamethasone and norethandrolone) and an antihistamine (promethazine) were compared in an effort to determine their effect on collagen production and tendon healing. Maximum collagen healing was achieved in the norethandrolone-treated group at 10 to 14 days after tendon repair, while the dexamethasone- and promethazine-treated groups demonstrated maximum synthesis between 14 and 28 days. A lathyrogenic agent, beta-aminoproprionitrile, which blocks the conversion of lysine in peptide linkages to an aldehyde, has also been investigated. Although it proved to inhibit adhesions after flexor tendon repairs in chickens, it was found to have untoward side effects in a clinical trial. Newer analogs of BAPN may prove useful since the toxic side effects have apparently been eliminated.

Nonsteroidal anti-inflammatory drugs (ibuprofen and indomethacin), may also reduce post-injury/repair adhesions and improve tendon excursion by blocking prostaglandin synthesis through the inhibition of the enzyme cyclooxygenase at the cell level. Ibuprofen has been shown to decrease adhesion formation after flexor tendon repairs in primates but there is also a significant reduction in repair strength. The effect of hyaluronate on

FLEXOR TENDON REPAIR METHODS

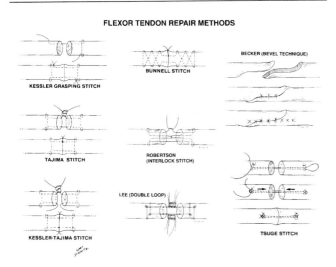

KESSLER GRASPING STITCH

BUNNELL STITCH

BECKER (BEVEL TECHNIQUE)

TAJIMA STITCH

ROBERTSON (INTERLOCK STITCH)

LEE (DOUBLE LOOP)

KESSLER-TAJIMA STITCH

TSUGE STITCH

Figure 13-6. End-to-end flexor tendon repair methods. The Robertson and Lee methods are four-strand repairs and approximately twice as strong as the two-strand methods.

monkey tendon healing has also been investigated with the finding that there was a 27% less flexion deformity than saline-treated controls without inhibiting the diffusion of nutrients. In a double blind clinical study, however, hyaluronate was found to have no statistically significant effect on total active motion. No drug has yet been clearly shown to diminish adhesions without delaying wound or tendon healing or increasing the incidence of infection.

An ultrastructural study of the effect of constant direct electrical current on the intrinsic healing of rabbit flexor tendons in vitro suggests that low amperage currents may suppress adhesion causing synovial proliferation in the epitenon and promote active collagen synthesis in the tenocytes.

Tendon Suture Methods

Numerous methods of tendon suture (Fig 13-6) have been advocated throughout the years in an effort to satisfy the following characteristics for an ideal repair: (1) sufficient strength throughout healing to permit the application of early motion stress to the tendon; (2) sutures easily placed in the tendon; (3) secure knots; (4) minimal gapping at the repair site; (5) minimal interference with tendon vascularity; and (6) smooth juncture of tendon ends with minimal bulk.

Most current repair methods employ the technique first described by Kirchmayr in 1917 and later popularized by Kessler in 1973, or one of its many variations. Evaluation of the relative strengths of several commonly used repair methods have been carried out both *in vitro* and *in vivo* in laboratory animals. Unfortunately it is difficult for one to draw any meaningful conclusions from these comparative studies because of the many differences in the experimental protocols, measurement methodology, animals selected, suture materials, the use of a peripheral epitenon suture, the diverse

definitions of tendon repair failure, (i.e. rupture, gapping of greater than 1mm, 2mm, or 3mm) and the technical skill of each investigator.

A thorough attempt to compare the findings of a number of investigations would lead to several general conclusions with regard to the strength of various tendon repairs. (1) Regardless of the method employed, the strength of a flexor tendon repair is roughly proportional to the number of suture strands that cross the repair site. (2) The repair strength in unstressed tendons probably decreases by 10% to 60% between five and 21 days after repair. (3) Repair strength increases more rapidly when the tendon is subjected to early motion stress. (4) Repair strength is not significantly altered by the caliber of the suture material. (5) Repairs usually rupture at the suture knots. (6) Locking loops contribute little strength to the repair and may actually collapse and lead to repair gapping at moderate loads.

The observation that the number of suture strands crossing the repair strongly influences the strength of the repair is best demonstrated by Savage, who found that a complex six-strand repair was three times stronger than a two-strand repair; and by two recently published four-strand repair methods that were found to be approximately twice the strength of two-strand methods *in vitro*. Assuming a 50% decrease in the strength of these four-strand methods during the first three weeks of healing, the repairs would still have sufficient tensile strength to withstand light active motion without the likelihood of rupturing. Some flexor tendon repair protocols are now adopting four-strand repair methods and controlled active post-repair motion programs with the hope of improving tendon excursion and digital motion.

The importance of the use of a peripheral circumferential epitenon suture has been demonstrated by experimental studies to provide a 10% to 50% increase in repair strength and a significant reduction in gapping between the tendon ends. These benefits have been further confirmed by experiments that apply both static and cyclic loads to the tendon repair. In addition, the running lock stitch, horizontal mattress, and epitenon/intrafiber methods have been shown to be the strongest of the peripheral suture techniques (Fig. 13-7). The gap-retarding quality of these peripheral epitendinous sutures is particularly important in light of the finding that gapping of flexor tendon repairs was associated with poorer clinical results.

In recent years, many surgeons have advocated repair of the flexor tendon sheath after tendon suture. The stated advantages of sheath repair are that it serves as a barrier to the formation of extrinsic adhesions, provides a quicker return of synovial nutrition, acts as a mold for the remodeling tendon, and results in better tendon sheath biomechanics. Disadvantages include the fact that sheath repair is often technically difficult to accomplish and that the repaired sheath may be narrowed and restrict tendon gliding. Even though an excellent, recent chicken experiment supported the concept that restoring the integrity of the flexor tendon sheath may ultimately reduce adhesions around traumatized flexor tendons, there are conflicting laboratory and clinical studies regarding the biologic and biomechanical benefits of sheath repair.

PERIPHERAL SUTURE TECHNIQUES

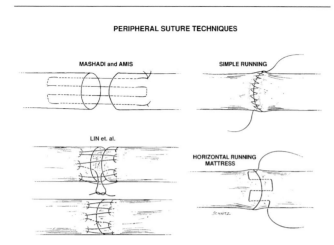

Figure 13-7. Peripheral circumferential suture methods. The "running locking loop" (Lin, *et al.*) technique and the intra-fiber continuous mattress (Mashada and Amis) method provide greater strength and resistance to gapping than simple and horizontal mattress running sutures.

Experiments have been conducted to determine the biomechanics of pulley reconstruction using mathematical theoretical models, cadaver studies, and clinical radiologic evaluations of many pulley combinations, in an effort to determine their optimum number and placement. Information from these experiments has led to the following recommendations: (1) Pulleys should be rebuilt proximal and distal to each joint. (2) The two pulleys should be balanced about the joint axis both in distance from the axis and in pulley height. (3) They should be positioned at the edge of the flare of the metaphysis. (4) The three individual joints can be balanced, one to another, by maintaining minimal bowstringing at all three joints.

Several autogenous and synthetic materials have been employed to restore sheath continuity including tendon, fascia, extensor retinaculum, peritenon, veins, silicone sheeting, and polytetrafluoroethylene. Morphologic studies on the reconstruction of annular pulleys with autogenous tendon in dogs have demonstrated marked degeneration of the collagen fibers and thinning of the pulleys, which increases with time.

Efforts have also been made to determine the best tendon suture materials; a polyfilament ensheathed by Caprolactan (Supramid™) was found by one investigator to be the strongest. Absorbable sutures have been developed for tendon repair and would seem advantageous because of low long-term foreign body tissue reaction and reduction of stress shielding effects of the host tissue. Unfortunately the optimal rates of material absorption and strength reduction are yet to be determined. In actual practice, 3-0 and 4-0 braided polyester sutures are the most commonly employed because of their ease of placement, adequate strength, and minimum extension at failure.

There has also been considerable debate regarding the appropriate management of partial tendon lacerations. Initial investigations created considerable controversy by recommending that partial flexor tendon lacerations should not be repaired. Recent studies have demonstrated that lacerations of less than 60% need not be sutured, but that those greater than 60% should be repaired since they may lead to entrapment, rupture, or triggering.

Post-repair Rehabilitation

Splints and exercise programs are now routinely implemented early in the post-tendon repair period in an effort to favorably influence the biological process of collagen synthesis and degradation. Favorable remodeling of the scar around a healing tendon is best accomplished by applying stress to the tendon, which in turn transmits the stress to the adjacent scar. It appears to be biologically effective to impart small but frequent forces in opposite directions in an effort to modify and elongate restrictive tendon adhesions. Although some excellent experimental studies are being carried out, adequate data is still not available concerning how much stress is appropriate, the optimum duration and frequency of stress application, and the most advantageous methods for the delivery of that stress to a finger following a tendon injury.

Numerous techniques and modifications have been advanced in an effort to mechanically alter the normal biological sequence of tissue healing and modify the formation of adhesions around a tendon repair. Imparting early post-repair motion stress to repaired flexor tendon repairs has been shown to be beneficial for a more rapid recovery of tensile strength, fewer adhesions, improved tendon excursion, and minimal repair-site deformation in a canine model. The load at failure of immediately mobilized tendons tested at three weeks was twice that of immobilized tendons, while the linear slope was almost three times greater; the differences continued through 12 weeks. There were also significant differences in the angle of rotation of the distal interphalangeal joints after the application of a small load. Apparently, the rapid reinstitution of tendon gliding and alternating stress and relaxation provides the stimulus for cellular activation of the epitenon. Alternatively, the ingrowth of cells from the tendon sheath in the proliferative stage may overwhelm the epitenon repair response and block the migration of tenocytes into the repair site. It would seem that greater magnitudes, frequencies, and durations of motion stress may have an acceleratory and/or magnifying effect, and almost all splinting and passive/active motion protocols now permit greater interdigital motion at more frequent intervals than was previously recommended.

While most *in vivo* studies of repaired and immobilized tendons indicate that there is a substantial weakening of the tensile strength of the repair from five days to three weeks, a recent examination of chicken flexor tendon repairs subjected to immediate controlled mobilization demonstrated that this loss of repair strength is not inevitable. In this study, controlled mobilization allowed progressive tendon healing without an intervening phase of tendon softening. Cellular examination of mobilized tendon repairs reveals an increased intrinsic healing response resulting in early healing without overwhelming scar formation. The benefits of extrasynovial flexor tendon healing following the use of continuous passive motion techniques has been demonstrated in rabbits, and a multicenter clinical study has shown modest benefits from the use of CPM for intrasynovial flexor tendon repairs.

Studies have been conducted in an effort to determine the amount of flexor tendon excursion resulting from increments of digital joint motion and, more importantly, the amount of excursion that occurs in the various post-tendon repair motion splints commonly employed following flexor tendon repair. It has been observed that passive metacarpophalangeal joint movement produces no relative motion of the flexor tendons; distal interphalangeal joint motion produces excursion of the flexor digitorum profundus of 1mm to 2mm of motion per 10° of flexion, while proximal interphalangeal joint motion produces excursion of both the flexor digitorum profundus and the flexor digitorum superficialis of about 1.5mm. Studies measuring tendon excursion following flexor tendon repair have demonstrated a substantial decrease in the excursion of the profundus to an average of 0.3mm per 10° of distal interphalangeal joint flexion (36%), while the proximal interphalangeal joint retained about 1.3mm (90%) of FDS and FDP excursion per 10° of flexion. The amount of tendon excursion that should occur for uninjured tendons in the original Kleinert-type splint, modifications of the Kleinert splint with a palmar bar pulley (Brooke Army Splint and others), and an experimental "synergistic" dynamic tenodesis splint that permits wrist extension (Mayo Clinic) have also been studied. The results of these studies have been summarized in Table 13-1 and demonstrate the improved excursion that can be expected from the use of a palmar bar and the even greater improved excursion by adding wrist extension.

Table 13-1.

Zone II Excursion (rounded)

	FDS	FDP	Differential
Kleinert (no palmar bar)	8	10	2.3
Brooke Army (palmar bar)	13	15	2.0
Synergistic splint (Mayo)	15	20	4.6

Table 13-1 reprinted with permission from Cooney WP, Lin An KN: Flexor tendon excursion in different splints. *J Hand Ther*, April, 1989.

Differential excursion between the two digital flexors was also dramatically increased by the "synergistic" splint. It has also been demonstrated that if an active post-flexor tendon repair motion protocol is selected, the wrist should be at 45° extension and the metacarpophalangeal joints at 90° in order to minimize the force across the repair site which is required to achieve or hold full active digital flexion.

Ongoing studies in these important areas will, it is hoped, provide more biologically effective methods of tendon repair and post-repair mobilization protocols, resulting in better and more predictable recovery of function following these difficult injuries.

Annotated Bibliography

Structure and Anatomy

Doyle JR: Anatomy of the finger flexor tendon sheath and pulley system. *J Hand Surg*, 13A:4:473-484, 1988.

Additions and changes in the anatomy of the finger are restudied by the author. Sixty-one fresh human cadaver fingers were dissected using the operating room microscope. The pulleys identified were the palmar aponeurosis pulley, five annular pulleys, and three cruciform pulleys. A significant addition to the pulley system is the palmar aponeurosis pulley described by Manske and Lesker.

Manske PR, Lesker PA: Palmar aponeurosis pulley. *J Hand Surg*, 8:3:259-263, 1983.

The transverse fascicular fibers and paratendinous bands of the palmar aponeurosis are positioned at the proximal margin of the flexor tendon sheath. These anatomic structures form a tunnel around the flexor tendon and appear to function as a palmar aponeurosis pulley in conjunction with the first and second annular pulleys of the digital flexor mechanism.

Nutrition

Manske PR, Lesker PA: Nutrient pathways of flexor tendons in primates. *J Hand Surg*, 7:436-444, 1982.

The perfusion and diffusion pathways to the flexor profundus tendons of 40 monkeys were investigated by measuring the uptake of tritiated proline by various tendon segments. In the absence of all vascular connections, the process of diffusion provides nutrients to all areas of flexor tendon and, in this study, the process of diffusion was greater.

Weber ER: Nutritional pathways for flexor tendons in the digital theca, in Hunter JM, Schneider LH, Mackin EJ (eds): *Tendon Surgery in the Hand*, St. Louis, CV Mosby Co, pp. 91-99, 1987.

A system of nonvascular channels has been demonstrated in the flexor tendons of the dog and chicken. The channels predominate on the volar surface of the tendon, which has the least vascular supply, and appear to be associated with nonparallel collagen fibers. Body fluid, as marked by fluorescein dye, penetrates the tendon from its least vascular area, and motion augments the penetration of this dye into the central portion of the tendon. Synovial fluid nourishes flexor tendons within the digital theca.

Biochemical Composition

Gelberman R, Goldberg V, An K, Banes A: Tendon. In, *Injury and Repair of the Musculo-skeletal Soft Tissues*, American Academy of Orthopaedic Surgeons Symposium. Woo S, Buckwalter J (eds), pp. 5-40, 1987.

This chapter discusses the structure and function of normal tendons, the mechanical environment of tendon injury, response in tendon repair, and the methods of improving the repair process, including repair techniques, rehabilitation, and tendon implants.

Biomechanical Properties

Hume EL, Hutchinson, DT, Jaeger SA, Hunter JM: Biomechanics of pulley reconstruction. *J Hand Surg,* 16A:4:722-730, 1991.

A mathematical theoretical model, confirmed by a cadaver model, and a clinical radiographic model were used to evaluate a variety of different joint and pulley combinations. Twenty-four sets of radiographs of 12 fingers in nine patients were examined for whom excursion was measured and predicted by the mathematical model. The 30 pulley combinations evaluated in the *in vitro* cadaver model showed statistical correlation with the biomechanical mathematical model.

Idler, RS: Anatomy and biomechanics of the digital flexor tendons. *Hand Clin,* 1:1:3-12, 1985.

The digital flexor system constitutes one of the most elegant and sophisticated systems of movement in the human body. Intimate knowledge of its anatomy and biomechanics is necessary for the surgeon who elects to care for acute flexor tendon injuries or to perform secondary reconstruction.

Schuind F, Garcia-Elias M, Cooney WP, An KN: Flexor tendon forces: *in vivo* measurements. *J Hand Surg,* 17A:291-298, 1992.

S-shaped force transducers were developed for measurement of the forces along intact tendons. After calibration, the transducers were applied to the flexor pollicis longus and flexor digitorum superficialis and profundus tendons of the index finger in five patients operated on for treatment of carpal tunnel syndrome. The tendon forces generated during passive and active motion of the wrist and fingers were recorded.

Tendon Healing

Gelberman RH, Khabie V, Cahill CJ: The revascularization on healing flexor tendons in digital sheath: a vascular injection study in dogs. *J Bone Joint Surg,* 73A:6:868-881, 1991.

To explore the exent to which intrasynovial flexor tendons revascularize after transsection and suture, a vascular injection study was carried out in a canine model. The tendons to the second and fifth digits of the forepaw in 12 adult mongrel dogs were transected and repaired. In the experimental tendons, longitudinal and transverse clarified sections showed consistent revascularization of the site of repair by proximal vessels in the absence of ingrowth of peripheral adhesions. Vessels in the epitenon progressively extended for a distance of 10mm, through normally avascular regions, to reach the site of repair by the 17th postoperative day. Intratendinous vessels about the site of repair

consistently originated from surface vessels, rather than from extensions of preexisting intratendinous vessels. New vessels penetrated all areas, including the normally avascular volar segments of tendon, irrespective of previous topical zones of avascularity.

Gelberman RH, Steinberg D, Amiel D, Ing D, Akeson W: Fibroblast chemotaxis after tendon repair. *J Hand Surg,* 16A:686-93, 1991.

Healing canine flexor tendons were treated with early controlled passive mobilization. The repair site and proximal and distal tendon stumps were stained for fibronectin and examined by light microscopy at three, seven, 11, and 17 days. Fibronectin production appears to be an important component of the early tendon repair process. Fibroblast chemotaxis and adherence to the substratum in the days after injury and repair appear to be related directly to fibronectin secretion. This study is the first to provide documentation of fibronectin localization in a clinically relevant tendon-repair model.

Soluble Factors Influencing Tendon Healing

Duffy FJ, Seiler JG, Hergrueter J, Kandel T, Gelberman RH: Intrinsic mitogenic potential of canine flexor tendons. *J Hand Surg,* 17B :275-277, 1992.

Healing canine flexor tendons were treated with early passive mobilization and the repair site analyzed at three, 10 and 17 days. Specimens were mechanically digested and subjected to a standard BALB/c3T3 mitogenic assay, which measures the capacity of tissue extracts to induce DNA synthesis and cell division in fibroblasts. Results revealed that both control and repaired flexor tendons possessed mitogenic activity, with the greatest activity observed in control specimens. Decreasing activity was noted as the time between repair and analysis increased. These data provide increasing evidence for the flexor tendon's active role in the healing process, and support the concept that mitogenic or growth-promoting factors are associated with flexor tendons and may be released following injury, during the early stages of healing.

Adhesion Formation and Control

Amadio PC, et al: The effect of vincular injury on the results of flexor tendon surgery in Zone 2. *J Hand Surg,* 10A:626, 1985.

From a consecutive series of 82 fingers (69 patients) that sustained flexor tendon lacerations in Zone 2, 47 fingers (39 patients) had the status of the vincular system determined during primary repair. The vincula were intact in 22 fingers and not intact in 25. Total active motion after rehabilitation and before a reconstructive procedure, such as a repair of a rupture, tenolysis, or grafting of a tendon, was the end point of the study. This study suggests that the integrity of the vincular system is a determinant of end result TAM and flexor tendon lacerations in Zone 2.

Carlstedt CA, Madsen K, Wredmark T: The influence of indomethacin on biomechanical and biochemical properties of the plantaris longus tendon in the rabbit. *Arch Orthop Trauma Surg,* 106: 157-160, 1987.

Sixty-eight New Zealand white rabbits were used for the experiment. Half were treated with indomethacin, 10mg/kg orally a day, and the other half with placebo. After four, eight, and 16 weeks of treatment, biomechanical and biochemical variables were determined and compared between the two groups. After 16 weeks there was a significant increase in tensile strength in the group treated with indomethacin.

Fujita M, Hukuda S, Doida Y: The effect of constant direct electrical current on intrinsic healing in the flexor tendon *in vitro. J Hand Surg,* 17B:94-98, 1992.

Light and electron microscopy were performed in a study of the effects of electrical stimulation upon the reparative processes in flexor tendons cultured *in vitro.* After one or two weeks of incubation, the unstimulated control tendons were covered with fibroblastic surface cells, thought to have originated from the epitenon. In contrast, the tendons subjected to electrical stimulation had no proliferation of the epitenon cells in the surface layer. The results indicate that electrical currents of low amperage suppress adhesion-causing synovial proliferation in the epitenon and promote active collagen synthesis in the tenocytes. This suggests the potential value of electrical stimulation in the control of adhesion formation after flexor tendon repair.

Gelberman RH, Woo SLY, Amiel D, Horibe S, Lee D: Influences of flexor sheath continuity and early motion on tendon healing in dogs. *J Hand Surg,* 15A:69-77, 1990.

The healing response of flexor tendons treated with either sheath reconstruction or sheath excision, and early passive motion rehabilitation was investigated in a canine model. Flexor sheath repair, sheath excision, and autogenous sheath grafting were compared for biomechanical characteristics, and biochemical and ultrastructural alterations at the repair site at intervals over a 12-week period. No significant differences could be found in tendons treated with either sheath repair or sheath excision by biomechanical, biochemical, or morphologic assessments. The findings demonstrate that reconstruction of the tendon sheath, either by suture or autogenous graft, does not significantly improve the biomechanical, biochemical, or morphologic characteristics of repaired tendons treated with early motion rehabilitation.

Hagberg L: Exogenous hyaluronate as an adjunct in the prevention of adhesions after flexor tendon surgery: a controlled clinical study. *J Hand Surg,* 17A:1:132-136, 1992.

In a prospective double-blind, randomized, clinical study, open therapeutic control sodium hyaluronate or physiologic saline solution was injected into the tendon sheath after completion of tenorrhaphy or tendon grafting in 120 digits. Sodium hyaluronate had no statistically significant effect as evaluated on total active motion at follow-up.

Kulick MI, Smith HS, Hadler K: Oral ibuprofen: evaluation of its effect on peritendinous adhesions and the breaking strength of a tenorrhaphy. *J Hand Surg,* 11A:110-120, 1986.

In a study of 21 primates, treatment with oral ibuprofen significantly reduced the force required for tendon gliding following flexor tendon injury in Zone II. Tendons that were partially lacerated but not repaired required less force for tendon motion than those repaired. Ibuprofen also reduced the breaking strength of completely divided and repaired extensor tendons.

Peterson WW, Manske PR, Dunlap J, Horwitz DS, Kahn B: Effect of various methods of restoring flexor sheath integrity on the formation of adhesions after tendon injury. *J Hand Surg,* 15A:48-56, 1990.

The effect of three different methods of restoring flexor sheath integrity on the formation of adhesions around traumatized flexor tendons was studied by use of a chicken model. The three methods were: I, primary sheath repair; II, a fascia patch; and III, a synthetic polytetrafluroethylene surgical membrane patch. These were compared with controls in which the flexor sheath was excised. At 12 weeks, all three methods of sheath reconstruction had similar tendon-gliding biomechanics, and all were significantly better than the controls.

Tendon Suture Methods

Bishop AT, Cooney WP, Wood MB: Treatment of partial flexor tendon lacerations: The effect of tenorrhaphy and early protected mobilization. *J Trauma,* 26:4:301-312, 1986.

In this study, a novel nonweightbearing canine model was developed in order to closely approximate human flexor tendon conditions. The relative effects of immobilization, early protected mobilization, tenorrhaphy, and no repair of flexor tendon healing were evaluated by paired comparisons of four experimental groups (24 animals). Parameters evaluated after a 35-day healing period included tendon excursion, breaking strength, energy absorption, and stiffness. Data analysis revealed statistically significant adverse effects on breaking strength, stiffness, and energy absorption when repaired by the modified Kessler technique. Early motion improved excursion and stiffness significantly, and resulted in more nearly normal tendon morphology than immobilized tendons. Thus, we conclude that partial flexor tendon lacerations of 60% cross-sectional area are optimally treated without tenorrhaphy and with early mobilization.

Ketchum LD: Suture materials and suture techniques used in tendon repair. *Hand Clin,* 1:1:43-53, 1985.

Various types of suture materials are discussed including stainless steel, absorbable, and nonabsorbable synthetic fibers – the most desirable materials available. Suture techniques include the lateral trap, end-weave, Bunnell, Kessler, and Mason-Allen. The less traumatic suture techniques facilitate closure of the tendon sheath, which helps to reestablish the continuity of the synovial fluid system, a major source of nutrition to the tendon. The simplest and least traumatic suture technique, although weakest at first, will allow tendon healing to proceed more rapidly. If such a repair is protected from tension by splinting the wrist and metacarpophalangeal joints in flexion during healing (while allowing controlled passive motion of the finger joints), there will be a rapid increase in tensile strength of the tendon juncture with minimal gap formation, as the repaired hand is progressively stressed until about 90 days post-repair. The less traumatic suture techniques facilitate closure of the tendon sheath, which not only acts as a mechanical barrier to the ingrowth of extra-sheath adhesion, producing fibroblasts, but also reestablishes the continuity of the synovial fluid system, which is a major source of nutrition to the tendon.

Lee H: Double loop locking suture: a technique of tendon repair for early active mobilization. Part I.
J Hand Surg, 15A:945-952 Part II. 953-958, 1990.

Part I: experimental study on human tendon specimens showed that the average tensile strength of tendon junctures was 4400 grams by double loop locking sutures and 2252 grams by Kessler's technique. The study also showed that the weakest point of the tendon juncture by double loop locking sutures was the sutures. Part II: tendons repaired by double loop locking sutures show sufficient strength to allow early active mobilization under protective splint. Clinical experience with 51 tendons repaired by this technique resulted in satisfactory functional recovery. Eleven flexors in zone II showed excellent results in 10 and good results in one by the Strickland formula. Early active mobilization of repaired tendons with double loop locking sutures seems to enhance their healing by the intrinsic mechanism and reduce extrinsic adhesion formation and stiff joints.

Lin GT, An KN, Amadio PC, Cooney WP: Biomechanical studies of running suture for flexor tendon repair in dogs. *J Hand Surg,* 13A:553-558, 1988.

A new running-locking loop suture technique has been developed to increase tendon repair strength and to provide better tendon edge inversion. Biomechanical analysis documented the failure mechanism and the failure strength of various circumferential repair techniques. When compared with two well-known techniques, the simple circumferential running suture and Lembert running suture, the locking suture technique was shown to have 3.77 and 1.68 times greater tensile failure strength and 1.73 and 1.26 times greater stiffness than these traditional suture methods. A running peripheral locking suture may help augment the strength of tendon repair.

Mashadi ZB, Amis AA: The effect of locking loops on the repair strength of tendon repair. *J Hand Surg,* 16B:1:135-139, 1991.

A multiple X-raying method was used to examine the locking loop tendon sutures, such as the modified Kessler, Verdan, and Ketchum techniques. Locking loops did not contribute towards the strength when small diameter sutures (5/0) of various materials were applied to the tendon, collapsing at 12. Larger diameter sutures (4/0) slightly reduced the risk of failure of locking loops, but they still collapsed at 15 or less, so suture techniques which depend on locking loops will often lead to gap formation at low loads and hence poor results.

McGeorge DD, Stilwell JH: Partial flexor tendon injuries: to repair or not. *J Hand Surg,* 17B:176-177, 1992.

The correct management of partially divided flexor tendon injuries is still in dispute. This study compares the results of repair with nonrepair in zone 2 injuries. The conclusion is that tendons divided by 60% or less in cross-sectional area should not be repaired.

Pruitt DL, Manske PR, Fink B: Cyclic stress analysis of flexor tendon repair. *J Hand Surg,* 16A:701-707, 1991.

A method of evaluating flexor tendon repair techniques with the use of cyclic testing is presented. This type of evaluation complements the presently used load-to-failure tests by providing more detailed information about gap formation at the repair site. An epitenon stitch placed circumferentially around the laceration site added strength in both load-to-failure and cyclic tests, and significantly reduced gap formation regardless of the core suture techniques.

Robertson GA, Al-Qattan MM: A biomechanical analysis of a new interlock suture technique for flexor tendon repair. *J Hand Surg,* 17B:92-93, 1992.

Using a computerized tensometer, both the gap producing and breaking forces of a new interlocking suture for flexor tendon repairs were compared to the modified Kessler and the Strickland techniques. Thirty porcine deep flexor tendons were used in each group and all repairs were performed with 3/0 polypropylene sutures. The interlock technique withstood gap producing and breaking forces significantly better than the modified Kessler and Strickland techniques. Also, the gap-producing force was closer to the breaking force with the interlock technique than with the other two techniques.

Savage R: *In vitro* studies of a new method of tendon repair. *J Hand Surg,* 10B:2:135-141, 1985.

The mechanical factors in tendon repair have been studied and physical principles applied to this unsolved problem. A new technique of tendon repair has been derived and tested in the laboratory. Compared to several well-known techniques, it has been shown to have three times the tensile strength and to allow one tenth the gap to form between the tendon ends under load. It has been designed not to constrict the blood supply of the tendon and

the tests indicate that it will be strong enough to allow early active mobilization even after inflammation has caused the tendon to soften.

Strickland JW: Review article: Flexor tendon surgery, Part II. *J Hand Surg,* 14B:4:368-382, 1989.

In those instances where flexor tendons divided in zone 1 or zone 2 have not been or cannot be directly repaired, conventional free-tendon grafting may represent the best procedure for restoring digital function. Conventional free-tendon grafting, staged flexor tendon reconstruction, flexor tenolysis, and flexor pulley reconstruction techniques are described.

Trail IA, Powell ES, Noble J: The mechanical strength of various suture techniques. *J Hand Surg,* 17B:1:89-91, 1992.

The mechanical strengths of five techniques of tendon repair have been evaluated using human cadaver tendons. A modified Kessler repair with a peripheral circumferential suture and the method of Becker were found to require the greatest load to produce gapping, but the Becker and Savage repairs withstood the highest load before failure.

Wade PJF, Wetherell RG, Amis AA: Flexor tendon repair: significant gain in strength from the Halsted peripheral suture technique. *J Hand Surg,* 14B:232-235, 1989.

A biomechanical study *in vitro* has evaluated a new modification of the core and peripheral suture technique for flexor tendon repair. Groups of repairs were conducted in cadaver tendons, using a core suture alone, a core suture with a simple running surface suture, and a new modification involving a "Halsted" horizontal mattress technique for the peripheral stitch.

Post-repair Rehabilitation

Brand PW: *Clinical Mechanics of the Hand.* St. Louis, CV Mosby, 1992.

The clinical management of adhesions is reviewed including conservative postoperative therapy and passive mobilization.

Cooney WP, Lin GT, An KN: Improved tendon excursion following flexor tendon repair. *J Hand Ther,* 2:102-6, 1989.

To evaluate the concept of passive motion of flexor tendons, and to determine differences in excursion between the flexor digitorum superficialis and flexor digitorum profundus, the Kleinert splint, the Brooke Army Hospital splint, and a new splint employing the concept of synergistic wrist motion were compared. Results indicate that synergistic wrist motion provided the largest tendon excursion for both the FDS and FDP tendons of the long finger.

Gelberman RH, Nunley JA, Osterman AL, Woo SLY: Influence of the protected passive mobilization interval on flexor tendon healing (a prospective randomized clinical study). *Clin Orthop,* 264:189-196, 1991.

A prospective multicenter clinical study was carried out to determine whether improved tendon gliding could be achieved with greater durations of daily passive-motion rehabilitation after flexor tendon repair. The data from this experiment indicate that the duration of the daily controlled motion interval is a significant variable insofar as post-repair flexor tendon function is concerned.

McGrouther DA, Ahmed MR: Flexor tendon excursions in "no man's land." *The Hand,* 13:129-141, 1981.

The excursions of the digital flexor tendons have been measured relative to the sheath and to one another at a point in no-man's land over the proximal phalanx, in fresh cadavers. The significance of these measurements is discussed in relation to the exploration of tendon injuries, the mechanism of failure after tendon repair, dynamic mobilization; and the anatomy of no-man's land.

Savage R: The influence of wrist position on the minimum force required for active movement of the interphalangeal joints. *J Hand Surg,* 13B:3:262-268, 1988.

Active and passive muscle tendon tension is discussed in relation to finger flexor and extensor tendons. Minimizing active tension required to produce finger movement is seen as an important part of postoperative finger mobilization following flexor tendon repair in which active movement is used. It is argued that "minimal active tension" in the flexors is equal to, or just exceeds, the passive tension in the extensors.

Silfverskiold KL, May EJ, Tornvall AH: Flexor digitorum profundus tendon excursions during controlled motion after flexor tendon repair in zone II: a prospective clinical study. *J Hand Surg,* 17A:122-131, 1992.

Intratendinous metal markers were used to study flexor digitorum profundus tendon excursions during early controlled motion with dynamic flexion traction and to evaluate their significance for results after flexor tendon repair in zone II. Compared to active motion, controlled motion of the distal interphalangeal joint mobilized the tendon with an efficiency of 36% and controlled motion of the proximal interphalangeal joint mobilized the tendon with an efficiency of 90%.

14

Flexor Tendon Injuries

Lawrence H. Schneider, MD

Flexor Tendon Zones of Injury

For purposes of treatment and prognosis, the flexor tendon system in the hand has been divided into zones which have specific anatomic characteristics. Zone 2 is the most difficult area in which to restore smooth, gliding tendon function since two tendons lie close together within an unyielding fibrous retinaculum. Now that primary repair is being performed at all levels, the zones may not be as important as previously believed.

Zone 1–Distal to the Superficialis Insertion

At this level, only the profundus is injured. Primary repair is preferred and end-to-end attachment is recommended over advancement of the tendon to its bony insertion unless the tendon is severed close to the insertion. Profundus advancement greater than 1 cm carries a risk of creating a flexion deformity in the finger and should be avoided.

Zone 2–Within the Finger Flexor Retinaculum (No-man's Land)

Both tendons are usually injured here but at times only the profundus is injured. This area is the most studied and the most difficult in which to obtain a good result.

Zone 3–the Palm

At this level, proximal to the finger flexor retinaculum but distal to the carpal ligament, one or both tendons may be injured and direct repair has a relatively good prognosis due to the absence of retinacular structures.

Zone 4–the Carpal Tunnel

Under the transverse carpal ligament, the flexor tendons are enclosed in synovial sheaths and held in a tight compartment where recovery of function is more difficult to achieve. In this zone, both flexors or the superficialis alone are subject to injury. Injury to the main trunks of the median and ulnar nerves greatly complicates rehabilitation at this level. Primary repair is best before significant muscle contracture develops.

Zone 5–the Wrist and Forearm

Proximal to the carpal ligament, the flexor tendons are less constrained and are surrounded by relatively mobile and loose areolar tissue so that repairs of the flexor tendons in this zone have a more favorable prognosis. Problems in rehabilitation are mainly related to associated injuries to the major nerves and vessels, which can have a significantly adverse effect on recovery of hand function.

Acute Injuries

Today, primary repair of flexor tendon lacerations is performed even when the injury is in Zone 2 (no-man's land). In the past, primary repair was advocated only in those injuries outside of Zone 2. Zone 2 injuries were treated by a delayed palm-to-fingertip free-tendon graft. The dictum against direct repair of flexor tendons in no-man's land originated with Sterling Bunnell, who wrote in 1928: "If the flexor tendons are severed in a finger in the usual place opposite the proximal phalanx, one cannot join them by suture with success, as the junction will become adherent in the narrow fixed channel and will not slip. It is better to remove the tendons entirely from the finger and graft in a new tendon smooth throughout its length." (*J Bone Joint Surg*, 10:1-28, 1928)

This concept dictated the care of the acutely lacerated flexor tendon through the years, although a few surgeons, and even Bunnell himself, did direct repairs in Zone 2 in selected cases. Those surgeons who did primary repairs placed severe time constraints on Zone 2 injuries since they believed that it was necessary to do the repair within two-to-four hours of the injury. In the 1950s and 1960s, Verdan and Kleinert demonstrated that primary repair was feasible and had obvious advantages over tendon grafting. At the present time, primary repair in Zone 2 is the accepted procedure. If wound conditions allow, the repair is done as soon after the injury as feasible. If repair is delayed (even as long as two to three weeks after the injury), it does not seem to compromise the end result.

Diagnosis

Active finger motion is the measure of flexor tendon function. The flexor digitorum profundus (FDP) flexes the DIP joint, and flexion against resistance at this joint proves the integrity of this structure. The superficialis tendon flexes the proximal interphalangeal joint. The presence of an isolated flexor superficialis tendon injury is difficult to diagnose because of the functional overlap by the profundus. To test for FDS integrity, it is necessary to immobilize the profundus tendons by holding all the uninvolved fingers in extension, thereby isolating superficialis function for the examination. Posture of the fingers also provides a clue to flexor tendon disruption in the uncooperative or anesthetized patient. In the relaxed state, the fingers with intact flexor tendons form a cascade of semi-flexion with the little finger more flexed compared to the index finger, which is least flexed. Partial tendon lacerations may be difficult to diagnose and delayed loss of function may occur when the remaining tendon fibers separate due to use of the hand. A high index of suspicion may prompt primary exploration of such injuries to avoid this phenomenon.

Prognostic Factors in Flexor Tendon Injury

Nature of the injuring agent
A sharp clean laceration (such as a knife injury) has a better prognosis than tendon laceration due to a crush injury. Associated injuries such as fracture, skin loss, joint or neurovascular injury also reduce the prognosis.

Level of Injury
Zone 2 injuries carry the worst prognosis.

Age of the Patient
Generally, younger patients have a better prognosis than older patients but the very young have problems in management due to the small size of the injured structures and their inability to cooperate.

Skin Laceration Level and Level of Tendon Injury
The level of the flexor tendon laceration does not always correlate with the skin laceration. Flexor tendons severed with the fingers in flexion are cut more distally in relation to the skin laceration while those cut in extension more closely parallel the skin laceration.

Suture Technique

Repair of the tendon is most frequently carried out using the Kessler or another grasping or locking type suture. The Bunnell crisscross suture, which was once more widely used, has several theoretical disadvantages (i.e., a threat to the tendon circulation as well as a built-in tendency to allow gap formation). Despite this, it is still used with success by some surgeons. These suture techniques are adequate to the demands made of them in the commonly used protected passive mobilization programs discussed below. The creation of a suture technique that is secure enough to allow immediate unprotected motion is an unrealized goal of the hand surgeon but is being vigorously pursued. There are many articles in the literature today showing newer suture techniques which are reported to produce repairs with superior tensile strength aimed at the prospect of immediate active postoperative motion. While these techniques, which are usually associated with some form of protected active mobilization program, show promise, caution is still recommended because of the risk of tendon rupture in the postoperative period. In early reports on these techniques this has not been a problem but time is still needed for further evaluation of these newer methods.

Experimental studies on resistance to gap formation or complete breakdown of a specific repair have suggested that the number of grasping loops is not as significant as the number of strands of suture that cross the repair site.

A circumferential suture is often added to the core suture to smooth the tendon surface, which promotes gliding of repairs in the finger flexor retinaculum. Although at one time this running suture was not believed to add strength to the repair, recent studies have shown that it can provide significant additional resistance to gap formation and suture failure in the postoperative period.

Relevant Issues in Flexor Tendon Repair

Repair of One or Both Tendons
Today the accepted treatment is to repair, when possible, both superficialis and profundus tendons. This is believed to result in better balance of the injured finger. In Zone 2 this technique can result in sparing of the long vinculum of the superficialis, which carries blood supply to the profundus and theoretically promotes its healing (provided the surgeon does not forcefully separate the tendons). Repair of the superficialis also prevents the occasional hyperextension deformity at the PIP joint, adds strength to the finger, and provides a smooth gliding bed for the profundus repair.

Sheath Repair
Sheath repair is a technique intended to take advantage of the synovial pathways of tendon nutrition of the healing tendon. Although closure of the sheath with the hope of lessening adhesions is commendable, it has not been conclusively proven to be of benefit in human flexor tendon healing or in the restoration of gliding. Manske and coworkers showed in animals that the sheath was not essential for the tendon to receive nutrition. In clinical studies, Saldana and coworkers and also Lister and Tonkin were not able to demonstrate a difference in the clinical results between tendon repairs done with and without sheath repair, although a later assessment of the Lister-Tonkin study changed the original impression of the authors, who reported that "closure of the tendon sheath decreases external adhesion formation and improves motion without increasing the risks of rupture." At the present time, sheath closure is still a controversial issue in primary tendon repair and further study is needed to assess its value in the final restoration of function. However, unnecessary sheath or pulley removal at the time of primary tendon repair is to be avoided. Sheath closure should be attempted but extraordinary attempts to repair the sheath using distant materials are not justified by our current state of knowledge.

Controlled Mobilization
Surgeons have long believed that protected motion after flexor repair would limit the formation of restricting adhesions, and consequently, programs for early mobilization of tendon repairs were developed. Laboratory studies by Matthews and Richards revealed that immobilization after repair was related to increased adhesion formation. Protected or passive mobilization programs utilized active extension to the limits of a posterior splint device with passive flexion supplied by elastic bands attached to the fingernail. Other techniques used passive motion alone applied by the patient at the involved joints. A series of

animal experiments by Gelberman and colleagues confirmed the beneficial effects of passive motion on flexor tendon repair. These studies showed that passive motion increased tensile strength, decreased adhesions, favored the restoration of a gliding surface, improved excursion, and provided better vascularization in repaired dog flexor tendons. Gelberman felt that "controlled passive mobilization augments the quality of repair and stimulates a flexor tendon's intrinsic (non-adhesion) healing capability." The best way to provide this motion in humans is still not agreed upon. Adding to the confusion are studies such as those by McGrouther which suggest that these passive motion techniques do not actually impart much motion to the repair itself. In summing up the issues in passive mobilization, Manske stated that the "benefits of this treatment are clear but the mechanism and how to apply these techniques is less clear."

In a clinical series, Strickland, and later Chow, showed that protected passive motion programs led to improved results in flexor tendon repair in Zone 2 injuries. These programs, and modifications, are widely used after flexor tendon repair and are regarded as one of the reasons for significantly improved results in flexor tendon surgery. When considering the mechanism by which this comes about, Manske felt that patients in the passive programs may, in fact, be actively moving their tendons and that this may be a factor in better results seen with so-called protected mobilization.

Partial Tendon Injuries

Does repair improve the results in treatment of partial flexor tendon lacerations? Animal studies have suggested that suture may not be needed in partial tendon lacerations and, in fact, ruptures were seen in a group of chicken flexor tendons in which suture was used for repair of partial tendon injuries while there were no ruptures seen in the nonsutured group. Kleinert and associates believed that repair of partial lacerations was necessary and cited three examples in which entrapment, rupture, and triggering occurred due to untreated partial tendon injury. Kleinert's group believed that if the lesion was 50% or less of the cross-sectional diameter, a 6-0 running suture around the periphery would suffice. When the injury involved more than 50% of the cross section, they recommended a core suture and a running circumferential stitch. Protected mobilization was then applied in both instances. Most authors agree that if only a small flap laceration is found (less than 25%), then only resection and protected mobilization is needed.

Secondary Repair and Reconstruction

Secondary repair is defined as delayed primary repair performed three or more weeks after injury. Delayed primary repair usually cannot be performed after about four weeks after injury unless the lacerated tendon remains in the finger due to an intact vinculum, which tethers the tendon. When this occurs it may be possible to carry out a delayed primary repair even after a considerable passage of time. When a delayed primary repair is attempted late, care must be exercised that the repair is not put up with too much ten-

sion. After the core suture is placed, the surgeon should examine the cascade of the fingers and look very critically at the tension in the flexor system. Contracture of the muscle-tendon unit may have occurred and the surgeon should be ready to abandon the repair and proceed with a tendon graft.

Flexor Tendon Grafting

The free flexor tendon graft is less frequently performed today because of the successful and widespread application of primary tendon repair. Tendon grafting is the indicated treatment when both flexor tendons have been injured in Zone 2 and when the indications for primary or delayed primary repair cannot be met. This need for tendon grafting would occur when repair was deferred because of intercurrent problems or when the extent of the injury was missed beyond the period suitable for primary repair. Ideally, prior to tendon grafting, the wound should be healed and the finger supple without extensive scarring and with full passive motion. The tendon graft is used to reconstruct the profundus tendon only, and transverses the difficult Zone 2 with junctures in the more forgiving Zone 3 proximally and Zone 1 distally. When an intact flexor superficialis is present, it is never sacrificed to perform a tendon graft. Stark and others have noted the hazards and risks of inserting a free-tendon graft through an intact superficialis in patients over 20 years of age. Postoperatively, the grafted extremity may be immobilized for three weeks and then an active motion program started. A protected mobilization program similar to that used in primary repair is advocated by some. While this postoperative motion technique may not have the same clear-cut rationale as in primary repair, it maintains the mobility of the joints and may reduce the formation of adhesions.

Source of Tendon Grafts

The palmaris longus is the favored source of tendon graft material and supplies sufficient material for one palm-to-fingertip tendon graft. Its presence is easily identified preoperatively, but it is absent from 25% of upper extremities. The average length of the palmaris longus tendon is 16 cm. The plantaris tendon or the long-toe extensors from the lower extremity provide a suitable source of tendon grafts if the palmaris longus is not present or if longer material is needed as in the staged flexor tendon reconstruction that is discussed later. The plantaris and toe extensor tendons can provide a tendon graft up to 40 cm long. The plantaris was absent in 19% of 240 lower extremities dissected by Wehbe. When multiple tendon grafts are needed, lower extremity sources are utilized. Occasional use of the proprius extensors is mentioned in the literature, but these are infrequently used as tendon grafts.

Tendon Graft in the Presence of an Intact Superficialis

The selection of late treatment for a finger with a ruptured or divided flexor profundus tendon in the presence of a normally functioning superficialis requires considerable judgment and experience. The impairment to the finger may not be great. For this reason the application of a free-tendon graft should not be taken lightly because of the risk of injury to the functioning superficialis. If the superficialis is injured in the process of restoring profundus function, the overall function of the finger may be reduced. The patient's age and functional needs should be considered. If functional loss is minimal, the finger may be accepted as is. If hyperextension or instability at the distal joint is a problem, then a tenodesis or arthrodesis of the DIP joint may be considered. Reconstruction of profundus function by a tendon graft is most often indicated in the little finger where the superficialis is frequently incompetent (about 34% of fingers). Ideally, as for all tendon grafts, the finger should have full passive motion. If possible, the graft should be threaded through the superficialis decussation and the junctures made distally at the distal phalanx and proximally to the profundus motor at the lumbrical origin in the palm. If passage of the graft through the decussation is prevented by scar tissue, then passage is made around the superficialis. The indication for surgical reconstruction is stronger in a finger with limited motion due to a partly defective superficialis. Such findings may be an indication for staged flexor reconstruction, which is described later.

Aftercare is as for a standard tendon graft except that active superficialis tendon motion may be started earlier.

Flexor Tenolysis

Regardless of the skill levels of surgeons and therapists, some flexor tendon primary repairs fail to achieve adequate gliding and become adherent to their beds. Tendon adhesions may occur whenever the surface of a tendon is damaged either through the injury itself, be it laceration or crush, or by surgical manipulation. Tenolysis, which is the release of nongliding adhesions that form along the surface of a tendon after injury or repair, is useful in the salvage of tendon function. Tenolysis is considered whenever these adhesions cannot be mobilized by therapy. Tenolysis is most appropriate when passive joint motion is complete but local adhesions prevent satisfactory active motion. Usually, the adhesions involve a long segment of the involved tendon and require extensive exposure for release. Joint contracture, which can occur secondary to the tendon fixation, may also require correction and this adversely affects the patient's recovery. Tenolysis is as demanding as tendon repair itself and should not be undertaken lightly.

Timing

It is suggested that tenolysis be deferred until it is established that progress in therapy has ceased. Tenolysis should rarely be performed until three months after a tendon repair and even longer after a graft. The procedure is a painstaking one in which the restricting adhesions are lysed while the surgeon tries to avoid injury to the involved tendon itself and to preserve as much of the retinacular pulley system as possible. This procedure is best done under local anesthesia, when possible, so that the functional result can be evaluated from time to time as the procedure progresses. If general anesthesia is required, an additional proximal incision is made in the distal forearm so that traction can be applied to the involved tendon to evaluate the potential pull through of the tendon. This method is not as desirable as evaluating active motion directly under local anesthesia. Postoperatively, it is imperative that the patient begin an immediate active motion program preferably under the supervision of a trained hand therapist. Prognosis is best in cases with limited adhesions in a vascularized finger with good passive motion and in a motivated patient. Combining tenolysis with certain procedures such as osteotomy, tendon repair, or pulley reconstruction reduces the prognosis for a good result.

Complications of tenolysis are not infrequent, the most serious being tendon rupture in the postoperative period. At the time of tenolysis, the repair may be found to be ruptured and not be salvageable by tenolysis. Therefore, patients who undergo tenolysis should be prepared to proceed with a staged tendon reconstruction if this is the case or if there is a major problem with the retinacular pulley system.

Staged Tendon Reconstruction

The placement of a silicone rubber tendon implant to induce the formation of a bed favorable for flexor tendon grafting at a second stage is an accepted procedure in the treatment of the severely damaged flexor system. Staged reconstruction is not required in tendon injuries that are characterized by minimal scarring, pliable joints, and an adequate retinacular pulley system. In such instances, a standard one-stage palm-to-distal phalanx tendon graft should be done. Nongliding adhesions, a scarred tendon bed, and contractures not corrected by therapy or disruption of the pulley system are conditions that would indicate the use of the staged tendon technique. Most of the cases that require staged tendon reconstruction are due to failed prior flexor tendon surgery. It must be noted that atrophic fingers with severe neurovascular deficiency have a poor prognosis and may be best treated by arthrodesis or amputation.

When the staged technique is elected at Stage I, the scarred tendon remnants are excised, joint contractures are released, nerves repaired, and a flexible silicone-Dacron reinforced tendon implant is inserted along with pulley reconstruction as required.

Active Tendon Implants

The development of a permanent flexor tendon prosthesis is in progress. While permanence is not yet established, an active silicone rubber tendon implant is available which has devices that allow for attachment distally to the distal phalanx and proximally to the motor tendon. This allows for active use of the digit soon after implantation. Although the implant will be removed, the period between Stage I and II in which the motor tendon unit is in active use may better prepare the motor and sheath system for Stage II. Stage II may be done electively or when the implant attachments break down. Complications were not infrequent in the salvage of these difficult cases. Research is continuing with the hope of designing a reliable permanent prosthesis that would not require tendon graft replacement.

Pulley Reconstruction

The ability to rebuild pulleys over the tendon implant is a major advantage of the two-stage tendon reconstruction over the single Stage I free-tendon graft and provides one of its strongest indications. While the ideal pulley system resembles the original, some compromises are necessary when reconstruction of this system is performed. As a minimum, the A2 and A4 pulleys are required but the surgeon should, where possible, preserve or reconstruct as much of the pulley system as possible. Indications for pulley reconstruction become obvious when, while pulling proximally on the distally attached implant, one can see whether the implant bowstrings on the palmar side of the underlying phalanx. Assuming that the joints are pliable and that there is a limited amount of available tendon excursion, joint range of motion depends upon the integrity of the pulley system. If longitudinal traction on the tendon implant is ineffective in pulling the finger into complete flexion, the relationship between tendon excursion and joint motion should be improved by pulley reconstruction.

To reconstruct a pulley, local damaged pulleys or their remnants can be used, as these do not adhere to the silicone rubber implant. One tail of the superficialis can be utilized at the A3 level by bringing it across the implant and suturing it to the fibrous rim on the other side. There are usually abundant tendon sources for pulley material when one is excising the damaged flexor tendon system. In addition to using the excised tendons, other sources of material include the palmaris longus or toe extensors. Retinacular material from the dorsal wrist retinaculum or even synthetic materials have their advocates. Pulley reconstruction may be performed using a length of discarded tendon woven through the remaining fibrous rim of the pulley and double and triple graft loops wrapped around the phalanges. In clinical situations, the most effective pulley at the critical A2 level (proximal phalanx) consists of two or three loops around the implant and beneath the extensor tendon system. The belt loop technique of Karev, which uses the volar plate of each of the joints, has its advocates, although it may lead to reduced joint motion due to its location just palmar to the joints.

Although tendon tissue is widely used in pulley reconstruction, it was disconcerting to note a recent report by Deffino and associates who found deterioration of this material in dogs when it was used as pulleys. While pulley rupture in the clinical situation may occur at times, it should not be unexpected in this study since the pulley sat passively against a silicone tube without any significant stresses. Such a reconstruction does better when used in an active and dynamic system.

In the passive staged tendon reconstruction program, only the distal end of the tendon implant is attached to the profundus stump distally, and the proximal end is left free in the distal forearm. A passive motion program is then begun in the postoperative period to regain passive range of digital motion and to move the implant while the soft tissues build a smooth new synovial-like sheath around it. Although studies suggest that six to eight weeks are adequate, three months should be allowed for complete soft-tissue healing prior to doing Stage II.

At Stage II a tendon graft is used to replace the implant with minimal disturbance to the newly formed sheath. The graft is attached distally to the base of the distal phalanx and proximally to the profundus motor, which is generally in the distal forearm and thereby bypasses a possibly scarred palm. Postoperative protected mobilization is used and active motion is delayed for approximately four weeks. If good gliding is found early on, active motion can be deferred for a longer time to avoid graft rupture.

Assessment of Results in Flexor Tendon Surgery

In spite of ongoing improvement in the results of flexor tendon repair, the restoration of normal function is difficult to achieve. Unfortunately, variation in the methods of assessment make it difficult for the student to compare the results in various studies in this field. The need for a consistent and comparable measurement system in the assessment of results of flexor tendon surgery is apparent when one reviews the extensive literature in this field.

A simple technique makes use of total active motion in which the total active flexion angle of all three joints of a finger are measured while attempting to make a full fist. Subtracted from this number was the total extension deficit in degrees for the same three joints. This provides one number for each injured finger. An average TAM is 260. While modifications of this system have been used, including removal of the MP joint from the equation, the great advantage is that it gives a single number for comparison to the TAM of the contralateral finger or to the 260 standard value for a finger. In a reconstructive case the TAM achieved may be compared to the preoperative total passive motion. The use of TAM has some limitations but in the search for a standardized method it is the simplest, the most direct and reproducible measurement technique.

Annotated Bibliography

Gelberman RH and Woo SY-L: The physiological basis for application of controlled stress in the rehabilitation of flexor tendon injuries. *J Hand Ther*, 2:66-70, 1989.

A review of the scientific basis for early motion programs.

Horii E, Lin GT, Cooney WP, Linscheid RL, An KN: Comparative flexor tendon excursion after passive mobilization: an *in vitro* study. *J Hand Surg*, 17A:559-66, 1992.

Passive motions techniques were studied to see what magnitude of flexor tendon excursion was obtained. Flexor tendon excursions due to passive joint motion were found to be much lower than predicted values. A postoperative splint that allows synergistic wrist motion was developed that may improve passive motion techniques.

Hunter JM, Salisbury RE: Flexor tendon reconstruction in severely damaged hands. *J Bone Joint Surg*, 53A:829-858, 1971.

This classic article reviewed the first 10 years of Hunter's work and established the two-stage reconstruction procedure as a viable treatment option in secondary flexor tendon reconstruction.

Hunter JM, Singer DI, Jaeger SH, Mackin EJ: Active tendon implants in flexor tendon reconstruction. *J Hand Surg*, 13A: 849-59, 1988.

A review of the results in 45 active flexor tendon implants in salvage fingers. Overall improvement was modest and complications were frequent in 27 fingers that had the implant replaced with a tendon graft. The feasibility of an active implant is demonstrated with a future possibility of a permanent prosthesis.

Leddy JP: Flexor tendon—acute injuries, In: Green DP, ed. *Operative Hand Surgery*, pp. 1935-1068. second ed. Churchill Livingstone, New York, 1988.

A review stressing indications and techniques in the acute flexor tendon injury.

Lee H: Double loop locking suture: a technique of tendon repair for early active mobilization. part II: clinical experience. *J Hand Surg*, 15A:953-958, 1990.

A clinical series using a new suture technique that is stronger than the Kessler suture. Results suggest that protected early active motion is a practical technique and deserves more study.

Lin GT, An KN, Amadio PC, Cooney WP: Biomechanical studies of running suture for flexor tendon repair in dogs. *J Hand Surg*, 13A:553-558, 1988.

A circumferential running-locking loop suture was tested *in vitro* on dog tendons and was found to have more tensile strength and stiffness than the traditional suture methods. It was felt that this suture, when added to a core suture, could add strength to tendon repairs.

Mashadi ZB, Amis M : The effect of locking loops on the strength of tendon repair. *J Hand Surg*, 16B:35-39, 1991.

Locking loops, as used in the Kessler type repair, were not effective in resisting gap formation and failure at the repair site. Adding additional loops did not help. It was noted that if newly designed repair techniques are to be stronger they should not make use of locking loops.

Matthews P: Early mobilization after tendon repair. *J Hand Surg*, 14B:363-367, 1989.

A current summary of the advantages and risks of early mobilization based on the science of flexor tendon surgery as it stands at this time. Motion will have a place in the management of these injuries but is adjunctive in nature to the meticulous surgery required. "No amount of movement can compensate for a badly done repair."

Matthews P, Richards H: Factors in the adherence of flexor tendons after repair. *J Bone Joint Surg*, 58B:230-236, 1976.

Splint, suture, and excision of the tendon sheath all contributed to dense adhesions in the repair of rabbit flexor tendons. The goal should be to minimize these factors as much as possible in the repair of flexor tendons. A classic article.

May EJ, Silfverskiold KL, Sollerman CJ: Controlled mobilization after flexor tendon repair in zone II: a prospective comparison of three methods. *J Hand Surg*, 17A:942-952, 1992

A new controlled motion technique in which all four fingers are put into the device was compared to two variations of the Kleinert technique. The results were significantly better and extension deficits were significantly less with this technique compared to the two variations of the Kleinert technique.

McCarthy JA, Lesker PA, Peterson WW, Manske PR: Continuous passive motion as an adjunct therapy for tenolysis. *J Hand Surg*, 11B:88-90, 1986.

The use of continuous motion after tenolysis of a flexor tendon in a chicken model was found to lead to poor results including decreased range of motion. There was increased granulation tissue formed around the tenolysed tendon.

McGrouther DA, Ahmed MR: Flexor tendon excursions in "no-man's land." *Hand*, 13:129-141, 1981.

The motion of the flexor tendons relative to each other and to the sheath was found to be much less than predicted during passive motion studies in fresh cadavers. In the clinical situation sutures and swelling would be expected to reduce this excursion further. This brought into question the source of the observed benefits of the protected passive mobilization programs.

Schneider LH, Hunter JM: Flexor tendons - Late reconstruction. In: Green DP, (ed.) *Operative Hand Surgery*, pp. 1969-2044. second ed. Churchill Livingstone, New York, 1988.

A review of reconstructive techniques used in late flexor tendon problems.

Schuind F, Garcia-Elias M, Cooney WP, An KN: Flexor tendon forces: *in vitro* measurements. *J Hand Surg*, 17A:291-298, 1992.

The tendon forces generated during passive and active motion of the wrist and fingers were measured with a special force transducer. It was shown that given the currently reported breaking strength of tendon repair, passive motion programs should not have a deleterious effect on tendon healing or cause tendon gap formation. However, active motion generated forces greater than the current strength of common flexor tendon repairs.

Silfverskiold KL, May EJ, Tornvall AH: Gap formation during controlled motion after flexor tendon repair in zone II: a prospective clinical study. *J Hand Surg,* 17A:539-546,1992

A general trend toward poor clinical results in elongation of the repair was present but in individual cases gap formation was a poor predictor of the clinical result. The results indicate that controlled motion is effective in restricting the formation of adhesions associated with gap formation during postoperative immobilization.

Savage R, Risitano G: Flexor tendon repair using a "six-strand" method of repair and early active mobilization. *J Hand Surg,* 14B:369-399, 1989.

Active mobilization after repair using a six-strand grasping suture gave excellent or good results in 81% of fingers.

Strickland JW: Biologic rationale, clinical application, and results of early motion following flexor tendon repair. *J Hand Ther,* 2:71-83,1989.

The history, development, and results of protected mobilization techniques are reviewed along with an evaluation of current methods of assessment in flexor tendon surgery.

Trail IA, Powell ES, Noble J: The mechanical strength of various suture techniques. *J Hand Surg,* 17B:89-91, 1992.

The mechanical strengths of five techniques were evaluated in cadaver tendons. The Becker and Savage repairs withstood the highest load before failure.

Wade PJF, Muir IFK, Hucheon LL: Primary flexor tendon repair: the mechanical limitations of the modified Kessler technique. *J Hand Surg,* 11B:71-76, 1986.

Postoperative active movement of the repaired tendon is of current interest. The Kessler suture was strengthened with a peripheral stitch that was found to be an important structural component of the suture. Cautious active postoperative movement may be possible using this combination of Kessler suture plus peripheral stitch.

Wade PJF, Wetherell RG, Amis A: Flexor tendon repair: significant gain in strength from the Halsted peripheral suture technique. *J Hand Surg,* 14B:232-235, 1989.

A cadaver study in which a core suture alone, a core suture with a simple running surface suture, or a Halsted horizontal mattress technique for the peripheral stitch were compared. It was felt that this last technique reduced the risks of technical failure after flexor tendon repair and allowed early active mobilization.

Wehbe MA: Tendon graft donor sites. *J Hand Surg,* 17A:1130-1132, 1992.

Dissection of 120 cadavers revealed that the palmaris longus was absent in 25% of upper extremities and the plantaris in 19% of lower extremities dissected.

Wehbe MA, Hunter JM, Schneider LH, Goodwyn BL: Two-stage flexor tendon reconstruction: ten year experience. *J Bone Joint Surg,* 68A:752-763, 1986.

A review of 150 fingers in which this technique was applied. Overall good salvage was obtained in difficult flexor tendon problems. Despite complications this is a useful technique and the only method to regain active tendon function in the severely damaged flexor system.

Widstrom CJ, Johnson G, Doyle JR, Manske PR, Inhofe P: A mechanical study of six digital pulley reconstruction techniques: part I. Mechanical effectiveness. *J Hand Surg,* 14A:821-825, 1989.

The belt-loop pulley of Karev was the most effective in transforming tendon excursion into finger flexion. This is because it is closer to the joint and not stretchable. Snug pulleys near the joint axis of rotation are the most mechanically effective. In this study a two pulley system was created. Factors other than mechanical effectiveness may relate to the clinical outcome of pulley reconstruction.

Widstrom CJ, Doyle JR, Johnson G, Manske PR, McGee R: A mechanical study of six digital pulley reconstruction techniques: part II. Strength of individual reconstructions. *J Hand Surg,* 14A:826-829, 1989.

The breaking strengths of six different pulley reconstructions were compared utilizing the Bunnell, Karev, Weilby, Lister, and two new reconstructions described by the authors. The new loop and one-half technique as described by the authors was significantly stronger than the other five reconstructions.

15

Extensor Tendon Injuries

James R. Doyle, MD

Introduction

Extensor tendon injuries are now accorded the same respect as flexor tendon injuries by experienced hand surgeons. The management of injuries to the extensor mechanism requires the same amount of skill and knowledge as flexor tendon injuries. Although traditional wisdom suggested that extensor tendon injuries seen and treated early and properly usually respond well to treatment, a retrospective analysis has suggested that this is not always true, especially in those patients with associated injuries such as fracture, dislocation, capsule, or flexor tendon injury.

Anatomy

Extension of the finger is a complex act and is considered to be more intricate than finger flexion. This mechanism is composed of two separate and neurologically independent systems—the radial nerve innervated extrinsic extensors and the intrinsic muscles supplied by the ulnar and median nerves. A composite depiction of the anatomy of the extensor mechanism is given in Figures 15-1 and 15-2. Variations in the morphology and distribution of the various tendons of the extensor mechanism are common. Although the tendons of the extensor digitorum communis (EDC) are usually single in the middle and ring fingers, they are occasionally multiple. The EDC to the little finger is present less than 50% of the time and when absent is almost always replaced by a junctura tendinum from the ring finger to the extensor aponeurosis of the little finger. Each hand has three juncturae tendinum which are of three types: fascia, ligament, and tendon as seen from the radial to the ulnar side of the hand.

The extensor digiti quinti proprius arises from a single muscle belly and usually divides into two slips beneath the extensor retinaculum but may have three or four slips.

The extensor indicis proprius is usually a single tendon but may be double. When double, the slips may be radial or ulnar to the EDC to the index or with one slip on each side of the EDC. When it is radial it may have a connection to the EPL. A junctura tendinum has also been reported between an otherwise normal index EDC and the EPL. The EIP is usually distinguished from the EDC by its ulnar location and absence of a junctura tendinum. Traditional knowledge suggested that independent extension of the index and little finger is due solely to the proprius tendon. Loss of independent extension of the index was said to be highly probable if the extensor index proprius (EIP) was transferred. This concept was disproved in a series of 27 patients who demonstrated independent index extension after transfer of the EIP.

Zones of Extensor Tendon Injury

The extensor mechanism can be injured from the DIP joint to the proximal forearm. As shown in Table 15.1, nine zones of injury (I-IX) have been identified to aid in classification and discussion of treatment.

Table 15.1

Zone	Finger	Thumb
I	DIP joint	IP joint
II	Middle phalanx	Proximal phalanx
III	PIP joint	MP joint
IV	Proximal phalanx	Metacarpal
V	MP joint	CMC joint/radial styloid
VI	Metacarpal	
VII	Dorsal wrist retinaculum	
VIII	Distal forearm	
IX	Mid and proximal forearm	

Evaluation of Results in Extensor Tendon Injuries

The results following extensor tendon injury and treatment may be evaluated by total active motion, extension lag, extension lag and flexion loss, and grip strength. Little has been published about the results after extensor tendon repair. Most authors have focused on the loss of extension as the most important parameter but recent studies have emphasized the importance of the ability to flex the digit and make a tight fist; this is in contrast to TAM and grip strength, which are accepted indicators of hand function after flexor tendon injuries. TAM and grip strength may not adequately reflect the loss of function at the PIP joint or the ability to use tools effectively. Based on these factors a rating system for extensor tendon injuries is as follows:

Excellent: full flexion and extension.
Good: 10° or less of extension lost, 20° or less of flexion lost.
Fair: 11° to 45° of extension lost, 21° to 45° of flexion lost.
Poor: 45° or more of both extension and flexion lost.

Dynamic Splinting for Extensor Tendon Injuries

Extensor tendon injuries have traditionally been managed by immobilization with the wrist in 40° to 45° of extension and the fingers in slight flexion for three to four weeks after surgical repair. However, in some instances this resulted in adhesions between the extensor mechanism and the sur-

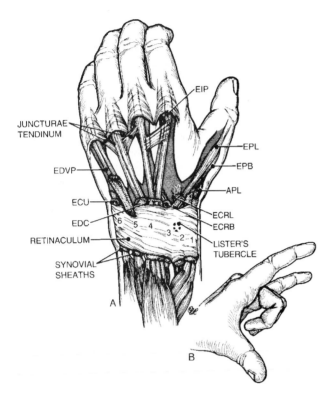

Figure 15-1.   (A) The extensor tendons gain entrance to the hand from the forearm through a series of six canals, five fibro-osseous and one fibrous (the fifth dorsal compartment, which contains the extensor digiti quinti proprius). The first compartment contains the abductor pollicis longus and extensor pollicis brevis; the second the radial wrist extensors; the third the extensor pollicis longus, which angles around Lister's tubercle; the fourth the extensor digitorum communis to the fingers, as well as the extensor indicis proprius; the fifth; the extensor digiti quinti proprius and the sixth the extensor carpi ulnaris. The communis tendons are joined distally near the MP joints by fibrous interconnections called juncturae tendinum. These juncturae are usually found only between the communis tendons and may aid in surgical recognition of the proprius tendon of the index. The proprius tendons are usually positioned to the ulnar side of the adjacent communis tendons. Beneath the retinaculum, the extensor tendons are covered with a synovial sheath. (B) The proprius tendons to the index and little fingers are capable of independent extension, and their function may be evaluated as depicted. With the middle and ring fingers flexed into the palm, the proprius tendons can extend the index and little fingers. Independent extension of the index, however, is not lost following transfer of the indicis proprius. ECRB, extensor carpi radialis brevis; ECRL, extensor carpi radialis longus.

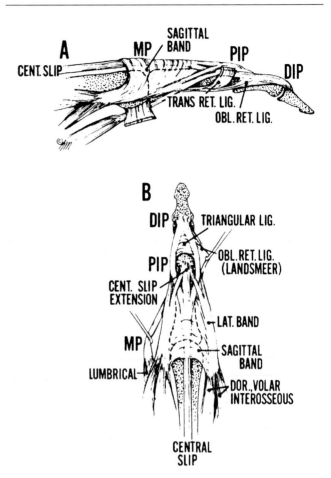

Figure 15-2.   The extensor tendon at the MP joint level is held in place by the transverse lamina or sagittal band, which tethers and centers the extensor tendons over the joint. This sagittal band arises from the volar plate and the intermetacarpal ligaments at the neck of the metacarpals. Any injury to this extensor hood or expansion may result in subluxation or dislocation of the extensor tendon. The intrinsic tendons from the lumbrical and interosseous muscles join the extensor mechanism at about the level of the proximal and midportion of the proximal phalanx and continue distally to the DIP joint of the finger. The extensor mechanism at the PIP joint is best described as a trifurcation of the extensor tendon into the central slip, which attaches to the dorsal base of the middle phalanx, and the two lateral bands. These lateral bands continue distally to insert at the dorsal base of the distal phalanx. The extensor mechanism is maintained in place over the PIP joint by the transverse retinacular ligaments.

rounding tissues. This is especially true when the tendon injury is associated with a crush injury, surrounding soft-tissue loss, infection, underlying fracture, joint capsule or flexor tendon injury. In flexor tendon injuries, controlled and early passive motion of the tendon suture site provided by dynamic splinting has proven a useful method to promote a well healed, smooth, nonadherent and gliding flexor tendon surface with improved tensile strength.

Several recent studies have reported on the application of this knowledge to extensor tendon injuries with improved results. Although absolute confirmation of the value of dynamic splinting awaits a controlled prospective study comparing dynamic vs. static splinting, the current trend is to use dynamic splinting especially in those cases with multiple extensor tendon injuries beneath the extensor retinaculum or with associated injuries. Anatomic studies have shown that, depending on the involved finger, 27.3° to 40.9° of MP joint flexion would produce 5mm of EDC glide in zone V, VI, and VII injuries. In the thumb, the EPL would glide 5mm at Lister's tubercle with 60° of IP joint flexion. Five millimeters of gliding was found to be safe (no repair-site disruption) as well as effective in limiting adhesions.

Typical postoperative management for finger zones V, VI, and VII and thumb zones IV and V begins with dynamic splinting at three days postoperative with the wrist at 40° to 45° of extension and the MP and IP joints supported at 0° in elastic traction slings attached to an outrigger device. A palmar block splint is positioned, which limits MP flexion to that arc of motion previously noted to result in 5mm of extensor tendon excursion. The patient actively flexes the MP joints but allows the dynamic traction on the outrigger devices to passively return the digital joints to 0°. These exercises are performed 10 times per hour (Fig.15-3). In thumb injuries involving zones IV and V, the EPL is splinted with the wrist extended and the CMC joint at neutral. Dynamic traction is maintained with the IP joint at 0° but allows 60° active flexion. This dynamic splinting is discontinued between the third and fourth weeks and active motion is started thereafter, which includes gentle active and active assistance exercises that emphasize extension at the MP joints with the wrist supported in extension. Between four and five weeks, individual finger extension and the claw position exercises are performed to direct controlled stress to the adhesions. At five to six weeks, finger flexion is emphasized. At seven weeks, resistance and functional electrical stimulation and dynamic flexion splinting are considered safe modalities to promote full finger flexion.

Dynamic splinting for extensor tendon injuries has been a useful method for the postoperative management of both complex and simple extensor tendon injuries in zones V-VIII. Its usefulness in zones II-IV is less apparent at this time. These techniques are most likely to yield a good result in a cooperative patient and when a skilled hand therapist is available to fabricate the splint and to monitor progress. More traditional forms of immobilization may be useful in children and uncooperative adults.

Extensor Tendon Injuries at Specific Zones

Zone I (DIP joint, Mallet finger)

Loss of continuity on the conjoined lateral bands at the distal joint of the finger results in the characteristic flexion deformity called mallet finger. The distal joint assumes varying degrees of flexion and active extension is lost, although full passive extension is usually present. Hyperextension of the middle joint may also be observed due to unopposed central slip tension at the PIP joint and PIP palmar plate laxity. The injury may be secondary to a variety of sports, occupational, or home activities. Open injuries may be due to sharp or crushing type lacerations

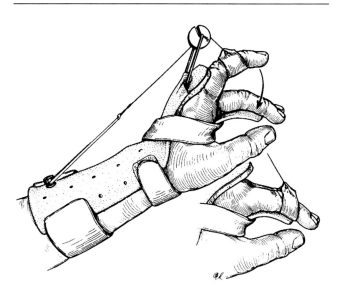

Figure 15-3. Dynamic Splint for Early Motion of Extensor Tendon Injuries. Elastic traction maintains the fingers in extension. Excursion of the repaired extensor tendon is achieved by active flexion. Splinting is started three to five days after surgery and is maintained for five weeks. Active flexion is performed 10 times an hour.

but closed injuries are more common. The usual mechanism of injury is sudden acute forceful flexion of the extended digit, which results in rupture of the extensor tendon or avulsion of the tendon with or without a small fragment of bone from its dorsal insertion. A torsion injury with associated rupture of one of the lateral bands in association with mallet finger has been reported but is very rare. Forced hyperextension of the distal joint may result in a fracture at the dorsal base of the distal phalanx involving one-third or more of the phalanx. Although a mallet deformity is associated with this injury the lesion should be considered as a fracture with a secondary mallet finger deformity.

The microvascular anatomy of the distal digital extensor tendon reveals an area of deficient blood supply in the region of insertion over the DIP joint, and this avascularity may have implications in the cause and treatment of mallet finger. This area of avascularity may explain the poor results with open suture of the ruptured tendon or an inappropriately applied splint that places too much external pressure over the DIP joint or places the DIP joint in excessive hyperextension.

Classification of Mallet Finger

Mallet finger deformities are classified as follows:

Type I: closed or blunt trauma with loss of tendon continuity with or without a small avulsion fracture.

Type II: laceration at or just proximal to the DIP joint with loss of tendon continuity.

Type III: deep abrasion with loss of skin, subcutaneous tissue and tendon substance.

Type IV: (a) transepiphysial plate fracture in children, (b) hyperflexion injury with fracture of articular surface of 20% to 50%, (c) hyperextension injury with fracture of the articular surface usually greater than 50% and with early or late volar subluxation of the distal phalanx.

Treatment of Mallet Finger

Type I injuries are the most common and are usually treated with a dorsal or volar or prefabricated splint such as the Stack splint. Excellent to good results can be anticipated in approximately 80% of these cases when treatment is provided early. Fair or poor results can be anticipated in those patients treated on a delayed basis or who wear the splints improperly. Continuous maintenance of the extended position of the DIP joint must be achieved for a minimum of six weeks for the splint to be effective. Some advocate eight weeks of splinting followed by two weeks of night splinting. Direct repair of type I injuries is to be avoided since the extensor tendon at this level is extremely thin and has a poor blood supply. Operative repair is not only unnecessary but is probably contraindicated in view of the more satisfactory results achieved with conservative treatment. A transarticular Kirschner wire may be utilized in patients such as health professionals, who cannot wear a splint for six weeks, but physical activities must be limited and a splint worn the majority of the time to protect the pin from breakage.

A recent study which reviewed the short- and long-term complications encountered in the treatment of mallet fingers revealed a high complication rate (45%) represented mostly by transient skin problems including dorsal maceration, skin ulceration, and tape allergy. Fifty percent of the skin ulcerations and 67% of the macerations appeared during the second week of treatment. Other complications included transverse nail grooves and pain from the splint, but these were less common. This study found that use of the dorsal aluminum foam splint had a higher rate of dorsal ulceration and maceration and incidence of nail grooves. Based upon the relatively high incidence of complications, the authors discouraged the use of a dorsal splint. If used, this study recommends the placement of tubular gauze or mole-skin beneath the splint. Others have reported full-thickness skin necrosis over the DIP joint after dorsal splint immobilization in hyperextension. Hyperextension is therefore to be avoided because of the relative avascularity it might produce.

A recent study of 66 fingers noted that the average total passive hyperextension of the DIP joint was 28.3° and that skin blanching occurred at approximately 50% of this total passive hyperextension. It is therefore recommended, that the distal joint be splinted with minimal hyperextension and that the amount of hyperextension that produces blanching not be exceeded. A greater than 50% complication rate was noted in patients treated surgically for mallet finger and these included permanent nail deformities, joint incongruities, infection, pin or pull-out wire failure, and radial or ulnar prominence or deviation of the DIP joint. Loss of surgical reduction, which required additional surgery, was noted in seven of 45 patients. Of these seven operated digits, four had an arthrodesis, one had an amputation, and one had a fixed flexion contracture and a mallet deformity more severe than before surgery. This study indicates the hazards associated with operative intervention in mallet finger deformity.

Although operative treatment has been recommended for type IV mallet finger injuries with fracture fragments involving greater than one-third of the articular surface, an accurate reduction is sometimes difficult to achieve. An accurate reduction has been advocated to prevent joint deformity with secondary arthritis and stiffness. The anatomic reduction and fixation of these mallet fractures is probably one of the most challenging operations in hand surgery. Various techniques have been advocated including fixation with a 0.028 diameter K-wire or a stainless-steel wire pull-out suture for fixation of the fracture. The joint must be maintained in extension until the fracture has healed.

In contrast to recommendations for open reduction, others have advised nonoperative treatment by splinting for all mallet fractures including the hyperextension type, even with subluxation of the distal phalanx. This study reflects the belief that restoration of joint congruity does not influence the end result since remodeling of the articular surface usually occurs and leads to a near-normal, painless joint in spite of persistent joint subluxation. Hyperextension mallet fractures with volar subluxation should not be placed in hyperextension since this would promote the tendency for subluxation of the major fragment. Encouraging results have been obtained using the Stack splint even with relatively large fracture fragments, and many authors have abandoned open reduction and internal fixation even with volar subluxation of the distal phalanx.

Treatment of Chronic Mallet Deformities

The management of chronic mallet deformities seen late include arthrodesis or secondary extensor tendon reconstruction. If the deformity of the DIP joint is fixed and does not respond to exercises and splinting, and if the joint surfaces are incongruous or significant degenerative arthritis is present, the only viable surgical option is arthrodesis. However, if the mallet finger deformity can be corrected and satisfactory joint congruity is present, reconstruction may be achieved by resection of a portion of the extensor tendon followed by repair under appropriate tension, or a tuck may be taken in the tendon. The third option relates to advancement of the tendon into the dorsal base of the distal phalanx. Only 2mm to 3mm needs to be excised. Following tendon repair, the distal joint is immobilized with a transarticular K-wire for four to six weeks and then a splint is used to immobilize the DIP joint at all times for a total of six to eight weeks. The patient is gradually weaned off the splint to promote gliding of the tendon without overstretching of the repair site. In cases where tendon substance is lost, a free-tendon graft may be required and must be firmly anchored to bone in order to achieve satisfactory continuity. Fowler's central slip release is favored by some practitioners and may be useful in rebalancing the extensor mechanism.

Swan Neck Deformity

Swan neck deformity is a classic manifestation of a dynamic imbalance that may occur between the extrinsic and intrinsic extensor mechanism. It is seen most commonly in the traumatic setting due to a mallet finger deformity. Coexistent volar plate laxity allows the PIP joint to hyperextend. The relative lengthening of the distal extensor mechanism secondary to disruption at the DIP joint allows dorsal migration of the lateral bands at the PIP joint and further accentuates the deformity. The deformity is complemented by the powerful flexor digitorum profundus, which becomes an unopposed deforming force at the DIP joint. Restoration of this balance by correction of the basic underlying problem (mallet finger deformity) usually corrects the problem and allows restoration of the critical balance between the profundus tendon, the distal insertion of the extensor mechanism, and the central slip at the PIP joint. Operative techniques for this problem encompass correction of the flexion posture at the DIP joint and the hyperextended posture at the PIP joint. These two deformities can be corrected by a tendon graft which mimics the dynamic function of the oblique retinacular ligament.

An accepted and proven technique for correction of this problem is the spiral oblique retinacular ligament reconstruction (Fig. 15-4). The palmaris longus or similar tendon graft is used to provide a tenodesis to correct the imbalance at both the DIP and PIP joints. The tendon graft is inserted in bone at the dorsal base of the distal phalanx and then is brought proximally and volarly across the mid-portion of the middle phalanx beneath the PIP joint to the opposite side of the base of the proximal phalanx where it is attached to bone using a pull-out wire technique. Tension is adjusted so that the PIP joint rests in 20° of flexion and the distal joint is at full extension. A transarticular K-wire is used across the PIP joint and is removed at four weeks; thereafter the involved digit is supported with a dorsal splint that holds the PIP joint in 20° of flexion and the DIP joint at full extension. Active PIP joint flexion exercises are then started; a 20° extension block is maintained and is gradually straightened over the next six to 10 weeks. A 5° to 10° persistent flexion contracture at the PIP joint is a reasonable goal and an attempt should not be made to obtain full extension at the PIP joint.

Zone II (Finger Middle Phalanx and Thumb Proximal Phalanx)

Injuries in zone II are usually secondary to a laceration or crush injury rather than an avulsion. Lacerations in this zone may produce partial division of the tendon due to its increased width and curved shape over the underlying osseous phalanx. Partial lacerations of less than 50% of the tendon can be treated by skin wound care followed by

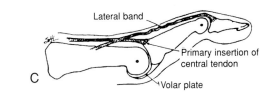

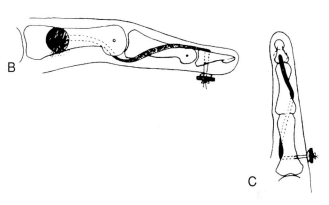

Figure 15-4. The palmaris longus or similar tendon is used for reconstruction of the oblique retinacular ligament for swan neck deformity and is called the spiral oblique retinacular ligament reconstruction.

active motion in seven to 10 days. Complete lacerations require suture and static splinting of the IP joint in full extension for six weeks. Dynamic splinting should be considered if associated injuries that might compromise the end result are present.

Zone III (Boutonnière Deformity)

Disruption of the central slip of the extensor tendon at the PIP joint with volar migration of the lateral bands will result in the so-called boutonnière deformity, which includes loss of extension at the PIP joint and compensatory hyperextension at the DIP joint. The lesion is most often secondary to closed blunt trauma with acute forceful flexion at the PIP joint. This produces avulsion of the central slip from its insertion on the dorsal base of the middle phalanx, with or without fracture and/or laceration of the extensor tendon at or near its insertion. Volar dislocation of the PIP joint may also result in avulsion of the central slip and subsequent boutonnière deformity. In closed injuries the characteristic boutonnière deformity may not be apparent at the time of injury and may not be noted until 10 to 21 days after injury. A painful, tender, swollen PIP joint that has recently been injured should alert the examiner that a boutonnière deformity may develop. A review of 43 of 71 patients treated in an emergency room with a diagnosis of jammed or sprained finger over a 14-month period revealed that two of the 43 patients developed a boutonnière deformity. Two diagnostic tests that are useful in early recognition of this lesion are: (1) a 15° to 20° or greater loss of active extension of the PIP joint when the wrist and MP joint are fully flexed and (2) extravasation of intra-articular radiopaque dye dorsal and distal to the PIP joint. Weak extension against resistance has also been noted to be a helpful diagnostic finding and is suggestive, if not diagnostic, of central slip injury. Disruption of the central slip and volar migration of the lateral bands are also associated with decreased flexion of the DIP joint. The boutonnière deformity illustrates the problem of imbalance in the finger, which is a chain of joints with multiple tendon attachments. This chain collapses into an abnormal postural deformity when there is an imbalance of the critical forces maintaining equilibrium.

Treatment of Boutonnière Deformity

Treatment of the closed acute boutonnière deformity is dependent upon restoration of the normal tendon balance and precise length relationships of the central slip and lateral bands. In acute cases before fixed contractures have occurred, this may be achieved by progressively splinting the PIP joint into full extension and at the same time performing active and passive flexion exercises of the DIP joint. Splinting of the PIP joint in full extension reduces the separation of the torn ends of the central slip of the extensor tendon, and active flexion of the DIP joint draws the lateral bands distally and dorsally. This allows repair by contracture of the disrupted central slip tendon to its anatomic length and migration of the lateral bands to their normal anatomic position above the joint axis of rotation at the PIP joint. A variety of means have been used to achieve extension of the PIP joint, including transarticular Kirschner wires, plaster casts, and various types of static or dynamic splints. In a closed boutonnière deformity operative intervention is indicated under two circumstances: (1) when the central slip has been avulsed with a bone fragment which is lying free over the PIP joint; and (2) a long-standing boutonnière deformity in a young person. Depending on its size the bone fragment is excised, or reattached. If the fragment is excised, the central slip should be reattached to the base of the middle phalanx and the joint transfixed with a K-wire for 10 days followed by dynamic or static splinting of the PIP joint in full extension and active flexion of the distal joint.

Open lacerations over the PIP joint are likely to enter the joint space and the first aim of treatment should be to prevent infection. Laceration of the central slip and/or lateral bands at the PIP joint level requires primary repair and splinting of the PIP joint in full extension for at least five to six weeks. During that time the distal joint is actively flexed to maintain balance between the central slip and the lateral bands. Care must be taken to restore the anatomic length of the lacerated tendon. Acute injuries that result in loss of significant substance in the extensor mechanism at this level may be treated by any method that restores substance to the extensor tendons such as a free-tendon graft or a flap of the extensor mechanism turned distally to restore continuity.

Treatment of Chronic Boutonnière Deformity

Dynamic splinting of the boutonnière deformity is useful even in chronic and fixed deformities. If it fails, then surgical intervention is required. Surgical treatment of chronic boutonnière deformity in which conservative treatment in the form of dynamic splinting and exercise has failed, consists of restoration of the balance between the extrinsic and intrinsic tendons. Any tendon procedure is best done after the joint has full passive mobility. In some cases this is not possible, and the stiff joint must be surgically corrected first, followed later on by tendon reconstruction. Secondary reconstruction is compromised if the joint architecture has been disturbed as in severe posttraumatic arthritis. The surgeon must be aware that flexion in the PIP joint must not be jeopardized in an attempt to gain extension. Secondary reconstruction for chronic boutonnière deformity falls into two categories: (1) soft-tissue release and (2) secondary tendon reconstruction. Several authors have described similar techniques for soft-tissue release which utilize the surgical principle of decreasing the extensor tone at the distal joint by transection of the extensor mechanism just distal to the PIP joint but leaving the oblique retinacular ligament intact. This allows the lateral bands of the extensor mechanism to slide proximally and increases their tone at the PIP joint. The extensor mechanism is divided transversely over the junction of the middle and proximal thirds of the middle phalanx just distal to the dorsal transverse retinacular fibers. The oblique retinacular ligament applies extension force to the distal joint. A favorable surgical result is predictable in the patient who has full passive extension preoperatively. Other methods of secondary tendon reconstruction include excision of redundant scar tissue in the central slip and direct repair of the extensor mechanism or a Y-V advancement. Care is taken to avoid any tension imbalance between the central slip and lateral bands. The lateral bands must be returned to their usual position dorsal to the PIP joint axis by soft-tissue release as needed. If the lateral bands are so contracted that they produce a fixed flexion deformity at the PIP joint, they may be released at the middle phalanx (except for the lumbrical and oblique retinacular ligaments). The lateral bands are then placed dorsally and sutured to the central slip. In some cases the central slip deficit is so severe that a free-tendon graft is required to restore continuity; this procedure should be done only when full passive extension of the PIP joint is present. The tendon graft must pass through the dorsal base of the osseous middle phalanx and be sutured under proper tension to the proximal remnants of the extensor mechanism. Variations of this free-tendon graft include utilization of the ulnar lateral band, which is cut over the distal end of the middle phalanx and then passed through the radial lateral band at the PIP joint and then through a hole at the dorsal base of the middle phalanx. All of these tendon procedures require that the PIP joint be stabilized with a transarticular K-wire for five to six weeks. During that time active extension of the distal joint is performed. Further splinting of the PIP joint is required until balance has been obtained between the extrinsic and intrinsic mechanism.

Zone IV (Proximal Phalanx of Finger and Thumb Metacarpal)

Injuries at zone IV are similar to zone II injuries in that they may be partial lacerations due to the tendon width and the underlying curvature of the osseous phalanx. Lacerations of an isolated lateral band are repaired and protected motion begun immediately after repair. Complete lacerations of the finger central tendon require repair to avoid relative lengthening of the tendon and resultant imbalance between the central slip and lateral bands. After repair, the PIP joint should be maintained in full extension for six weeks. Thumb zones III and IV tendon lacerations involve easily distinguished EPB and EPL tendons which are sutured with a buried core type suture, and postoperative management includes maintaining the wrist in 40° extension and the thumb MP joint in full extension for three to four weeks. Dynamic traction may be used in selected cases for controlled active flexion of the MP and IP joints.

Zone V (MP Joint)

Injuries to the extensor mechanism at the MP joint are often secondary to human bite wounds. A high index of suspicion should be present when examining lacerations in this area. Most if not all patients will deny this mechanism of injury. This is a contaminated wound and the organisms involved are capable of producing a significant wound infection with the potential for joint-space infection and destruction of the articular cartilage. The incidence of complications of this type are directly related to the virulence of the organisms and the time span from injury to treatment. A radiograph should be obtained to note the presence or absence of fracture or foreign body. The wound must be extended proximally and distally to permit inspection of the joint and a culture should be taken. The wound is debrided, irrigated, and left open. Appropriate antibiotics should be started immediately and precautions taken to culture for the usual organisms as well as Eikenella corrodens. Under no circumstances should a human bite wound be closed. Most tendon injuries associated with this type of wound are partial and need not be repaired immediately. The hand is splinted with the wrist in 40° to 45° of extension and the MP joints in 15° to 20° of flexion. The soft-tissues including the capsule and extensor hood are allowed to seek their own position over the joint. Partial or even complete lacerations are seldom if ever associated with significant retraction at this level. The tendon laceration may be repaired secondarily as needed in five to seven days or even later depending upon the nature of the wound at the time of inspection. Dynamic splinting should be started when the infection is under control.

Simple lacerations of the extensor mechanism or hood at the MP joint should be repaired using simple sutures of nonabsorbable material followed by dynamic splinting. Lacerations of the hood or sagittal bands at this level must be repaired so that the extensor tendon will remain centralized over the dorsum of the joint. Failure to repair this type of injury may result in subluxation of the extensor tendon and associated loss of extension.

Traumatic Dislocation of Extensor Tendon (Rupture of Sagittal Bands)

Subluxation or dislocation of the extensor tendon may occur at the MP joint following laceration of the hood, or may occur following forceful flexion or extension injury of the finger. In traumatic dislocation without laceration, the middle finger is most commonly involved. The lesion is secondary to a tear of the sagittal band and oblique fibers of the hood, usually on the radial side. Ulnar dislocation usually occurs and is associated with incomplete finger extension and ulnar deviation of the involved digit. Acute tears can be satisfactorily repaired by primary suture of the defect. There have been case reports of successful treatment by plaster cast immobilization with the MP joints in full extension for four weeks. Conservative treatment is more likely to be successful if the diagnosis and treatment occur immediately after the injury. If diagnosis or treatment is delayed and delayed primary suture is not possible, some type of reconstructive procedure is required to centralize the tendon by first restoring it to its central location and then providing a soft-tissue anchor. Reefing of the radial fibers over the hood along with release of the ulnar side of the hood may provide an acceptable repair, but if the radial portion of the hood is absent or not suitable for repair, then a tether must be made to centralize the tendon (Fig. 15-5).

Zone VI (Metacarpal Level)

Zone VI injuries have been noted to have a better prognosis than more distal lesions involving zones II to V. This may be due to the fact that zone VI injuries are unlikely to have associated joint injuries, and that decreased tendon surface area in zone VI lessens the potential for adhesion formation. There is also increased subcutaneous tissues in zone VI along with greater tendon excursion. Extensor tendons in this zone have sufficient substance to accept substantial buried core-type sutures, and dynamic splinting

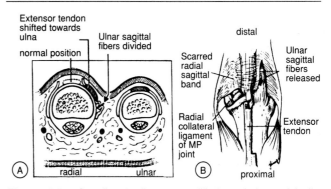

Figure 15-5. Carroll and colleagues modified a technique originally described by Kilgore, and associatedl for stabilizing the extensor tendon by forming a distally based loop of tendon from the ulnar side of the extensor digitorum communis and wrapping it around the radial collateral ligament and then suturing it back to itself under appropriate tension.

can be performed with the assurance that disruption of the suture site is unlikely. Postoperative management includes dynamic splinting beginning three to five days after repair with the wrist in 40° to 45° of extension and the MP joints in 0° to 15° of flexion for five weeks.

Zone VII (Wrist Level)

Injuries to the extensor mechanism at the wrist level are associated with injuries to the retinaculum. The retinaculum prevents bowstringing of the extensor tendons, and lacerations of the extensors at this level are said to be associated with subsequent adhesions to the overlying retinaculum. For this reason many authors in the past have advised that portions of the extensor retinaculum located over the site of tendon repair should be excised to prevent adhesions. However, a recent study has noted no statistical differences in the results when comparing zones VI, VII, and VIII. This study reported on primary repair of extensor tendons in zones VI, VII and VIII and used traditional postoperative immobilization. The excellent results with early dynamic splinting reported by several authors suggest that excision of portions of the retinaculum over the tendon repair site may not be as important as previously believed. However, limited excision of portions of the retinaculum does no harm and may facilitate tendon exposure and gliding; it should be considered, especially in repairs in which there might be impingement between the suture site and the adjacent retinaculum. If the surgeon is concerned about maintaining the anatomic integrity of the retinaculum, the traumatic openings in the retinaculum may be extended distally and proximally at each end of the retinacular lacerations to facilitate tendon repair and then reapproximated. Multiple tendon injuries at this level may be dealt with by appropriate excision of the retinaculum as needed, but portions of the retinaculum should always be preserved either proximal or distal to the suture line to prevent bowstringing. Although it has been previously recommended that complete excision of the extensor retinaculum be performed with lacerations at multiple levels in this area, recent findings suggest that complete excision of the retinaculum is seldom, if ever, necessary. Some portion of the retinaculum can usually be preserved and adhesions that limit function are unlikely, especially if early dynamic splinting is utilized.

Zone VIII (Distal Forearm)

Zone VIII injuries at the muscle tendon junction require careful reapproximation of the separated parts. Although the distal tendon accepts and holds sutures well, the proximal muscle belly does not and reapproximation of the separated parts is facilitated by multiple nonabsorbable sutures that join the tendon and muscle together. Tendons characteristically originate from a fibrous tissue raphe in the substance of the muscle belly several centimeters proximal to the area where the tendon is recognizable as a distinct structure. A septa can usually be identified. Sutures are placed in this fibrous tissue as much as possible, with the knots buried between the tendon and the muscle in order to

keep the sutures from pulling out. Care is taken, however, to avoid strangulation of the muscle with these coaptation sutures. Postoperative management includes static immobilization of the wrist in 40° to 45° of extension and the MP joints in 15° to 20° of flexion for four to five weeks. Flexion of the MP joints may be started at two weeks against elastic traction resistance. A static night splint that maintains the wrist in extension is used for an additional two weeks.

Zone IX (Proximal Forearm Level)

The wrist and common finger extensors as well as the little finger proprius arise from the region of the lateral epicondyle at the elbow. The thumb extensors and abductors along with the proprius tendon of the index finger arise from the forearm below the elbow. Injuries at this level are usually due to a penetrating wound secondary to a knife or a piece of broken glass. The size of the skin wound may give little indication as to the magnitude of the injury. The demonstrated loss of function may be due to a muscle injury, nerve injury or both. Accurate preoperative diagnosis may be impossible. The radial nerve at the level of the distal forearm gives branches to the brachialis, brachioradialis, and extensor carpi radialis longus. A major division of this nerve then occurs into the sensory branch and posterior interosseous nerve (motor branch). The superficial (sensory) branch continues distally under cover of the brachioradialis into the forearm, wrist, and hand areas. The posterior interosseous nerve gives branches to the extensor carpus radialis brevis (ECRB) and supinator which it penetrates, supplies, and then innervates the remainder of the extensor muscle group.

Penetrating wounds in this area should be evaluated by careful physical examination and then explored to determine the exact etiology of any losses noted. Under tourniquet control and appropriate anesthesia the wound margins are debrided and then extended proximally and distally and the extent of damage noted. If the injury involves muscle belly only, a careful repair of the muscle belly is performed with multiple figure-of-eight sutures of polyglactin (Vicryl-Ethicon). Experimental data on repaired muscle lacerations in laboratory animals reveals that useful, but not complete function, can be restored with adequate repair of skeletal muscle. A muscle segment totally isolated from its motor point may not contribute to the contractile function of the innervated muscle. In a recent series of patients with forearm muscle lacerations, it was noted that tendon grafting was an effective method of repair to overcome extensive defects. The indications for this technique were lacerations of two or more muscles with at least 50% of the muscle substance lacerated. The palmaris longus or toe extensors were utilized and passed through the superficial epimysium, muscle belly, and deep epimysium proximally and distally and sutured to themselves with a Pulvertaft side-weave technique. One to three grafts were used as required. The limb was immobilized for three weeks with the elbow at 90°. Protected motion was started at three weeks and progressive motion at six weeks.

If evidence of nerve injury is noted, the appropriate branches are identified and traced out to their insertions. Penetrating wounds often injure the nerve at or near its entrance to the muscle belly and retraction of the distal nerve stump into the muscle belly may occur, complicating its location and subsequent repair. Immediately after an injury it is often impossible to determine if functional loss is due to muscle or nerve damage. However, after seven to 10 days a denervated muscle will spontaneously contract for several minutes under the influence of succinylcholine during induction of general anesthesia. Additional information may be gained by electrodiagnostic studies three to four weeks after injury. The decision for secondary nerve repair or reconstruction vs. tendon transfer will depend on the judgment and experience of the surgeon. If the lesion is confined to the muscle belly, definitive repairs are performed using sutures or tendon graft as previously described.

Immediately after injury the muscle is usually quite hemorrhagic and muscle planes are difficult to identify. Identification is aided by evacuation of the hematoma, irrigation, and gentle sponging of the cut muscle ends. Postoperatively, the extremity is supported in a plaster splint that maintains the wrist in 45° of extension and the MP joints in 15° to 20° of flexion. The elbow is immobilized at 90° of flexion if the muscles involved arise at or above the lateral epicondyle. Immobilization is continued for four weeks after injury and then protected range of motion started, but a night splint is used to maintain the wrist in extension for another two weeks.

Annotated Bibliography

Anatomy

Godwin Y, Ellis H: Distribution of extensor tendons on the dorsum of the hand. *Clin Anat,* 5:394-403, 1992.

Extensor digitorum tendons are usually single except for the middle and ring fingers, which are occasionally multiple. The EDC of the little finger may be fused to the ring finger EDC or absent. Extensor digiti minimi usually has two tendons but may have three to four. Extensor indicis (EI) varies in the number of its tendons, in its position relative to the EDC of the index, and in its connection to the extensor pollicis longus.

Moore JR, Weiland AJ, Valdata L: Independent index extension after extensor indicis proprius transfer. *J Hand Surg,* 12A:232-236, 1987.

In 27 cases of EIP transfer the authors noted independent and full extension of the index finger after transfer of the EIP tendon.

Steichen JB, Petersen DP: Junctura tendinum between extensor digitorum communis and extensor pollicis longus. *J Hand Surg,* 9A:674-76, 1984.

This is a documented (intraoperative) case of a junctura tendinum between an otherwise normal index EDC and the EPL. The lesion was probably bilateral since the patient lacked independent extension of the thumb and fingers in both hands.

Wehbe M: Junctura anatomy. *J Hand Surg,* 17A:1124-1129, 1992.

Three types of junctura were identified: fascia, ligament, and tendon. Each hand had three juncturae with the most frequent presentation being fascia-ligament-tendon as observed from the radial to the ulnar side of the hand.

Results After Extensor Tendon Injuries

Newport ML, Blair WF, Steyers CM, Jr: Long-term results of extensor tendon repair. *J Hand Surg,* 15A:961-966, 1990.

This retrospective study of 62 patients with 101 digits revealed (1) 60% of all fingers had an associated injury such as fracture, dislocation, joint capsule, or flexor tendon injury which resulted in 45% of good to excellent results in contrast to 64% good to excellent results in patients without associated injuries; (2) distal zone injuries (I-IV) had a less favorable result than proximal zone injuries (V-III); and (3) the average loss of flexion was greater than the average loss of extension.

Dynamic Mobilization Of Extensor Tendon Injuries

Browne EZ, Jr. Ribik CA: Early dynamic splinting for extensor tendon injuries. *J Hand Surg,* 14A:72-76, 1989.

In a review of 52 patients the authors verified the efficacy of early dynamic splinting started at three to five days after repair in well motivated and reliable patients. Dynamic splinting was discontinued after five weeks and was followed by an extension night splint for one month.

Evans RB, Burkhalter WE: A study of the dynamic anatomy of extensor tendons and implications for treatment. *J Hand Surg,* 11A:774-779, 1986.

This pilot study reported on 66 digits with controlled passive motion in untidy extensor tendon injuries. The authors noted, depending on the digit tested, that 27.3° to 40.9° of MP joint flexion would yield 5mm of EDC tendon glide in zones V, VI, and VII. Dynamic splinting was discontinued between the third and fourth week followed by active motion.

Hung LK, Chan A, Chang J, Tsang A, Leung PC: Early controlled active mobilization with dynamic splintage for treatment of extensor tendon injuries. *J Hand Surg,* 15A:251-257, 1990.

The authors of this prospective study of 38 patients with 48 digit injuries noted that controlled active mobilization is a reliable and effective means of rehabilitating extensor tendon injuries. Although this method was expensive and labor intensive, the authors noted that average return to work in 8.5 weeks indicated money and effort well spent.

Mallet Finger

Bowers WH, Hurst LC: Chronic mallet finger: the use of Fowler's central slip release. *J Hand Surg,* 3A:373-376, 1978.

Fowler's release was used in five patients with failed mallet finger. The authors noted excellent results in four out of five patients and reemphasized Fowler's advice that this is a salvage procedure. The procedure, however, is an alternative to reconstruction in some types of chronic mallet deformity.

Crawford GP: The molded polythene splint for mallet finger deformities. *J Hand Surg,* 9A:231-237, 1984.

The author has obtained encouraging results with nonoperative treatment of mallet fractures using the Stack splint even with relatively large fracture fragments.

Rayan RA, Mullins PT: Skin necrosis complicating mallet finger splinting and vascularity of the distal interphalangeal joint overlying skin. *J Hand Surg,* 12A:548-552, 1987.

In a series of 66 fingers the authors noted that average total passive hyperextension of the DIP joint was 28.5° and that skin blanching occurred at approximately 50% of the total passive hyperextension. They advised that the degree at which the dorsal skin begins to blanch must be determined and the amount of hyperextension should not exceed that degree.

Stern PJ, Kastrup JJ: Complications and prognosis of treatment of mallet finger. *J Hand Surg,* 13A:329-334, 1988.

Fifty-three percent of 45 surgically treated patients developed complications and of these 76 were long-term. Complications included nail deformities, joint incongruities, infection, pin or pull-out wire failure, or joint deviation. Loss of surgical reduction which required reoperation occurred in seven digits: four had an arthrodesis, one an amputation, one a fixed flexion contracture, and one a mallet deformity more severe than the original.

Warren RA, Kay NRM, Norris SH: The microvascular anatomy of the distal digital extensor tendon. *J Hand Surg,* 13B:161-163, 1988.

The relative avascularity of the extensor tendon at the DIP joint probably explains the tendency for rupture in this area as well as the poor results that can be anticipated with primary repair or an inappropriately applied splint which applies too much external pressure over the DIP joint.

Wehbe MA:, Schneider LH: Mallet fractures. *J Bone and Joint Surg,* 66A:658-669, 1984.

The authors treated 44 mallet fractures in 160 mallet injuries of which 13 had volar subluxation of the distal phalanx. All were treated by splinting since the authors believe that restoration of joint congruity does not influence the end result. Remodeling of the joint occurred, which led to a near-normal painless joint in spite of persistent joint subluxation.

Swan Neck Deformity

Thompson JS, Littler JW, Upton J: The spiral oblique retinacular ligament. SORL. *J Hand Surg,* 3:482-487, 1978.

This tenodesis procedure using a palmaris longus graft can correct the two components of swan neck deformity, PIP joint hyperextension, and DIP joint flexion.

Boutonnière Deformity

Burton RI: The Hand, pp. 137-190. In Goldstein LA, Dickerson RC (eds): *Atlas of Orthopedic Surgery,* Second ed, CV Mosby, St. Louis, 1981.

The author describes the technique of Eaton and Littler, which releases the extensor mechanism just distal to the dorsal transverse retinacular fibers over the middle phalanx allowing the extensor mechanism to slide proximally. The oblique retinacular ligaments are preserved. A favorable result is associated with full passive preoperative extension.

Carducci AT: Potential boutonnière deformity. Its recognition and treatment. *Orthop Rev,* 10:121-123, 1981.

The author reviewed 43 of 71 patients treated in an emergency room for jammed or sprained fingers over a 14-month period and noted that two of the 43 developed boutonnière deformity. He noted that two diagnostic tests were useful in early recognition: (1) a 15° to 20° degree or greater loss of extension at the PIP joint with the wrist and MP joints fully flexed and (2) extravasation of intra-articular radiopaque dye dorsal and distal to the PIP joint.

Doyle JR: Extensor tendons—acute injuries. In Green DP (ed): *Operative Hand Surgery,* ed2, Churchill Livingstone, New York, 1988, pp. 2055-2060.

The author reviews the nonsurgical and surgical methods for management of the acute boutonnière deformity.

Lovett WL, McCalla MA: Management and rehabilitation of extensor tendon injuries. *Orthop Clin North Am,* 14:811-826, 1983.

The authors noted that weak extension of the PIP joint against resistance was an excellent diagnostic sign for central slip injury.

Human Bite Wounds

Rayan GM, Putnam JL, Cahill SL, Flournoy DJ: Eikenella corrodens in human mouth flora. *J Hand Surg,* 13A:953-956, 1988.

The authors noted 100% susceptibility of E. corrodens to second and third-generation cephalosporins and suggested that the use of these drugs only was appropriate empiric therapy for human bite wounds. However, follow-up culture and susceptibility testing should always be done to detect resistant organisms.

Traumatic Dislocation of Extensor Tendon

Carroll C, Moore JR, Weiland AJ: Posttraumatic ulnar subluxation of the extensor tendons: a reconstructive technique. *J Hand Surg,* 12A:227-231, 1987.

The authors report four cases of ulnar subluxation treated successfully by six weeks of splinting of the MP joint in 0° of extension. These four cases were compared to five fingers diagnosed late which required secondary reconstruction. The authors described a secondary reconstructive procedure using a portion of the extensor tendon as a sling placed around the radial collateral ligament.

Muscle Repair

Botte MV, Gelberman RH, Smith DB, Silver MA, Gellman H: Repair of severe muscle belly lacerations using a tendon graft. *J Hand Surg,* 12A:406-412, 1987.

The authors describe their technique for restoration of continuity of significant muscle belly lacerations using free-tendon grafts.

Garrett WE, Jr, Seaber AV, Boswick J, Urbaniak JR, Goldner JL: Recovery of skeletal muscle after laceration and repair. *J Hand Surg,* 9A:683-692, 1984.

The authors noted useful but not complete recovery of muscle function in rabbits following repair of skeletal muscle lacerations.

16

Tendon Transfers

H. Relton McCarroll, MD

Principles

Tendon transfers replace lost motor function when repair of an injured nerve/muscle/tendon unit is impossible. A tendon transfer can restore the balance between the flexors and extensors and thus reduce deformity. Stronger transfers can replace the lost power needed for strong grasp.

Motor Selection

A motor unit selected for transfer must be expendable and have sufficient excursion and adequate strength to replace the lost function. Excursion is measured directly in centimeters, or indirectly by the mean fiber length with which there is a direct relationship. Relative strength is measured by the mass fraction or the tension fraction. The mass fraction (the volume of an individual muscle compared to the total volume of all hand/forearm muscles) is appropriately used if muscle work is the most important consideration. The tension fraction (the cross-sectional area of the muscle compared with the area of all muscles) is used when isometric strength (i.e. pinch) is more important (Table 16-1).

Table 16-1. Normal values for muscles pertinent to radial nerve palsy.

Muscle	Tension fraction (%)	Mass fraction (%)	Fiber length (cm)
FCU	6.7	5.6	4.2
PT	5.5	5.6	5.1
ECU	4.5	4.0	4.5
ECRB	4.2	5.1	6.1
FCR	4.1	4.2	5.2
ECRL	3.5	6.5	9.3
FDS (middle finger)	3.4	4.7	6.0
FDS (index finger)	2.0	2.9	7.2
FDS (ring finger)	2.0	3.0	7.3
EDC (middle finger)	1.9	2.2	6.0
EDC (ring finger)	1.7	2.0	5.8
EPL	1.3	1.5	5.7
PL	1.2	1.2	5.0
EDC (index finger)	1.0	1.1	5.5
EDQ	1.0	1.2	5.9
EIP	1.0	1.1	5.5
EDC (little finger)	0.9	1.0	5.9
FDS (little)	0.9	1.3	7.0

Table 16-1 modified and reproduced with permission from Brand PW, et al: Relative tension and potential excursion of muscles in the forearm and hand. *J Hand Surg,* 6A:209-219, 1981.

The excursion can be less than that of the normal motor unit if the transfer is assisted by the tenodesis effect of a mobile wrist. Prior to transfer, the strength of any motor unit must be good or normal (four or five) by the usual rating scale. Because motion of the wrist or fingers against gravity is relatively easy compared to an elbow or knee, a motor unit that produces a full range of motion against gravity (grade three or fair) is useful only when the extremity is uniformly and generally weak. The standard grading scale (absent, trace, poor, fair, good, normal) overemphasizes weak, nonfunctional muscles. Semiquantitative grading of motor-unit strength would be more useful if done as a percentage of the normal strength.

Synergistic muscles are easier to retrain to perform their new function after transfer. Normal hand function coordinates wrist extension with finger flexion and wrist flexion with finger extension. This link makes it easier for a patient to use a wrist flexor as a finger extensor as opposed to a wrist extensor. Tendon transfers can be retrained to perform nonsynergistic functions, but it is a more difficult chore for the patient. Some individuals are not especially good at adapting muscles to new functions; they are more apt to fail with nonsynergistic transfers.

Prerequisites

Tendon transfers should be performed at the conclusion of the reconstructive program. Bone alignment should be restored and passive range of motion regained prior to tendon transfer. A tendon transfer will never produce better motion than the preoperative passive range. Most individuals will not use an insensitive hand; thus, reconstruction is contraindicated in the absence of sensibility. The exceptions to this rule are those with bilateral involvement who do not have a normal extremity and individuals with tetraplegia or Hansen's disease.

Surgical Principles

With time patients learn to substitute a functioning muscle for one that is paralyzed, for example by using the finger flexors to flex the wrist. Children are especially adept at such tricks. If there is any question about the capacity of a proposed donor muscle, it should be inspected at surgery to ensure that the color of the muscle is normal. The excursion of the muscle should be checked and, in some instances, increased by appropriate dissection. The muscle must be mobilized in a manner that preserves the neurovascular bundle.

Several guidelines are recommended to adjust the tension of a transfer appropriately. One technique is to maximally approximate the donor tendon to its proposed insertion by motion of the intervening joints. The sutures are inserted without maintaining any tension on the donor muscle. This can be technically difficult if the situation requires suturing on the palmar surface of a flexed wrist. An alternate method permits suturing an opponensplasty with the wrist in neutral position and the thumb passively held in opposition. The donor motor unit is passively stretched and allowed to recoil while observing the donor tendon. The midpoint of the tendon's excursion at the proposed suture site represents appropriate tension. If there is still an art of tendon transfer surgery, it is in deciding how tight to suture the transfer.

In most instances the tendon should be rerouted in a straight line through subcutaneous tissue. Pulleys change the direction of action but reduce the efficiency of the muscle; they should be avoided if possible. Tendons are most likely to adhere to bone, small fascial windows, and scar. Tendon transfers usually tolerate crossing narrow scars; they do not tolerate resting in scar over a distance or in any dense scar.

Function

A tendon transfer can exert pull in only one direction at a time and, therefore, performs a single function. Transfers with a split or double insertion will pull on whichever insertion is the tightest. A yoke (Y-shaped) insertion can be useful in preventing subluxation of the transfer or help keep the transfer centralized over the powered joint. For example, an opponensplasty can be inserted into both the abductor pollicis brevis and the adductor pollicis. The ulnar insertion into the adductor pollicis prevents the transfer from slipping palmarward and becoming a deforming flexor of the MP joint. It does not make the transfer both an abductor and an adductor. Success of a given transfer may require other procedures, such as arthrodesis, or a second tendon transfer to complete a complicated function.

Radial Nerve Palsy

Deficit

Radial nerve paralysis involves loss of the wrist and finger extensors. The major functional loss is the inability to extend the wrist; this places the hand in a poor functional position and weakens the ability to grasp. Both wrist and finger extension need to be replaced, but one extensor motor unit can power all four ulnar digits.

Transfers: Types and Goals

A very strong, single motor unit is needed to replace wrist extension. The pronator teres is most frequently selected; it is strong enough, it will reach the extensor carpi radialis brevis without prolongation, and the muscle still assists pronation after transfer (Table 16-1).

There are two approaches to powering the ulnar finger extensors: transfer of a wrist flexor or transfer of the flexor digitorum superficialis.

The most common transfer for finger extension is rerouting of the flexor carpi ulnaris around the ulnar border of the forearm to insert into all four digital extensors. The flexor carpi radialis is preferred by some surgeons for its greater excursion, especially in carpenters or those who require forceful ulnar deviation of the wrist.

The most common operation for thumb extension is to route the extensor pollicis longus tendon over the basal joint of the thumb to the palmar surface of the forearm and power it with the palmaris longus. In this manner one transfer combines abduction at the basal joint and extension of the distal joint; this is usually adequate.

An alternative approach is transfer of two flexor digitorum superficialis tendons, one to motor the index finger and thumb, and one to extend the ulnar three digits. These transfers are passed through the interosseous membrane, a site for potential scarring. To be successful, the transfer must be inserted under greater-than-average tension. Since three of the superficialis are digastric (index, ring, and little fingers), this extra tension ensures that the muscle pulls on the transferred tendons and not on the remaining, untransferred tendons.

A final possibility relies on the fact that the long finger superficialis does not share the proximal muscle belly with the other three superficialis. Since it has completely independent function, it can be used for extension of the ulnar digits without interference with the flexor power of the other superficialis muscles. The palmaris longus is used to extend the thumb.

Special Considerations

Because the wrist flexors have a shorter excursion than the finger extensors, transfer of a wrist flexor to the finger extensors limits the ability to maintain a fist and flex the wrist simultaneously. A fisherman may find his fingers extend as he flicks the wrist, and his rod and reel sail into the lake.

Pitfalls

It is important to remember that one wrist flexor is needed in all but the weakest extremities. Without a good wrist flexor the wrist tends to rest in exaggerated dorsiflexion. In addition, it is difficult to obtain good finger extension without the tenodesis effect produced by wrist flexion. As a general principle, always leave one strong wrist flexor in place.

Low Median Nerve Palsy

Deficit

The muscles innervated by the median nerve in the hand are the superficial thenar muscles that provide opposition of the thumb, specifically the opponens pollicis and the abductor pollicis brevis. The superficial head of the flexor pollicis brevis is most often innervated by the median nerve but in some instances it is innervated by the ulnar nerve. When the superficial head of the flexor pollicis brevis is paralyzed, opposition of the thumb is lost; when it remains functional, adequate opposition may persist. Thus, not all patients with a low median nerve palsy need a tendon transfer.

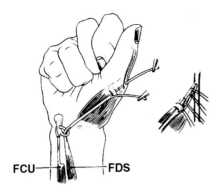

Figure 16-1. Riordan's procedure to restore thumb opposition when the ADP and deep head of the FPB are present, as in patients with isolated median nerve lesions. The insertion is into the APB tendon and the EPL tendon over the proximal segment. Figure 16-1 reproduced with permission from Riordan DC: Tendon transfers in hand surgery. *J Hand Surg,* 8A:748-753, 1983.

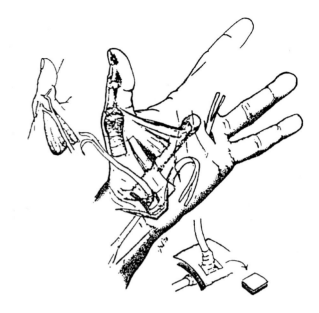

Figure 16-2. The ring finger FDS is brought through a transverse carpal ligament window, which acts as a pulley to restore opposition to the thumb. Insets show the distal juncture and the rerouted FDS tendon with a sleeve of mesentery prolapsing through the window. Figure 16-2 reproduced with permission from Snow JW, Fink GH: Use of a transverse carpal ligament window for the pulley in tendon transfers for median nerve palsy. *J Plast Reconstr Surg,* 48A:238-240, 1971.

Transfers: Types and Goals

The most reliable opponens transfer, especially by surgeons who perform only an occasional tendon procedure, is transfer of the ring finger flexor digitorum superficialis to the abductor pollicis brevis tendon (Fig. 16-1). The motor has adequate power, more than sufficient excursion, and requires only slight change of direction by a pulley. The tension does not need to be perfect for an adequate functional result.

Good results follow use of either a tendon loop pulley at the wrist crease, made from half of the flexor carpi ulnaris tendon, or a window cut in the volar carpal ligament (Figs. 16-1 and 16-2). Both of these pulleys result in a line of pull directed from the pisiform toward the thumb MP joint, which is the same as the abductor pollicis brevis.

The tendon is sutured over the axis of the MP joint into the tendon of the abductor pollicis brevis with enough tension to cause opposition of the thumb when the wrist is dorsiflexed. A yoke insertion will prevent subluxation of the transfer and excessive MP joint flexion power.

When minimal power of abduction is needed or muscle recovery is likely, as in advanced carpal tunnel syndrome with thenar atrophy, the palmaris longus is an accessible, usually available, transfer (Camitz procedure). The tendon is prolonged with a strip of palmar fascia, dissected in continuity with the tendon. The transfer is tunneled in a straight line to the tendon of the abductor pollicis brevis where it is sutured. Without benefit of a pulley, it provides abduction but no pronation.

The experienced hand surgeon may prefer to use the extensor indicis proprius or one slip of the extensor digiti minimi, which do not reduce the available flexion power. Neither transfer requires construction of a pulley as the ulnar border of the forearm redirects the pull of the transfer. The surgeon must choose the tension carefully for neither muscle has power or excursion to spare.

In children with congenital anomalies the abductor digiti minimi is useful as an opponensplasty. The addition of a muscle belly, rather than a tendon, improves the bulk and appearance of the thenar eminence. The width of the muscle provides some fibers which recreate the line-of-pull of the abductor pollicis brevis along with some fibers which are in the line of a flexor pollicis brevis. Thus, the muscle transfer can assist both abduction and flexion.

Special Considerations

The median nerve provides sensibility to the thumb, index, long, and radial one-half of the ring finger. The sensibility provided by the ulnar nerve alone is insufficient for good function of the hand. Thus, every effort is justified to regain sensibility in the median nerve distribution, even when there is no hope of muscle regeneration.

Pitfalls

Although an opponensplasty can position the thumb appropriately for grasp and pinch, an active thumb adductor or short flexor is required to facilitate this function. If the ulnar innervated deep thenar muscles are absent, the long extensor acts as an accessory adductor and pulls the thumb back alongside the index ray. An opponensplasty may fail if this is not recognized.

When the number of available motors is limited (frequent after poliomyelitis or Guillain-Barré syndrome), the surgeon may need to perform one transfer to replace all of the thenar muscles. If a long or ring finger flexor digitorum superficialis is available, it can be transferred across the other flexor tendons distal to the volar carpal ligament to the abductor pollicis brevis (Royal-Thompson transfer). This will reproduce the line-of-pull of the flexor pollicis brevis. Functionally the transfer provides some, but not complete, abduction with power for key-type pinch, but limited pulp-to-pulp pinch.

High Median Nerve Palsy

Deficit

Loss of the median nerve at the elbow results in significant loss of flexor function in the forearm, wrist, and hand: only the flexor carpi ulnaris and the ring and little finger flexor digitorum profundus motors remain. None of these is available for transfer. The critical functions that must be restored are finger flexion, thumb interphalangeal joint flexion, and usually, thumb opposition.

Transfers: Types and Goals

Finger flexion is usually achieved by connecting the functioning profundus tendons to the nonfunctional index and long finger tendons. This is done by transfer of a slip from the ring finger tendon without detaching the muscles. If some muscle activity should return, it will still be able to provide function. This transfer borrows power from the remaining two active profundus tendons and shares that power with the index and long fingers.

Another possibility is transfer of the extensor carpi radialis longus to the index and long finger profundi. This approach adds to the total finger flexion power, but is limited by the small excursion of the wrist extensors in comparison to the profundus.

The brachioradialis is often transferred to the flexor pollicis longus to provide thumb interphalangeal joint flexion. The excursion of the brachioradialis must be maximized by freeing it from its fascial envelope up to the proximal forearm. The tendon is sutured in place with the elbow in 90° of flexion.

Opposition of the thumb is usually provided by transfer of either the extensor indicis proprius or a slip of the extensor digiti minimi around the ulnar border of the wrist.

Low Ulnar Nerve Palsy

Deficit

Loss of the ulnar nerve at the wrist paralyzes all of the intrinsic muscles except the superficial thenar muscles. This deficit causes an imbalance between the long flexors and extensors with secondary clawing, weakened grasp from loss of MP joint flexion power, and weak pinch from loss of thumb adduction.

The intrinsic muscles are critical for precision, coordinated functions but are too numerous to replace individually. Some transfers are designed to balance the hand; others are

intended to provide strong power across a specific joint. All fall short of reproducing the precision patterns of normal intrinsic muscle function.

Transfers: Types and Goals

The ulnar digits can be rebalanced by a relatively weak transfer inserted into one lateral band of each finger. The transfer can originate from either the palmar or dorsal surface. On the palmar side, one flexor digitorum superficialis can be divided into two slips. The ring and little fingers each receive a slip inserted into one lateral band or the flexor retinaculum (Fig. 16-3). Since the remaining index and long finger lumbrical muscles provide weak MP joint flexion, insertion of the transfer into all four digits may provide better grasp.

On the dorsal surface of the hand a number of different muscles are capable of balancing an intrinsic minus digit. The extensor indicis proprius, the ulnar slip of the extensor digiti minimi, and the palmaris longus prolonged with a tendon graft, can be transferred palmarward through the lumbrical canal to the appropriate lateral band. These transfers are designed to balance the hand and eliminate clawing of the ulnar two digits.

When strong grasp is needed, a powerful MP joint flexor is created by using a tendon graft to extend a radial wrist extensor through the lumbrical canals to insert on the proximal phalanges. The transfer is most easily attached by suturing it to part of the digital flexor retinaculum. The patient must have normal extension power at the MP joints or a flexion deformity is likely. All transfers from the dorsal surface must be routed palmar to the MP joint axis.

Special Considerations

When pinch power is deficient, thumb adductor function is replaced by transfer of the prolonged extensor carpi radialis brevis or the extensor indicis proprius through the index-long intermetacarpal space (Fig. 16-3D). Considerable disagreement exists as to whether replacement of the first dorsal interosseous is useful.

Pitfalls

Insertion of strong intrinsic transfers into the lateral bands of the fingers will, with time, cause a swan neck deformity. This regularly occurs if a superficialis tendon is used for a single digit and explains why one superficialis is usually divided.

High Ulnar Nerve Palsy

Deficit

The only additional functional loss, as compared with a low ulnar nerve palsy, is the absence of ring and little finger flexion.

Transfers: Types and Goals

The paralyzed profundi are usually sutured to the functioning index and long finger motors, providing finger flexion.

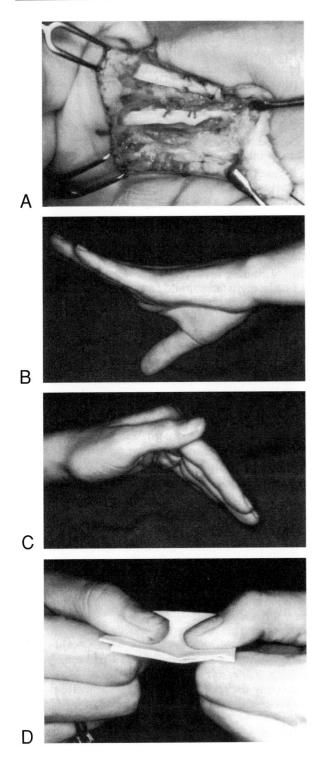

Figure 16-3. **(A)** Transfer of the long finger FDS to the A1 pulleys of the ring and little fingers. **(B)** Correction of the claw deformity. **(C)** Ability to assume intrinsic-plus position after transfer. **(D)** Improved key pinch with mild, but improved, Froment's sign after ECRB adductor transfer and MP joint fusion. Figure 16-3 reproduced with permission from Hastings II H, Davidson S: Tendon transfers for ulnar nerve palsy. *Hand Clin,* 4:167-178, 1988.

Special Considerations

With a high lesion, the dorsal ulnar sensory branch is involved. If there is no sensibility in the distribution of the ulnar nerve, the little finger will be anesthetic. If the digit sustains repeated trauma, amputation may be the best treatment.

Combined Palsies

Combined nerve palsies are frequently associated with severe stiffness and scarring. The same laceration that divides the nerves often lacerates multiple muscles and tendons. If the scar is severe, it will jeopardize the function of tendon transfers that pass through it. The goal of reconstruction is a helping hand that is better than a prosthesis.

Median and Ulnar Nerves

Absence of all intrinsic muscles from median and ulnar lesions at the wrist severely impairs hand function. The loss of balance between the extrinsic flexors and extensors produces clawing of all four fingers and "window-shade" flexion when making a fist. The thumb and hand flatten, and the thumb loses both opposition and pinch power. The absence of the interossei causes significant loss of grip power.

Transfers: Types and Goals

Clawing of the four fingers is frequently controlled by a single flexor digitorum superficialis tendon, split into four slips, with a separate insertion into each finger. On the dorsum, available small muscles (such as EIP and EDQP) can be used with each transfer activating two fingers.

The thumb is best reconstructed with two transfers, if there are sufficient motors available. A ring finger flexor digitorum superficialis or extensor digiti minimi transfer provides opposition. The extensor indicis proprius transferred through the index/long intermetacarpal space provides balancing adduction. It should be inserted into the radial side of the thumb MP joint to ensure that the thumb pronates, as there is no certainty the opponensplasty will be the stronger transfer.

If very powerful pinch power is needed, a radial wrist extensor can be prolonged with a tendon graft and used to replace the adductor pollicis.

Median and Radial Nerves

Combined radial and median nerve lesions leave only the intrinsic muscles, the ulnar two flexor digitorum profundus, and the flexor carpi ulnaris functioning. Although it is generally best to preserve the tenodesis effect of wrist motion, this devastating injury leaves too little power to control both the wrist and fingers. The wrist should be arthrodesed. The functioning ulnar flexor digitorum profundi are transferred to the radial flexor digitorum profundi, and the flexor carpi ulnaris is transferred to the finger and thumb extensors. The adductor pollicis insertion can be rerouted to the radial side of the thumb MP joint to simulate flexor pollicis brevis function.

Hansen's Disease

Deficit

The ulnar and median nerve palsies that are common in patients with Hansen's disease were the stimulus for much of the early use of tendon transfers and remain a significant clinical concern in developing countries. Physicians practicing in the continental United States will occasionally have the opportunity to evaluate a patient with Hansen's disease and should be alert to the unique problems that accompany the disease.

The loss of sensibility in all of the fingers that is part of combined median and ulnar nerve impairment frequently leads to fingertip trauma and swelling. The eventual sequelae are short digits and stiff joints. As medical treatment of the disease improves, these end-stage problems should decrease in frequency.

Transfers: Types and Goals

The transfers used in patients with Hansen's disease are those suitable for other median and ulnar nerve palsies. There are, however, special factors that influence the choice of motor and insertion. It is important to consider the flexibility of the joints that will be powered by the transfer. If the joints are tight or contracted, a more powerful motor will be needed; if the hand is very supple and pliable, a weaker motor may be used. If the PIP joint is supple, or tends to hyperextend, any transfer inserted into the lateral bands may, over time, create a swan neck deformity. In such a case, insertion as an MP joint flexor (i.e. into the proximal phalanx or digital flexor retinaculum) is likely to be the best choice.

In a supple hand current transfer, recommendations include extensor indicis proprius opponensplasty and a prolonged palmaris longus, passed through the carpal canal, for intrinsic replacement in all four digits. In a stiff or contracted hand, the more powerful flexor digitorum superficialis is needed. The ring finger flexor digitorum superficialis serves to provide opposition, and the long finger flexor digitorum superficialis provides intrinsic replacement.

Special Considerations

Hansen's disease tends to affect both hands and impairs sensibility as well as motor function. Even though the patient must use vision to substitute for sensibility, reconstruction of both hands is usually indicated in an attempt to circumvent progressive contractures.

Pitfalls

Hansen's disease tends to progress slowly. Until medication controls the intraneural infection, progression is due to active disease. Even with control of the infection, scarring can lead to increasing neurological deficit. Finally, long-standing muscle imbalance tends to cause joint deformity. The surgeon must consider this possibility when designing a scheme of tendon transfers. The best motor for tendon transfer may be the most likely to be paralyzed as the disease advances. As with the severe forms of Charcot-Marie-Tooth disease, the surgeon must think about the future course of the disease.

The Elbow

Deficit

Loss of elbow flexion severely limits the ability to position the hand in space. A tendon transfer to replace elbow flexion must be a very strong muscle. Adequate power is available from the shoulder girdle or by transfer of groups of forearm muscles.

Transfers: Types and Goals

The modified Steindler flexorplasty moves the origin of the flexor-pronator muscle mass proximally and laterally from the medial epicondyle to the anterior humerus. This increases the moment arm across the elbow joint and enhances these muscles as elbow flexors. The flexor-pronator mass must have near-normal strength for the procedure to be successful. The various recommendations for preoperative tests that ensure adequate power include the ability to maintain elbow flexion at 90°, the ability to flex the elbow with gravity eliminated, and demonstration of normal wrist flexion power. The procedure reliably provides elbow flexion from 30° to 90° and lifting capacity of one to two pounds.

Bipolar transfer of either the latissimus dorsi or the pectoralis major muscle will provide strong elbow flexion power. Because they are transposed on a neurovascular pedicle, the procedures are technically more difficult than older operations that move only one end of the motor. The latissimus transfer is cosmetically more acceptable as the pectoralis. The pectoralis transfer results in significant change in the chest wall contour. Either procedure can improve shoulder stability by crossing the glenohumeral joint to attach to the acromion.

Active elbow extension is very important to quadriplegic patients. Their low position in a wheelchair makes activities at and above shoulder height common. The triceps are needed for crutch walking and propelling a wheelchair. Moberg's transfer of the posterior deltoid to the triceps is generally agreed to provide excellent function. Fascia lata and the anterior tibial tendon have been used to extend the deltoid in addition to the toe extensors reported by Moberg. If the brachioradialis is transferred to the flexor pollicis longus, the triceps transfer stabilizes the elbow and increases pinch power.

Quadriplegia

Deficit

The severe motor deficits in the arms of quadriplegics are characterized by the limited number of functioning motors in the forearm and hand which are rated as good or better. The pattern of muscles available with lower levels of cervical spine injury is consistent but correlates only roughly with the level of injury. The remaining functional muscles listed by decreasing likelihood of useful function are the brachioradialis, the extensor carpi radialis longus, the extensor carpi radialis brevis, the pronator teres, and the flexor carpi radialis. With this very limited source of power, the goal of tendon transfers is a primitive pinch mechanism.

Transfers: Types and Goals

When only one to three motors are functioning, key pinch can be restored in highly motivated patients by tenodesis of the flexor pollicis longus to the radius so that active dorsiflexion of the wrist causes flexion of the thumb to the side of the partially flexed index finger. Associated procedures include stabilization of the interphalangeal joint of the thumb with a Kirschner wire, and release of the proximal pulley of the flexor retinaculum to increase the moment arm of the flexor pollicis longus across the MP joint. Refinements include transfer of the brachioradialis to the wrist extensors for added dorsiflexion power, tenodesis of the thumb extensors to the metacarpal to prevent hyperflexion of the MP joint, and tenodesis of the index finger flexor digitorum superficialis to assist index finger flexion.

Patients with four or more available motors will benefit from a more complex scheme of reconstruction. One method includes transfer of the extensor carpi radialis longus to the four profundus tendons, the pronator teres to the flexor pollicis longus, and prolongation of the brachioradialis by the ring finger flexor digitorum superficialis rerouted like a Royal-Thompson opponensplasty. In a separate procedure, extension is regained by multiple tenodeses of the thumb and finger extensors. A second protocol includes prepositioning of the thumb by carpometacarpal joint fusion and transfer of the brachioradialis to the finger and thumb extensors. Flexion is again provided by extensor carpi radialis longus and pronator teres transfers. Some patients have sufficient automatic extension to forego the tenodeses (Fig. 16-4).

Patients who have experienced the results of both protocols find the different transfers maximize different functions. Rather than express a preference for one protocol or the other, patients prefer to have one hand of each type.

Special Considerations

Severely affected quadriplegics have little or no sensibility remaining in their fingertips. In order to complete any function with the hand, they must use their eyes for feedback. Since they can only look at one hand at a time, reconstruction of both upper extremities may not prove useful. Less affected patients will have useful sensibility and will need vision only for supplemental feedback.

Pitfalls

Quadriplegics develop adaptive uses for their extremities

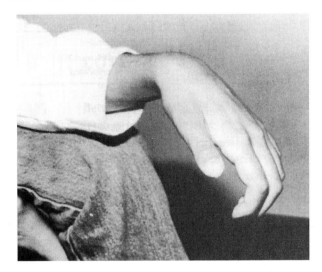

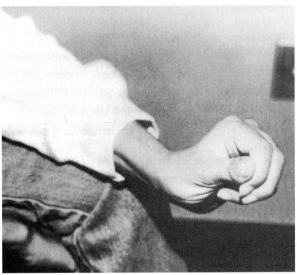

Figure 16-4. A quadriplegic patient with strong residual wrist extension treated by transfer of the BR to the FDP and the ECRL for opposition. **(Top)** With the hand open. **(Bottom)** Key pinch and ability to make a fist. Figure 16-4 reproduced with permission from Freehafer AA: Tendon transfers in patients with cervical spinal cord injury. *J Hand Surg,* 16A:804-809, 1991.

even in the face of severe deficits. Meticulous preoperative planning is important to ensure that no function is lost after the procedure.

It is very difficult to separate function of the two radial wrist extensors clinically. Some experienced surgeons prefer to leave the radial wrist extensors in place and make no attempt to determine if the extensor carpi radialis longus is available for transfer. An error in assessment can result in disastrous loss of all wrist dorsiflexion.

Annotated Bibliography

Brand PW, Beach RB, Thompson DE: Relative tension and potential excursion of muscles in the forearm and hand. *J Hand Surg,* 6A:209-219, 1981.

Defines the concepts of mass fraction and tension fraction with values for all forearm/hand muscles. Discusses the significance of the concepts in designing tendon transfers.

Smith RJ: *Tendon transfers of the hand and forearm.* Little, Brown and Company, Boston, 1987.

This monograph reviews the entire universe of tendon transfers. The author's logic is clear and his advice sound.

White WL: Restoration of function and balance of the wrist and hand by tendon transfers. *Surg Clin North Am,* 40:427-459, 1960.

The principles of tendon transfers about the hand have not changed since this classic paper and are clearly presented with an underlying foundation of common sense. Some specific recommendations for transfers have changed; eg, both wrist flexors should not be transferred dorsally to correct a radial palsy.

Zajac FE: How musculotendon architecture and joint geometry affect the capacity of muscles to move and exert force on objects: a review with application to arm and forearm tendon transfer design. *J Hand Surg,* 17A:799-804, 1992.

The architecture of a muscle is defined by measurement of its muscle fiber length, pennation angle, tendon length, muscle length, and physiologic cross-sectional area. This review discusses how these parameters determine the functional capacities of force, speed, and excursion.

Radial Nerve Transfers

Agee J, McCarroll HR, Hollister A: The anatomy of the flexor digitorum superficialis relevant to tendon transfers. *J Hand Surg,* 16B:68-69, 1991.

A brief review of the anatomy of the flexor digitorum superficialis muscle. The discussion relates the anatomy to use of the superficialis for synergistic and nonsynergistic tendon transfers.

Brand P: Biomechanics of tendon transfers. *Hand Clin,* 4:137-154, 1988.

An excellent short course in the biomechanical principles that determine the success or failure of tendon transfers. Balance, strength, excursion, and synergism are discussed. The author's selection of transfers for a radial nerve palsy is covered in detail.

Median Nerve Transfers

Anderson GA, Lee V, Sundararaj GD: Extensor indicis proprius opponensplasty. *J Hand Surg,* 16A:334-338, 1991.

After EIP opponensplasty 87% of 40 hands had an excellent or good result. The series includes a variety of pathologies including Hansen's disease and trauma. The authors use the palmar fascia near the pisiform as a pulley.

Foucher G, Malizos C, Sammut D, Marin Braun F, Michon J: Primary palmaris longus transfer as an opponensplasty in carpal tunnel release. *J Hand Surg,* 16A:56-60, 1991.

Seventy-three Camitz-Littler opponensplasties performed for carpal tunnel syndrome with thenar atrophy provided good results in 90%. The procedure is reliable and simple to perform. It does not provide the pronation component of opposition.

Riordan DC: Tendon transfers in hand surgery. *J Hand Surg,* 8A:748-753, 1983.

A review of frequently used tendon transfers for isolated nerve palsies and combined intrinsic palsy. The ring finger FDS opponensplasty is described as well as a number of transfers for clawing.

Snow JW, Fink GH: Use of a transverse carpal ligament window for the pulley in tendon transfers for median nerve palsy. *J Plast Reconstr Surg,* 48:238-240, 1971.

Describes substitution for the APB by transfer of the ring FDS through a window in the volar carpal ligament. The details of technique that help avoid adhesions are emphasized.

Ulnar Nerve Transfers

Brown PW: Reconstruction for pinch in ulnar intrinsic palsy. *Orthop Clin North Am,* 5:323-342, 1974.

The basic types of normal pinch are summarized. The discussion of how the deficits associated with ulnar nerve palsy produce different pathological pinch mechanisms is excellent. The EIP adductorplasty is described.

Hastings H, Davidson S: Tendon transfers for ulnar nerve palsy. *Hand Clin,* 4:167-178, 1988.

The standard transfers are described, and the results are compared. The varied goals of different transfers are clearly described. The differences between transfers for balance and those for strength are emphasized.

Combined Nerve Palsies

Eversmann WW: Tendon transfers for combined nerve injuries. *Hand Clin,* 4:187-199, 1988.

Recommended schemes for tendon transfers are described for common and rare combinations of nerve deficit. The limited goals anticipated for these severe injuries are emphasized. The logic implicit in the planning is excellent and makes this article valuable reading for all surgeons who undertake tendon transfers.

Omer GE: Tendon transfers in combined nerve lesions. *Orthop Clin North Am,* 5:377-387, 1974.

Tendon transfer schemes are recommended for all pairs of forearm nerve injuries. The recommendations are based on the author's experience with 204 extremities with combined nerve lesions. The associated factors that complicate treatment of these severe injuries are emphasized, including scarring, stiffness, and contractures.

Hansen's Disease

Anderson GA, Lee V, Sundararaj GD: Opponensplasty by extensor indicis and flexor digitorum superficialis tendon transfer. *J Hand Surg,* 17B:611-614, 1992.

Review of 175 opponensplasties (136 with Hansen's disease) suggests that the EIP provides the best results in supple hands. In stiffer hands the FDS benefits from its added force. Harvesting the FDS through a palmar oblique incision is recommended to minimize complications in the donor finger.

Brandsma JW, Brand PW: Claw-finger correction. *J Hand Surg,* 17B:615-621, 1992.

The authors review the subtle details of the techniques used for intrinsic replacement. The difference between the claw-finger deformity, the curled posture with attempted extension, and the claw-finger disability, the abnormal, "window-shade" flexion is emphasized. Replacement of active MP flexion is encouraged. In Hansen's disease patients, passing a tendon transfer through the carpal tunnel has not jeopardized the median nerve.

Brandsma JW, Ottenhoff-de-Jonge MW: Flexor digitorum superficialis tendon transfer for intrinsic replacement: longterm results and the effect on donor fingers. *J Hand Surg,* 17B:625-628, 1992.

Fifty-nine of 76 FDS claw-hand reconstructions and 68 of 82 FDS opponensplasties gave excellent or good results. Problems in the donor finger included swan neck deformity, DIP flexion, PIP flexion contracture, and loss of active flexion. The causes of these complications are discussed.

The Elbow

Brys D, Waters RL: Effect of triceps function on the brachioradialis transfer in quadriplegia. *J Hand Surg,* 12A:237-239, 1987.

Quadriplegic patients who have no active elbow extension increase their pinch power from 1.20 kg to 3.04 kg when the elbow is passively stabilized. Transfer of the posterior deltoid to the triceps not only provides active elbow extension but also increased pinch power.

Lacey SH, Wilber RG, Peckham PH, Freehafer AA: The posterior deltoid to triceps transfer: a clinical and biomechanical assessment. *J Hand Surg,* 11A: 542-547, 1986.

Length-tension curves of the posterior deltoid muscle show a large range of effective strength. The available amplitude of the posterior deltoid muscle is 7.31cm, which is more than is needed to replace triceps function. The transfer is very useful in quadriplegic patients.

Stern PJ, Caudle RJ: Tendon transfers for elbow flexion. *Hand Clin,* 4:297-307, 1988.

A review of flexorplasties including indications, techniques, results, and problems.

Wadsworth TG, Brooks DM: Neurological disorders. In Wadsworth, TG: *The Elbow.* Churchill Livingstone, Edinburgh, 1982.

A review of flexorplasties including a modification of Steindler's procedure that includes transposition of the extensor muscle mass as well as the flexor-pronator mass.

Quadriplegia

Moberg E: Surgical treatment for absent single-hand grip and elbow extension in quadriplegia. Principles and preliminary experience. *J Bone Joint Surg,* 57A:196-206, 1975.

With few functional motors the brachioradialis is best transferred to the extensor carpi radialis brevis to increase dorsiflexion power. The goal of reconstruction is a primitive lateral or key pinch.

House JH, Shannon MA: Restoration of strong grasp and lateral pinch in tetraplegia: a comparison of two methods of thumb control in each patient. *J Hand Surg,* 10A:22-29, 1985.

Two schemes of reconstruction are presented for patients with four or more motors. Both worked well and each had distinct advantages for the patients.

Hentz VR, Brown M, Keoshian LA: Upper limb reconstruction in quadriplegia: functional assessment and proposed treatment modifications. *J Hand Surg,* 8A:119-131, 1983.

Forty limbs of 30 patients who had lateral pinch reconstructed by the technique of Moberg encountered a number of problems. Only highly motivated patients with one to three grade-four muscles should have the reconstruction. Modifications of the Moberg procedures for lateral pinch and elbow extension are proposed.

Freehafer AA: Tendon transfers in patients with cervical spinal cord injury. *J Hand Surg,* 16A:804-809, 1991.

Reviews 124 tendon transfers in 32 patients. Emphasizes the need to provide active flexion by simple transfers. Extensor tenodeses were not required.

IV

Inflammatory Disorders

17

Rheumatoid Arthritis

Paul Feldon, MD

General Characteristics

Rheumatoid arthritis is a chronic, systemic, autoimmune, inflammatory disease with an unknown cause. It affects joints and periarticular tissue causing synovitis and tenosynovitis; these result in progressive joint and/or tendon destruction and deformity. Inflammatory reactions in other tissues can cause neuropathy, vasculitis, nodule formation, myositis, and chronic anemia.

The biochemistry of rheumatoid arthritis is complex. Cellular and chemical changes occur from antigen-antibody and antibody-antibody reactions. The antigen-antibody reaction in the joint tissues includes the complement sequence causing reduced complement levels in the synovial fluid, increased vascular permeability, and the influx of white cells. Neutrophils ingest the immune complexes and release hydrolytic enzymes, oxygen radicals, and arachidonic acid metabolites. These metabolites include prostaglandins, thromboxanes, and leukotrienes, which promote the inflammatory reaction and the release of degradative enzymes such as collagenases, gelantinases, and proteoglycanases, which damage articular cartilage, ligaments, tendon, and bone.

Early in the rheumatoid process there is microvascular injury, edema of subsynovial tissues, and synovial cell proliferation. As the disease progresses, the synovium becomes more edematous, with hypertrophy and hyperplasia of the synovial lining cells. There is venous distention, capillary obstruction, focal thrombosis, and perivascular hemorrhage. Aggregations of lymphocytes with a peripheral layer of plasma cells accumulate in the subsynovial tissues. The proliferation of fibroblasts, small vessels, and inflammatory cells results in pannus (granulation tissue) formation. The pannus itself destroys cartilage by producing collagenase and prostaglandins.

Articular cartilage and joint ligaments are damaged by increased joint fluid volume and pressure, as well as the mechanical forces of weightbearing and muscle pull, resulting in joint deformity.

Nonoperative Treatment of Rheumatoid Arthritis

Rheumatoid arthritis is a disease with many systemic manifestations. The severity and course of the disease varies from patient to patient; not all patients will require surgical treatment. The goals of nonsurgical treatment include pain relief, reduction of inflammation, limitation of side effects, and preservation of muscle and joint function. Early and mild disease is treated with a basic program including patient and family education, rest, controlled exercise and diet, pain relief with salicylates and/or minor analgesics, and psychological support. Aspirin is used in high doses (blood levels of 20 to 30 mg/ml) if these levels can be tolerated without tinnitus or gastric symptoms. Nonacetylated salicylates such as salasate and choline magnesium trisilicate can be used in some patients who are sensitive to aspirin.

If the patient's rheumatoid symptoms cannot be controlled on the therapy described above, nonsteroidal anti-inflammatory medication and/or antimalarial medication, as well as intra-articular steroid injections of selected joints can be added. Physical therapy, occupational therapy, and splints to rest and support inflamed joints may also be useful at this stage.

Patients with progressive disease and aggressive synovitis may require the next level of medical treatment, which includes gold, penicillamine, methotrexate, azathioprine, cyclophosphamide, and oral corticosteroids. All of these medications have serious side effects and must be monitored carefully. Corticosteroids are used much less frequently than in the past because of their significant side effects after long-term use, and because they are not curative and do not prevent progressive joint destruction.

Surgical Treatment of Rheumatoid Arthritis

The treatment priorities to be considered by the hand surgeon in treating rheumatoid arthritis are (1) pain control; (2) retardation of progression of the disease; (3) restoration or improvement in function; and (4) cosmetic improvement. The surgical treatment options can be classified as preventive, corrective, and salvage. Preventive procedures include tenosynovectomy and in some cases, synovectomy. Corrective surgical procedures include tendon transfer, nerve decompression, soft-tissue reconstruction, and again sometimes synovectomy. Synovectomies usually are performed when there is mild disease with good medical control and persistent synovitis in only one or two joints. Contraindications for synovectomy include rapidly progressive disease or disease that is under poor medical control, multiple joint involvement, or joints that are already destroyed by the arthritic process. The last surgical options, which include joint arthroplasty and joint fusion, are salvage procedures.

Rheumatoid Nodules

Nodule formation occurs in 20% to 25% of patients with rheumatoid arthritis and is usually associated with strong seropositivity and aggressive disease. Rheumatoid nodules cause symptoms because of their size and/or location. They occur frequently around the olecranon and posterior surface of the forearms where they are subjected to pressure and may become tender. Less frequently, they occur on the volar surfaces of the digits where they can be sensitive to pressure or compress digital nerves. Clusters of nodules frequently form on the dorsal surfaces of the hands where they are exposed to view and become cosmetically unacceptable.

In all of these circumstances, treatment is warranted. While a steroid injection can cause some nodules to regress, it may also stimulate ulceration of the nodule. During surgical resection, care must be taken to obtain meticulous hemostasis when nodules around the forearm and elbow are removed to avoid postoperative hematoma formation. Such hematomas can lead to a chronic draining sinus, which is difficult to control. In the digits, the nodules must be dissected from the skin carefully to avoid skin deficits and, when nodules are present near digital nerves, the nerves must be identified and protected. Nodules can recur after resection.

A condition called "rheumatoid nodulosis" is a separate clinical entity in which multiple rheumatoid nodules form and intermittent polyarthralgias are present, but joint destruction is minimal.

The Rheumatoid Wrist

Pathomechanics

Synovitis of the distal radioulnar joint stretches and attenuates the ligaments holding the radius to the ulna. Progressive destruction of this ligament supporting complex allows volar subluxation of the ulnar side of the carpus away from the ulnar—so-called "carpal supination." This results in dorsal prominence of the ulna. Attenuation and destruction of the volar wrist ligaments (radiocapitate and radioscapholunate) allow progressive vertical rotation of the scaphoid and subsequent carpal collapse with loss of carpal height. The supination deformity from the combined loss of ligament support on both the ulnar and volar/radial sides of the wrist decreases the mechanical advantage of the extensor carpi ulnaris tendon as this tendon subluxates volar to the flexion/extension axis of the wrist, and increases the mechanical advantage of the radial wrist extensors. This results in radial deviation of the metacarpals and aggravates the ulnar deviation deformities at the metacarpophalangeal joints.

Carpal collapse decreases the efficiency of the long finger flexors and extensors, and the resulting tendon imbalance can cause a relative "intrinsic plus" deformity and thereby, swan neck deformities of the fingers. Wrist deformities must be corrected before MP and/or PIP joint reconstructions are done. Failure to address deformity at the wrist first will prevent optimal surgical results and frequently lead to failure of the finger reconstructions. Surgical treatment of the rheumatoid wrist depends on the type and severity of the deformity, and will vary from patient to patient.

Tendon Transfer

Soft-tissue reconstruction by relocation of the subluxated ECU tendon and transfer of the ECRL tendon to the ECU tendon insertion is effective if done before fixed deformities occur.

Synovectomy

Synovectomy of the wrist joint can be done in combination with dorsal tenosynovectomy or carpal tunnel release. While wrist synovectomy may relieve pain, there is no evidence that synovectomy alone will prevent progressive wrist joint deformity. Several long-term studies have shown that wrist synovectomy results in infrequent recurrence of synovitis and good pain relief. Grip strength is preserved, but carpal collapse and ulnar translocation are not prevented. A functional range of wrist motion is maintained, but the overall wrist range of motion is decreased following synovectomy.

Soft-Tissue Stabilization

Stabilization procedures that realign the wrist and preserve some motion are an alternative to wrist arthrodesis. These procedures resect enough bone to allow the wrist deformity to be corrected and intentionally induce a pseudoarthrosis of the wrist joint which maintains the correction, yet allows at least some wrist motion. Follow-up studies show a high rate of unintended wrist fusion in spite of attempts to prevent this. Nonetheless, when pseudoarthrosis was obtained, pain was relieved and some wrist motion was preserved. The correction of preoperative volar subluxation was maintained, but ulnar subluxation tended to recur.

Partial Wrist Fusion

Radiolunate or radioscapholunate fusion is another alternative to total wrist arthrodesis when the radiocarpal joint is destroyed but the midcarpal joints are minimally affected. This technique can be used to prevent progressive ulnar translocation, but radiolunate fusion is not indicated in rapidly progressive disease. Radioscapholunate arthrodesis has been combined with a resection/interposition arthroplasty of the capitolunate joint in selected patients.

Wrist Fusion

Wrist fusion remains the predictable standard salvage procedure for wrists affected by advanced rheumatoid arthritis by providing a stable and pain-free wrist. There remains some controversy about the appropriate position for fusion of the rheumatoid wrist. Ulnar deviation of 5° to 10° is acceptable, and radial deviation is to be avoided. Neutral to slight wrist extension is acceptable for the patient with a unilateral wrist fusion. In bilateral wrist fusions, some authors recommend fusing one wrist in 20° to 30° of volar flexion to facilitate personal hygiene. Internal fixation using single intramedullary or single or dual intermetacarpal-intramedullary rods is rapid, effective, and minimizes the surgical exposure and soft-tissue dissection. The nonunion rate using this method is low. Internal fixation with plates and screws also can be used to provide rigid stabilization of the wrist fusion. This technique usually requires a more extensive surgical exposure. New plates specifically designed for wrist fusions are being developed.

Silicone Implant Arthroplasty

Resection arthroplasty using a silicone implant can be done in patients with a need to preserve wrist motion. These must be patients with low-demand requirements who do not need to use assistive devices for ambulation, who have adequate bone stock to support the implant, and who have minimal, if any, tendon imbalance. The postoperative range of motion should be deliberately limited to a total arc of 70° to 80° of combined flexion and extension. Several studies have shown high failure rates in long-term follow-up studies. Recession of the implant into bone has been a consistent problem with these implants. The use of metal grommets to protect the implant stems is under study as a method to minimize both recession and breakage.

Total Wrist Arthroplasty

Total wrist arthroplasty using metal-plastic prostheses remains an alternative to wrist fusion in selected patients at some centers. Loosening and progressive imbalance have occurred in several series. Revision may be difficult because of the need to remove cement in some cases.

The Distal Radioulnar Joint

Synovitis of the distal radioulnar joint stretches the joint capsule and attenuates the ligamentous supporting structures of the joint including the TFCC and the extensor carpi ulnaris tendon, and erodes the articular surfaces of the joint. The combination of distal radioulnar joint swelling and instability, pain, and limitation of pronation and supination, subluxation of the ECU tendon, and, frequently, erosion and attrition rupture of the long extensor tendons of the fingers has been termed the caput ulnae syndrome.

There is agreement that early surgical intervention is desirable to minimize joint destruction and instability by synovectomy, ECU tendon relocation, and ECRL to ECU tendon transfer to limit supination of the carpus away from the ulna.

Resection Arthroplasty

Reconstruction of advanced rheumatoid destruction of the DRUJ traditionally has included resection of the distal ulna. While removing the distal ulna reduces pain, this procedure may not enhance function and may allow or even contribute to carpal collapse and/or instability of the remaining ulna. Such instability frequently is symptomatic and is difficult to treat. No more than two centimeters of distal ulna should be resected when doing the Darrach procedure.

Hemiresection Techniques

Variations of the standard Darrach resection arthroplasty have been described for the DRUJ affected by rheumatoid arthritis. In the hemiresection interposition technique the articular surface of the distal ulna is resected, but the length of the ulna is preserved by leaving the styloid process and fovea of the ulna intact. This preserves the ligaments attached to the ulna for stability. A soft-tissue interposition is used to prevent impingement of the ulna against the radius. This technique can be used only in patients with mild to moderate rheumatoid involvement of the DRUJ, as it depends on the integrity of the TFCC. If the TFCC has been destroyed or cannot be reconstructed, another resection technique should be used.

A similar hemiresection procedure has been termed a "matched" resection. In this procedure, the distal ulna is resected to match the contour of the radius, thereby preserving the length of the ulna but removing the joint in such a way that the ulna and radius remain parallel to one another (without contact) throughout the full range of pronation-supination. The remaining distal ulna is decorticated to promote scar formation between the end of the ulna and the soft-tissue structures to maintain or restore stability. In both variations of hemiresection arthroplasty, careful attention to surgical detail is necessary to contour the ulna to avoid corners which might impinge the radius during forearm rotation.

Sauve-Kapandji Procedure

Fusion of the DRUJ combined with a segmental resection of the ulna to allow forearm rotation is more popular recently. This operation is now known as the Sauve-Kapandji procedure, and has been advocated for the rheumatoid wrist, particularly in younger patients, as it preserves the support for the ulnar side of the wrist. It provides a broad stable base, which is helpful if implant or total wrist arthroplasty is to be done. Instability of the stump of the ulna still can be problematic and a tethering procedure using the pronator quadratus detached from the ulna, brought through the ulna resection site, and sutured to the dorsal capsule should be done at the time of the original procedure.

Tendons in Rheumatoid Arthritis

Tenosynovitis

Tenosynovitis is a hallmark of the hand affected by rheumatoid arthritis. Tenosynovectomy is consistently effective in controlling tenosynovitis that cannot be controlled by medication. In addition, tenosynovectomy has been shown to prevent subsequent tendon rupture in multiple studies. Recurrent tenosynovitis after tenosynovectomy is rare.

The most common site of tenosynovitis is beneath the extensor retinaculum. Tenosynovitis occurs less frequently on the volar side of the wrist and in the digits. Tenosynovitis in the ulnar bursa (midpalm, carpal tunnel, and distal forearm) causes loss of finger motion and carpal tunnel syndrome. Flexor tendon ruptures can occur by direct invasion of the tendons by tenosynovium. Direct invasion of the tendon has been found in up to 50% of tendons at the time of tenosynovectomy.

In the digits, tenosynovitis can cause triggering, decreased active finger flexion, nodule formation, and occasionally tendon rupture.

Tenosynovectomy

Dorsal tenosynovectomy is effective in preventing extensor tendon rupture. It should be done in those rheumatoid patients with moderate to severe dorsal tenosynovitis that does not respond to medical management within six months. The distal ulna should be debrided or resected at the same time if the ulna is prominent dorsally and bone spikes have eroded through the dorsal capsule or if this is imminent. All or part of the extensor retinaculum can be placed volar to the extensor tendons after tenosynovectomy to provide a smooth bed for gliding and/or to reinforce the dorsal wrist/DRUJ capsule. If there is concern about bowstringing of the extensor tendons, the retinaculum can be divided transversely into proximal and distal portions. One half of the retinaculum can be passed volar to the tendons to enhance the bed and the other half retained dorsal to the tendons to restrict bowstringing.

When doing a flexor tenosynovectomy, the carpal tunnel is released as well. This requires a more extensive incision than that usually used for idiopathic carpal tunnel syndrome. Care must be taken when performing tenosynovectomies, as adherent tendon encased in a mass of fibrotic tenosynovium may mask tendon ruptures. If this is not recognized and each tendon has separated out from the adherent masks, loss of function may ensue and an extensive tendon reconstruction may be necessary.

In the digits, a tenosynovectomy without release of the annular pulleys is preferable to incising the A-1 pulley, which may allow ulnar shift of the flexor tendons and thereby increase ulnar drift of the finger(s). If a tenosynovectomy alone does not provide adequate decompression of the flexor tendon sheath, resection of one slip of the sublimis tendon effectively decompresses the tendon while preserving FDS function. Direct synovial invasion of the tendon within the fibro-osseous canal can form nodules within the tendon and cause triggering or tendon rupture. The nodules should be excised through longitudinal incisions in the tendon substance, and the tendon repaired.

Flexor Tendon Ruptures

Flexor tendon rupture in rheumatoid arthritis is much less common than extensor tendon rupture. It may be hard to detect ruptures of the sublimis tendons if the profundus tendons are intact. Tendon rupture should be considered when patients with volar wrist fullness complain of weakness and/or carpal tunnel syndrome symptoms, when physical examination shows restriction of active finger flexion, and particularly when there is a discrepancy between active and passive finger motion.

Attritional ruptures of the flexors occur in the carpal canal, usually from osteophytes arising from the volar aspects of the carpal bones. Rupture of the flexor pollicis longus on a volar scaphoid osteophyte is the most common flexor tendon rupture and is known as the "Mannerfelt" lesion or syndrome. After the FPL tendon ruptures from attrition, the flexor tendons of the index, long, ring, and small finger can rupture sequentially. Other common sites of flexor tendon rupture are at the trapezium, the distal radius, the hamate hook, and the distal ulna. Tendon rupture by direct invasion by the tenosynovium can occur as well.

The treatment of flexor tendon ruptures includes tenosynovectomy and removal of the source of attrition if present, followed by tendon reconstruction by adjacent tendon suture, bridge grafting, or tendon transfer. Primary repair usually is not possible because of the loss of tendon substance over a relatively wide area. The prognosis is better for flexor tendon ruptures occurring from attrition than for those occurring from prolific tenosynovitis with direct invasion. Tendon ruptures from invasive tenosynovitis within the fibro-osseous canal have a generally poor prognosis for restoration of function. When tendons rupture within the fibro-osseous canal, tendon repair is rarely possible. Tendon transfer, tendon advancement, adjacent tendon suture, bridge grafting, and joint fusion are options for treatment. The findings at surgery combined with the preoperative assessment of the patient's requirements for function will determine which procedure or combination of procedures is done.

Extensor Tendon Rupture

Synovitis of the DRUJ with erosion of the dorsal aspect of the ulna leaves sharp spikes on the ulna that erode through the joint capsule and eventually through the extensor tendons on the ulnar as part of the wrist (fifth and fourth extensor compartments). It is important to recognize and treat the caput ulnae syndrome before tendon rupture occurs. An isolated rupture of the EDQ tendon may be the first sign of impending rupture of the EDC tendons. Function of the EDQ is tested by holding the index, long, and ring fingers in flexion to nullify the action of the EDC tendons and asking the patient to extend the small finger. Inability to do this signals a rupture of the EDQ tendon and is an indication for urgent surgical treatment by DRUJ synovectomy, tenosynovectomy, and distal ulna resection. It is important to differentiate extensor tendon rupture from posterior interosseous nerve dysfunction, extensor mechanism subluxation, and MP joint dislocation.

The treatment of extensor tendon ruptures depends on how many tendons have ruptured. Direct repair of extensor tendons in rheumatoid arthritis is usually not possible. Adjacent tendon suture (side-to-side transfer), tendon transfer, and bridge grafting are the treatment alternatives. Single tendon ruptures usually involve either the EPL or the EDQ. EIP transfer is used for EPL rupture. An isolated rupture of the EDQ does not require treatment if the EDC (5) is intact. If both EDC (5) and EDQ are ruptured, it is preferable to transfer the EIP to EDC (5) than to suture the short distal stump of the small finger extensor to the adjacent intact extensor tendon of the ring finger; the latter will result in excessive abduction of the small finger. Multiple tendon ruptures are treated by bridge grafting or by a combination of tendon transfer and adjacent tendon suture. The prognosis for restoration of function is better for single or double ruptures than for triple or quadruple ruptures.

Finger Deformities

The treatment of finger joints affected by rheumatoid arthritis varies from joint to joint. At the DIP joint, the recommended surgical treatment option usually is fusion. At the PIP joint, isolated PIP joint synovitis can be treated by synovectomy. This may prevent progressive deformity and has little morbidity associated with it. For PIP joints destroyed by the rheumatoid process, arthroplasty and fusion are the salvage options available. At the MP joint, synovectomy, extensor mechanism relocation, intrinsic tendon release, and extensor intrinsic tendon release are the available soft-tissue procedures. For destroyed joints, MP joint arthroplasty has been effective in alleviating pain, improving function, and improving cosmesis. However, subluxation and ulnar drift at the MP joints are not an absolute indication for performing MP arthroplasties if satisfactory function and strength are present.

Metacarpophalangeal Joint Deformities

MP joint deformities in rheumatoid arthritis occur as synovitis distends and stretches the joint capsule, and synovial invasion of the collateral ligament attenuates these ligaments. The volar and ulnar forces on the joint result in subluxation and may be caused or augmented by radial deviation of the wrist as a result of tendon imbalance about the wrist and/or wrist joint destruction. Attenuation of the radial sagittal band will allow the extensor mechanism to subluxate ulnarward, causing inability to extend the MP joint. Intrinsic contractures contribute to MP joint deformities.

Using Nalebuff's and Millender's staging system for the MP joints, Stage I disease is marked by synovitis. Medical management of the synovitis and splinting is used at this stage.

In Stage II MP joint disease, there is joint-space narrowing with bony erosions. Medical management, splinting, and surgical synovectomies are the treatment options.

In Stage III MP joint disease, there is moderate joint destruction with volar subluxation and ulnar deviation of the joints. Moderately good hand function may be present. Splinting and assistive aids are used at this stage of disease, although soft-tissue reconstruction without joint reconstruction has been shown to be effective as long as some articular cartilage remains on both sides of the MP joint. Soft-tissue reconstruction by division of the junctura tendineae, synovectomy, crossed intrinsic transfer, capsular reefing, and extensor tendon relocation, but without metacarpal head resection, was found to provide good pain relief, correction of ulnar drift, and range of MP motion (average 56°) in a five-year follow-up study.

In Stage IV disease, there is advanced joint destruction on radiographs with fixed MP joint deformities and loss of hand function. MP arthroplasties should be considered for Stage IV deformities. It is necessary to correct fixed wrist deformities before reconstructing the MP joints. At the time of arthroplasty, soft-tissue releases are performed as necessary and the radial-side collateral ligament of the MP joint is reconstructed. It may be necessary to release the intrinsic tendons and/or relocate the extensor tendons at the time of arthroplasty. Postoperative splinting and hand therapy are very important in achieving maximum function after MP joint arthroplasties. Late recurrence of the deformities can occur if there has been inadequate soft-tissue reconstruction or if there is progressive wrist disease with secondary radial deviation at the metacarpals. In one recent five-year

(average) follow-up study comparing the early and late results of silicone rubber implant MP arthroplasty, ulnar drift was corrected from a preoperative average of 25° to a postoperative average of 5° at four months, with recurrence to an average of 12° at five years. The extensor lag of the MP joint was improved from a preoperative average of 56° to a postoperative average of 10° at four months, and 22° at five years. MP joint flexion increased from a preoperative average of 17° to a postoperative average of 51° at four months, with a decrease to 39° at five years. Pain relief and patient satisfaction were high in spite of the recurrent drift and loss of motion over time. The bone on either side of the MP joint has been shown to tolerate silicone rubber implants well. Bone remodeling rather than bone resorption occurs around the implant stem. The shape of the cortical bone is preserved, and the thickness of bone in the metaphyseal area of both the metacarpals and proximal phalanges increases with time.

Boutonnière Deformity

Boutonnière deformities (PIP joint flexion with DIP hyperextension) occur as the result of PIP joint synovitis. The deformity begins with PIP flexion as synovitis causes central slip elongation and/or rupture. Rupture of the central slip allows volar subluxation of the lateral bands beneath the PIP joint axis of rotation. The increased tension on the lateral bands of the extensor mechanism causes DIP joint hyperextension and limited DIP flexion. Contracture of the transverse and oblique retinacular ligaments causes the deformity to become fixed. Long-standing boutonnière deformities result in joint stiffness as the volar plate and collateral ligaments contract.

The treatment of boutonnière deformities depends on the stage of the disease. In Stage I disease, there is PIP joint synovitis and mild deformity. This can be corrected by synovectomy, splinting, lateral band reconstruction with relocation of the lateral bands dorsal to the axis of rotation, or by terminal tendon tenotomy.

In the Stage II boutonnière deformity, there is moderate deformity of the PIP joint. There may be a 30° to 40° flexion contracture of the joint, but passive extension is possible. The joint space is preserved on radiographs. The surgical alternatives include synovectomy combined with central slip reconstruction, lateral band reconstruction, and/or terminal tendon tenotomy. In Stage III boutonnière deformities, there is a fixed PIP joint flexion contracture with joint stiffness such that the flexion deformity cannot be corrected passively. The alternative treatments here are limited to arthroplasty or fusion. Arthroplasty is effective but provides an improvement in the functional arc of motion rather than improving overall joint motion. A review of the results of PIP arthroplasty in rheumatoid boutonnière deformities showed a change in the average preoperative arc of PIP motion of -59° of extension and 91° of flexion to an average postoperative arc of -8° of extension to 54° of flexion.

Swan Neck Deformities

There are various causes for swan neck deformities. The terminal tendon can rupture or attenuate, causing a mallet deformity with secondary hyperextension of the PIP joint as a result of tendon imbalance. PIP joint hyperextension also can occur if the volar capsule stretches and becomes incompetent as a result of prolonged synovitis. Rupture of the flexor digitorum superficialis tendon can result in loss of the dynamic stabilization of the PIP joint and a secondary hyperextension deformity, particularly if there is concomitant PIP joint synovitis. Intrinsic tightness from MP joint subluxation also can result in tendon imbalance and a swan neck deformity. Swan neck deformities have been classified by their degree of severity.

In the Type I deformity, there is full passive motion of the PIP joint, regardless of the position of the MP joint. These can be treated by splinting, DIP joint fusion, or soft-tissue reconstruction to limit PIP joint hyperextension.

In Type II swan neck deformities, the PIP joint flexion is limited with the MP joint in certain positions, usually as a result of MP joint deformity with secondary intrinsic tightness. Treatment of the Type II deformity may require intrinsic tendon release or reconstruction of the MP joint.

In the Type III swan neck deformity, PIP joint flexion is limited regardless of the position of the MP joint, but the PIP joint is preserved on radiographs. Treatment for the Type III deformity includes joint mobilization under anesthesia by manipulation with or without temporary pin fixation and/or dorsal skin release. If the joint cannot be mobilized under anesthesia, lateral band mobilization, which surgically separates the central tendon from the lateral bands by parallel incisions, can provide significant improvement. Again, pin fixation and/or skin release may be necessary. In one series, average postoperative motion from -10° of extension to 55° of flexion was maintained over a two-year period after surgical lateral band mobilization.

In Type IV swan neck deformities, the PIP joint is not only stiff, but there is joint destruction on radiographs. PIP joint fusion should be considered for the index and/or middle fingers if stability is important for pinch or if the MP joint requires an arthroplasty. PIP joint fusion is almost always mandatory if there is a concomitant flexor tendon rupture. A PIP joint arthroplasty can be considered for the ring and small fingers if the surrounding soft-tissue structures and the flexor and extensor tendons are intact. However, in a large series of PIP arthroplasties, the highest complication rate occurred in the swan neck group. There was a 21% recurrence rate of deformity, and an average of only 39° of PIP joint flexion was obtained.

Thumb Deformities

The Nalebuff Type I thumb or "boutonnière" thumb has a flexion deformity of the MP joint and a hyperextension deformity of the interphalangeal joint. This occurs as synovitis attenuates the extensor hood, allowing volar and ulnar displacement of the EPL tendon. The displaced EPL tendon acts as an MP joint flexor, rather than as an extensor. Hyperextension of the IP joint occurs as volar subluxation of the proximal phalanx (also caused by MP joint synovitis) places increased tension on the thumb intrinsic mus-

cle insertions. In the early stages, the MP and IP joints are passively correctable and there is minimal joint destruction on radiograph. The surgical treatment is by synovectomy and extensor tendon reconstruction. EPL rerouting (transection of the EPL tendon over the distal phalanx to decrease IP hyperextension and transfer of the tendon to the base of the proximal phalanx to increase MP joint extension) is recommended in patients with early joint involvement with full passive correction and normal radiographs. However, a review of this procedure (MP synovectomy and EPL rerouting) showed a 64% recurrence rate that required additional reconstructive surgery at an average of six years. Therefore, while the procedure is effective in the short term, the patient should understand that an additional procedure may be needed later.

In moderately advanced boutonnière thumbs, there is a fixed MP joint flexion deformity with passively correctable IP joint deformity. MP joint fusion and MP joint arthroplasty are the surgical alternatives at this stage. MP joint fusion is reliable and is the procedure of choice for durability and function, as long as the CMC and IP joints are functional. This is particularly so in the high-demand or younger patient in whom lateral instability of the MP joint may become problematic with time. While MP arthroplasty has been effective in preserving motion and improving stability, this procedure also has a higher incidence of subsequent IP joint collapse and may be more suited for the low-demand patient.

In the advanced thumb boutonnière there are fixed MP and IP joint deformities. The surgical alternatives include interphalangeal joint fusion and MP joint arthroplasty or both IP and MP joint fusions. The latter can be done only if the thumb CMC joint is mobile and functional.

The Nalebuff Type III thumb deformity or "swan neck" deformity occurs when CMC joint disease allows dorsal and radial subluxation of the CMC joint with a secondary flexion and adduction contracture of the metacarpal. This results in hyperextension of the MP joint. In early thumb swan neck deformities, there is minimal CMC joint deformity and minimal, if any, MP joint deformity. At this stage, the CMC joint subluxation can be treated either by splinting or by CMC joint arthroplasty. In moderately advanced swan neck deformities of the thumb, the CMC and MP joint deformities are correctable passively. The treatment alternatives include CMC joint arthroplasty combined with MP joint tenodesis or fusion. In the advanced thumb swan neck deformity, there is CMC joint dislocation with a fixed MP joint deformity and fixed metacarpal adduction. This deformity requires CMC joint hemiarthroplasty, MP joint fusion, and a first web release.

The Nalebuff Type IV thumb deformity is similar to a "gamekeeper's thumb." There is an abduction deformity of the thumb MP joint with secondary adduction of the first metacarpal which occurs as the ulnar collateral ligament of the MP joint is stretched by synovitis. The treatment alternatives include synovectomy, collateral ligament reconstruction, and adductor fascia release in mild deformities, or MP joint arthroplasty with ulnar collateral ligament reconstruction or MP joint fusion in more advanced disease.

The Nalebuff Type II deformity is rare and is a combination of Type I (boutonnière) deformity with CMC joint subluxation or dislocation.

The Nalebuff Type V deformity is described as a combination of MP and IP joint destruction with lateral deformity at the MP joint and a hyperextension deformity at the IP joint.

Complex Rheumatoid Hand Deformities

Rheumatoid deformities rarely occur in isolation; multiple joints usually are involved. One deformity may cause or aggravate another deformity. Complex deformities with involvement in multiple levels require an organized and systematic approach during treatment.

With combined wrist and MP joint deformities, the wrist deformity must be corrected either by tendon transfer or partial or complete wrist fusion before or during MP joint reconstruction. MP joint function depends on a stable wrist without significant deformity.

Combined MP and PIP joint deformities are difficult to treat. PIP and MP joint ("double row") arthroplasties compromise function of both levels and are rarely indicated. Retaining motion at the MP joint level is a greater priority than retaining motion at the PIP joint level. Mild to moderate PIP joint deformities can be accepted or treated by manipulation and pinning, in combination with MP joint arthroplasty. In severe deformities at both levels, a PIP joint fusion combined with MP joint arthroplasty may be the preferable alternative. Isolated PIP joint deformities in a single finger can be reconstructed as indicated at the same time MP joint arthroplasties are performed.

When tendon ruptures are present in the face of either MP or wrist deformity, one must decide whether to attempt a single-stage reconstruction or do a staged reconstruction. If a staged reconstruction is elected, the MP joint deformities are corrected before tendon transfers are done. In this case, MP joint motion is maintained by passive exercises and splinting after the arthroplasties have been completed and prior to performing the tendon reconstruction. In general, a staged reconstruction is the more conservative choice.

Annotated Bibliography

Rheumatoid Arthritis/General Characteristics

Schumacher HR: *Primer on the Rheumatic Diseases-Ninth Edition.* Arthritis Foundation.
1-170, Atlanta, 1988.

A concise but detailed overview of the current concepts of the pathophysiology and treatment of rheumatoid arthritis and its variants.

Nonoperative Treatment

Ferlic DC, Smyth CJ, Clayton ML: Medical considerations and management of rheumatoid arthritis.
J Hand Surg, 8:662-666, 1983.

Reviews the basic principles of the medical management of rheumatoid arthritis as well as the appropriate interrelationship of medical and surgical treatment in the overall care of the rheumatoid patient.

Rheumatoid Nodules

McGrath MH, Fleischer A: The subcutaneous rheumatoid nodule. *Hand Clin,* 5:127-135, 1989.

Review of the subcutaneous nodule in rheumatoid arthritis including its prognostic significance and treatment.

Rheumatoid Wrist

Brase DW, Millender, LH: Failure of silicone rubber wrist arthroplasty in rheumatoid arthritis. *J Hand Surg,* 11A:175-183, 1986.

Seventy-one wrist replacements were done in 61 patients. The failure rate was 25% (18 wrists), with failure defined as implant breakage or revision for pain and deformity. Implant arthroplasty should be used only for patients with adequate bone stock and reasonable wrist alignment with low-demand requirements for wrist use and motion.

Brumfield R Jr, Kuschner SH, Gellman H, Liles DN, Van Winckle, G: Results of dorsal wrist synovectomies in the rheumatoid hand.
J Hand Surg, 15:733-735, 1990.

One hundred and two dorsal wrist tenosynovectomies with distal ulna resection and wrist synovectomy were done in 78 patients followed for an average of 11 years. Pain decreased in 83%. Synovitis recurred in 16%. Motion decreased an average of 13°. Revision surgery was necessary in 28%.

Dennis, DA, Ferlic DC, Clayton ML: Volz total wrist arthroplasty in rheumatoid arthritis: a long term review.
J Hand Surg, 11A:483-490, 1986.

Thirty Volz arthroplasties were done in 23 patients with follow-up ranging from 36 to 106 months. Sixty percent rated as good or excellent, 27% fair, and 13% poor. Eighty-six percent of patients reported little or no pain, 13.8% had moderate pain, and no patients had severe pain. However, there were 16 complications in 12 arthroplasties. Single-prong metacarpal prostheses gave better results than double-pronged prostheses; this was attributed to wrist imbalance. Bone resorption of the distal radius and radiolucency around the metacarpal component were seen frequently.

Fatti JF, Palmer AK, Mosher JF: Long-term results of Swanson silicone rubber interpositional wrist arthroplasty. *J Hand Surg,* 11A:166-175, 1986.

Fifty-three arthroplasties in 42 patients, 31 for rheumatoid arthritis. Pain was the most common indication. In 36 followed for longer than 2.5 years, 61% rated as excellent or good, and 39% fair or poor.

Kobus RJ, Turner RH: Wrist arthrodesis for treatment of rheumatoid arthritis. *J Hand Surg,* 15:541-546, 1990.

Eighty-seven wrist fusions in 79 patients with six-year average follow-up using Millender-Nalebuff single-rod technique. Complications occurred in 23%, half of which were related to hardware. Discusses bilateral wrist fusions. Overall, wrist fusion resulted in high patient satisfaction.

Taleisnik J: Rheumatoid arthritis of the wrist. *Hand Clin,* 5:257-278, 1989.

Comprehensive review of the pathomechanics and treatment of the rheumatoid wrist.

Distal Radioulnar Joint

Clawson MC, Stern PJ: The distal radioulnar joint complex in rheumatoid arthritis: an overview. *Hand Clin,* 7:373-381, 1991.

A review of the treatment options for the distal radioulnar joint affected by rheumatoid disease.

Newman RJ: Excision of the distal ulna in patients with rheumatoid arthritis. *J Bone Joint Surg,* 69-B:203-206, 1987.

Thirty-five wrists in 25 patients had distal ulna resection for pain. With average follow-up of 3.7 years, 88% were rated as excellent or fair. The pain relief obtained after excision of distal ulna was not necessarily associated with improved arm function.

Posner MA, Ambrose L: Excision of the distal ulna in rheumatoid arthritis. *Hand Clin,* 7:383-390, 1991.

Review of the methods of resecting and stabilizing the distal ulna in rheumatoid arthritis.

Tenosynovitis

Brown FE, Brown M-L: Long-term results after teno-synovectomy to treat the rheumatoid hand. *J Hand Surg,* 13-A:704-708, 1988.

One hundred-seventy three tenosynovectomies were done in 125 patients. Follow-up averaged 70 months. One hundred seventeen were done prophylactically because of persistent synovitis despite six months of medical treatment. In these, only one of 42 tendons was found to be invaded by tenosynovium and one of 44 tendons which were not invaded at the time of surgery ruptured subsequent to the surgery. Seven patients had recurrent tenosynovitis. Fifty-six procedures were done in patients with tendon rupture present at the time of surgery.

Ertel AN, Millender LH, Nalebuff EA, McKay D, Leslie B: Flexor tendon ruptures in patients with rheumatoid arthritis. *J Hand Surg,* 13:860-866, 1988.

One hundred fifteen flexor tendon ruptures in 45 hands with rheumatoid arthritis or rheumatoid variants were reviewed. Seventy-nine percent had ruptured at the wrist, 3.5% in the palm, and 17.5% in the digits. Patients with attrition ruptures had better results after reconstruction than did those with ruptures caused by

invasion. The worst results occurred in patients with multiple ruptures within the carpal canal and in those with ruptures in the fibro-osseous canals. Overall, the motion gained after surgery was poor. Prevention of rupture by tenosynovectomy and spur removal is recommended.

Leslie BM: Rheumatoid extensor tendon ruptures. *Hand Clin,* 5:191-202, 1989.

A concise review of the pathology and treatment of extensor tendon ruptures caused by rheumatoid disease.

Mannerfelt LG: Tendon transfers in surgery of the rheumatoid hand. *Hand Clin,* 4:309-316, 1988.

Reviews the principles of tendon transfers and specific tendon transfer techniques for rheumatoid tendon ruptures as well as for rheumatoid deformities of the wrist and hand.

Finger Deformities

Bieber EJ, Weiland AJ, Volenec-Dowling S: Silicone-rubber implant arthroplasty of the metacarpophalangeal joints for rheumatoid arthritis. *J Bone Joint Surg,* 68-A:206-209, 1986.

Forty-six patients with MCP arthroplasties on 210 finger joints in 55 hands were followed an average of five years, three months. Ulnar drift improved following surgery, as did MCP joint extension lag and overall MCP range of motion. The gains obtained immediately after surgery declined with time. Grip strength and prehension were not improved significantly in either the long or short term. Implant fractures and silicone synovitis were not found.

Kirschenbaum D, Schneider LH, Adams DC, Cody RP: Arthroplasty of the metacarpal phalangeal joints with use of silicone-rubber implants in patients who have rheumatoid arthtitis. *J Bone Joint Surg,* 75-A:3-12, 1993.

Review of 144 arthroplasties at 8.5-year average follow-up. Flexion/extension arc of motion improved to a more functional range and did not deteriorate. Ulnar drift was corrected to 0° to 6° and was maintained. PIP joint function continued to deteriorate over the course of follow-up.

Oster LH, Blair WF, Steyers CM, Flatt AE: Crossed intrinsic transfer. *J Hand Surg,* 14A:963-971, 1989.

Thirty-one hands in 22 patients followed for an average of 12.7 years had crossed intrinsic transfers. Correction of ulnar drift was obtained and maintained with average postoperative ulnar drift of 5°. However, MCP and PIP joint motion decreased.

Swanson AB, Poitevin LA, Swanson GdG, Kearney J: Bone remodeling in flexible implant arthroplasty in the metacarpophalangeal joints. *Clin Orthop,* 205:254-267, 1986.

Thirty-one hands in 29 patients who had implant MCP arthroplasty of 120 fingers and 13 thumb MP joints with follow-up of at least five years. Bone remodeling occurs to form a cortical bony shell around the implant stems with thickening of the cortical bone at the metacarpal and phalangeal metaphyses and midshafts of the phalanges. There was a decrease in the metacarpal midshaft cortical thickness that was permanent and was attributed to surgical reaming. There was no shortening of the proximal phalanx and an average of 9.1% shortening of the metacarpal.

Wilson RW, Carlblom ER: The rheumatoid metacarpophalangeal joint. *Hand Clin,* 5:223-237, 1989.

Review of the anatomy, pathomechanics, and treatment of finger MP joints in rheumatoid arthritis.

Wood VE, Ichtertz DR, Yahiku H: Soft-tissue metacarpophalangeal reconstruction for treatment of rheumatoid hand deformity. *J Hand Surg,* 14A:163-174, 1989.

Long-term follow-up of soft-tissue MP joint reconstruction without joint resection. Sixteen hands in 12 patients followed for an average of 81 months. Results were classified as excellent in six hands, good in seven, fair in one, and poor in two. Complete pain relief was reported by 88% of patients. There was only one recurrence of MP joint synovitis. Swan neck deformities worsened in two patients. The results were considered comparable to silicone replacement arthroplasty.

Thumb Deformities

Figgie MP, Inglis AE, Sobel M, Bohn WW, Fisher DA: Metacarpal phalangeal joint arthroplasty of the rheumatoid thumb. *J Hand Surg,* 15:210-216, 1990.

Fifty-nine silicone-rubber implants in 50 patients with rheumatoid deformity. All patients had less pain after surgery. Average active motion was 25°. Average key pinch strength was four pounds. Only one MP joint fusion was required for instability after arthroplasty.

Terrono A, Millender LH, Nalebuff, EA: Boutonnière rheumatoid thumb deformity. *J Hand Surg,* 15:999-1003, 1990.

Review of treatment of 53 patients who underwent 74 procedures for rheumatoid boutonnière deformity of the thumb. Mild deformity treated with synovectomy and EPL rerouting had a 64% recurrence rate. MP fusion is recommended for moderate deformity; MP arthroplasty is recommended for low-demand patient; MP arthroplasty combined with IP joint fusion is recommended for severe deformity.

Complex Rheumatoid Hand Deformities

Miller-Breslow A, Millender LH, Feldon P: Treatment considerations in the complicated rheumatoid hand. *Hand Clin,* 5:279-289, 1989.

Discussion of the systematic evaluation and the treatment principles of patients with advanced or complicated deformities of the hand from rheumatoid arthritis. Seven illustrative cases are presented.

Nalebuff EA: Factors influencing the results of implant surgery in the rheumatoid hand. *J Hand Surg,* 15B:395-403, 1990.

Review of planning and important considerations in rheumatoid patients selected to undergo implant arthroplasty of the hand. Emphasizes the importance of the status of the adjacent joints to the outcome of the arthroplasty. Recommendations for appropriate staging of procedures in patients with complex deformities.

18

Osteoarthritis

Vincent D. Pellegrini, Jr., MD

Introduction

In contrast to the true inflammatory arthritides such as rheumatoid disease, osteoarthritis refers to a degenerative condition of diarthrodial joints that is characterized by a primary disorder of hyaline cartilage. This condition has been referred to as osteoarthrosis by our British colleagues, implying the absence of a prominent inflammatory component when compared to rheumatoid arthritis. However, recent research concerning cartilage metabolism in osteoarthritis has demonstrated the importance of synovially derived inflammatory mediators in this disease, justifying the "-itis" suffix in its proper name.

The term "osteoarthritis" has been rather loosely used to refer to all degenerative conditions of articular cartilage other than the classically described inflammatory arthropathies such as rheumatoid disease and the seronegative spondyloarthropathies. However, conditions that are the obvious result of previous trauma, developmental skeletal abnormalities, crystalline deposition diseases, infection, or other known causes are better described as specific entities based on their etiology. Terms such as posttraumatic arthritis, degenerative arthritis secondary to developmental hip disease, and gouty arthritis might be more appropriately used to name these conditions. Osteoarthritis is best reserved to describe the degeneration of articular cartilage occurring without clear etiology, and indeed "primary idiopathic osteoarthritis" has been suggested as a more descriptive name for this condition. The clinical and radiographic examination of the hand is fundamental to any physician in making the diagnosis of primary idiopathic osteoarthritis.

Epidemiology of Primary Idiopathic Osteoarthritis

Within this nomenclature two main variants of osteoarthritic disease have been described. Primary generalized osteoarthritis, as originally described by Kellgren and Moore in 1952 and characterized by involvement of the terminal interphalangeal joint (Heberden's nodes), has long been recognized as the hallmark of familial osteoarthritic disease. The clinical finding of Heberden's nodes has since been repeatedly shown to be a strong predictor of radiographic involvement of multiple sites by osteoarthritis. Conversely, the absence of Heberden's nodes is nearly as strong a predictor of the absence of significant osteoarthritic disease in the hand. Of the 120 clinical cases Kellgren and Moore analyzed from one year of rheumatologic practice, 85% had radiographic involvement of the distal interphalangeal joints, 65% involved the trapeziometacarpal joint (carpometacarpal or CMC joint), and 46% affected the proximal interphalangeal joints of the hand. Involvement of the weightbearing joints of the lower extremity was far less common, despite their more frequent appearance on the modern operating schedule, with 62% of knees, 38% of great toe metatarsophalangeal joints, and 30% of hips demonstrating disease. More recent epidemiologic studies have confirmed the only weak association of hip disease and primary generalized osteoarthritis as manifest in the hand. While the early course of disease is marked by inflammatory involvement of the DIP joints and frequent transient elevation of the sedimentation rate, as a rule symptoms at the terminal joints spontaneously subside leaving behind the characteristic appearance of the painless Heberden's node. Ultimately, the greatest functional impairment in these patients occurs with advanced disease of the basal joints of the thumb, limiting forceful lateral pinch activities and breadth of grasp.

Nearly 15 years later erosive osteoarthritis was described by Peter, Pearson, and Marmor to emphasize the bony erosions underlying the deformity seen in the finger interphalangeal joints. (Fig 18-1) Ehrlich in 1968 coined the term inflammatory osteoarthritis to describe a clinical syndrome in women around the age of menopause with osteoarthritis of the radial aspect of the hand characterized by marked swelling and redness of the fingers and a peculiar propensity for involvement of the MCP joints. Finger DIP joints were involved in 75%, PIP joints in 50%, the trapeziometacarpal joint in 40%, and the index MCP joint was involved in 12% of the 170 patients studied with this condition. While terminal joint disease was common, only 9% of patients developed mucous cysts. The knees were involved in 40% and the hips in only 20% of patients.

Of greatest interest, 15% of patients ultimately developed a clinical syndrome indistinguishable from rheumatoid arthritis with an indolent course characterized by dorsal wrist tenosynovial swelling, ulnar carpal erosions, prolonged morning stiffness, and periarticular osteopenia. The primary functional limitation in this patient population occurs from PIP joint disease; painful limitation of motion in the ulnar fingers impairs power grip and instability of the index finger hinders lateral pinch.

Apart from this clinical presentation of these two subsets of osteoarthritic disease, distinctive surgical phenotypes exist among patients requiring reconstructive procedures on the hand for advanced osteoarthritis. While the prevalence of clinical and radiographic disease is greatest in the DIP joints followed by the trapeziometacarpal, PIP, and MCP joints, the frequency of surgical reconstruction is greatest in the trapeziometacarpal joint followed by the PIP joints and, rarely, the DIP joints. In nearly 200 procedures performed on the osteoarthritic hand, of those having primary operation on the basal joints of the thumb, only 10%

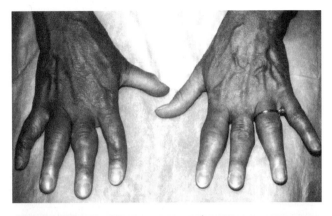

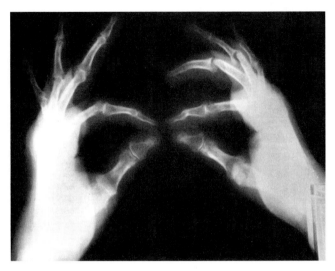

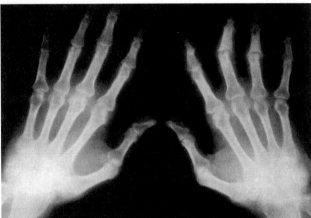

Figure 18-1.   (Top Left)
Characteristic appearance of hand
with erosive OA. PIP joint involvement
with swelling and angular deformity is
most prominent. Inflammatory
component with soft-tissue swelling,
warmth, and local tenderness about
the PIP joint is characteristic.

(Bottom Left and Top Right)
Radiographic appearance with
subchondral erosive lesions.

required procedures on the DIP joints and 2% on the PIP joints. Conversely, of those patients operated on for primary PIP joint impairment, half required procedures on the DIP joints and only 3% on the basal joints of the thumb. Therefore, patients with primary generalized osteoarthritis present to the hand surgeon with different functional problems from those with erosive osteoarthritis, and each group usually requires different surgical procedures to address their respective impairment. Indeed, the need for surgical treatment of trapeziometacarpal joint and PIP joint osteoarthritic disease in the hand would appear to be nearly mutually exclusive.

Beyond the poorly understood familial predisposition to primary generalized osteoarthritis that is manifest most prominently in women and their female children, there are considerable population differences in the prevalence of this disease. The major factors accounting for these differences in the upper extremity would appear to be both environmental and heritable in nature. Kellgren and Lawrence studied the occurrence of disease in populations of coal miners, farmers, and office workers in England and demonstrated a significantly greater prevalence of OA at the thumb carpometacarpal joint and a similar trend in the DIP joints of male cotton workers. However, all men with severe trapeziometacarpal osteoarthritis also had prominent

Heberden's nodes, suggesting that their disease was at least as likely related to a systemic diathesis as to trauma. Other population studies from the United Kingdom have demonstrated significantly greater prevalence of OA in the elbows of male pneumatic drill operators and the shoulders of male bus drivers.

Geographic and racial differences among populations also appear to have a strong influence on osteoarthritis in the hand, as evidenced by the differences in prevalence of trapeziometacarpal disease among Asian and Caucasian populations. Caucasian postmortem material has consistently demonstrated a prevalence of severe disease with eburnation of joint surfaces in 50%, chondromalacia in 25%, and grossly normal hyaline cartilage in 25% of specimens. In contrast, a review of published studies in the Japanese literature accounting for over 500 specimens provides data suggesting eburnation in only 8%, chondromalacia in 48%, and normal joint surfaces in 44% of specimens. Some evidence suggests that anatomic differences such as flattening of the Asian joint may in part account for this variation in disease. Anatomic variation is most apparent in the preserved skeletons of the ape ancestors of modern man and fossil specimens of hominid hands. The chimpanzee trapeziometacarpal joint is characterized by a prominent dorsovolar concavity of the metacarpal base which provides greater bony constraint than that found in the human joint. Notably, postmortem chimpanzee material has failed to demonstrate any evidence of severe osteoarthritic disease. Against this backdrop, the configuration of modern man's trapeziometacarpal joint would appear to represent an evolutionary design compromise. It has been suggested that as a result of anatomical evolution insufficient to keep pace with changing functional demands, selected joints are relatively underdesigned and suffer from eventual osteoarthritic disease secondary to overuse. Nonetheless, we must conclude that the development of osteoarthritis is dependent upon a complex interaction between a generalized systemic diathesis and local mechanical abnormalities peculiar to each specific joint.

Pathophysiology of Disease

The recognition of different types of osteoarthritis allows formulation of a continuum of arthritic disease to aid in the broader understanding of arthritic conditions in general (Fig. 18-2).

Figure 18-2.

Rheumatoid Arthritis	Erosive OA RA convert	Erosive OA	Primary GOA	Traumatic Arthritis

Inflammatory--Mechanical
The Spectrum of Arthritic Disease

At the far end of the spectrum are the true inflammatory arthropathies such as rheumatoid disease, and at the opposite extreme are the trauma and developmentally induced arthritic conditions secondary to a mechanical disturbance of the joint. Primary generalized osteoarthritis lies closer to the mechanical end of the spectrum but, as recent research has demonstrated, it is more appropriately placed slightly to the inflammatory side of true posttraumatic degenerative joint disease. Similarly, erosive osteoarthritis and the subset of 15% of patients with EOA who undergo seroconversion to rheumatoid disease are characterized by an even more prominent inflammatory component and may provide a conceptual link between rheumatoid arthritis and osteoarthritis as they are classically understood.

Current research into the general etiology of osteoarthritis has advanced our understanding of the interplay between biomechanical and biochemical factors in the production of clinical disease. Recognition of early proteoglycan loss and late preservation of collagen, increased proteoglycan synthesis characterized by relatively increased amounts of chondroitin sulfate, and relative insufficiency of link protein have all been demonstrated in osteoarthritic cartilage in the anterior cruciate-deficient animal knee model. Synovially derived cytokines such as interleukin-1, formerly known as catabolin, have been shown to activate degradative enzyme synthesis in the chondrocyte, which results in breakdown of the proteoglycan matrix components. Neutral proteases and metalloproteoglycanases play a

central role in catabolism of the matrix, resulting in a lesser fixed charge density, decreased hydrophilic properties, and a smaller volume of hydration of the cartilage. These biochemical events significantly alter the mechanical properties of hyaline cartilage, making it more susceptible to failure under load and less effective in buffering the subchondral trabeculae from impact loading and fracture. Preliminary data suggest that hyaline cartilage and the surrounding collagenous tissues may be sensitive to estrogen-related compounds, potentially clarifying our understanding of the gender predisposition of this disease.

Beyond these investigative findings germane to all joints afflicted by osteoarthritis, the trapeziometacarpal joint provides a valuable opportunity to study this disease process in the hand. The prevalence of trapeziometacarpal disease, its frequent need for surgical treatment, and the compact anatomy of the joint allowing *en bloc* resection of diseased articular surfaces (Fig. 18-3) make this joint uniquely suited for the study of regional changes in osteoarthritic disease. Study of both surgical and postmortem specimens has established the chondromalacic nature of the articular cartilage in the dorsal compartment, but more importantly the palmar joint surfaces were often found to be polished to eburnated bone. (Fig. 18-3). Eburnation always began on the most palmar perimeter of the joint and spread dorsally with progressive disease, sparing only a small peripheral rim of pitted and softened cartilage in the dorsal compartment of end-stage joints. Palmar cartilage surface degeneration was closely associated with degeneration of the beak ligament from the articular margin of the metacarpal (Fig. 18-4). In all cases of eburnation there was frank detachment of the ligament from its normal position confluent with the joint surface, effectively reducing its mechanical efficiency in checking dorsal migration of the metacarpal on trapezium during dynamic flexion-adduction of the thumb. Patterns of articular degeneration identical to those found in the surgical arthritic joints were observed in two-thirds of post-mortem specimens, attesting to the previously reported discrepancy between radiographic prevalence of degenerative changes and symptomatic disease. Variation in the subjective appreciation of pain plays a central role in determining which patients with trapeziometacarpal disease ultimately seek medical care for disabling symptoms.

Joint surface contact pressure patterns in a cadaver model simulating lateral pinch have confirmed the primary loading areas to be in the same palmar regions of the joint as the eburnated surfaces in diseased joints. Division of the beak ligament in specimens with healthy cartilage surfaces altered the contact patterns and reproduced the topography of the eburnated lesions observed in the arthritic joints. Furthermore, contact patterns in specimens with end-stage arthritic disease were notable for pathologic congruity with total contact of joint surfaces, hypertrophic marginal osteophytes, and diffuse eburnation.

Biochemical analysis of hyaline cartilage from arthritic trapeziometacarpal joints has noted preferential loss of glycosaminoglycan from the extracellular matrix with relative sparing of the collagen framework in the palmar regions of the joint where osteoarthritic lesions first appear. This is

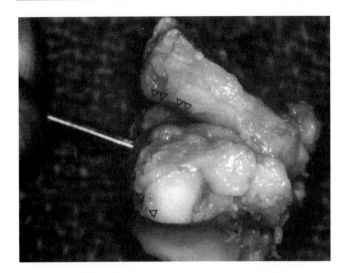

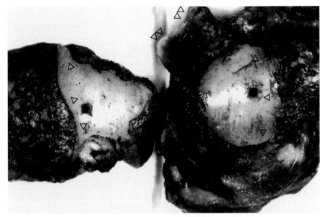

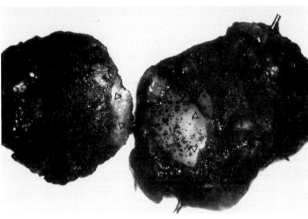

Figure 18-3. **(Top Left)** Trapeziometacarpal specimen removed at time of basal joint arthroplasty; *en bloc* trapezium and metacarpal articular surface. Articulated specimen of right thumb viewed from ulnar aspect demonstrating index metacarpal facet (single arrow) and dorsal metacarpal overhang in noncontact zone (double arrows). **(Bottom Left)** Stained specimen with early disease. Metacarpal left and trapezium right of right thumb with palmar surfaces adjacent to one another in center of picture. Eburnation in well circumscribed areas of palmar surfaces without staining (arrows), greater on trapezium. **(Top Right)** Stained specimen with advanced disease. Same orientation as bottom left photo. Extensive pale areas of eburnation (single arrows) involve entire trapezium and spare only the dorsal noncontact zone of the metacarpal. Prominent trapezial osteophyte (double arrows) apparent along palmar margin of eburnated surface.

consistent with the aforementioned studies of osteoarthritic cartilage suggesting a selective biochemical degradation of the extracellular matrix. The unique feature of this observation in the trapeziometacarpal joint is the localization of this process to the palmar contact areas of the joint where mechanical abrasion and shear are most severe. Scanning electron microscopy of trapeziometacarpal surfaces has demonstrated disruption of the protective superficial cartilage lamina in these same palmar contact regions where glycosaminoglycan loss and eventual osteoarthritic disease is known to occur.

A unifying hypothesis for the etiology of trapeziometacarpal osteoarthritis might posit initial attritional changes in the beak ligament culminating in eventual detachment with destabilization of the thumb metacarpal. Dorsopalmar metacarpal translation generates increased shear forces in the palmar contact areas of the joint and damages the protective surface layer of the hyaline cartilage, allowing regional access of synovially elaborated inflammatory mediators to the cellular elements in the deeper cartilage layers. Stimulation of chondrocyte enzyme production then results in selective biochemical degradation of the glycosaminoglycan component of the extracellular matrix, leaving a compromised collagen infrastructure vulnerable to the continued effects of abrasive wear in the palmar contact regions of the joint. Eventually, complete loss of the hyaline cartilage results from the combined effects of both abnormal biomechanical forces and biochemical breakdown of the matrix. Such a mechanism of osteoarthritis predicated upon instability of the trapeziometacarpal joint is consistent with the empirical clinical observations of amelioration of synovitis and retardation of the progression of arthritic disease in young women with symptomatic hypermobile joints following palmar beak ligament reconstruction procedures.

Management of Clinical Disease

Nonoperative

The initial management of osteoarthritic disease in the hand consists of a sequence of rest of the affected part in the form

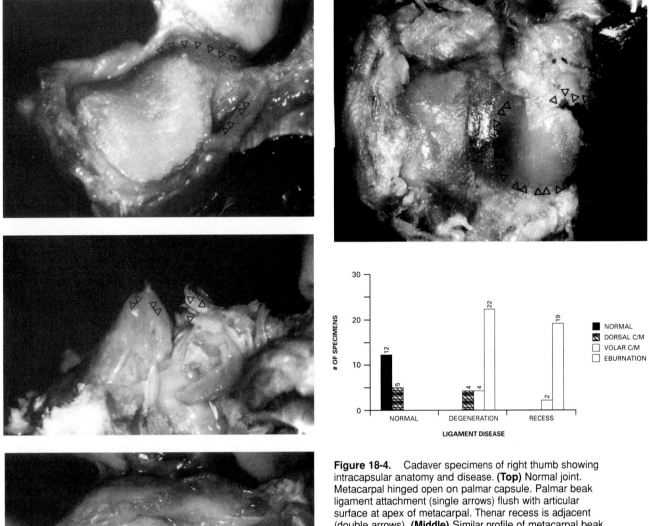

Figure 18-4. Cadaver specimens of right thumb showing intracapsular anatomy and disease. **(Top)** Normal joint. Metacarpal hinged open on palmar capsule. Palmar beak ligament attachment (single arrows) flush with articular surface at apex of metacarpal. Thenar recess is adjacent (double arrows). **(Middle)** Similar profile of metacarpal beak (double arrows) in specimen with advanced OA and beak ligament detachment (single arrows). **(Bottom)** Metacarpal articular surface with palmar region chondromalacia (double arrows) and adjacent degeneration of the beak ligament (single arrows) with early separation. Thenar recess is adjacent (triple arrows). **(Top Right)** Metacarpal surface with advanced disease and palmar eburnation (double arrows) and frank detachment of the adjacent beak ligament (single arrows). **(Bottom Right)** Relationship of palmar ligament degeneration and severity of articular disease. More severe ligament degeneration and detachment predicts increasing frequency of end-stage disease.

of activity restriction and splinting, use of anti-inflammatory medication, and a gentle strengthening program to functionally stabilize the involved joint prior to resumption of activities.

Numerous nonsteroidal anti-inflammatory drugs have been brought to market in the recent decade, but due to similar pharmacological properties and performance in clinical trials no single compound has been found to be singularly more effective than the rest. While there is no good evi-

dence that these medications alter the natural course of the disease and may be no more effective than acetaminophen, they offer the attractive feature of symptomatic control via alleviation of synovitis and effusion. Selection of an agent for a particular patient is therefore largely driven by the convenience of dosing interval as it affects compliance and the tolerance of gastrointestinal and renal side effects. Indeed, endoscopically visible gastric mucosal ulcers are apparent in 20% of patients using NSAIDS for six months and 1% to 2% will develop complications of these ulcers in the form of hemorrhage or perforation. Healing of uncomplicated lesions occurs in 90% of patients in four to six weeks following discontinuation of the drug in conjunction with use of H2 blockers and a coating agent such as sucralfate. More recently, a prostaglandin E1 analogue, misoprostol has been shown to prevent gastric ulcers related to NSAID use but critical analysis suggests cost efficacy only in high-risk older patients or those with a previous history of NSAID-related ulcer disease or hemorrhage.

Operative

Distal Interphalangeal Joint

Indications for surgical treatment of DIP joint disease include intractable pain refractory to medicinal agents, deformity, painful instability secondary to end-stage arthritic disease, and the existence of a problematic mucous cyst. In the early to intermediate stages of disease, pain at the terminal interphalangeal joints in most patients is satisfactorily managed with anti-inflammatory medication. Deformity of the distal joint in the form of nodular enlargement about the joint line, or Heberden's nodes, occurs after the initial inflammatory phase and is often painless. Surgical intervention at the patient's request solely to improve cosmesis in this setting is fraught with eventual patient dissatisfaction and is mentioned only to be discouraged. However, painful instability, particularly into radial or ulnar deviation in the index and long fingers, precludes effective tip pinch with the thumb and is reliably remedied by fusion. Flexion of the terminal joint to 10° to 15° in the index finger, increasing to 30° in the small finger, results in a functional arthrodesis. While intramedullary screw fixation obviates skin problems from protruding pins, it limits the arthrodesis position to near-complete extension and the author prefers the time-honored method using K-wires. In view of the associated risks of complication and failure, there remain no good indications for implantation of one of the currently available prosthetic devices to preserve motion at the distal joint.

Progressive enlargement with eventual drainage, vulnerability to repeated local trauma, ridging of the nail, pain, and complicating infection are indications for surgical treatment of the mucous cyst. Most worrisome is the cyst with recurrent cellulitis and pain on motion of the joint; a communicating septic arthritis is suspected in this setting and must be ruled out. While small lesions may be followed and frequently spontaneously recede, management of the significant mucous cyst is by debridement of the associated osteophyte and synovial tissue. In the event of advanced arthritic disease and limited motion of the affected joint, arthrodesis may be a preferable treatment. If the cyst has recently drained or there is reason to suspect past or current infection, a two-stage approach may be indicated with open debridement and antibiotic treatment followed by definitive closure after resolution of the infectious process.

Proximal Interphalangeal Joint

The indications for surgery on the PIP joint include pain refractory to medicinal management, deformity interfering with function, and painful instability or restriction of motion-limiting daily activities. Surgical intervention to improve cosmesis of the PIP joint with painless deformity and a functional range of motion is to be condemned. This is even more true of the proximal than the distal interphalangeal joint. The shoulders of the commonly implanted silicone prosthesis frequently protrude beyond the bone surfaces and result in a widened contour of the knuckle, not dissimilar from the preoperative appearance, that can continue to prevent wearing rings on the operated finger. Functional considerations dictate that radioulnar stability is of primary importance on the radial side of the hand where the fingers must withstand the forceful contact of the thumb in lateral pinch. In contrast, restoration of flexion arc takes priority in the ulnar digits where power grip is dependent upon full closure of the fingers into the palm to optimize function.

While numerous prosthetic devices have been introduced over the years to preserve and restore motion to the arthritic PIP joint, only the silicone interpositional materials are currently available for implantation in a noninvestigational setting. Most recently the Biomeric device, a cemented constrained implant with titanium stems and a synthetic rubber hinge, was reported to have a 100% failure rate at a mean of less than 2.5 years after implantation in the radial fingers. Failure was via fatigue and disintegration of the synthetic hinge without evidence of loosening of the cemented titanium stems. Revisional salvage was by either conversion to a silicone interposition arthroplasty in the ulnar digits or arthrodesis, which required use of distant bone graft material, in the radial digits.

Silicone interpositional arthroplasty offers the prospect of a functional range of motion approximating 55° and maximal flexion approaching 60° with modest lateral stability in osteoarthritic joints. Surgical results are generally good over the short and intermediate term. Restoration of a painless arc of motion in a more functional range is largely responsible for the satisfactory outcome that ensues in over 90% of patients. Traditionally, a dorsal approach has been advocated but this usually necessitates takedown and repair of the central tendon insertion and an obligatory period of postoperative splinting and avoidance of active flexion to protect the extensor mechanism. While this approach is useful in the finger with boutonniére deformity in need of central tendon reconstruction, reestablishment of perfect extensor balance is a difficult proposition. This is evidenced by a nearly equal frequency of PIP joint resting posture in neutral, slight flexion, and slight hyperextension in our own series of silicone implant arthroplasty. Alternatively, a volar surgical approach in fingers without boutonniére deformity may minimize the risk of extensor lag by avoiding interference with the extensor mechanism and allowing active motion in the early postoperative period. Additionally, this approach affords the opportunity for lysis of adhesions between the superficial and deep flexor

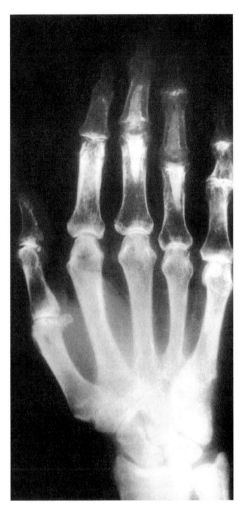

Figure 18-5. Three years following silicone interposition arthroplasty, these implants in the long and ring fingers are surrounded by a favorable sclerotic rim and lack of erosions representative of the typical favorable host bone response seen at early and intermediate term follow up.

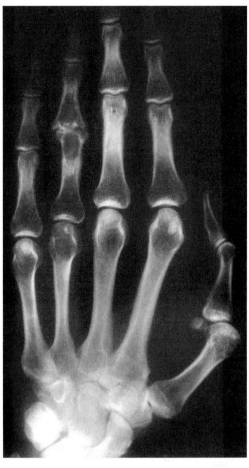

Figure 18-6. Nine-year follow-up of silicone interposition arthroplasty in ring finger of dominant hand. Advanced changes of bone erosion adjacent to fragmented and fractured implant, loss of arthroplasty space, and scalloping of the endosteal surface adjacent to implant stem are apparent. The portions of the implant stem most distant from the joint space in each phalanx remain surrounded by a benign sclerotic interface, attesting to the centrifugal progression of the erosive process commencing in the region of the flexible hinge.

tendons as are commonly found in the stiff osteoarthritic finger.

At intermediate term follow-up of 5.1 years, Swanson reported a need for revision of the prosthesis in 10.9% of fingers, implant fracture in 5.2%, and recurrent ulnar deviation in 3.7%. While 95% of fingers demonstrated a favorable host bone response to the implant (Fig. 18-5), bone overgrowth was seen in 4% and bony resorption in 1% of fingers. However, long-term follow-up suggests that silicone at the PIP level is subject to the same wear and fragmentation over time as seen in carpal implants, and may provoke destructive changes in the adjacent bone. A recent report of 26 implants noted radiographic bony erosions appearing first at the periarticular margin in 27% of fingers at a mean of four years postoperatively. These ultimately progressed to involve the intramedullary canals adjacent to the prosthetic stems in 8% of devices at a mean of six and one-half years after implantation (Fig. 18-6). While flexible silicone interpositional materials represent the best available prosthetic device for the PIP joint at this time, they are not without identified problems of a progressive nature and accordingly warrant close routine follow-up. Use of a silicone device in the most radial finger engaged in lateral pinch with the thumb is not advisable due to the significant radial deviation forces at the PIP joint tending to disrupt the integrity of the implant.

Arthrodesis in a functional position remains the best surgical treatment for the painful, unstable PIP joint in the index or long finger subjected to the repeated lateral stress of the thumb in key pinch. Arthrodesis improved lateral pinch strength more than any arthroplasty procedure improved any other objective strength parameter in one report. A stable index PIP joint would allow silicone implant arthroplasty of the adjacent long finger PIP joint, but careful consideration must be given to fusion of this joint if the index is unstable, even if asymptomatic, to lateral stress. Even arthrodesis of the ipsilateral DIP and PIP joints of the index finger is functionally well tolerated and restores pinch strength in spite of some degree of shortening. Arthrodesis of the ulnar digits is less desirable due to the need for flexion in gripping activities, but it remains the procedure of choice for the young manual laborer with end-stage arthritic disease in whom optimal function may be more dependent upon durability and strength than maximal flexion arc.

Trapeziometacarpal Joint

Indications for surgical treatment of basal joint disease of the thumb are almost exclusively pain or deformity that interferes with daily function including grip and breadth of palm. The trapeziometacarpal joint is overwhelmingly the most common site in need of surgical reconstruction in the osteoarthritic upper extremity.

In Stage I disease the most appropriate surgical treatment is reconstruction of the palmar beak ligament with a slip of flexor carpi radialis tendon as described by Eaton and Littler. However, for this stabilizing procedure to provide pain relief, the joint surfaces must be free of eburnation and demonstrate only the earliest changes of chondromalacia in the contact areas of the palmar compartment. Such a complete assessment of the articular surfaces is best afforded intraoperatively by the exposure gained through a Wagner approach detaching the origin of the thenar musculature to reveal the membranous capsule between the abductor pollicis longus and the palmar beak ligament. Hence the plan to perform ligament reconstruction without an arthroplasty procedure must always be contingent upon intraoperative confirmation of satisfactory articular surfaces, and both surgeon and patient must be prepared to exercise an alternative treatment option should this not be the case. More advanced disease of only the most palmar periphery of the joint may still allow isolated ligament reconstruction if debridement of this marginal palmar eburnation or osteophyte can be accomplished in conjunction with the stabilization procedure. Intermediate to long-range follow-up suggests that ligament reconstruction in the symptomatic hypermobile joint may retard the progression of degenerative articular changes leading to frank trapeziometacarpal osteoarthritis.

Slightly more advanced disease of radiographic Stage II usually demonstrates eburnation of cartilage in the contact areas of the palmar compartment of the joint. This pathology eliminates isolated ligament reconstruction as a treatment option and demands consideration of a procedure to address the articular surface disease. Traditionally, these procedures would include arthrodesis or arthroplasty with either synthetic or biologic implant material. Alternatively, Wilson has described metacarpal osteotomy for advanced trapeziometacarpal osteoarthritis with satisfactory results. Recent reports claim significant pain relief and increased

breadth of web with notable absence of any favorable radiographic changes as seen after successful osteotomy about the hip or knee. Unfortunately, there is not good documentation of intraoperative status of the joint as it relates to postoperative outcome or other selection criteria to assist in identifying patients most appropriate for this procedure. Laboratory investigations have not demonstrated significant unloading of the palmar contact areas when osteotomy is performed in postmortem specimens with advanced Stage III radiographic disease with extensive articular eburnation. The pain relief afforded by osteotomy in this clinical setting might be attributed to a biological decompression of the medullary canal, whose effect would be transient and unreliably reproduced from patient to patient. In contrast, a 30° closing wedge extension osteotomy effectively unloaded the palmar compartment when eburnation involved less than one-half, and optimally only one-third, of the palmar joint surfaces. Osteotomy in this setting shifted the contact areas to the intact dorsal articular cartilage and could reasonably be expected to provide longer symptomatic relief in the patient with Stage II disease without involvement of the dorsal compartment. Osteotomy might be most appropriate in the high-demand hand of a young laborer with Stage II disease, and in whom the limitations of motion imposed by arthrodesis and the concerns over durability of an arthroplasty leave doubt as to the appropriateness of either of these procedures. Furthermore, performance of an osteotomy does not preclude conversion to either arthrodesis or arthroplasty at a later date in the event of progression of arthritic disease.

Stage III disease implies end-stage degeneration of the trapeziometacarpal joint salvageable only by a procedure that removes or replaces the entire articular surface. Cemented arthroplasty has been associated with an unacceptably high loosening rate and has fallen from favor. Recently the de la Caffiniere prosthesis has undergone design revisions intended to reduce the incidence of early metacarpal loosening by enlarging the stem diameter, adding a circumferential collar, and providing a modular head-neck segment. The polyethylene trapezial component remains unchanged. Meaningful results using this new component design will not be available for several years. Arthrodesis, partial or complete trapezium resection, and implant arthroplasty with synthetic or biologic materials remain the appropriate treatment alternatives.

Trapeziometacarpal fusion has been widely employed in the past and its frequency of selection as a primary surgical intervention is inversely proportional to the availability and expected durability of alternative arthroplasty procedures. While achievement of a sound radiographic arthrodesis has not been universally successful, with failure rates in published series of 5% to 50%, the clinical result is not severely compromised by a solid fibrous union. Fusion does impose some limitations in function, however, and the resulting stress transfer to adjacent diseased joints can accelerate progression of degenerative changes. Loss of motion, the inability to manipulate the hand into restricted areas or onto flat surfaces, progression of arthritis in neighboring joints, distal thumb joint involvement requiring arthrodesis, and the excellent results of motion-preserving procedures have all contributed to this procedure's decline in popularity.

Gervis introduced excisional arthroplasty in 1949 and eventually submitted to this procedure for his own basal joint arthritis. The weakness and instability he noted have been echoed in subsequent reports as the major drawbacks of this operation. Additionally, proximal migration of the metacarpal with resultant shortening of the thumb ray presents both a cosmetic and functional problem. While for these reasons it is no longer a commonly chosen primary surgical intervention, excisional arthroplasty does offer a viable solution to the difficult problem of the failed infected implant arthroplasty.

In the early 60s, prior to the availability of prosthetic implants, the concept of fascial or tendon interposition was pursued as an alternative to simple trapezium excision in an effort to reduce thumb shortening and improve pinch strength. Froimson first reported on the use of a rolled flexor carpis radialis "anchovy" spacer following total trapeziectomy in 1970. While pain relief was universal, he subsequently described a 30% reduction in pinch strength relative to the unoperated hand and a 50% loss of the arthroplasty "space" secondary to metacarpal settling at a mean (range two to 20 years) follow-up of six years. He concurrently recommended hemitrapeziectomy for Stage III disease in hopes of minimizing thumb shortening and loss of pinch strength. Several other authors have suggested use of other tendons, fascia lata, banked fascia, and gelfoam as interpositional materials. Although some reports have offered that performance of simple tendon interposition arthroplasty is comparable to that of silicone implant arthroplasty at short-term follow-up, most have suggested that the addition of fascial interpositional material may reduce shortening of the thumb but does not significantly improve function over that achieved by simple trapezial excision. Reports of key pinch and grip strengths after traditional tendon interposition arthroplasty have been varied but often show values at or below the lower end of normal. Usually strengths are reported relative to the opposite unoperated hand because of insufficient preoperative data. With an incidence of bilateral disease of 20% to 30% in most reported series and an additional prevalence of more than 20% with asymptomatic disease, the validity of comparative strength determinations relative to the "normal" hand is questionable. While restoration of totally normal pinch strength is neither necessary nor expected after arthroplasty for basal joint arthritis in most patients, reconstruction of critical capsular and ligamentous supports would seem central to maximizing postoperative strength and function in a disease where pathologic instability is responsible for articular cartilage degeneration.

Swanson has been primarily responsible for the popularization and success of silicone implant arthroplasty since its inception in 1965. Replacement of the arthritic trapezium with a silicone prosthesis alleviated pain, preserved length of the thumb, and restored a functional range of motion. The introduction of silicone as an interpositional material initiated a new era in arthritis surgery of the hand. Since then numerous sizes, shapes, and composites of silicone have been exchanged for painful arthritic joints. While dramatic relief of pain and restoration of motion ensued in most cases, early complications of implant instability focused attention on adequate bony resection for implant seating and capsular reconstruction with or without augmentation by tenodesis. Swanson's follow-up of 147 of 150 cases at average 3.5 years postoperatively indicated significant subluxation (one-third or more of prosthesis) in 14.5%, dislocation in 6%, and "purposeful radial articulation" in 5.5% with a reoperation rate of 3.3%. Overall more than one-quarter of implants failed to satisfactorily seat in the trapezium fossa. Implant fractures of the original design were infrequent but became less common following development of the high-performance silicone elastomer in 1974. Eaton addressed the instability problem by designing a cannulated silicone trapezium implant to allow incorporation of beak ligament reconstruction by tenodesis with the abductor pollicis longus to the base of the index metacarpal as an integral part of the arthroplasty procedure. For all practical purposes, this modified device eliminated instability as a troublesome problem in silicone implant arthroplasty of the basal joint. Inevitably, with longer-term follow-up of stable silicone implants, the issue of host tolerance of the silicone material has emerged as a major clinical concern. Associated with the widespread use of high-performance silicone material, but not restricted to it, was the increasingly frequent observation of implant wear, cold flow, and erosive bony changes both adjacent to carpal bone implants and at distant sites in the carpus and distal radius (Fig. 18-7). While this process was typically painless at the outset, revisional procedures performed for progressive bony changes and implant mechanical failure demonstrated an aggressive membrane and associated synovitis with histologic characteristics of a foreign body reaction to particulate silicone debris. This "silicone synovitis" has been subsequently reported with increasing frequency to be associated with all configurations of silicone as longer follow-up of these devices becomes available. At a mean four-year follow-up of silicone trapezial implants, a clinical failure rate of 25% has been observed in association with a mean subluxation of 35% of the width of the prosthesis and 50% loss of vertical implant height along the ulnar margin. An inverse relationship existed between implant instability and material wear; that is, ligament reconstruction reduced implant subluxation but increased material wear and cold flow. The Swanson devices with an average subluxation of 60% of the implant width lost only 25% of vertical height whereas the clinically and radiographically more stable cannulated implants lost an average of 50% of vertical ulnar height. Associated dynamic tendon transfers did not prevent implant subluxation and had no effect on the magnitude or location of implant wear. Perhaps most worrisome is the progressive nature of asymptomatic carpal erosions reported with an incidence of 51% to 84% at 4.5- to 12-year follow-up of silicone arthroplasty in osteoarthritic thumbs.

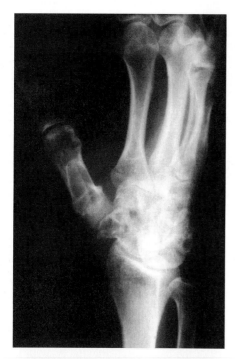

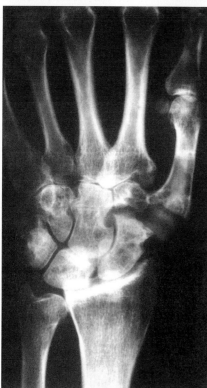

Figure 18-7. **(Top)** Unstable fractured Swanson silicone implant with progressive carpal bone erosions, symptomatic after six years, immediately prior to revision surgery. **(Bottom)** Worn ulnar margin of Eaton silicone implant with progressive adjacent carpal bone erosions, asymptomatic at five years.

Smaller and more stable implants have likewise been associated with a greater incidence of erosive cysts. The clinically silent yet progressive nature of this reactive bone resorption has led to the recommendation of regular radiographic and clinical follow-up of all *in situ* trapezium implants and suspension of further silicone implantation at the base of the osteoarthritic thumb.

The more recent combination of beak ligament reconstruction with tendon interposition arthroplasty has become the preferred procedure for osteoarthritis of the thumb basal joint complex and addresses the need for stabilization of the diseased trapeziometacarpal joint while eliminating concern for host tolerance of a synthetic implant device. Support of the palmar metacarpal cortex by the ligament reconstruction maintains thumb length and prevents proximal metacarpal migration (Fig. 18-8). Only distal hemitrapeziectomy is required for Stage III disease (without scaphotrapezial involvement), but complete trapeziectomy facilitates performing the procedure by providing broad distal exposure of the flexor carpi radialis tendon and maximal correction of the contracted first web with optimal projection of the reconstructed thumb. By definition, Stage IV disease requires total removal of the trapezium. Serial follow-up of patients at early (two-year), intermediate (six-year), and late (nine years, four month) intervals following LRTI arthroplasty has been encouraging. Aggregate pinch and grip strengths improved nearly 20% from preoperative levels at two-year follow-up. Continued interval improvement was noted from two-year to six-year follow-up with increases from 4.8kg to 5.6kg in key pinch and 17.3kg to 24kg in grip strength. Grip and pinch strengths plateaued thereafter and at nine years, four month follow-up there was a 92.5% improvement in grip and 50% aggregate improvement in pinch strengths compared to preoperative values. Over the same intervals, radiographic assessment was notable for insignificant increases in metacarpal subluxation from 7% to 8% to 11% and loss of arthroplasty space from 11% to 11% to 13% (Fig. 18-8). Overall, clinical and radiographic results have been shown to maintain functional improvements through the available period of follow-up. No intercarpal instability has been observed following complete trapeziectomy for this procedure. One revisional operation has been necessary to repair a herniation of the interpositional tendon material through a defect in the capsular reconstruction. No instances of metacarpal impingement on the scaphoid or remaining trapezium have occurred when ligament reconstruction was performed. However, reoperation for symptomatic impingement has been necessary after simple interpositional arthroplasty, with successful conversion to LRTI arthroplasty by suspension of the thumb metacarpal. Variations on this operation have been described with similarly satisfactory results at shorter-term follow-up. The common features of all these procedures suggest that the essential elements of contemporary trapeziometacarpal arthroplasty include use of a suitable biological interpositional material and reconstruction of the beak ligament to provide both mobility and stability to the base of the thumb.

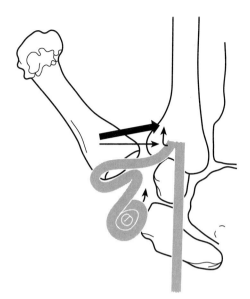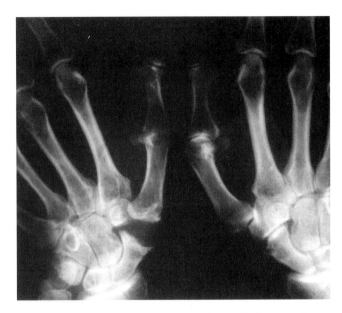

Figure 18-8. **(Left)** Ligament reconstruction—tendon interposition arthroplasty with suspension of palmar metacarpal cortex by flexor carpi radialis and interposition of remaining tendon material. **(Right)** Four years following LRTI arthroplasty with total trapeziectomy, asymptomatic and stable on stress radiograph.

Scaphotrapeziotrapezoid Joint

Slightly more proximal along the thumb axis, degenerative arthritis is seen much less commonly at the distal pole of the scaphoid unaccompanied by trapeziometacarpal osteoarthritis. The consideration of this condition as a manifestation of primary osteoarthritis is somewhat controversial, however, as its association with intercarpal instability and crystalline calcium pyrophosphate deposition disease has been frequently reported. Nonetheless, there remain infrequent cases not associated with these conditions that would appear to represent idiopathic osteoarthritic disease.

Watson has suggested that 95% of all degenerative disorders of the wrist are centered about the scaphoid and 26% affect the scaphoidtrapeziumtrapezoid joints in the absence of intercarpal instability. Carstam, Eiken, and Andren have noted the association of volar wrist ganglia and degeneration at the trapezioscaphoid joint. They attributed this to the proximity of the flexor carpi radialis tendon sheath to the joint and demonstrated a common communication between these structures by arthrography. Crosby, Linscheid, and Dobyns observed an abnormally vertical position of the scaphoid unique to this condition, with scapholunate angles of less than 45° in 84% of wrists, implying dorsal rotation of the scaphoid and volar subluxation of the thumb axis on the distal scaphoid articular surface. Nearly all patients had tenderness localized to the volar surface of the scaphotrapezial joint and a decrease in strength and range of motion was evident in 50% of patients.

Beyond the customary initial nonoperative management with anti-inflammatory medication, protective splinting, and avoidance of bothersome activities, surgical treatment has been varied. Joint debridement, silicone interposition arthroplasty, limited resection and tendon interposition arthroplasty, arthrodesis, and total trapeziectomy in the setting of concurrent trapeziometacarpal disease have all been described without clear consensus as to a superior method. Complications associated with silicone and stiffness with late secondary degeneration of other joints associated with arthrodesis have contributed to the decline in popularity of these procedures. Conservative joint resection, preferably from the trapezial surface to avoid destabilization of the distal pole of the scaphoid, with tendon interposition provides satisfactory symptomatic relief with the expectation of fewer long-term complications and is the author's preferred method of treatment.

Future Trends

The most immediate need in surgical treatment of osteoarthritic disease in the hand is in development of a reliable prosthetic or biological arthroplasty for the end-stage proximal interphalangeal joint. Research in this area is in progress.

Nonetheless, the real future of our understanding and treatment of osteoarthritis lies in the biological sphere rather than on the bench of prosthetic design engineers. Biological resurfacing of diseased joints with osteochondral segments will become more reliable as the immunologic basis for tissue rejection is elucidated, but the application of this procedure remains limited by our ability to control the transmission of disease via tissue transplantation. Ultimately, advances in molecular biology, genetic engineering, and the biochemistry of connective tissue, combined with the techniques of tissue culture, will allow artificial repair and synthesis of cartilage elements and provide meaningful strides in the treatment and prevention of osteoarthritic disease.

Annotated Bibliography

Epidemiology of Primary Idiopathic Osteoarthritis

Bagge E, Bjelle A, Eden S, Svanborg A: Factors associated with radiographic osteoarthritis: results from the population study 70-year-old people in Goteborg. *J Rheumatology,* 18:1218-22, 1991.

Swedish epidemiological data on prevalence of OA. Confirmation of the association of male obesity with GOA as seen in the hands of men, resembling the pattern commonly seen in women.

Cobby M, Cushnaghan J, Creamer P, Dieppe P, Watt I: Erosive osteoarthritis: is it a separate disease entity? *Clin Radiology,* 42:258-263, 1990.

Update on the radiographic diagnosis of EOA indicating that many more radiographically abnormal joints were present than in controls, due largely to an increase in both distal and proximal interphalangeal joint involvement. Erosions were associated with more severe hand disease but not a distinct disease entity.

Ehrlich G: Inflammatory osteoarthritis—I. The clinical syndrome, and II. The superimposition of rheumatoid arthritis. *J Chronic Dis,* 25:317-328 and 635-643, 1972.

Description of the clinical syndrome of erosive or inflammatory OA and the relationship to PIP joint disease and 15% rheumatoid conversion at mean age of 63 years. Relatively benign rheumatoid course.

Fujisawa K: Arthrosis of the carpometacarpal joint of the thumb (the third report)—a comparative radiographic and anatomical study. *J Japanese Society Surg Hand,* 5:412-415, 1988.

Forty-five of 48 postmortem specimens were radiographic Stage I or II and gross inspection of the joint surfaces demonstrated only 19% of metacarpals and 25% of trapeziums with pathologic chondromalacia or eburnation.

Hutton C: Generalized osteoarthritis: an evolutionary problem? *Lancet,* June 27:1463-1465, 1987.

The concept of functional underdesign and overdesign, based on evolution of joint-specific tasks and anatomy, is introduced as it relates to osteoarthritis.

Kellgren J, Lawrence J: Osteoarthrosis and disk degeneration in an urban population. *Ann Rheum Dis,* 17:388-397, 1958.

Epidemiologic data base from English towns allowing analysis of environmental factors as they relate to prevalence of osteoarthritis.

Kellgren J, Moore R: Generalized osteoarthritis and Heberden's nodes. *Br Med J,* 1:181-187, 1952.

Original description of clinical features of GOA in 120 cases.

Kihara H: Anatomical study of the normal and degenerative articular surfaces on the first carpometacarpal joint. *J Japanese Orthop Assoc,* 66:228-239, 1992.

Only 13 of 138 postmortem trapeziometacarpal specimens demonstrated eburnation of advanced osteoarthritis. The concave and convex dimensions of the joint were found to be more shallow in female specimens.

Marzke M: Evolutionary development of the human thumb. *Hand Clin,* 8:1-8, 1992.

Comparative anatomy of fossil hominid hands and ancestral apes to modern human hands relative to contour of the trapeziometacarpal joint.

VanSaase J, VanRomunde L, Cats A, Vandenbroucke J, Valkenburg H: Epidemiology of osteoarthritis: Zoetermeer survey. Comparison of radiological osteoarthritis in a Dutch population with that in 10 other populations. *Ann Rheum Dis,* 48:271-280, 1989.

OA prevalence in a Dutch village. DIP joint disease appeared in 64% of men and 76% of women.

Pathophysiology of Disease

Dingle JT: Catabolin—a cartilage catabolic factor from synovium. *Clin Orthop Rel Res,* 156:219-231, 1981.

Original description of catabolin identified as a synovially elaborated messenger molecule stimulating chondrocyte enzyme synthesis.

Hamerman D: The biology of osteoarthritis. *N Engl J Med,* 320:1322-1330, 1989.

Current status of the biochemistry of osteoarthritis and cartilage metabolism.

Knowlton R, Katzenstein P, Moskowitz R, Weaver E, Malemud C, Pathria M, Jimenez S, Prockop D: Genetic linkage of a polymorphism in the type II procollagen gene (COL2A 1) to primary osteoarthritis associated with mild chondrodysplasia. *N Engl J Med,* 322:526-530, 1990.

Identification of a genetically transmitted abnormal collagen predisposing to osteoarthritic disease.

Nojima T, Towle C, Mankin H, Treadwell B: Secretion of higher levels of active proteoglycanases from human osteoarthritic chondrocytes. *Arthritis Rheum,* 29:292-295, 1986.

Evidence for increased metabolic activity in chondrocytes of osteoarthritic cartilage, with elevated levels of chondroitin sulfate and degradative enzymes.

Pellegrini VD, Jr: Osteoarthritis of the thumb trapeziometacarpal joint: a study of the pathophysiology of articular cartilage degeneration. I. Anatomy and pathology of the aging joint. *J Hand Surg,* 16A:967-974, 1991.

Correlation of beak ligament degeneration and articular cartilage disease in postmortem trapeziometacarpal specimens.

Pellegrini VD, Jr: Osteoarthritis of the thumb trapeziometacarpal joint: a study of the pathophysiology of articular cartilage degeneration. II. Articular wear patterns in the osteoarthritic joint. *J Hand Surg,* 16A:975-982, 1991.

Trapeziometacarpal wear ratios demonstrate greater areas of eburnation on trapezium than metacarpal, implying translational movement of metacarpal on trapezium.

Smith RL, Allison A, Schurman D: Induction of articular cartilage degradation by recombinant interleukin 1 a and 1 b. *Connective Tissue Research,* 18:307-316, 1989.

Induction of chondrocyte enzyme synthesis is demonstrated by interleukin messenger molecules.

Management of Clinical Disease

Bradley J, Brandt K, Katz B, Kalasinski L, Ryan S: Comparison of an anti-inflammatory dose of ibuprofen, an analgesic dose of ibuprofen, and acetaminophen in the treatment of patients with osteoarthritis of the knee. *N Engl J Med,* 325:87-91, 1991.

Comparable efficacy of relief of arthritic pain is reported with acetaminophen as compared with high- or low-dose ibuprofen in the treatment of osteoarthritis of the knee.

Brooks P, Day R: Nonsteroidal anti-inflammatory drugs—differences and similarities. *N Engl J Med,* 324:1716-1725, 1991.

A current review of the therapeutic and adverse effects of the available classes of NSAIDS.

Burton RI, Pellegrini VD, Jr: Surgical management of basal joint arthritis of the thumb. Part II. Ligament reconstruction with tendon interposition arthroplasty. *J Hand Surg,* 11A:324-332, 1986.

Description of soft-tissue interposition arthroplasty combined with ligament reconstruction at a two-year follow-up.

Eaton R, Lane L, Littler JW, Keyser J: Ligament reconstruction for the painful thumb carpometacarpal joint. A long-term assessment. *J Hand Surg,* 9A:692-699, 1984.

Follow-up at seven years after ligament reconstruction for instability and early arthritic disease suggests lack of disease progression after stabilization.

Eaton R, Littler JW: Ligament reconstruction for the painful thumb carpometacarpal joint. *Br J Surg,* 55A: 1655-1666, 1973.

Original rationale and technique description for ligament reconstruction for symptomatic trapeziometacarpal instability.

Edelson J, Tosteson A, Sax P: Cost-effectiveness of misoprostol for prophylaxis against nonsteroidal anti-inflammatory drug-induced gastrointestinal tract bleeding. *JAMA,* 264:41-47, 1990.

The significant cost of cytotec combined with the low (1%) incidence of GI bleeding in patients taking NSAIDS for six months makes use of this new drug reasonable only as a secondary prevention in patients with a history of GI bleeding.

Molitor P, Emery R, Meggitt B: First metacarpal osteotomy for carpometacarpal osteoarthritis. *J Hand Surg,* 16B:424-427, 1991.

Osteotomy relocates functional arc of motion by a 15° shift into abduction and is accompanied by improvement in fatigue of grip strength and pain relief.

Pellegrini VD, Jr, Burton RI: Surgical management of basal joint arthritis of the thumb. Part I. Long-term results of silicone implant arthroplasty. *J Hand Surg,* 11A:309-324, 1986.

Trapezial implant instability and cold flow are related to erosive bone lesions and silicone synovitis at intermediate range follow-up.

Pellegrini VD Jr, Burton, RI: Osteoarthritis of the proximal interphalangeal joint of the hand: arthroplasty or fusion? *J Hand Surg,* 15A:194-209, 1990.

Failures of Biomeric prostheses are analyzed and erosive bone lesions are identified as they relate to silicone implants at intermediate and long-term follow-up.

19

Other Arthritides

Leonard K. Ruby, MD

Juvenile Rheumatoid Arthritis

Juvenile rheumatoid arthritis is by definition an inflammatory arthritis affecting the prepubertal age group. It is of unknown etiology, but may have a genetic disposition. It is characterized by chronic synovial inflammation and hyperplasia. Diagnosis is based on clinical findings and can only be confirmed by biopsy, although this is usually not necessary. Laboratory studies are not diagnostic. Twenty percent of patients have positive rheumatoid factor and 30% to 40% of patients have positive antinuclear antibodies. The sedimentation rate is usually elevated and is helpful in monitoring the course of the disease. There are three clinical subgroups based on appearance at presentation. They are: (1) systemic type or Still's disease; (2) polyarticular; and (3) pauciarticular (Table 19-1).

Hand involvement is most common in the polyarticular variant. The usual manifestations are wrist flexion and ulnar deviation deformity with accompanying stiffness of the metacarpophalangeal joints and proximal interphalangeal joints in extension (Fig. 19-1). There may also be significant flexor tenosynovitis and occasionally there is extensor tenosynovitis present. Because of the open epiphyses in these patients and the danger of growth arrest, nonoperative measures are recommended as the primary treatment in a high percentage of these patients. Hand therapy mobilization techniques, splinting (especially of the wrist) in the corrected position, as well as treatment with nonsteroidal anti-inflammatory drugs are the standard of care. Surgical measures should be considered only if the patient fails to improve or worsens in spite of good medical care. Synovectomy can provide pain relief but seldom improves motion. Tenosynovectomy especially on the flexor side may improve motion. Flexor tendon ruptures rarely occur.

Table 19-1. Modes of Onset of Juvenile Rheumatoid Arthritis

	SYSTEMIC	POLYARTICULAR		PAUCIARTICULAR	
Presentation	Extra-articular manifestations (fever, rash, organomegaly serositis, myalgia, hematologic changes) and arthritis	Symmetric arthritis involving large and small joints		Asymmetric arthritis involving few joints, usually large	
		Five or more joints affected		Less than five joints affected, frequently only one joint	
		RF negative	**RF positive**	**Type I**	**Type II**
Percent of patients	20%	25%-30%	10%	25%	15-20%
Age at onset (median)	5 years	3 years	>8 years	2 years	10 years
Sex distribution	M=F	F>M	F>M	F>M	M>F
Rheumatoid factor	Generally negative	Negative	Positive	Generally negative	Generally negative
Antinuclear antibodies	Generally negative	Positive in 25%	Positive in 75%	Positive in 50%	Generally negative
Course	Systemic manifestations are self-limited; arthritis may become chronic, with 25% of patients developing severe destructive arthritis	Majority do well, 10% develop severe sequelae, particularly hip and temporomandibular joint problems	Resembles adult rheumatoid disease, severe destructive arthritis in 50% of cases	Arthritis mild; morbidity associated with ocular problems (eg, iridocyclitis)	Course variable; patients may develop ankylosing spondylitis pattern

Table 19-1 reproduced with permission from Jay S, Helm S, Wray BB: Juvenile rheumatoid arthritis. *Am Fam Physician,* 26(2):139-147, 1982.

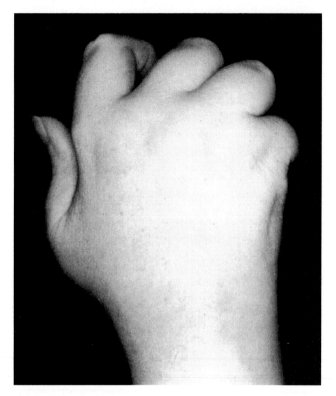 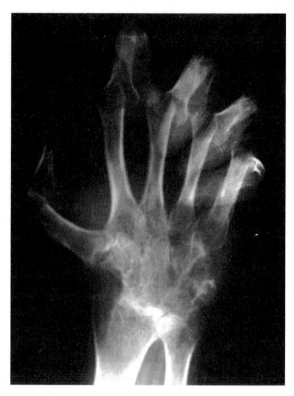

Figure 19-1.   (Left) Juvenile rheumatoid arthritis.   **(Right)** Juvenile rheumatoid arthritis.

The Wrist

These patients tend to have a high incidence of spontaneous fusion at the carpometacarpal and intercarpal joints. The radial carpal joint, although often spared, usually exhibits limited motion (Fig. 19-1). The best course is to allow this ankylosis to occur in a functional position and therefore long-term splinting or corrective casts are the mainstay of treatment. If, however, ankylosis occurs in a poor position, i.e. ulnar deviation and flexion, then corrective osteotomy of the radius can be performed. The ulna often is short, and this contributes to the ulnar deviation deformity. If this is also a painful problem then one can perform a limited distal radial ulnar joint arthroplasty such as the hemiresection arthroplasty described by Bowers.

The Digits

Metacarpophalangeal and proximal interphalangeal joint stiffness is best treated nonoperatively with therapy, as neither synovectomy nor capsulotomy usually improves motion. Arthroplasties are contraindicated in this young age group. Flexor tenosynovectomy may improve motion in those patients where passive flexion is greater than active flexion. This should be considered if local steroid injections fail.

Psoriatic Arthritis

Psoriatic arthritis is defined as an inflammatory arthritis associated with past or present psoriatic skin lesions. Rheumatoid factor and antinuclear antibody studies are negative. HLADR7 and HLADR4 studies are often positive. The clinical manifestations are onychodystrophy, with distal phalanx acrolysis, proximal interphalangeal joint fusion; metacarpophalangeal joint erosions of a characteristic "pencil and cup" type; and wrist fusion usually in good position (Fig. 19-2). Usually the skin findings precede the joint involvement by several years, although both manifestations may present simultaneously. There are four clinical subgroups: (1) pseudorheumatoid psoriatic arthritis; (2) oligoarthritis; (3) spondyloarthropathy; and (4) distal interphalangeal joint psoriatic arthritis.

The pseudorheumatoid form of psoriatic arthritis is distal and symmetric. Different from rheumatoid arthritis, the condition is less destructive. Nodules are absent except in those patients who take Methotrexate. There may be a prominent tenosynovitis involving the digital flexor sheaths and the FCR and FCU.

The oligoarticular form of the disease involves one to three joints. The process tends to be subdued, but progressive digital deformity, (usually boutonniére) often develops.

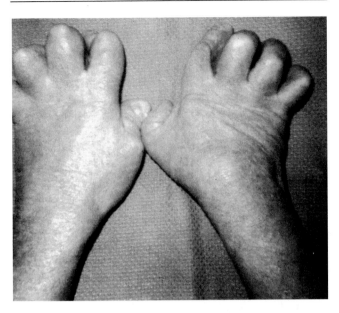

Figure 19-2. Psoriatic arthritis. The PIP and MP joints are most involved in this patient. The thumbs show osteolysis.

Arthritis mutilans, a rare manifestation of the disease, tends to occur in patients with oligoarthritis or the pseudorheumatoid type. The total percentage is approximately 5%. The mutilans form of psoriatic arthritis is clinically characterized by progressive painless shortening of one or more digits as a result of osteolysis of the PIP joints. Curiously the involved joints remain mobile, tendons tend to be spared, and passive stretching can restore the digits to their pre-erosion length. There is relative absence of periarticular osteopenia, and there is a tendency to both osteolysis and bony fusion.

The spondylarthropathy form primarily affects the spine and is relatively uncommon. Since the hand is not affected, it is mentioned only for completeness.

The distal interphalangeal joint form is characterized by swelling, pain, and redness at the distal interphalangeal joints. Clinical and radiographic changes may be difficult to differentiate from degenerative arthritis, although centripetal erosion of the joint often occurs, resulting in pseudo widening rather than collapse, with lack of bone on bone contact at the joint spaces. The lesion may progress to a "pencil and cup" deformity in which there is a whittling of the middle phalanx and expansion of the base of the distal phalanx. Recent reports have highlighted the association between HIV infection and this very destructive type of arthritis. Rapidly progressing joint deformities should alert the hand surgeon to this entity.

Nonoperative Treatment

Initial treatment of psoriatic arthritis in its various forms is with nonsteroidal anti-inflammatory drugs in association with hand therapy. Many patients become asymptomatic with this program. Sulfasalazine is usually added in patients who fail to improve and a favorable response is obtained in approximately 50% of these cases. Resistant cases are treated with Methotrexate and the response is excellent. An additional advantage of Methotrexate treatment is that the skin is also improved. One of the unfortunate side effects of Methotrexate is hepatic cirrhosis, and so these patients must abstain from alcohol ingestion. In patients who cannot take Methotrexate or Azathioprine, injectable gold may be used. Azathioprine is less effective than Methotrexate on the skin, and gold has no effect on psoriatic plaques. Psoriatic tenosynovitis responds well to corticosteroid infiltration and intra-articular steroid injections usually result in prolonged disease remission in the injected joint. Systemic corticosteroids are seldom used in psoriatic arthritis as the psoriasis may become worse.

Operative Treatment

The Wrist

If the wrist does not spontaneously fuse in a functionally adequate position then surgical arthrodesis with or without ulnar head resection can be performed.

The Digits

Metacarpophalangeal joints infrequently require surgical treatments as patients often have sufficient mobility without pain with the typical "pencil and cup" erosion. However, in those patients where pain and stiffness is a problem, arthroplasty can be considered. The standard silicone rubber arthroplasties can be difficult because of the severe erosion of the proximal phalanges, and the Tupper volar plate arthroplasty may be technically superior in these cases.

The proximal interphalangeal joints often become stiff in a functional position and no surgery is necessary. However, in those cases in which there is severe flexion deformity, arthrodesis with sufficient bone resection to improve the position can be helpful. In those patients who have arthritis mutilans with significant bone loss, arthrodesis with bone graft will arrest further erosion and restore stability and some length to the digits. Tenosynovitis is very rare in psoriatic arthritis.

Scleroderma

Scleroderma or systemic sclerosis is a multisystem disease which often affects the hand. There are several manifestations of this disease in the hand, including Raynaud's phenomenon, flexion deformities of the PIP joints, symptomatic calcific deposits in the soft tissues, skin ulcers, and septic arthritis.

Raynaud's phenomenon is seen in over 90% of patients with scleroderma, occurring equally in the disseminated cutaneous and the limited cutaneous, or CREST forms of the disease. The acronym CREST stands for Calcinosis, Raynaud's phenomenon, Esophageal involvement, Sclerodactyly, and Telangiectasia. While 40% to 50% of patients with disseminated disease exhibit the Sclero-70 antibody, 80% of patients with CREST test positive for the anticentromeric antibody. The Raynaud's phenomenon of scleroderma is usually associated with painful fingertip ulcers leading to pitted scars. By contrast, Raynaud's disease, a common condition of young women, does not usually cause permanent changes in the digits. Angiograms of the hand reveal occlusion of individual digital arteries, both proper and common, as well as vasospasm. The ulnar artery and superficial arch are often involved and the deep arch is often spared. Treatment for the Raynaud's phenomenon consists initially of supportive measures such as cold avoidance with mittens, warm gloves, hat, and scarves. Good skin care including moisturizers should be employed. If this fails then calcium channel blockers such as Nifedipine 40 mg per day are reported to be effective in approximately 60% of patients. If this too fails and local care is ineffective in resolving the ulcers, then digital sympathectomy, and even superficial arch reconstruction has been recommended by some authors. Before these vascular procedures are undertaken, however, it is recommended that patients undergo cold stress testing and/or a trial of chemical sympathectomy, such as carpal tunnel injection with dilute Lidocaine or Mepivicaine to elicit temporary improvement. If necrosis does occur then autoamputation or delayed surgical amputation is best to preserve the maximal amount of tissue.

Flexion deformities of the proximal phalangeal joints, if severe, i.e. 90° or more, are best treated by arthrodesis with generous bony resection to correct the flexion deformity to 40° to 50°. Kirschner wires and interosseous wiring have been reported as effective, resulting in 94% union rate.

For the calcific deposits (calcinosus circumscripta) (shown in Fig. 19-3) debridement should be done if these lesions become painful or erode through the skin, with or without infection. Surgical drainage, and debulking of the calcific lesions, leaving the wounds open, provides symptomatic relief.

Systemic Lupus Erythematosus

Over 90% of patients with SLE have arthritis, often involving the hand in a rheumatoid-like pattern, sometimes with prominent tenosynovitis, but these patients are unlikely to be referred to the hand surgeon because the inflammation is short-lived and has no residue. In some patients, however, important rheumatoid-like deformities appear, characteristically without pain or erosions on radiograph. These patients have marked laxity of the joints, especially the metacarpophalangeal articulations, which is known as Jaccoud's Arthritis (Fig. 19-4). Cardiac, pulmonary, and renal involvement are common in systemic lupus erythematosus.

Diagnosis can be suspected on clinical grounds, especially if the patient has the classical facial butterfly rash, or the various organ systems manifestations. The antinuclear antibody test is almost always positive and high titers of anti-DNA antibodies are quite specific. In the hand the major manifestations include Raynaud's phenomenon, hypermo-

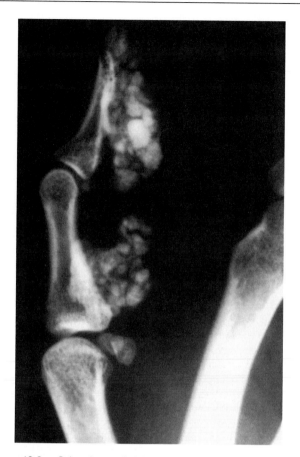

Figure 19-3. Scleroderma. Calcinosis circumscripta in the thumb of this patient.

bile joints with dorsal subluxation of the ulna (i.e. palmar subluxation of the radius), ulnar subluxation of the extensor tendons at the metacarpophalangeal joints with consequent extensor lag and ulnar deviation of the metacarpophalangeal joints, and swan neck deformities of the proximal interphalangeal joints. In the thumb there is instability of the carpometacarpal joint, metacarpophalangeal joint flexion deformity, and interphalangeal joint hyperextension deformity. Initially these malalignments are passively correctable, but with time they become fixed.

Treatment is primarily medical and consists of systemic corticosteroids. Splinting has not been shown to be of long-lasting value but may be tried as a temporizing measure. Surgical experience with this disease has been limited; however, various procedures have been attempted. In the wrist, ulnar head resection can be utilized if there is a painful distal radial ulnar joint subluxation or extensor tendon erosion secondary to the prominent ulnar head. Although intercarpal instability is common, surgery is usually not indicated, as most of these patients are asymptomatic. If they do become symptomatic, then arthrodesis is more likely to be successful than a soft-tissue reconstruction. For the metacarpophalangeal joints, soft-tissue reconstruction may

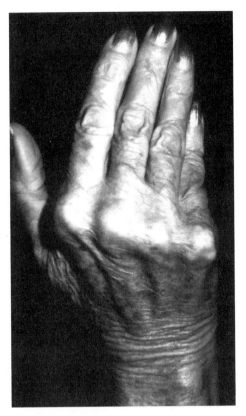

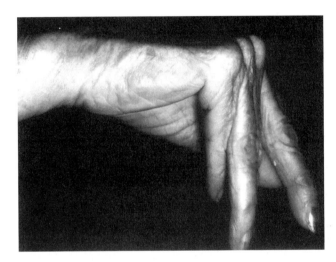

Figure 19-4.   (Left and Right) Systemic lupus erythematosus. Severe involvement of the MCP joints of this patient.

have a role, but must include more than simple extensor relocation, as this has proven to be inadequate by itself. Silicone rubber arthroplasty has been useful if the joints are still passively correctable. It has not been shown to be a reliable procedure in those joints with fixed deformities. Shortening osteotomies of the metacarpals with soft-tissue reconstruction have also been recommended. For the thumb, reconstruction of the carpometacarpal joint is the key to correcting the metacarpophalangeal and interphalangeal joint deformities. Although performed in only a few cases, both ligament reconstruction with a slip of FCR and first metacarpal trapezial arthrodesis have been performed successfully.

Crystal-induced Arthritis

Two types of crystals—sodium urate and calcium pyrophosphate—cause arthritis and most crystal-induced arthritides may involve the upper extremity joints, particularly the hand and wrist. Different from other rheumatic conditions, some forms of crystal-induced arthritis have specific treatment. Furthermore, these conditions have a wide clinical range; while acute cases may closely mimic suppurative arthritis, chronic cases may resemble rheuma-

toid arthritis and other forms of chronic arthritis. The importance of accurate diagnosis can therefore not be overemphasized.

Gout

Gout, an arthropathy that results from tissue deposition of monosodium urate crystals, is the result of sustained hyperuricemia. Only about one in five patients with chronic hyperuricemia ever develop gout. Because it is not possible to predict among hyperuricemic patients the ones who will develop gout, and because raised serum uric acid levels per se lack deleterious effects, treatment of silent hyperuricemia is not warranted. As suggested by the nearly constant finding of synovial microtophi (aggregates of closely packed MSU crystals) when the first attack of gout develops, plus the occasional finding of tophi during arthroscopies performed for unrelated conditions in patients who never experienced gout, tissue deposition of MSU crystals appears to be a prerequisite for the development of acute gout. To understand the effects of MSU crystals on joints, one must differentiate the acute inflammatory reaction that results from crystal phagocytosis by PMNs, leading to cell lysis and the release of lysosomal enzymes from the

eroding effect of tophi. It is believed that the release of collagenase and stromelysin by cells in the periphery of tophi
are responsible for the bone erosions seen in chronic gout.
Thus, the mechanism responsible for the excruciatingly
painful gout attack differs from the one leading to chronic
destructive synovitis, erosive tophi, and visceral deposits.
Hyperuricemia is either a result of increased synthesis or a
raised kidney threshold for uric acid elimination. The latter,
which occurs in 90% of patients with primary gout, may
also be a result of nephropathy, arterial hypertension,
chronic use of diuretics, exposure to toxic substances such
as lead and beryllium, and the use of cyclosporine, an
immunosuppressive agent extensively used in organ transplantation that currently is a leading cause of refractory
gout seen in tertiary hospitals. Alcohol abuse, which has
traditionally and rightfully been associated with a predisposition to gout, increases serum uric acid by increasing
production and decreasing renal excretion.

Clinical Types of Gout

Acute Gout

Although acute gout most often occurs in the first
metatarsal phalangeal joint (podagra) or the knee, involvement of upper extremity joints is common. Frequently
involved joints include wrists, MCPs, PIPs, and DIPs
(Fig. 19-5), particularly in older individuals with
Heberden's nodes, the so-called nodal gout. As in pseudogout, when gout occurs in the wrist in the geriatric group,
diffuse hand edema may be prominent. Isolated tenosynovitis is relatively rare in acute gout. In contrast, gouty olecranon bursitis is common and different from other forms
of acute bursitis, in that it may occur bilaterally, concurrently or in sequence. Although tophi are highly suggestive
of the correct diagnosis, it is not possible to clinically distinguish gout from other types of acute arthritis, tenosynovitis, or bursitis affecting the upper extremity. Thus, joint
aspiration and examination of the sample under polarizing
microscopy is essential for diagnosis. The diagnosis is
proven by the finding of intracellular, strongly negative
birefringent needle-shaped crystals in polymorphonuclear
leucocytes. Since gout and septic arthritis may co-exist, all
aspirates should be cultured.

Chronic Gout

The signs of chronic gouty arthritis may closely resemble
rheumatoid arthritis, including symmetric MCP and PIP
swelling, ulnar deviation of digits, tenosynovitis and the
presence of subcutaneous nodules (tophi). Many such
errors (a wrong diagnosis of RA in patients with gout) have
been seen by the author over the years. This is unfortunate
because the joint destruction of chronic tophaceous gout is
completely preventable. Clues that should alert the clinician include the male sex of the patients, a negative rheumatoid factor test (low-titer positive results are common in
elderly patients without RA), an antecedent episode of
podagra, the hard consistency of the swelling, and more
importantly, a pebbly yellow appearance of the nodules

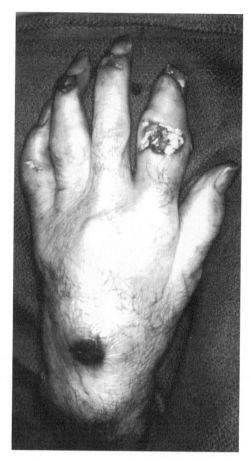

Figure 19-5. Chronic gout. Tophi have eroded the skin in this
advanced case.

when overlying skin is stretched. Diagnosis of these cases
is quite easy once gout is suspected. A large bore needle
aspiration of a tophus is performed. The sample is examined under a polarizing microscope. The MSU crystals are
usually extracellular in these lesions.

Radiographic Findings

Pathognomonic of gout is the association of an erosive
bone lesion adjacent to a relatively radiodense soft-tissue
mass due to calcification of the tophus, which is often partially covered by overhanging margin. This finding is late,
however, and may take years to develop. Indeed, in this day
and age it should not appear. The only radiographic finding
in acute gout is soft-tissue swelling.

Treatment of Acute Gout

Treatment of acute gout is best accomplished with a single
intramuscular injection of ACTH, 40 U. If less than 50%
improvement occurs within 24 hours, the injection may be

repeated once. Alternatively, patients may be treated with indomethacin. Other NSAIDs are also effective, but their action may be slower. Oral colchicine is less favored because of the high frequency of diarrhea (70%) as a side effect. Intravenous colchicine is contraindicated because it has resulted in deaths and safer alternatives are available.

Prevention of Recurrent Gout

Because approximately 20% of gout patients experience only a single attack, prophylactic treatment is not routinely prescribed following the first episode. Infrequent attacks may be treated acutely (provided the case is not tophaceous and that evidences of chronic joint involvement are lacking). When prophylaxis is deemed necessary, it may be accomplished with colchicine 0.6-1.2 mg per day, or with the use of probenecid or allopurinol. Because they cannot mount an acute attack, patients treated prophylactically with colchicine should be watched for the possible occurrence of silent tophaceous joint damage. If the use of a uric acid lowering agent is deemed necessary, allopurinol or

probenecid may be used. The choice of uric acid lowering agents depends on the 24-hour uric acid excretion, kidney function, presence of tophi, etc. The frequency of gout attacks increases in the first months of uric acid lowering agents. Prophylactic colchicine 0.6 mg once or twice a day should therefore be used in the initial six months.

Surgical Treatment

In addition to diagnosing gout, the hand surgeon may be involved in treating patients with acute inflammatory episodes of a joint or other soft tissues such as the finger pulp. Also, gouty tenosynovitis, including tendon rupture, carpal tunnel syndrome, and destructive arthritis may require surgical intervention. Operative management is undertaken when medical treatment has failed. Depending on the clinical problem, surgery consists of debridement of the urate crystal deposit, tenosynovectomy, or rarely, tendon reconstruction after rupture from gouty crystal involvement. On occasion, arthrodesis or arthroplasty to treat destroyed joints, such as the distal interphalangeal or prox-

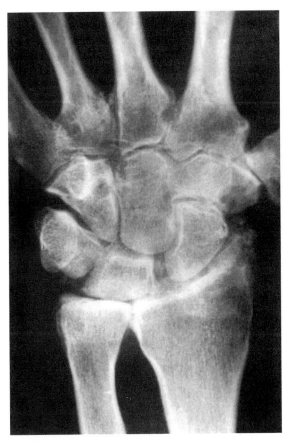 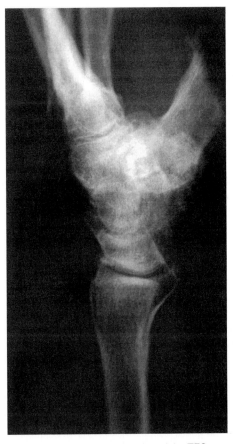

Figure 19-6.   Pseudogout. **(Left)** Note calcification of the scapholunate interosseous ligament and faint calcification of the TFC. **(Right)** Note DISI often seen in pseudogout.

imal interphalangeal joint, or even the wrist, may be indicated and has been performed.

Pseudogout (Calcium Pyrophosphate Deposition Disease, or CPPD)

This condition is of interest to the hand surgeon because pseudogout has a predilection for the wrist and easily resembles septic arthritis. In contrast to patients with gout, there are no detectable biochemical abnormalities in the blood of patients with pseudogout. On the other hand, CPPD may be the presenting syndrome in some patients with underlying hyperparathyroidism, hemochromatosis, and possibly hypothyroidism. Wrist pseudogout is an acute arthritis associated with diffuse dorsal edema. Carpal tunnel syndrome may be the most prominent symptom. Finger joints may be affected bilaterally and symmetrically in the "pseudorheumatoid" form of the disease in which recurrent episodes are the rule. This entity, which is rare, should be suspected in cases of "acute RA" with a negative rheumatoid factor test. Patients with pseudorheumatoid CPPD pseudogout tend to be older and radiographs reveal generalized chondrocalcinosis. Tenosynovitis may occur in pseudogout but it is quite rare and CPPD tophi are exceptional.

Radiographic findings in CPPD pseudogout include stippled or continuous calcification most commonly involving the triangular fibrocartilage of the wrist as well as the hyaline cartilage between carpal bones. In more advanced cases there is narrowing of the radiocarpal joint and degenerative changes in the carpal bones (Fig. 19-6 Left). Scapholunate dissociation is a particularly common finding in pseudogout (Fig. 19-6 Right). Patients with hemochromatosis, on the other hand, exhibit cystic-like erosions in the index and middle metacarpal phalangeal joints involving primarily the volar aspect of the metacarpal heads. Treatment for patients with pseudogout is splinting and ACTH, 40 U intramuscularly. Recurrent cases may be suppressed with the chronic use of colchicine 0.6 mg, once or twice per day. The diagnosis is confirmed by aspiration of the involved joint and observation of negative or weakly positive birefringent crystals under the polarizing microscope. Synovial biopsy is also definitive, but rarely necessary. Of primary concern to the hand surgeon is the possibility of confusing this entity with septic arthritis, especially of the wrist. These patients are best treated with anti-inflammatory medications and splinting and rarely require surgical treatment.

Annotated Bibliography

Askew LJ, Beckett VL, Kai-nan An A, Chao YS: Objective evaluation of hand function in scleroderma patients to assess the effectiveness of physical therapy.
Br J Rheumatoloay, 22:224-232, 1983.

This documented paper shows significant improvement in hand function in 12 patients with scleroderma, after a single treatment of physical therapy.

Belsky MR, Feldon P, Millender LH, Nalebuff EA: Hand involvement in psoriatic arthritis. *J Hand Surg,* 7:2, 203-207, 1982.

The authors describe the results of hand surgery in 25 patients with psoriatic arthritis. The characteristics of these patients were spontaneous fusion of the wrist in a functional position, severe involvement of the proximal interphalangeal joints (often with marked flexion contractures), and severe erosion of the distal interphalangeal joints, with spontaneous fusion. No improvement in motion and a significant rate of infection were also noted after arthroplasty surgery.

Bleifel CJ, Inglis AE: The hand in systemic lupus erythematosis. *J Bone Joint Surg,* 56A: 1207-1215, 1974.

This is a large-scale study of the hand in systemic lupus. This paper emphasizes the fact that hand deformity is due to laxity of the supporting soft tissues, and not an articular destruction, as occurs in rheumatoid arthritis. Swan neck deformities without intrinsic tightness and hyperextension deformities of the thumb and interphalangeal joint were noted to be characteristic. There was also a 50% incidence of Raynaud's phenomenon.

Dray GJ: The hand in systemic lupus erythematosis. *Hand Clin,* 5:145-155, 1989.

Further description of the characteristic deformities of the hand in lupus is provided, as is a description of treatment options.

Dray GJ, Millender LH, Nalebuff EA, Phillips C: The surgical treatment of hand deformities in systemic lupus erythematosis. *J Hand Surg,* 6:339-345, 1981.

The authors describe their experience in 10 patients, pointing out a failure rate of 70% in soft-tissue procedures for 30 metacarpophalangeal joint deformities, a fair result in 16 patients with metacarpophalangeal joint arthroplasties, and a good result in 17 patients who had metacarpophalangeal joint arthroplasties with passively correctable deformities. They also describe their experience with thumb instabilities in four patients, and had a good result with first carpometacarpal joint soft-tissue stabilization.

Gahho SF, Ariyan S, Fraser WH, Cuono CB: Management of Sclerodermal Finger Ulcers. *J Hand Surg,* 9A:320-327, 1984.

This study included 59 patients who had scleroderma about the hand. Ninety-three percent had Raynaud's phenomenon, and 65% developed fingertip ulcers within four years of the diagnosis. They also describe a sclerodactyly distal phalangeal resorption, calcinosis cutis, and flexion contractures of the PIP joints. The authors recommended early sympathectomy to relieve the vasospastic disease, but this did not affect the course of the ulcers. They recommended conservative fingertip amputation for nonhealing ulcers to control the pain.

Granberry WM, Magnum GL: The hand in the child with juvenile rheumatoid arthritis. *J Hand Surg,* pp. 105-113.

These authors performed a clinical examination of 100 children and showed frequent loss of wrist extension and ulnar deviation. They also noted flexion and radial deviation deformities of the metacarpophalangeal joints more frequently than in the adult. Chart and radiographic review of 200 patients showed that all had ulnar shortening up to 9mm, but no correlation with ulnar deviation or metacarpophalangeal joint radial deviation. These authors recommended nonoperative treatment, and stated that surgery was rarely indicated.

Higgins CB, Hayden WG: Palmar arteriography in acronecrosis. *Radiology,* 119:85-90, 1976.

This was a radiographic study of seven patients, all of whom had arteriography. This demonstrated a high incidence of incomplete arches, multiple occlusions, and stenosis (most severe in the proper digital arteries), in those patients with atherosclerosis complicating collagen vascular disease.

Jones NF, Imbriglia JE, Steen VD, Medsger TA: Surgery for scleroderma of the hand. *J Hand Surg,* 12A:391-400, 1987.

A total of 31 patients who had one or more surgical procedures involving the hand were retrospectively reviewed. This was out of a total series of 813 patients examined with scleroderma. The authors recommended nonoperative treatment for Raynaud's phenomenon and digital tip ulcerations, but recommended digital amputation when nonoperative treatment failed. They also described digital sympathectomy and microsurgical revascularization in several patients. They also recommended arthrodesis of the proximal interphalangeal joints in 44° to 55° of flexion, stating that this improved hand function and allowed primary healing of PIP ulcers in 12 patients.

Moore JR, Weiland AJ: Gouty tenosynovitis in the hand. *J Hand Surg,* 10A:291-295, 1985.

Patients are described who had extensive urate deposition in the extensor tendons of the wrist and the digits, in addition to involvement of the flexor tendons and the carpal canal. The authors felt that nonoperative treatment may not lead to the best management in these conditions, and favored operative treatment to debulk the tophaceous deposits to improve tendon gliding, decompress nerves, allow increased range of motion, and ameliorate pain.

Resnick CS, Miller BW, Gelberman RH, Resnick D: Hand and wrist involvement in calcium pyrophosphate dihydrate crystal deposition disease. *J Hand Surg,* 8:856-863, 1983.

This was a retrospective study of the clinical records and radiographs of the hand and wrist in 51 patients with calcium pyrophosphate and hydrate crystal deposition disease. The study describes the classic radiographic findings, including cartilage and synovial calcification, an arthropathy at the metacarpophalangeal joints, and radiocarpal joint of the wrist, including scapholunate dissociation. The study found many patients with radiographic signs who were asymptomatic, and symptomatic patients who had normal radiographs.

Rodeheffer RJ, Rommer JA, Wigley F, Smith CR: Controlled double blind trial of Nifedipine in the treatment of Raynaud's phenomenon. *NEJ Med,* 4:880-882, 1983.

The authors described a prospective study with Nifedipine for treatment of Raynaud's phenomenon and showed a 60% positive response.

Rose JH, Belsky MR: Psoriatic arthritis in the hand. *Hand Clin,* 5:137-144, 1989.

This was an updated report of the experience with psoriatic arthritis in the hand.

Schneller S: Medical considerations and perioperative care for rheumatoid surgery. *Hand Clin,* 5:115-126, 1989.

The nonoperative treatment, including drugs, splinting, and therapy, is described for patients with rheumatoid arthritis of the hand. This includes the preoperative and postoperative care.

Simmons BP, Nutting JT: Juvenile rheumatoid arthritis. *Hand Clin,* 5:157-168, 1989.

The authors reviewed the manifestations and treatment of patients with juvenile rheumatoid arthritis involving the hand, with a description of the operative options.

Waters PM, Simmons BP: Unusual arthritic disorders in the hand, Part I. *Surgical Rounds for Orthopaedics,* pp. 15-20.

This is a survey of all the unusual arthritides of the hand, reasonably describing the diagnosis and treatment of patients with systemic lupus, psoriasis, scleroderma, and gout. The authors discuss surgical options available for treating these conditions.

V
Nerve

20

Peripheral Nerve Biology

Thomas M. Brushart, MD

Functional Anatomy

Epineurium

The external epineurium is a layer of collagenous connective tissue that forms the outer covering of peripheral nerve (Fig. 20-1). The internal epineurium, an extension of this tissue, surrounds individual fascicles within the nerve. Internal epineurium cushions the fascicles from external pressure, and allows movement of one on another; both layers absorb longitudinal stress before it is transmitted to the perineurium. The percentage of nerve cross-sectional area occupied by epineurium varies along each nerve, from nerve to nerve, and from individual to individual. Near joints, where extra padding is needed, as much as 75% of the nerve is epineurium. Epineurial fibroblasts respond vigorously to injury; much of the scar formed after nerve transection results from brisk proliferation of these cells.

Perineurium

Perineurium is the tissue layer surrounding individual fascicles (Fig. 20-1). As many as 10 concentric layers of flattened cells with prominent basement membranes are "dovetailed" together and linked with tight junctions. Longitudinally and obliquely oriented collagen fibers occupy the space between layers. The perineurium is an extension of the blood-brain barrier, controlling the intraneural environment by limiting diffusion, blocking the ingress of infection, and maintaining a slightly positive intrafascicular pressure. The perineurium is also the neural component most resistant to longitudinal traction; as long as it remains intact, the elastic properties of the nerve are retained.

Endoneurium

The endoneurium is the collagenous packing that surrounds individual axons within the perineurium (Fig. 20-1). Endoneurium also participates in the formation of the "Schwann Cell Tube" (or "endoneurial tube"), the cylindrical structure that contains the myelinated axon and its associated Schwann cells. Larger myelinated axons are surrounded by two layers of collagen; the outer is longitudinally oriented and the inner is arranged randomly and associated with carbohydrate-rich reticulin. Small myelinated axons possess only the outer, longitudinal layer.

Vascular Supply

Segmental nutrient vessels supply longitudinally oriented vascular plexi in the epineurium (Fig. 20-1). These in turn feed similar plexi within the perineurial lamallae. Perineurial vessels often enter the endoneurium at an oblique angle, placing them at risk for occlusion if endoneur-

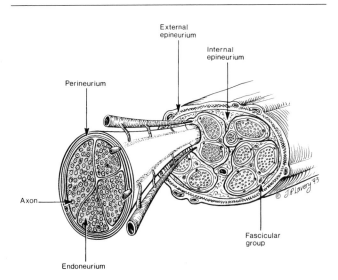

Figure 20-1. The macroscopic and gross microscopic organization of peripheral nerve.

ial pressure is raised. The endoneurial space is devoid of lymphatics. A longitudinal network of capillaries, arterioles, and venules extends throughout the endoneurium of each fascicle; the direction of flow in any portion can be rapidly changed in response to injury. The longitudinal orientation and dynamic flexibility of its vascular supply allows the uninjured peripheral nerve to be mobilized over long distances without risk of ischemia.

Fascicles

A fascicle is a group of axons packed within endoneurial connective tissue and contained by a sleeve of perineurium. It is the smallest unit of nerve structure that can be manipulated surgically. The number of fascicles within a nerve varies throughout its course, the median nerve containing as few as three and as many as 36. Fascicles are interconnected to form an intraneural plexus. Plexus formation is most prominent in nerves to the proximal extremity, such as the musculocutaneous, but is less frequent in the distal median and ulnar nerves. In many areas of peripheral nerves, fascicles are clustered into "fascicular groups" of three to six fascicles bound together by condensations of the inner epineurium (Fig. 20-1). Fascicular groups can be isolated over much greater distances than can individual fascicles, and may still be identified and matched after several centimeters of nerve substance are lost. Although fascicular interconnections may be frequent within a group, they are much less common among separate groups.

The degree to which axons destined for a terminal nerve branch are grouped together in proximal portions of the nerve has been the subject of recent controversy. Studies based on anatomical dissection have not detected functional localization at proximal levels. However, these studies are inherently limited by assumptions that are forced upon the dissector. The dissector functionally identifies a fascicle by its distal termination, then works proximally, separating the fascicle from its neighbors (Fig. 20-2). However, when an intrafascicular plexus is encountered, it must be assumed that all proximal components contribute equally to the single distal fascicle being traced. As fascicular interconnections are repeatedly encountered, a large number of fascicles are traced, most of which do not actually contribute to the fascicle under study. Maps based on dissection thus represent the sum of all potential axon sources; their failure to detect localization cannot be used as evidence that it does not exist. Greater precision has recently been achieved by histochemical tracing of primate axons and by intrafascicular microstimulation studies in awake humans. Primate digital nerve axons were traced with horseradish peroxidase, and were found to occupy only one-third to one-sixth of the median nerve cross section as it entered the brachial plexus. Early microstimulation studies found that 42% of human median nerve fascicles in the upper arm projected only to skin, and of these, 67% projected only to a single digital interspace. At the wrist level, 87% of fascicles projected even more discretely to a single digital nerve. With refinements in technique, somatotopic arrangement of axons has also been demonstrated within individual fascicles. These two bodies of evidence strongly suggest that axons terminating in a peripheral median nerve fascicle travel near one another even at proximal levels; they are not widely separated by interfascicular plexus formation, as suggested by earlier dissection studies. The long-accepted picture of intraneural chaos, which reflects the limitations of dissection technique, is thus replaced by a view of partial localization of distal function at proximal levels.

Longitudinal Excursion

Peripheral nerve is loosely anchored by nutrient vessels and terminal branches, and rarely crosses a joint at the axis of motion; limb movement therefore results in sliding of the nerve along its bed. The resulting longitudinal excursion of upper extremity peripheral nerves has been studied electrophysiologically and anatomically. Study of action potentials showed wrist and digital flexion/extension to produce 7.4 mm of median nerve excursion, with an additional 4.3 mm resulting from elbow flexion. Displacement of the median nerve during wrist and digital flexion was two to four times greater at the wrist than in the upper arm. Anatomical dissection revealed a brachial plexus excursion of 15 mm in the frontal plane during abduction of the arm. The median and ulnar nerves moved an average of 7.3 mm and 9.8 mm respectively through a full range of elbow motion. Full wrist flexion/extension produced the greatest excursion, 15.5 mm of the median nerve and 14.8 mm of the ulnar as measured at the proximal edge of the carpal tunnel. The excursion was much lower in the palm and digits.

Cellular Components

The Neuron

The "wires" in peripheral nerve are the axonal processes of parent neurons, associated with Schwann cells as they course distally (Fig. 20-3). Motor neurons lie in the anterior horn of the spinal cord, sensory neurons within the dorsal root ganglia, and autonomic neurons within paravertebral ganglia. Synthesis of structural components and transmitters occurs within the neuron, the location of ribosomes, endoplasmic reticulum, and the Golgi apparatus. In con-

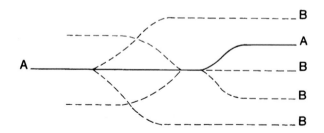

Figure 20-2. The formation of interfascicular plexi within peripheral nerve. Distal is to the left, proximal to the right. The solid line labeled "A" represents the true course of a group of axons through this segment of nerve, which can be determined by histochemical or electrophysiologic tracing. The fascicles labeled "B" on the proximal end will all be identified by the dissector as potential sources of the axons in "A" distally because of interfascicular connections. Dissection produces a map of all potential axon sources. Its failure to reveal localization cannot be used to deny that localization exists.

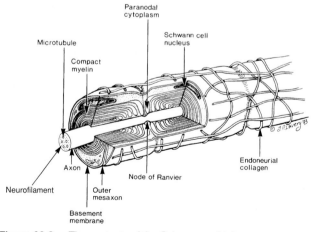

Figure 20-3. The contents of the Schwann cell tube.

trast, the axon contains mostly axoplasm, neurofilaments, and microtubules. Neurofilaments, polymers of cytokeratin protein, are approximately 10 mm in diameter, are longitudinally oriented, and form the major skeletal component of the axon. Microtubules are cylindrical polymers of tubulin, 25 to 30 mm in diameter and up to 0.1 mm long. They are also arranged longitudinally, but are found in only one-third to one-tenth the concentration of neurofilaments. They participate in axoplasmic transport.

Products of synthesis originate within the neuron but must be transported to the periphery within the axon. Three major types of axoplasmic transport have been described. Fast anterograde (away from the neuron) transport moves membrane-enclosed subcellular organelles, such as synaptic vesicles, down the "railroad track" of microtubules at speeds up to 400 mm/day. The motor for this process is kinesin, an ATPase which links the traveling organelles to the underlying microtubules. Slow anterograde transport, in contrast, carries cytoskeletal elements and soluble proteins at 0.2 to 5 mm/day. The volume of neurofilament components being transported in this way helps determine the caliber of the axon. Material is also transported from the periphery back to the neuron. Fast retrograde (to the neuron) transport is linked to microtubules in a fashion similar to that in the anterograde direction. However, it is driven by the ATPase dynein, and travels only about half as fast as the anterograde transport driven by kinesin. Retrograde transport returns scavenged components to the cell body for recycling, and also carries messages from the periphery to the cell body regarding end-organ connections. The best-characterized of these "messages" is nerve growth factor, a protein manufactured by the targets of developing sensory and sympathetic axons. Axons that make end-organ contact take up NGF and transport it back to the cell body, where it promotes neuronal survival. This relationship is termed "neurotrophic," or nutritive, and NGF is termed a "neurotrophic factor." Axons without appropriate connections cannot provide NGF to their neurons, which may subsequently die.

The Schwann Cell

The Schwann cell is the glial cell of the peripheral nervous system. Its phenotype is largely determined by the type of axon it encircles. The nonmyelinating phenotype is expressed when the Schwann cell envelops several small (<1u diameter) axons within invaginations of its cytoplasm. In this state, the Schwann cell expresses NGF receptors and the adhesion molecules L1 and N-CAM. Myelinating Schwann cells, in contrast, are each associated with a single axon. During development, this axon is surrounded by a tongue of Schwann cell membrane, the mesaxon (Fig. 20-3), which progressively elongates as it spirals around the axon in concentric circles. The cytoplasm is squeezed from between these layers, which condense into the lamallae of compact myelin. The larger the axon, the thicker the myelin sheath. Myelin is 70% lipid, largely cholesterol and phospholipid, closely resembling the composition of the cell membrane from which it is made; the remaining 30% is protein. The adhesion molecule MAG, a

member of the immunoglobulin superfamily, is found predominately at the edge of the developing myelin sheath and is thought to participate in the process of myelin formation. Po, also a member of the immunoglobulin superfamily, is the major structural protein of myelin. It bridges the adjacent layers of membrane, and may play a role in myelin compaction by interacting with receptors on the opposing surfaces. Additional protein constituents include the family of myelin basic proteins. The myelinating Schwann cell thus expresses MAG, Po, and MBP.

Electrical Properties

Ion Channels

The electrical activity of peripheral nerve is mediated by ion channels and glycoprotein molecules that bridge the inner and outer surfaces of the cell membrane and provide a pathway for movement of ions in and out of the cell. Channels are specific for a particular ion. Those that remain open at all times are termed "non-gated," and are responsible for the cell membrane's passive electrical properties. Other channels can be opened selectively, or "gated," and participate in rapid ion fluxes during impulse conduction. Gated channels open in response to a change in voltage, the presence of a chemical transmitter, or mechanical deformation.

Resting Potential

The neural membrane functions as a capacitor, separating a positive charge on its external surface from a negative internal charge. The result of this charge separation, the "resting membrane potential," is normally between -60 and -70 millivolts, and is determined by the relative concentration of ions on both sides of the membrane. Na^+ and Cl^- are more concentrated outside the cell, and K^+ and organic ions are more concentrated inside. The organic ions, largely organic acids and proteins, cannot diffuse through the membrane, and are permanently contained within the cell. The resting potential is determined by the relative concentration of nongated channels for K^+, Na^+, and Cl^-. The more numerous the channels, the more rapid the diffusion of a specific ion across the membrane. Nongated K^+ channels far outnumber those for Na^+ and Cl^-, so the resting membrane potential is largely determined by the activity of the K^+ ion. K^+ tends to diffuse down its concentration gradient and out of the cell, leaving the large, nondiffusable organic anions (- charge) inside. However, as the outside of the cell becomes more positively charged, the resulting electrical potential tends to drive K^+ back into the cell, against its diffusion gradient. The membrane potential at which the two factors reach equilibrium was first calculated by Nernst in 1888 and is termed the Nernst potential. If nongated channels permitted only K^+ to pass, this potential would be -75mV. However, the membrane is also permeable to Na^+, which follows its concentration gradient into the cell, and is driven into the cell by the positive external charge established by K^+. The resting potential is thus slightly more positive than the Nernst potential of K^+

alone. Equilibrium is maintained by the Na+/K+ pump, which expends ATP to counteract the K+ and Na+ fluxes.

The Action Potential and its Conduction

The interaction of gated axon channels to produce the action potential was described by Hodgkin and Huxley in 1952. Voltage-gated Na+ channels open, allowing Na+ to move down its concentration gradient into the cell. The resulting decrease in membrane potential produces the rising phase of the action potential. The falling phase is then produced by two simultaneous events; the Na+ channels are closed, halting the influx of Na+, and voltage-gated K+ channels are opened, allowing more K+ to diffuse out of the cell. The membrane potential then returns to its resting value. The action potential generated in one segment of membrane supplies the depolarizing current to the adjacent segment, activating the voltage-gated channels and depolarizing the membrane. However, the depolarization of adjacent membrane, and thus axon conduction, is slowed by the electrical resistance of the axoplasm. The time required for spread of depolarization varies inversely with the product of axon resistance and capacitance over a given length. Two strategies are thus available for speeding axonal conduction. Increasing axon diameter, and thus volume, will increase the supply of available ions (charge carriers) and decrease the resistance to current flow. Use of this strategy is limited by the large number of axons that must be contained within peripheral nerve.

Production of myelin to decrease capacitance is a more efficient solution to the problem. Myelin dramatically increases effective thickness of the membrane, thereby decreasing its capacitance, and making it easier for a small amount of current to discharge the membrane and propagate the action potential passively. However, myelin also interferes with the flux of ions across the cell membrane, blocking the normal mechanism for active propagation of the action potential. If the myelin sheath were continuous, the action potential would eventually die out. This problem is solved by the Node of Ranvier (Fig. 20-3), the small exposed portion of axonal membrane at the juncture between Schwann cells. This area contains a high concentration of voltage-gated Na+ channels, and amplifies the signal by generating a strong inward Na+ current when stimulated by the more passive spread of depolarization from within the myelinated segment. The brief slowing of conduction during this amplification process at the Node of Ranvier results in a relative jumping of the impulse from node to node, or "saltatory" conduction.

Neuromuscular Transmission

As the motor axon potential nears muscle, it is distributed to several terminal axon branches, each ending in a synaptic bouton (Fig. 20-4). The bouton is specialized for transmitter release. Acetylcholine, the neuromuscular transmit-

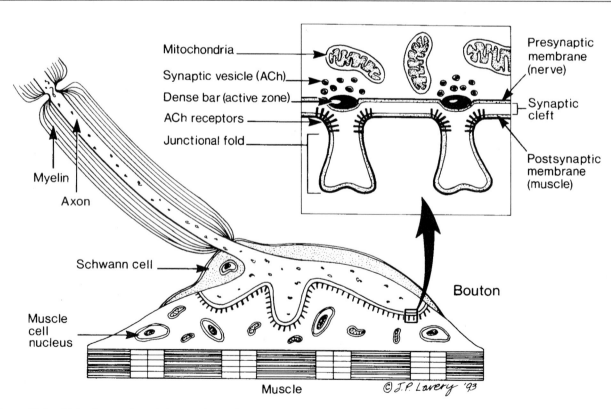

Figure 20-4.   Lightmicroscopic and electronmicroscopic views of the motor end plate.

ter, is contained within synaptic vesicles which have been transported from the neuron by rapid axoplasmic transport. The active zone, the distal portion of the bouton membrane, is designed for transmitter release. The terminal portion of the bouton also contains voltage-gated Ca+ channels. These respond to the action potential by allowing influx of Ca+, which triggers fusion of synaptic vesicles and release of their contents. The ACh released from the bouton diffuses across the synaptic cleft to interact with specific ACh receptors in the muscle basement membrane. These receptors are transmitter-gated ion channels that respond to ACh by opening and allowing passage of Na+ ions across the muscle membrane. Na+ influx depolarizes the membrane, resulting in a small "end-plate potential." Its magnitude is limited by the volume of ACh released. However, Na+ influx also activates voltage-gated Na+ channels adjacent to the end plate. The additional Na+ is sufficient to depolarize the membrane and result in an action potential and muscle contraction.

The Motor Unit

In 1925, Liddell and Sherington introduced the term "motor unit" to describe the smallest unit of neuromuscular function, a single motoneuron and the muscle fibers innervated by it. The number of muscle fibers in the motor unit is described as the "innervation ratio." This varies from 80 to 100 in the intrinsic muscles to 1,000 to 2,000 in the large muscles of the leg. Smaller innervation ratios allow more precise muscular control. Muscle fibers, initially classified as either "slow" (Type I) or "fast" (Type II) on the basis of contractile properties, have been further characterized on both functional and histochemical grounds. Slow fatigable muscle (Type I) contracts slowly and is highly resistant to fatigue. It is histochemically identified as slow oxidative, with high concentrations of mitochondria, oxidative enzymes, and the myoglobin responsible for its dark color. However, it can generate only one-tenth the force of the most powerful fibers. These are represented by the fast fatigable fibers (Type IIB), which contract and relax quickly, but are also quick to fatigue. Histochemically identified as fast glycolytic, high levels of myosin ATPase correlate with their rapid contraction rate. High concentrations of glycogen and glycolytic enzymes, and a paucity of mitochondria, similarly reflect their anaerobic metabolism. These extremes are bridged by fast fatigue resistant (Type IIA, histochemically fast oxidative-glycolytic) and fast fatigue intermediate (Type IIC, fast intermediate), representing relatively slow and intermediate types of fast muscle. It is important to realize that these functional and histochemical grades overlap significantly, and correlate generally, but not precisely, with one another. Each muscle contains a mixture of the various fiber types, which are present in varying proportions depending upon the muscle's function. Slow units are usually deep within the muscle while fast units are superficial. The individual fibers of each motor unit are dispersed within the muscle rather than directly adjacent to one another.

Within an individual motor unit, neuronal properties correlate effectively with muscle fiber characteristics. Fast fatigable fibers are supplied by large, rapidly conducting axons from large motoneurons and slow fatigable fibers are supplied by smaller, slower axons from smaller motoneurons, so that conduction speed and contraction speed are matched. Motor units are recruited in an orderly, reproducible pattern as increasing increments of force are required of a muscle. The smallest motoneurons are discharged first because they have the lowest threshold for activation. Motoneurons serving a given muscle are grouped together in a "motoneuron pool" within the anterior horn of the spinal cord. As the impulse to the motoneuron pool increases in strength, progressively larger motoneurons with larger axons and faster muscle fibers are activated. This "size principle," formulated by Henneman, is a basic concept of neuromuscular integration. A direct consequence is simplified control of muscular force, as progressively stronger input to the motoneuron pool as a whole will result in progressively stronger force generation without the need for specific activation of different fiber types.

Touch

Peripheral Receptors

Glabrous (nonhairy) skin is supplied with three types of mechanoreceptors that transduce components of touch into neural action potentials: the Merkel cell complex, the Meissner corpuscle, and the Pacinian corpuscle. All three transmit these action potentials through A-beta, or small myelinated fibers of 6-12u diameter. The Merkel cell complex is clustered around the sweat duct as it enters the undersurface of the intermediate dermal ridge. It consists of several receptors served by branches of a single axon. In each, the axon terminal synapses directly with an epithelial cell transducer. The receptor is slowly adapting; it continues to fire as long as the stimulus is present. The receptive field, the area of skin through which appropriate stimuli will fire the receptor, is well circumscribed at 2-4 mm. The Merkel cell is thus equipped to respond to small areas of steady skin indentation and is the principal mediator of static two-point discrimination.

The Meissner corpuscle is located at the sides of the intermediate ridge, to which it is attached by thin strands of connective tissue. The encapsulated receptor contains stacks of flattened discs, the lamellar cells, and is served by two to eight terminal axon branches. In contrast to the Merkel cell, the Meissner corpuscle is rapidly adapting; it fires briefly at the beginning of a stimulus, and occasionally at the end, but not throughout. The maximum sensitivity "flutters" at 30cps and it too has a small receptive field. The Meissner corpuscle is thus suited to the analysis of motion and participates in moving two-point discrimination.

The Pacinian corpuscle lies within subcutaneous tissue. It is visible to the naked eye during surgery, resembling a small grain of rice. A single axon is surrounded by 40 to 60 concentric lamallae, giving it the appearance of an elliptical onion on cross section. The Pacinian corpuscle is rapidly adapting, responding maximally to vibration at 250cps. However, it cannot precisely localize these stimuli because of its large receptive field, often several centimeters in diameter.

Central Transmission and Processing

The action potential from a digital cutaneous mechanoreceptor passes through the dorsal root ganglion, the location of its cell body, up the ipsilateral dorsal column of the spinal cord, and through a series of intermediate nuclei (relays) on its way to the contralateral cerebral cortex. The first synapse occurs in the nucleus cuneatus of the brainstem, the second in the VPL nucleus of the thalamus, and the third in the cortex itself. Along this pathway, the location of the original stimulus is conveyed by the area of fiber termination on a precise somatotopic map within each nucleus. The intensity of the stimulus is coded by the frequency of neuron firing and by the number of neurons discharged. However, the impulse does not pass unchanged from one level to the next. Within each nucleus, it activates both inhibitory and excitatory interneurons. One such consequence of interneuronal activity is crucial to two-point discrimination. Two distant points each discharge a separate population of cutaneous receptors. As the resulting signals are processed within the nucleus, each point is topographically represented by a central excitatory zone and a concentric inhibitory surround. As the points are brought closer together, the inhibitory surrounds overlap, further accentuating and separating the central excitatory zones. Were all signals given equal weight, the points would rapidly blend together as the edges of their excitatory zones overlapped. Two-point discrimination is thus a property of the relay nuclei, which is encoded before signals reach the cortex.

The body surface is mapped separately onto each of four cortical areas within the postcentral gyrus of the parietal lobe. Most input from the thalamus is received by areas 3a and 3b, and is then passed on to areas 1 and 2 after further processing. Area 3a responds primarily to muscle stretch, area 3b (Fig. 20-5) to cutaneous receptors, area 1 responds to RA cutaneous receptors, and area 2 to deep pressure receptors. Areas 3a and 3b respond largely to simple, punctate stimuli. However, areas 1 and 2 contain specialized neurons which are able to integrate this unitary information. These neurons may be motion-sensitive and able to integrate information about a moving stimulus regardless of its direction; direction-sensitive and more responsive to stimuli moving in a certain, specific direction; and orientation-specific and sensitive to stimuli arrayed along a specific axis. The information processed by these complex neurons combines to provide stereognosis, the appreciation of three-dimensional contours, as well as awareness of the direction of stimulus movement. Not only is the cortex topographically mapped along its surface, it also possesses six distinct cellular layers arrayed vertically, perpendicular to the surface. Vertical columns of cells encompassing all six layers respond to the same stimulus from the same body area, and form the basic unit of cortical organization. Each layer then sends projections on to other brain areas for further integration.

The mapping of body areas onto cortex has traditionally been viewed as a dynamic phenomenon in juvenile primates. The superior results of nerve repair in young children have been attributed to this plasticity, with novel peripheral inputs resulting in cortical reorganization. Inherent in this theory is the assumption that cortical projections are fixed in adults. However, recent electrophysiologic investigations have shown dramatic flexibility in the organization of adult cortex in response to peripheral manipulation (Fig. 20-5). These findings, especially in view of recent evidence that peripheral regeneration specificity is enhanced in juvenile animals, mandate a reappraisal of the mechanisms underlying sensory recovery in children.

Sensory Examination

Constant touch is detected by the Merkel cell receptor, which is slowly adapting. Its threshold, the minimum stimulus required to produce a single action potential, is tested with Semmes-Weinstein monofilaments. Its innervation density, the measure of distance between receptors, is tested by determination of static two-point discrimination. The transducers of moving touch are the Meissner corpuscle (30cps) and the Pacinian corpuscle (250cps), both of which are rapidly adapting. Their threshold is tested with a vibrometer, and their innervation density by determination of moving two-point discrimination. Stereognosis, the complex integration of unitary sensory information within the cortex to provide knowledge of texture, form, and motion, is more difficult to quantify. The best approximation at this time is obtained with the Moberg pick-up test.

Sensory testing is most often applied by the hand surgeon to determine if a nerve is transected, to detect nerve compression, and to monitor the progress of regeneration after nerve repair. Complete denervation by nerve transection results in absent two-point discrimination within the autonomous zone of the nerve, that area served only by the nerve in question without overlap from adjacent nerves. Nerve compression is most readily detected by tests of threshold, Semmes-Weinstein monofilaments for the SA receptors, and the vibrometer for the RA fibers. As individual receptors fail to conduct impulses centrally, the threshold in the area they serve will increase. However, two-point discrimination will remain intact, in spite of the drop-out of many individual receptors, as long as the somatotopy of receptor representation is preserved within the CNS. The converse applies during regeneration after peripheral nerve transection. Soon after fibers return to the periphery, threshold activity will be detectible, albeit at elevated levels. Two-point discrimination returns late, if at all, because the somatotopy of receptor projections has been completely rearranged (Fig. 20-6).

Degeneration and Regeneration

Wallerian Degeneration

When the axon is severed, the distal stump undergoes Wallerian degeneration (Fig. 20-6). This process clears degraded myelin and axoplasm from the Schwann cell tube, and provides an environment that is attractive to regenerating axons. The sequence begins with breakdown of axoplasm

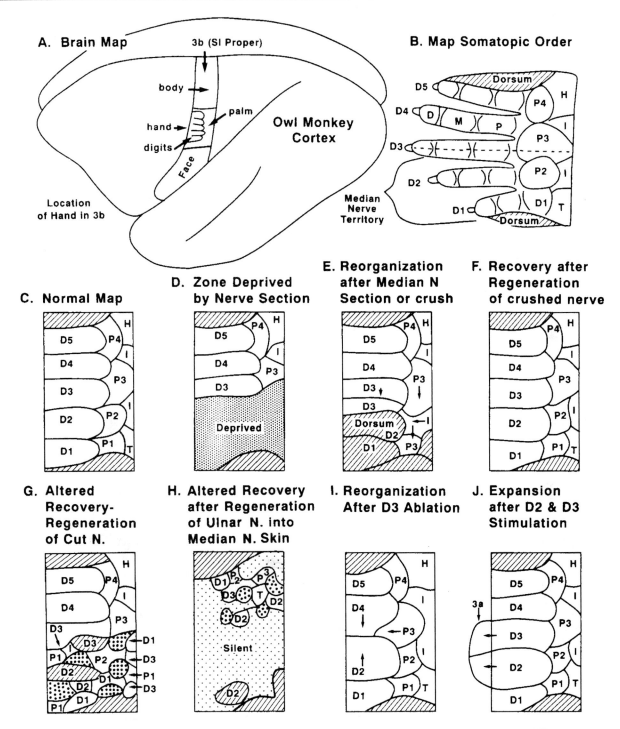

Figure 20-5. The reorganization of primary somatosensory cortex (area 3b) of monkeys after experimental manipulation. **(A)** The location of area 3b in the owl monkey brain. **(B)** The topographic order of the digits and pads is largely preserved in the cortex. **(C)** The actual cortical map of digits (D1-D5) and pads (P1-P4). **(D)** Section of the median nerve deprives most of the radial half of the hand representation of normal activation. **(E)** After long-term denervation the map is reorganized by expansion of remaining territories. **(F)** After crush and regeneration, a normal map is restored. **(G)** After median nerve repair, parts of the deprived territory remain responsive to other inputs, and parts become responsive to median inputs in a somatotopically disorganized pattern. **(H)** After reinnervation of the distal median nerve with ulnar nerve axons, some regions of cortex lack input and remain unresponsive. The cortical area of the ulnar nerve is partially activated in a somatotopically disorganized manner by ulnar axons which have reinnervated median skin. **(I)** After removal of digit 3, cortex formerly devoted to that digit becomes activated by the glabrous skin of D2, D4, and adjoining palm. **(J)** Tactile stimulation of D2 and D3 results in expansion of their cortical territories. Figure 20-5 reproduced with permission from Kaas JH: Plasticity of sensory and motor maps in adult mammals. *Annu Rev Neurosci,* 14:137-167, 1991.

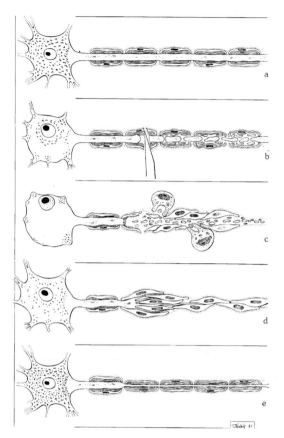

Figure 20-6. Degeneration and regeneration of a myelinated nerve fiber: **(a)** normal appearance. **(b)** axon transection is followed by disintegration of the cytoplasm. The cell body swells and the nucleus becomes eccentric. **(c)** Macrophages enter the distal segment, and phagocytose myelin along with the dividing Schwann cells. **(d)** Schwann cells have proliferated to form the band of Bunger, now the principal contents of the Schwann cell tube. The proximal axon sends out multiple sprouts, the "regenerating unit," which course distally between basement membrane and Schwann cells within the Schwann cell tube. **(e)** At the completion of regeneration a single nerve fiber remains. It is smaller in diameter, less well myelinated, and conducts less rapidly than the axon it replaces. Figure 20-6 reproduced with permission from Lundborg G: *Nerve Injury and Repair,* p. 151, Churchill Livingstone, New York, 1988.

and cytoskeleton into granular material, an event triggered by injury-induced calcium influx. This "granular disintegration" occurs within 24 to 48 hours in rodents, the source of most experimental evidence. However, the events of granular disintegration in humans can be inferred from electrophysiologic studies. Motor amplitudes decrease by 50% three to five days after injury, and are absent by nine days. Sensory amplitudes are reduced by 50% at seven days, and are absent by 11 days.

A major advance in the understanding of Wallerian degeneration has been the identification of the macrophage as the primary phagocyte of myelin. Some macrophages are recruited from the small resident population, but most originate in the circulation. They are present in the endo-

neurium in significant numbers two to three days after injury, when they express 1a, the major histocompatability marker, and complement receptor 3. They lose these markers as they pass through the basement membrane of the Schwann cell tube, but continue to express interleukin 1, a potent stimulus to Schwann cell NGF production. Macrophages and Schwann cells then break down myelin, first into ovoids, then into disorganized whorls, after which it is removed from the Schwann cell tube. Individual Schwann cells become metabolically active and proliferate, forming a continuous chain of cells, the band of Bunger, which remains within the confines of the original Schwann cell tube. These Schwann cells produce the neurotrophic (nourishing) factor NGF and its receptor, needed to display NGF on the cell surface where it may be contacted by regenerating axons. They also express L1 and NCAM, as they did in the nonmyelinating state. These adhesion molecules provide a favorable surface for axon elongation. Conversely, MAG, Po, and MBP, components of mature myelin, are downregulated. Additional cellular changes include leaking of endoneurial capillaries, resulting in endoneurial edema and breakdown of the blood-nerve barrier, and proliferation of endoneurial fibroblasts.

A potent tool for the analysis of Wallerian degeneration has recently become available. In the Ola mutant of the C57Bl6 mouse, the distal stump of transected peripheral nerve survives intact for several weeks. This observation indicates that Wallerian degeneration is not an immediate consequence of axotomy. The defect in the Ola results from delayed axonal recruitment of macrophages. Understanding its mechanism may lead to clinical strategies for the modification of Wallerian degeneration.

The Cell Body Reaction

The neuron responds to axotomy by returning to its developmental program. Production of growth-associated proteins is increased 100-fold. These axonally transported phosphoproteins, found on the inner surface of the developing and regenerating neuronal membrane, are substrates for protein kinase C, and are thought to participate in growth cone extension. Production of actin, another protein crucial to growth cone function, and tubulin, a component of microtubules, also increased after axotomy. Neurofilament protein, the skeletal subunit normally made in development only after axons have contacted their targets, is downregulated. The volume of available neurofilaments can regulate axon caliber; regenerating axons are thus smaller than the axons they replace. The stimulus for the neuronal response to axotomy is probably the interruption of trophic support from the periphery. In NGF-dependent neurons, the neuron reaction to axotomy is blocked by NGF administration and mimicked by administration of antibodies to NGF.

The Axon

Transected axons form regenerative sprouts within hours of injury. The initial sprouts are often resorbed; more durable ones, with internal cytoskeletons, are present after the first 24 hours. Sprouts are generated at the most distal Node of Ranvier which remains intact. This will be directly adjacent to a sharp transection, but may be far proximal after more diffuse trauma with crush or blast components. Multiple collateral sprouts from each axon advance distally as the "regenerating unit." As a result, myelinated axon counts in the distal stump are elevated by a factor of 1.5 to five for several months after nerve transection and repair. In a recent sequential study of rat sciatic nerve regeneration, the number of myelinated distal stump axons was almost twice normal at three months, then gradually diminished until normal numbers were reached at 24 months. The collateral sprouts from a single regenerating unit may enter separate, and often unrelated, Schwann cell tubes in the distal nerve stump. Once entered, these pathways usually confine axons and guide them to the end organ served by the original axon. Collaterals of a single motoneuron may reinnervate separate muscles, and collaterals of a single sensory axon may supply separate receptive fields. Ultimately, collateral survival is determined by successful reestablishment of end-organ contact. Even in the final survivors, axon caliber, and thus conduction velocity, will not return to normal. The myelin sheath will also be thinner, reflecting Schwann cell response to the shorter internodal distance in regenerated axons.

The rate of axon elongation within the environment of the distal stump is species dependent. Rodent axons may reach speeds of 2 to 3.5 mm/day, while the maximum human rate is 1 to 2 mm/day. This rate slows progressively as the periphery is neared. The rate of axon outgrowth may be increased by a prior "conditioning" lesion. By seven days after an initial injury, slow transport of structural protein in the rat sciatic nerve is increased from 3.6 ± 0.5 mm/day to 5.1 ± 0.5 mm/day, and this correlates directly with an increased outgrowth rate. Changes in fast transport do not appear to be involved. Conditioning was initially described in response to axon transection, but has subsequently been found to result from a variety of insults including crush, chronic nerve compression, freeze, or inflammation in the area of the parent neuron. So far, conditioning has not been found to influence the final outcome of axon regeneration.

Injury and regeneration also affect the proximal axon, adjacent to the neuron. Neurofilament protein synthesis controls axonal caliber and is downregulated during regeneration. As neuronal supplies of neurofilament are depleted, the proximal axon shrinks, and this atrophy spreads distally from the neuron at the speed of slow axoplasmic transport. It is later reversed when contact with the periphery is reestablished.

Growth Cone and Pathway

The growth cone, the tip of the regenerating axon, is the locomotive of regeneration. It is designed to sample the surrounding terrain, integrate its findings, and pull the axon into the most suitable environment. Fingerlike extensions, the filopodia, actively extend and sample; they are followed by lamellipodia, larger expansions of the membrane. These processes extend on a framework of actin filaments, backed by microtubules which enter the base of the growth cone. The growth cone membrane is rich in GAP-43, imported by fast axoplasmic transport. It is active in the

endocytosis of molecules from the environment such as NGF, which is transported back to the cell body to perform its neurotrophic function.

The Schwann cell is crucial to peripheral growth cone elongation. Acellular environments, such as tubular "nerve guides" or muscle basement membrane grafts, must be populated with Schwann cells before axons can pass. If Schwann cell migration is blocked by cytotoxins, regeneration will not occur. Several Schwann cell products contribute to growth cone elongation. Schwann cell basement membrane contains neurite-promoting factors, such as laminin, for which there are specific receptors on the growth cone; antibodies to laminin inhibit growth of neurites on peripheral nerve sections in culture. The adhesion molecules L1, N-cadherin, NCAM (and others) are also present on the Schwann cell membrane. They appear to act in concert; antibodies to an individual adhesion molecule will reduce axon growth on Schwann cells, but antibodies to several must be administered together before growth is blocked altogether. The Schwann cell also produces NGF. Little NGF or NGF receptors are present in a normal nerve. After injury, levels of NGF, NGF receptors, and their mRNA's are increased in the distal stump in association with Schwann cells. This production is probably stimulated by interleukin from macrophages. Growth cones are also known to ascend gradients of NGF in culture, turning towards the NGF source as it is moved. However, in recent experiments sensory nerves of adult rats were found to regenerate and restore sensory function independently of NGF; our understanding of even the most thoroughly characterized neurotrophic factor is thus incomplete. Other growth factors may also participate in PNS regeneration. Brain-derived neurotrophic factor, insulin-like growth factor, ciliary neuronotrophic factor, fibroblast growth factor, and others are currently under investigation, and may play crucial roles.

Regeneration Specificity

The specificity of axon regeneration has profound functional consequences. Axons may regenerate in normal numbers, but little or no useful function will result if they reach inappropriate targets. For instance, motor axons may enter sensory Schwann cell tubes and be directed to skin, while cutaneous axons may enter motor Schwann cell tubes and be directed to muscle. These misdirected axons will usually fail to establish functional connections and may exclude appropriate axons from the pathways they occupy.

The specificity of axon regeneration may be viewed in a hierarchical framework, proceeding from gross through progressively finer discriminations. The most basic form of specificity involves growth of regenerating axons to other nervous tissue (instead of bone or tendon), and is termed "tissue specificity." Known since the time of Ramon y Cajal, it probably reflects the action of neurotropism (not to be confused with neurotrophism), or directed axon growth up a gradient of a diffusable substance produced by the target. The action of neurotropism can only be proven if the axons are seen en route to the target; once target contact is made, specificity may be generated by selective neurotrophic support of these axons at the expense of those that have reinnervated other, inappropriate targets.

Several experiments in the last decade have been interpreted as showing specificity at the level of the nerve trunk. This work, largely performed in the rat sciatic nerve model, involved preferential growth of tibial or peroneal nerve axons back to the appropriate distal stump. However, this would occur only in a "Y" tube, and when only one stump was present as axon source. Recently, it has been shown that the size of the distal fascicle, not its specific identity, is responsible for the number of axons attracted to it. There appears to be no inherent nerve trunk specificity.

Recent work has evaluated the possibility of sensory/ motor specificity. This has demonstrated that motor axons regenerating in mixed nerve preferentially reinnervate distal motor branches and/or muscle, a process termed preferential motor reinnervation. Collaterals of a single motor axon often enter both sensory and motor Schwann cell tubes of the distal stump; specificity is generated by pruning collaterals from sensory pathways while maintaining those in motor pathways, even when the pathway ends blindly in a silicon tube. Motor pathways thus differ from sensory pathways in ways that survive Wallerian degeneration, and can be used by regenerating motor axons as a basis for collateral pruning and specificity generation. The carbohydrate epitope L2/HNK-1 is present in motor pathways, but not in sensory pathways, and selectively enhances motor axon regeneration in tissue culture. The interaction of motor axons with this molecule to produce regeneration specificity *in vivo* is currently under investigation.

Within both sensory and motor systems, there is a potential for topographic and/or end-organ specificity. Topographic specificity describes reinnervation of the correct muscle within the motor system or the correct patch of skin within the sensory system; end-organ specificity involves reinnervation of the correct type of sensory end organ within the sensory system, and the correct fiber type (fast vs.

slow, motor end plate vs. muscle spindle) in the motor system. In the sensory system, topographic specificity can be generated only by surgical axon alignment. The consequences of failure to control topographic specificity are readily apparent when the cortical projections of reinnervated skin are mapped (Fig. 20-5). Early experiments on end-organ reinnervation were interpreted as providing evidence for inherent end-organ specificity. However, they were performed in the sural nerve, where a limited receptor population made appropriate reinnervation likely. In a larger mixed nerve, where more receptor types are available, sensory end-organ reinnervation was found to be random. The topography of motor innervation is not restored in adult mammals after most nerve lesions. However, reinnervation of the diaphragm and serratus anterior, muscles innervated by multiple spinal levels, is topographically specific in the adult rat. This is consistent with recent observations that muscles display surface markers of their spinal level of origin. Motor axons do not selectively reinnervate muscle fiber types in the adult. Instead, the motoneuron converts the muscle fiber type (*vide supra,* the motor unit). This conversion is accomplished to varying degrees, however, so that a reinnervated motor unit will contain an admixture of hybrid myofiber types. In neonatal rats, in contrast, soleus motoneurons selectively reinnervate slow muscle fibers, providing evidence for a developmental cue present on neonatal muscle that is lost (or to which axons become insensitive) in the adult.

Overall, there is only limited evidence for inherent regeneration specificity of sufficient magnitude to influence the outcome of nerve repair. The principal exception is preferential motor reinnervation, which shapes the outcome of routine nerve suture and is sufficiently strong to overcome the effects of stump malalignment or an interstump gap. Mechanical alignment of proximal and distal stumps by the surgeon remains the only determinant of topographic specificity in both motor and sensory systems, and end-organ specificity remains an elusive goal.

Annotated Bibliography

Bixby JL, Harris WA: Molecular mechanisms of axon growth and guidance. *Annu Rev Cell Biol,* 7:117-159, 1991.

This review discusses proteins that promote neurite outgrowth, receptors for growth promoters, second messengers implicated in neurite growth, and molecules that guide axons.

Brushart TM: Central course of digital axons within the median nerve of Macaca mulatta. *J Comp Neurol,* 311:197-209, 1991.

HRP-WGA was used to continuously trace digital nerve axons throughout the median nerves of monkeys. These axons were more tightly grouped than the dissection studies of Sunderland would suggest, occupying one-third to one-sixth of the cross section of the nerve at the entrance to the brachial plexus. Axon-tracing techniques map actual axon location, while dissection can only infer location, and is limited in its accuracy by interfascicular plexus formation.

Brushart TM: Motor axons preferentially reinnervate motor pathways. *J Neurosci,* 13:2730-2738, 1993.

Motor axons regenerating after transection of mixed nerve preferentially reinnervate distal motor branches and/or muscle, a process termed preferential motor reinnervation. Collaterals of a single motor axon often enter both sensory and motor Schwann cell tubes of the distal stump; specificity is generated by pruning collaterals from sensory pathways while maintaining those in motor pathways. This occurs even if the pathways end blindly. Motor pathways thus differ from sensory pathways in ways that can be used by regenerating motor axons as a basis for collateral pruning and specificity generation.

Chaudhry V, Cornblath DR: Wallerian degeneration in human nerves: serial electrophysiological studies. *Muscle & Nerve,* 15:687-693, 1992.

Motor-evoked amplitudes were reduced by 50% at three to five days after injury; the response was absent by day nine. Sensory-evoked amplitudes were reduced by 50% at seven days after injury; the response was absent by day 11. Wallerian degeneration proceeds more slowly in humans than in rodent experimental models.

Dahlin LB, Kanje M: Conditioning effect induced by chronic nerve compression. *Scand J Plast Reconstr Hand Surg,* 26:37-41, 1992.

Silicon tubes were chronically implanted around the sciatic nerves of rats. After a subsequent nerve crush, regeneration as measured by the pinch reflex test was more rapid in nerves that had been compressed than in those that had only been mobilized and crushed. Chronic compression may thus serve as a conditioning lesion.

Diamond J, Foerster A, Holmes M, Coughlin M: Sensory nerves in adult rats regenerate and restore sensory function to the skin independently of endogenous NGF. *J Neurosci,* 12:1467-1476, 1992.

The ability of crushed axons to regrow and to restore functional recovery of three sensory modalities in adult rat skin (A-alpha-mediated touch, A-delta-mediated mechanonociception, and C-fiber-mediated heat nociception) was totally unaffected by anti-NGF treatment. NGF clearly affects axon regeneration in culture, but its presumed role in sensory axon regeneration *in vivo* must be questioned.

Glass JD, Brushart TM, George EB, Griffin JW: Prolonged survival of transected nerve fibers in C57BL6/Ola mice is an intrinsic characteristic of the axon. *J Neurocytol,* 22:311-321, 1993.

The onset of Wallerian degeneration is markedly retarded in the C57BL6/Ola mouse. Nerve segments were exchanged between standard C57BL6 and C57BL6/Ola mice, allowing regeneration of host axons through grafts containing donor Schwann cells. These nerves were then transected and the time course of axonal degeneration was observed. Fast or slow degeneration was found to be a property of the host axon, not the graft Schwann cells.

Griffin JW, Hoffman PN: Degeneration and regeneration in the peripheral nervous system. Chapter 22 in: Dyck PJ, Thomas PK, Griffin JW, Low PA (eds): *Peripheral Neuropathy,* third ed., Saunders, Philadelphia, 361-376, 1992.

A current and thorough review of the cellular and molecular events of Wallerian degeneration and axon regeneration.

Hallin RG: Microneurography in relation to intraneural topography: somatotopic organization of median nerve fascicles in humans. *J Neurol Neurosurg Psych,* 53:736-744, 1990.

Recordings were made from the proximal median nerves of awake humans with a new, concentric needle electrode. Myelinated axons are not randomly distributed within a fascicle, but are arranged somatotopically into "microbundles" which supply limited areas of skin.

Jessen KR, Mirsky R: Schwann cell precursors and their development. *Glia,* 4:185-194, 1991.

An homogeneous pool of embryonic Schwann cells gives rise to two adult phenotypes. Myelin-forming Schwann cells are associated with axons of larger diameter, and express Po, MAG, and myelin basic protein. Nonmyelin-forming Schwann cells are associated with smaller-diameter axons, and express N-CAM, L1, GFAP, and NGF receptor. *In vivo,* the timing of myelination appears to be linked to signals that suppress proliferation and increase Schwann cell cAMP levels.

Kaas JH, Nelson RJ, Sur M, Lin C-S, Merzenich MM: Multiple representations of the body within the primary somatosensory cortex of primates. *Science,* 204:521-523, 1979.

Microelectrode mapping experiments revealed that primary somatic sensory cortex contains four separate body representations rather than just one.

Kaas JH: Plasticity of sensory and motor maps in adult mammals. *Annu Rev Neurosci,* 14:137-167, 1991.

This review discusses recent experimental evidence about the capacity of sensory and motor maps in the brains of adult mammals to change in response to peripheral nerve injury. Cortical plasticity, once thought to be an exclusive attribute of youth, is clearly present in adults.

Kandel ER, Schwartz JH, Jessell TM: *Principles of Neural Science,* third ed, Elsevier, New York, 1991.

Chapters five through 10 provide a current and highly readable discussion of ion channels, membrane potential, conduction of the action potential, and synaptic transmission.

Loughlin SE, Fallon JH: Neurotrophic factors. Academic Press, San Diego, 1993.

A current, comprehensive review of all aspects of neurotrophic factor activity.

Lundborg G: The intrinsic vascularization of human peripheral nerves: structural and functional aspects. *J Hand Surg,* 4:34-41, 1979.

Fascicles are vascularized segmentally by epineurial vessels, and each fascicle presents a well defined vascular organization composed of endoneurial and perineurial microvascular systems in combination.

Mackinnon SE, Dellon AL, O'Brien JP: Changes in nerve fiber numbers distal to a nerve repair in the rat sciatic nerve model. *Muscle & Nerve,* 14:1116-1122, 1991.

Myelinated axon counts in the distal rat sciatic nerve were evaluated between one and 24 months after proximal repair. Axon counts were highest at three months and did not return to normal until 24 months. Even in the rat, notorious for its rapid regeneration, two years must pass before the truly "final" results of nerve repair are obtained.

Martini R, Xin Y, Schmitz B, Schachner M: The L2/HNK-1 carbohydrate epitope is involved in the preferential outgrowth of motor neurons on ventral roots and motor nerves. *Euro J Neurosci,* 4:628-639, 1992.

The L2/HNK-1 carbohydrate molecule selectively labels peripheral motor pathways. In tissue culture, motor neurites preferentially elongate on sections of the femoral motor branch as opposed to sections of sensory branch. This preferential elongation is abolished by addition of antibodies to L2/HNK-1 to the culture system.

Mountcastle VB: Neural mechanisms in somesthesis. Chap 12 in Mountcastle VB, *Medical Physiology.* Mosby, St. Louis, 1980.

Vernon Mountcastle pioneered study of the electrophysiologic basis of sensibility. This chapter summarizes much of his work.

Scheidt P, Friede RL: Myelin phagocytosis in Wallerian degeneration: properties of millipore diffusion chambers and immunohistochemical identification of cell populations. *Acta Neuropath,* 75:77-84, 1987.

Mouse nerve, within millipore filters that did not allow passage of macrophages, were placed in the peritoneal cavity. Schwann cells did not proliferate, and myelin was not phagocytosed. When the pores were large enough to let macrophages in, these macrophages actively consumed myelin. The macrophage, not the Schwann cell, is the primary myelin phagocyte.

Skene HP, Jacobson RD, Snipes GJ, McGuire B, Norden JJ, Freeman JA: A protein induced during nerve growth (GAP-43) is a major component of growth cone membranes. *Science,* 233:783-786, 1986.

Axonal development and regeneration are both accompanied by high levels of the "growth associated protein" GAP-43. This protein has been found to be a major component of growth cone membranes. The growth cone is a specialized structure at the tip of growing axons which is essential for their elongation and guidance.

Totosy JE, Zung HV, Erdebil S, Gordon T: Motor-unit categorization based on contractile and histochemical properties: a glycogen depletion analysis of normal and reinnervated rat tibialis anterior muscle. *J Neurophysiol,* 67:1404-1415, 1992.

There is reasonable, but not complete, correspondence in normal muscle between physiological classification of motor units and histological classification of fiber types. In reinnervated muscle there is less correspondence between the two classifications, consistent with incomplete respecification of muscle fiber properties by the motoneurons that reinnervate them.

Vallee RB, Bloom GS: Mechanisms of fast and slow axonal transport. *Annu Rev Neurosci,* 14:59-92, 1991.

Fast anterograde transport is carried along microtubules by kinesin at up to 400 mm/day. Fast retrograde transport, also linked to microtubules, occurs more slowly, and is driven by dynein. Slow transport proceeds at <5mm/day and only in the anterograde direction; the responsible transport molecule remains the subject of controversy.

Wilgis EFS, Murphy R: The significance of longitudinal excursion in peripheral nerves. *Hand Clin,* 2:761-766, 1986.

Study of fresh cadaver arms documented mean longitudinal excursion of nerves to be brachial plexus 15.3 mm; median nerve proximal to carpal tunnel 14.5 mm; radial sensory nerve at wrist 5.8 mm; common digital nerves 7.0 mm; digital nerves proximal to PIP 3.1 to 3.6 mm. Interference with this mobility by scar tethering can focus longitudinal stress on the injured and often painful area.

Zhao Q, Dahlin LB, Kanje M, Lundborg G, Lu S-B: Axonal projections and functional recovery following fascicular repair of the rat sciatic nerve with Y-tunnelled silicon chambers. *Restor Neurol & Neurosci,* 4:13-19, 1992.

The Y-chamber model has been used previously to provide evidence for the existence of regeneration specificity at the nerve trunk level. This paper demonstrates that the size of the distal inserts, not their nerve of origin, determines the path of regeneration. There does not appear to be specificity at the nerve trunk level.

21

Nerve Compression Syndromes

Robert M. Szabo, MD

Epidemiology

Twenty years ago the typical presentation of an upper extremity compression neuropathy was either posttraumatic or a gradual onset of paresthesias and pain in a late middle-age patient, typically female. Although these two presentations are still common, in the last decade they have been surpassed by another presentation—the younger industrial worker of either sex who develops apparent compressive neuropathic symptoms at work in relation to repetitive motions, one of a group of ambiguous conditions termed "cumulative trauma disorders." Frequently, workers compensation litigation and labor-management hostilities are part of the picture. This group of patients has come to be the hand surgeon's equivalent of those with industrial low back pain; psychological and economic factors are an important part of the picture, and unequivocal, objective demonstration of specific nerve pathology becomes critical before surgical intervention can be considered.

Industry continues to seek a screening tool to identify patients at risk for carpal tunnel syndrome. Pre-employment screening is controversial and can lead to discriminatory practices. A small carpal tunnel area has been found not to be a risk factor. The only clearly documented intrinsic risk factors appear to be female sex, pregnancy, diabetes, and rheumatoid arthritis. The common task-related factors that contribute to occupational-related carpal tunnel syndrome are repetitiveness, force, mechanical stresses, posture, vibration, and temperature. These factors, however, appear to be inconsistent and the mechanisms by which they produce neuropathy are not well known.

The change in epidemiology to a work-related context requires a compensatory change in the physician's approach to managing the condition. The hand surgeon must at the outset subjugate his surgeon persona (the injury is in the arm; treat the arm) to his physician persona (the injury is in the patient; treat the patient). This approach may be best realized by working with a team that includes a physical therapist, occupational therapist, psychologist, kinesiologist, and most importantly, the patient. A successful outcome is more likely if the patient is not allowed to be passive, but rather takes an active role in his or her rehabilitation. Progress toward correction of obesity, alcohol abuse, or tobacco abuse is good evidence of the patient's commitment. As with industrial low back pain, if specific objective evidence of a compression neuropathy is lacking, it may be best to institute a trial of nonoperative management, and to let other members of the team assume the primary role in treatment.

Etiology

The term "compression neuropathy" implies an etiology; the nerve is compressed by some adjacent anatomic structure. Between the cervical spine and the wrist there are a number of specific sites where nerve compression is common, and these give rise to various well known nerve compression syndromes. A careful history and physical examination can distinguish these, and for most, surgical procedures to decompress the nerve have been established. This concept of the etiology of nerve compression syndromes, however, is too simple; other factors enter into the clinical picture. In idiopathic carpal tunnel syndrome, the pathology is related to a fibrous hypertrophy of the flexor tendon synovium probably due to repeated mechanical stresses inducing local necrosis with edema and collagen fragmentation. The principle that chronic tenosynovitis is the underlying cause of idiopathic carpal tunnel syndrome has been challenged. Fuchs and associates biopsied tenosynovium from 177 wrists undergoing carpal tunnel release and found inflammatory cells in only 10%. Instead they found edema and vascular sclerosis to be present consistently (98%).

Systemic Conditions

Diabetes, alcoholism, hypothyroidism, or exposure to industrial solvents may cause a systemic depression in peripheral nerve function that lowers the threshold for manifestation of a compression neuropathy. In many people, aging has a similar systemic effect. The importance of systemic conditions may be noted by the high prevalence of bilateral occurrence or multiple-nerve involvement, even if only one extremity is used in an activity that provokes symptoms. Children with mucopolysaccharidosis or mucolipidosis, a rare group of disorders, frequently have carpal tunnel syndrome and benefit from early carpal tunnel release.

Ischemia/Mechanical

The dramatic reversal of symptoms that sometimes occurs following surgical decompression suggests an ischemic etiology to many compression neuropathies. The earliest manifestation of low-grade peripheral nerve compression is reduced epineurial blood flow, which occurs at 20 mm to 30 mm mercury compression. Axonal transport becomes impaired at 30 mm mercury and with extended pressure at this level endoneurial fluid pressure becomes increased. Neurophysiological changes and symptoms of paresthesias have been induced in human volunteers with 30 mm to 40 mm mercury compression on the median nerve. Experimental compression at levels of 50 mm mercury for two hours causes epineurial edema and axonal transport block. Pressures greater than 60 mm mercury cause complete intraneural ischemia with complete sensory block followed by complete motor block. Morphologic examination after severe compression in animals has shown nodal displacement with invagination of compressed areas towards uncompressed nerve segments. In long-standing cases of nerve compression, recovery following decompression may be very slow, or progression of the condition may halt but without improvement of symptoms. In these cases, the initial vascular etiology is superseded by other mechanical processes, particularly fibrosis of the nerve, which diminish potential for recovery. These findings have led to the opinion that nerve compression lesions occur as a spectrum that can be divided into early, intermediate, and late categories. Early stages of low-grade compression respond most favorably to conservative management such as steroid injection and splinting in the case of carpal tunnel syndrome. Intermediate stages of nerve compression comprise patients who have persistent interference of intraneural microcirculation with symptoms of constant paresthesias and numbness. These patients respond best to decompression of the nerve; in the case of carpal tunnel syndrome, these patients predictably do well with carpal tunnel release. In advanced cases, long-standing endoneurial edema induces fibroblast invasion and endoneurial fibrosis. Patients in this stage of carpal tunnel syndrome, for instance, have permanent sensory loss and thenar atrophy, and carpal tunnel release alone may not eliminate all symptoms. These patients were once thought to benefit from internal neurolysis, but several recent studies have shown that neurolysis does not offer any benefits.

Traction Injuries

Nerves of the upper extremity have considerable mobility throughout their lengths. Compression may tether the nerve, restricting its mobility, and thereby cause traction (stretching) in response to joint motion. Traction alone can cause conduction block. It is likely, though not yet demonstrated, that many upper extremity compression neuropathies include traction on the nerve as an element of pathophysiology.

Double Crush Phenomenon

The nerve cell body synthesizes enzymes, polypeptides, polysaccharides, free amino acids, neurosecretory granules, mitochondria, and tubulin subunits which are necessary for survival and normal function of the axon. These substances travel distally along the axon and breakdown products return in a proximal direction by fast and slow axoplasmic transport mechanisms. Any disruption of the synthesis or blockage of the transport of these materials increases susceptibility of the axons to compression. A compression lesion at one point on a peripheral nerve lowers the threshold for occurrence of a compression neuropathy at another locus, distal or proximal, on the same nerve, possibly by restricting axonal transport kinetics. In such a case, the outcome of surgical decompression may be disappointing,

unless both entrapments are treated. For instance, less compression of the median nerve at the carpal tunnel level, as manifested by distal sensory latency, is found to produce symptoms when a proximal cervical lesion is present. Coexistent cervical root compression is one of the reasons for persistent residual symptoms following carpal tunnel release.

Clinical Presentation Diagnosis

Rarely, an upper extremity nerve compression syndrome develops rapidly in the context of trauma. An acute presentation, which is analogous to a compartment syndrome, should be considered an emergency requiring prompt surgical decompression. For instance, an acute carpal tunnel syndrome may be seen following a distal radius fracture or spontaneous bleeding in a patient on anticoagulation therapy. Such a patient requires immediate carpal tunnel release.

Much more commonly, upper extremity nerve compression is gradual in onset and chronic. In general, these conditions may be divided into two groups: those that are dynamic or exertional, i.e., with symptoms appearing in response to a specific provocative activity and resolving when the activity is stopped; and those that are insidious, with symptoms developing gradually, with no notable relationship to activity, and often worse at night. It is important to distinguish these by obtaining a careful history.

The diagnosis of an upper extremity compression neuropathy consists of two parts: the first is demonstrating the presence of a specific nerve lesion; the second is determining the underlying cause. Although the cause may be purely mechanical, frequently it is potentiated by a coexisting systemic disorder or a more proximal lesion of the same nerve (double crush phenomenon). It is important not to develop "tunnel" vision early in the diagnostic process, but rather to consider the possibility of additional causes. Some of the factors associated with development of carpal tunnel syndrome are listed in Outline 21-1. The author saw a patient whose Pancoast tumor was compressing the brachial plexus mimicking ulnar nerve symptoms, again pointing out the importance of casting a wide diagnostic net.

A number of diagnostic tests are available for characterizing nerve compression syndromes in the upper extremity. Those relevant to diagnosis of carpal tunnel syndrome are listed in Table 21-1. Recently, a carpal tunnel compression test was described, which its advocates claim is more sensitive and specific than the traditional provocative tests of nerve percussion (Tinel) and wrist flexion (Phalen). Direct compression of the median nerve at the carpal tunnel is performed with both thumbs of the examiner. If paresthesias are elicited within 30 seconds, the test is positive. In general, there is a trade-off between tests that have only modest accuracy but which are easily performed (eg, Phalen's test) and tests that have a high accuracy but which are difficult, expensive, or invasive (eg, electrodiagnostic tests). The use of liquid crystal thermography gets occasional attention, but sensitivity is quite low and it is not a useful test in the diagnosis of nerve compression.

Sensibility testing is an important part of the workup of a

Table 21-1. Diagnostic Tests for Carpal Tunnel Syndrome

Name of Test	How Performed	Condition Measured	Positive Result	Interpretation of Positive Result
Phalen's Test	Patient places elbows on table, forearms vertical, wrists flexed	Paresthesias in response to position	Numbness or tingling on radial side digits within 60 seconds	Probable CTS (sensitivity 0.75, specificity 0.47)
Percussion Test (Tinel's)	Examiner lightly taps along median nerve, at the wrist, proximal to distal	Site of nerve lesion	Tingling response in fingers at site of compression	Probable CTS if response is at the wrist (sensitivity 0.60, specificity 0.67)
Carpal Tunnel Compression Test	Direct compression of median nerve by examiner	Paresthesias in response to pressure	Paresthesias within 30 seconds	Probable CTS (sensitivity 0.87, specificity 0.90)
Hand Diagram	Patient marks sites of pain or altered sensation on the outline diagram of the hand	Patient's perception of site of nerve deficit	Signs on palmar side of radial digits without signs in the palm	Probable CTS (sensitivity 0.96, specificity 0.73), negative predictive value of a negative test = 0.91
Hand Volume Stress Test	Measure hand volume by water displacement. Repeat after seven-minute stress test and 10-minute rest	Hand volume	Hand volume increased by 10 mL or more	Probable dynamic carpal tunnel syndrome
Direct Measurement of Carpal Tunnel Pressure	Wick or infusion catheter is placed in carpal tunnel; pressure measured	Hydrostatic pressure: resting and in response to position or stress	Resting pressure 25mm Hg or more (this number is variable and may not be valid in and of itself)	Hydrostatic compression at wrist is cause of probable CTS
Static Two-point Discrimination	Determine minimum separation of two points perceived as distinct when lightly touched to palmar surface of digit	Innervation density of slowly adapting fibers	Failure to discriminate points more than 6mm apart	Advanced nerve dysfunction
Moving Two-point Discrimination	As above, but with points moving	Innervation density of quickly adapting fibers	Failure to disseminate points more than 5mm apart	Advanced nerve dysfunction
Vibrometry	Vibrometer head is placed on palmar side of digit; amplitude at 120 Hz increased to threshold of perception; compare median, ulnar nerves, both hands	Threshold of quickly adapting fibers	Asymmetry with contralateral hand or radial vs. ulnar	Probable CTS (sensitivity 0.87)
Semmes-Weinstein Monofilaments	Monofilaments of increasing diameter touched to palmar side of digit until patient can tell which digit is touched	Threshold of slowly adapting fibers	Value greater than 2.83 in radial digits	Median nerve impairment (sensitivity 0.83)
Distal Sensory Latency and Conduction Velocity	Orthodromic stimulus and recording across wrist	Latency, conduction velocity of sensory fibers	Latency greater than 3.5mm/sec or asymmetry of conduction velocity greater than 0.5mm/sec vs. contralateral hand	Probable CTS
Distal Motor Latency and Conduction Velocity	Orthodromic stimulus and recording across wrist	Latency, conduction velocity of motor fibers of median nerve	Latency greater than 4.5mm/sec or asymmetry of conduction velocity greater than 1.0mm/sec	Probable CTS
EMGs	Needle electrodes placed in muscle	Denervation of thenar muscles	Fibrillation potentials, sharp waves, increased insertional activity	Very advanced motor median nerve compression

Outline 21-1.

Factors in the Pathogenesis of Carpal Tunnel Syndrome

I. Anatomy
  A. Decreased size of carpal tunnel
    1. Bony abnormalities of the carpal bones
    2. Thickened transverse carpal ligament
    3. Acromegaly
  B. Increased contents of canal
    1. Neuroma
    2. Lipoma
    3. Myeloma
    4. Abnormal muscle bellies
    5. Persistent median artery (thrombosed or patent)
    6. Hypertrophic synovium
    7. Distal radius fracture callus
    8. Posttraumatic osteophytes
    9. Hematoma (hemophilia, anticoagulation therapy)
II. Physiology
  A. Neuropathic conditions
    1. Diabetes
    2. Alcoholism
    3. Proximal lesion of median nerve (double crush syndrome)
  B. Inflammatory conditions
    1. Tenosynovitis
    2. Rheumatoid arthritis
    3. Infection
    4. Gout
  C. Alternations of fluid balance
    1. Pregnancy
    2. Eclampsia
    3. Myxedema
    4. Long-term hemodialysis
    5. Horizontal position and muscle relaxation (sleep)
    6. Raynaud's disease
    7. Obesity
  D. Congenital
    1. Mucopolysaccharidosis
    2. Mucolipidosis
III. Position and use of the wrist
  A. Repetitive flexion/extension (manual labor)
  B. Repetitive forceful squeezing and release of a tool, or repetitive forceful torsion of a tool
  C. Finger motion with the wrist extended
    1. Typing
    2. Playing many musical instruments
  D. Vibration exposure
  E. Weightbearing with the wrist extended
    1. Paraplegia
    2. Long-distance bicycling
  F. Immobilization with the wrist flexed, ulnarly deviated
    1. Casting after Colles' fracture
    2. Awkward sleep position

patient with a nerve compression lesion. Much of the misunderstanding over which test is better at detecting an abnormality has been cleared up with our understanding the fundamental nature of what each test is measuring. Four sensory tests are available which test different fiber populations and receptor systems. Touch fibers (Group-A beta) can be divided into slowly and quickly adapting fiber systems. A quickly adapting fiber signals an on-off event and a slowly adapting fiber continues its pulse response throughout the duration of the stimulus. Static two-point discrimination and Semmes-Weinstein monofilament tests evaluate the slowly adapting fibers whereas vibration and moving two-point discrimination tests evaluate the quickly adapting fibers. Each fiber system is associated with a specific sensory receptor. Each clinical test of sensibility is related to a receptor group and is classified as either a threshold test or a test of innervation density. A threshold test measures a single nerve fiber innervating a receptor or group of receptors. An innervation density test measures multiple overlapping peripheral receptive fields and the density of innervation in the region being tested. Static and moving two-point discrimination are innervation density tests which require overlapping of different sensory units and complex cortical integration. These are reliable tests in assessing functional nerve regeneration after nerve repair where brain input is radically altered, but are not sensitive to the gradual decrease in nerve function seen in nerve compression. Cortical organization is intact in compression neuropathy as the integrity of the sensory relay system remains uninterrupted. Two-point discrimination may remain intact even if only a few fibers are conducting normally to their correct cortical end points. Semmes-Weinstein monofilament and vibration tests are threshold tests and are more likely to detect a gradual, progressive change in nerve function as a greater proportion of nerve fibers is lost while others maintain their normal central connections. Clinically, threshold tests are clearly more sensitive in evaluating compressive neuropathies. At present, Semmes-Weinstein monofilament testing is simpler, less expensive, and as reliable and sensitive as vibration testing. However, more accurate computerized vibratory testing devices are under development and may become more popular.

For dynamic (exertional) nerve compression disorders, provocative testing is essential. Often these patients are asymptomatic when at rest, and manifest symptoms only after a period of a specific activity. For this reason, diagnostic tests made in an office setting may produce false negative results. Braun and coworkers have shown that one can provoke symptoms of carpal tunnel syndrome and objectively measure a physiologic change such as the volume of water displaced by the hand. If the history suggests a dynamic condition, have the patient simulate the provocative activity (eg typing, shoveling, playing the violin) in the office until symptoms are felt; then proceed with the diagnostic tests. For instance, sensory testing with Semmes-Weinstein monofilaments can be performed before and after the wrist is maintained in flexion for 60 seconds in order to detect early sensibility changes.

Electrodiagnostic testing remains the diagnostic gold standard, yet it entails a number of pitfalls. It is highly operator dependent, and so should be done with the same equipment and operator each time. Nerve conduction velocities and latencies can be compared to published population norms, to the contralateral nerve, to other nerves in the same extremity, or to previous tests in the same patient. Systemic conditions (including age-dependent alterations in nerve conduction) may confound the comparisons. Studies of a particular nerve repeated on several occasions can document progression or resolution of a neuropathy. Inching techniques are useful to localize a lesion. The value of nerve conduction studies is that often they provide the only objective evidence of the neuropathic condition.

In general, radiographic information is of only modest value in diagnosis of upper extremity compression neuropathies. Plain radiographs in two orthogonal planes should be obtained to rule out posttraumatic deformity, neoplasm, cervical ribs, or other possible bony causes of the nerve condition. A chest radiograph should be obtained whenever a history of smoking, ulnar nerve symptoms, and shoulder pain is given by the patient. MRI and CT seldom have a role in the workup of these conditions, although MRI can be helpful in assessing the extent of a soft-tissue mass in a posterior interosseous nerve syndrome.

Median Nerve

Carpal Tunnel Syndrome

Compression of the median nerve at the wrist is the most common and best known of the compression neuropathies of the upper extremity. The clinical picture—pain and paresthesias on the palmar-radial aspect of the hand, often worse at night, and/or exacerbated by repetitive forceful use of the hand—is readily recognized. A variety of diagnostic tests are described in Table 21-1. Threshold tests such as Semmes-Weinstein monofilament or vibrometry tests, which measure a single nerve fiber innervating a group of receptors, are most sensitive. Nerve conduction studies can provide objective evidence of impaired conduction. Phalen's wrist flexion test, Tinel's nerve compression test, and a hand diagram in which the patient marks on an outline of the dorsal and palmar aspects of the hand the location of pain, numbness, or tingling, are easily performed tests that can support the diagnosis.

It is important not to focus too early on the mechanical problems at the wrist, but to consider the carpal tunnel syndrome in the context of the patient's overall health. Particularly if the condition is bilateral, metabolic abnormalities or other systemic causes should be sought. Be alert to the possibility of coexisting nerve compression more proximal, particularly cervical radiculopathy, thoracic outlet compression syndrome, and pronator syndrome. Patients with poliomyelitis or other paralysis that leads to the use of wheelchairs and other ambulatory aids are predisposed to carpal tunnel syndrome. This group of patients is particularly difficult to treat as surgery is less predictable and recurrent problems are common.

Conservative therapy includes splinting the wrist in neutral position, oral anti-inflammatory drugs to reduce synovitis, diuretics to reduce edema, and management of underlying systemic diseases. Steroid injection will offer transient relief to 80% of patients; however, only 22% will be symptom-free 12 months later. Those likely to benefit the most have had symptoms for less than one year, diffuse and intermittent numbness, normal two-point discrimination, no weakness, thenar atrophy, or denervation potentials on EMG exam, and only one to two millisecond prolongation of distal motor and sensory latencies. Forty percent of this group will remain symptom-free for longer than 12 months.

The great interest in pyridoxine (vitamin B6) for treatment of carpal tunnel syndrome has faded, as it does not appear to modify the natural history of this disease.

Failure of nonoperative treatment is an indication for surgical release of the transverse carpal ligament. The reliability and good visualization of an open procedure indicate that this is still the preferred technique, especially for the surgeon who does not do a large volume of these surgeries. Long-term data is still not available as to the recurrence rate in patients with endoscopic release. Cadaver studies have shown evidence of incomplete release in as many as 50% of specimens, yet, clinically, patients are experiencing symptomatic relief. The safety, efficacy, and increased cost are issues still under scrutiny.

Nevertheless, several new devices are available for endoscopic ligament release. Proponents of this technique cite a smaller scar and possible transient acceleration of rehabilitation as advantages. Pillar pain has not been reduced and palmar tenderness has not been eliminated. Grip strength has been shown by Gellman to return to preoperative level by three months after open release and pinch strength by six weeks. Endoscopic carpal tunnel release has shortened this period minimally. The gain from endoscopic carpal tunnel release in no way parallels the gains witnessed from arthroscopic joint surgery or endoscopic cholecystectomy. These small benefits must be weighed against the significant disadvantage of poor or absent visualization with the attendant risk of iatrogenic injury to the neurovascular structures. Incidentally, Gellman's study on pinch and grip strength after carpal tunnel release is the first data available that is useful in predicting "when" patients ought to be able to return to their previous level of occupation-related activity. Too many studies use "return to work" as a parameter of comparing treatment options without clearly stated goals of when a patient should be able to return to activities.

Routine reconstruction of the transverse carpal ligament has been proposed as insurance against bow-stringing of the flexor tendons when the wrist is flexed. However, bow-stringing of the tendons postoperatively is not usually a problem, and a short period of immobilization allows sufficient intrinsic repair of the transverse carpal ligament to prevent bow-stringing as a late complication when mobilization is initiated. As described, the operation requires considerably more dissection with release of Guyon's canal and mobilization of the ulnar nerve and artery. Until prospective randomized studies confirm any benefits, this procedure should be reserved for situations where repair of the ligament is necessary. Repair of the ligament is indicated when it is necessary to immobilize the wrist in some flexion after releasing the carpal tunnel, such as if a flexor tendon were repaired.

Previously, internal neurolysis was a commonly used adjunctive procedure in surgery of the carpal tunnel syndrome. Several clinical studies have failed to demonstrate any benefit to neurolysis, and it is no longer recommended.

The etiology of pillar pain, pain at the base of the hand after carpal tunnel release, is still unknown. While theories persist, Seradge described a syndrome called "pisotriquetral pain syndrome" which he noted in about 1% of his patients after carpal tunnel release. Release of the transverse carpal ligament alters pisotriquetral joint alignment producing persistent pain. If injection with anesthetic relieves symptoms, then pisiform excision seems to be a valuable therapeutic option.

Sometimes patients with carpal tunnel symptoms have sensory symptoms in the little finger and surgeons have recommended release of Guyon's canal. This is no longer recommended. Recent MRI evidence shows that the dimensions of Guyon's canal enlarge with carpal tunnel release alone. Clinically this finding has been substantiated as patients' ulnar nerve symptoms, if truly coming from Guyon's canal compression, will get better after carpal tunnel release alone.

Pronator Syndrome

The median nerve is vulnerable to compression at several sites around the elbow including between a supracondylar process and a ligament of Struthers; beneath the bicipital aponeurosis; deep to the arch of origin of the pronator teres; and under the origin of the flexor digitorum superficialis. The principal symptoms of numbness in the radial three and one-half digits and thenar weakness may be mistakenly attributed to a carpal tunnel syndrome. Sensory symptoms may also be present over the thenar eminence in the distribution of the palmar cutaneous nerve. Diagnostic features of pronator syndrome include pain in the anterior aspect of the proximal forearm, a positive nerve percussion sign in the forearm, and a negative Phalen's test. In addition, symptoms of pronator syndrome are typically absent at night, unlike carpal tunnel syndrome. Specific provocative maneuvers that reproduce the pain and distal paresthesias are used to localize the site of compression. Resisted elbow flexion with the forearm in supination implicates compression by the bicipital aponeurosis. Resisted forearm pronation with the elbow in full extension suggests compression between the two heads of the pronator. Isolated proximal interphalangeal joint flexion of the middle finger producing paresthesias in the radial three digits suggests entrapment under the fibrous origin of the flexor digitorum superficialis. Palpation of the medial humeral condyle and distal diaphysis may reveal a bony prominence which is a supracondyloid process; before surgery, anteroposterior, lateral, and oblique radiographs of the elbow should be obtained to rule out its presence. Few patients need surgery. Surgical decompression through the four sites mentioned above, however, eliminates the cause of compression in most cases. When surgery is done, full recovery is not always seen in all patients.

Anterior Interosseous Nerve Syndrome

Compression of the anterior interosseous nerve results in a loss of motor function without sensory involvement. The patient is unable to end-pinch between index finger and thumb and often complains of a nonspecific aching pain in the anterior forearm. In this syndrome, the index finger extends at the distal interphalangeal joint with compensatory increased flexion at the proximal interphalangeal joint during pinch. The thumb hyperextends at the interphalangeal joint and displays increased flexion of the metacarpophalangeal joint. Involvement of the pronator quadratus can be evaluated by testing the strength of resisted forced supination with the elbow maximally flexed. This eliminates the effect of the humeral head of the pronator teres, which is responsible for 75% of the rotational strength of this muscle. Bilateral involvement should alert one to think about Parsonage-Turner syndrome (brachial neuritis) or symmetrical polyneuropathy; however, at least one bilateral case has been attributed to anatomical nerve compressive lesions. On surgical exploration in each extremity of his patient with bilateral anterior interosseous nerve palsy, Braun found enlarged communicating veins directly compressing the median nerve in the distal arms. The onset of symptoms is usually spontaneous, and electrophysiological examination is valuable in confirming the diagnosis.

It is important to realize that if a patient presents with a history of acute spontaneous pain in the forearm, followed within a few days or weeks by anterior interosseous nerve palsy, that a Parsonage-Turner syndrome is likely and observation for three months is warranted. Failure of conservative management indicates surgery. Any of a variety of anomalous structures may be the mechanical cause of compression, so exploration of the full length of the nerve is appropriate with release of all encountered constricting structures.

At times the presentation of the syndrome is incomplete, with only one finger involved; in such a case a misdiagnosis of tendon rupture to the affected finger is a risk.

Ulnar Nerve

Pathologic compression of the ulnar nerve occurs most commonly at the elbow (cubital tunnel syndrome) or at the wrist where the ulnar nerve passes through the confines of the canal of Guyon (ulnar tunnel syndrome). With either of these conditions the patient may present with numbness along the little and ulnar half of the ring fingers, often accompanied by weakness of grip, particularly in activities in which torque is applied to a tool, and rarely by wasting of the intrinsic musculature in the hand. The site of the compression may be determined by a careful physical examination; pain at the medial aspect of the elbow, a positive percussion test at the cubital tunnel, or exacerbation of symptoms by full flexion of the elbow suggests cubital tunnel syndrome. Sensory involvement on the ulnar dorsal aspect of the hand also suggests cubital tunnel syndrome, as the dorsal cutaneous branch of the ulnar nerve originates proximal to the canal of Guyon. Weakness of the deep flexors to the ring and little fingers as well as weakness of the flexor carpi ulnaris signals proximal ulnar nerve entrapment.

A worrisome occurrence is the unanticipated onset of ulnar neuropathy following an unrelated surgery, suggesting improper patient positioning as a cause. Alvine and Schurrer have shown that most patients in this category had a preexisting neuropathy.

Cubital Tunnel Syndrome

Cubital tunnel syndrome may be caused by constricting fascial bands, soft-tissue structures (hypertrophied synovium, tumor, ganglion, anconeus epitrochlearis muscle), bony abnormalities (cubitus valgus, bone spurs), or by subluxation of the ulnar nerve over the medial epicondyle with elbow flexion. About half of such patients improve spontaneously.

Options for operative treatment of cubital tunnel syndrome include simple decompression, subcutaneous transposition, intramuscular transposition, submuscular transposition, or medial epicondylectomy; any of these techniques may be expected to provide 80% to 90% good results, with most return of function occurring within six months. Simple decompression, achieved by releasing the arch of origin of the flexor carpi ulnaris, is appropriate if a localized nerve percussion sign suggests isolated entrapment at this site, or in an older patient in whom the nerve is vulnerable to iatrogenic injury during transposition. Anterior transposition is preferred for cases with bony deformity, subluxation or dislocation of the nerve, or severe cases with motor involvement, especially in a younger patient. The sites of compression that should be explored and released from proximal to distal include the Arcade of Struthers, the medial intermuscular septum, the medial epicondyle, the cubital tunnel, and the deep flexor-pronator aponeurosis. Anterior submuscular transposition is the most popular procedure for reoperation of a previous failed attempt at decompression or transposition. Some surgeons routinely perform a medial epicondylectomy for cubital tunnel syndrome; however, medial epicondylectomy's best indication may be chiefly for nonunion of an epicondyle fracture with ulnar nerve symptoms. If a medial epicondylectomy is performed, it is important to extend the dissection proximally and distally to ensure mobility of the nerve.

Dellon reviewed 50 published reports between 1898 and 1988 and concluded that little more than personal bias is available for guidance in selecting treatment. On interpreting published data based on contemporary concepts of the pathophysiology of chronic nerve compression, Dellon concluded that for minimal compression, excellent results can be achieved in 50% of patients nonoperatively, and in nearly 100% by any of the accepted surgical approaches. For moderate compression, the anterior submuscular transposition yields the most excellent results with the fewest recurrences. For severe compression, the anterior intramuscular/transposition yielded the fewest excellent results with the most recurrences; the submuscular transposition gave the best results.

Failure may often be traced to inadequate decompression, inadequate mobilization of the nerve distally and proximally with the creation of new iatrogenic compression, or scarring in the surgical bed causing traction neuropathy. Intraoperatively, mobility of the nerve should be verified for 10 cm to 12 cm proximal to the cubital tunnel to clear the Arcade of Struthers, and 5 cm to 10 cm distally to clear the deep flexor-pronator aponeurosis. Failure due to tethering of the nerve in its new bed may be avoided by instituting early mobilization. Even a very limited arc of elbow motion with the forearm pronated and the wrist flexed is adequate to prevent tethering of the transposed nerve. For a failed decompression of the ulnar nerve at the elbow, reoperation with anterior submuscular transposition of the nerve may be expected to result in improvement, though with residual symptoms, in 75% of cases.

Ulnar Tunnel Syndrome

Entrapment at this level may present with pure motor, sensory, or mixed symptoms depending on the precise location of entrapment. Pain is usually a less significant aspect of the presentation than in carpal tunnel syndrome. Space occupying bony or soft-tissue lesions may be causative; ganglia arising from the triquetrohamate joint are responsible for more than 85% of the nontraumatic causes of ulnar tunnel syndrome. The distal ulnar tunnel is divided into three zones to allow more accurate localization of ulnar nerve compressive lesions. Zone 1 is the area proximal to the bifurcation of the nerve. Beginning at the edge of the palmar carpal ligament, it is about 3 cm in length. Compression in Zone 1 causes combined motor and sensory deficits and is most likely due to ganglions or fractures of the hook of the hamate. Zones 2 and 3 travel alongside each other from the bifurcation of the ulnar nerve to just beyond the fibrous arch of the hypothenar muscles. Zone 2 surrounds the deep motor branch and compression in this region will produce motor deficits without sensory disturbances. Again, ganglions and fractures of the hook of the hamate are the most likely causes. Zone 3 surrounds the superficial branch of the ulnar nerve and compression in this zone produces pure sensory deficits. Synovial inflammation has been reported to cause compression in Zone 3; more frequently, however, compression in Zone 3 is due to a vascular lesion resulting from thrombosis or aneurysm of the ulnar artery. The Allen test and Doppler studies are useful in making this diagnosis. Fractures of the hook of the hamate causing compression of the ulnar nerve in the ulnar tunnel can best be identified by computerized tomographic scans; however, carpal tunnel radiographs and oblique view of the wrist are frequently diagnostic.

Radial Nerve

Radial Nerve Entrapment in the Arm

Although rare, the radial nerve can be compressed proximal to the elbow. Reported cases have been both acute and chronic in onset. Frequently, the condition occurs after strenuous muscular activity. Compression is associated with a fibrous arch from the lateral head of the triceps. Clinical examination will reveal weakness in muscles innervated by the posterior interosseous nerve and in radially innervated muscles proximal to the PIN. Additionally, radial sensory symptoms may be present. Electromyography helps establish the diagnosis. Observation is warranted in acute cases. Typically, recovery occurs in one month. If there are no signs of recovery in three months, surgical decompression is indicated.

Posterior Interosseous Nerve Compression Syndrome

The radial nerve bifurcates proximal to the elbow, and the posterior interosseous nerve is vulnerable to entrapment just distal to this point where it passes between the two heads of the supinator muscle. As the PIN lacks sensory nerve fibers, the symptoms of this syndrome involve weakness and pain, but not sensory disorders. The muscles innervated by the posterior interosseous nerve are the extensor carpi radialis brevis, supinator, extensor carpi ulnaris, extensor digitorum communis, extensor indicis proprius and digiti quinti, abductor pollicus longus, and the extensor pollicus longus and brevis. The onset is typically insidious and the patient may not notice until late weakness of finger and wrist extension, or a tendency toward radial drift of the hand with wrist extension. Active wrist extension in radial deviation is still possible, because the extensor carpi radialis longus is innervated proximally by the radial nerve. In rheumatoids, rupture of the extensor communis tendons may present a picture similar to PIN syndrome. To add to the confusion, chronic proliferative rheumatoid synovitis can distend the elbow capsule and compress the posterior interosseous nerve. The first fibers to be affected are those to the extensors of the little and ring fingers, the same fingers affected first by extensor tendon ruptures. A careful examination will distinguish these; electromyographic studies are usually diagnostic as well. Routine elbow radiographs should be taken to rule out unreduced radial head dislocations that may have happened in childhood as well as fractures of the proximal radius or radial head pathology.

Gradual, painless loss of function may be due to a slow-growing mass (typically a lipoma or ganglion) at the elbow. A preoperative MR image is useful in planning surgery in these cases.

If there is failure to improve after four to 12 weeks of observation from the onset, surgical decompression of the PIN may be undertaken, with an expectation of good to excellent results in 85% of patients. The possible anatomical sites of compression include thickened fascial tissue superficial to the radiocapitellar joint, a leash of vessels from the radial recurrent artery known as the leash of Henry, the fibrous edge of the extensor carpi radialis brevis, the proximal edge of the supinator known as the Arcade of Frohse, and the distal edge of the supinator. All actual or potential sites should be released. Recovery may continue progressing for up to 18 months.

Radial Tunnel Syndrome

Radial tunnel syndrome is often work-related, with repetitive elbow extension or forearm rotation as an inciting factor. A typical presenting complaint is pain on the lateral aspect of the elbow which is deep and aching in character. Passive pronation and wrist flexion and active supination and wrist extension against resistance aggravate symptoms. Night pain may be a significant complaint in some patients. The chief differential diagnosis is lateral epicondylitis. These conditions can coexist, and 5% of patients with lateral epicondylitis also have radial tunnel syndrome. In radial tunnel syndrome, tenderness is more distal, over the radial tunnel rather than over the lateral epicondyle. A "middle finger test" is performed with the elbow and middle finger completely extended with the wrist in neutral position. Firm pressure is applied by the examiner to the dorsum of the proximal phalanx of the middle finger. The test is positive if it produces pain at the edge of the extensor carpi radialis brevis in the proximal forearm. Electrodiagnostic studies are not useful in this syndrome. In the author's opinion localized injection of anesthetic into the site of the radial tunnel, which produces a complete posterior interosseous nerve palsy and relieves the patient's symptoms, confirms the diagnosis. Release all the same structures described above in the PIN syndrome section. Reviewing their 10-year experience at the Mayo Clinic, Ritts and associates had only 51% good results with surgery and noted that worker's compensation cases were often unsatisfactory.

Wartenburg's Syndrome

The sensory branch of the radial nerve may be compressed by a scissors-like action of the tendons of the extensor carpi radialis longus and the brachioradialis as the forearm is pronated. The affected patient complains of pain, numbness, or tingling over the dorsal radial aspect of the hand, exacerbated by wrist movement or making a tight pinch with the thumb and index finger. Elicitation of symptoms within 30 to 60 seconds of forcefully pronating the forearm is a useful provocative test. A positive nerve percussion sign is found over the radial sensory nerve as it exits the deep fascia in the forearm in 96% of patients. Relief of symptoms by injection of anesthetic dorsal to the musculotendinous junction of the brachioradialis confirms the diagnosis. This test, plus careful sensory testing, can distinguish Wartenburg's syndrome from De Quervains' stenosing tendovaginitis. Differential anesthetic blocks are also useful to distinguish entrapment of the sensory branch of the radial nerve from compressive neuropathy of the lateral antebrachial cutaneous nerve. Nonoperative treatment including splinting, anti-inflammatory drugs, and changes in work activities are tried before recommending surgical decompression.

Lateral Antebrachial Cutaneous Nerve Compression

The lateral antebrachial cutaneous nerve is vulnerable to compression at the level of the elbow as it emerges lateral to the bicipital tendon and medial to the brachioradialis muscle. This is a sensory nerve, and motor deficits are not involved. Typical symptoms are pain and dysesthesias of the radial forearm incited by repetitive forceful hand motions with the elbow extended. Nerve block with local anesthetic and sensory conduction velocity studies between the elbow and axilla aid in the diagnosis. Failure of nonoperative treatment may indicate surgical decompression in selected patients by removing a wedge of the lateral edge of the biceps tendon. Note that this is a rare condition, and other articular, tendinous, or nerve compression pathologies must be scrupulously eliminated in arriving at the decision for surgical decompression.

Thoracic Outlet Syndrome

There are two types of thoracic outlet syndrome: vascular and neurogenic. The vascular variety is secondary to large vessel disease, leads to subclavian artery intimal damage or aneurysm, and is easily diagnosed by clinical and imaging studies. The neurogenic variety is infrequent and diagnosis is usually clinical, substantiated by physical findings. Electrophysiologic studies are rarely helpful. Symptoms include headaches; neck pains; and disabling pain, weakness, and paresthesias of the upper extremity. Patients often develop, or have, a strong underlying emotional component to their illness displayed as depression or changes in personality. Psychological testing and psychotherapy have been as controversial as surgery in the treatment of this disorder.

Physical findings manifested by arterial compression include a decrease or absence of the radial pulse or a drop of blood pressure of 20 mm mercury on extension and abduction of the shoulder. Unfortunately, 92% of people obliterate their radial pulse in at least one asymptomatic extremity. Adson's test is performed palpating the radial pulse with the head turned toward the affected side. Obliteration of the pulse means compression from the scalenus anticus muscle.

A costoclavicular maneuver, upward and backward shrugging of the shoulders, may obliterate the radial pulse by compression from the pectoralis minor, clavicle, or scalenus medius muscle in symptomatic individuals. The elevation test is performed while the patient abducts the shoulders and arms to 90°, and opens and closes the hand slowly for three minutes. A positive result occurs if the patient cannot complete this task due to pain.

Physical therapy is prescribed to include active strengthening of the upper extremity and neck, shoulder shrugging to strengthen the trapezius, shoulder and scapula adduction and abduction exercises, instruction on proper body mechanics, and posturing and relaxation techniques. If a true congenital anomaly is causing TOS, then exercises may actually aggravate symptoms. There are advocates of supraclavicular, infraclavicular, and transaxillary approaches for scalenotomy, scalenectomy, resection of fibrous bands, and cervical or first rib resections. Transaxillary first rib resection seems to be the favored procedure with 90% good to excellent results. Complication rates are significant, however, including irreversible injury to the brachial plexus, causalgia, intercostal brachial nerve pain, painful snapping scapula, and recurrent symptoms.

Annotated Bibliography

Epidemiology/Etiology

Dahlin LB, B Rydevik: Pathophysiology of nerve compression. *Operative Nerve Repair and Reconstruction*, p. 847-866, JB Lippincott, Philadelphia, 1991.

This is a comprehensive review of the basic pathophysiology of acute and chronic nerve compression lesions by two major contemporary contributors in this field.

Louis DS: Evaluation and treatment of median neuropathy associated with cumulative trauma. *Operative Nerve Repair and Reconstruction*, p. 957-961, JB Lippincott, Philadelphia, 1991.

Louis presents a summary of the psychosocial factors involved in treating the workers' compensation carpal tunnel syndrome.

Osterman AL: Double crush phenomenon; the double crush syndrome. *Orthop Clin North Am*, 19(1):147-155, 1991.

These studies show that, given a more proximal root compression, less involvement of the median nerve across the carpal tunnel is required to produce symptoms. Surgical outcome of carpal tunnel release in the double crush group is worse than in the group with isolated carpal tunnel involvement.

Carpal Tunnel Syndrome

Braun RM, K Davidson et al: Provocative testing in the diagnosis of dynamic carpal tunnel syndrome. *J Hand Surg* 14A:195-197, 1989.

This study measured the effects of provocative testing on a series of 40 patients with latent symptoms of carpal tunnel syndrome. Change in hand volume and loss of sensibility after stress were demonstrated and patients were considered to have dynamic carpal tunnel syndrome.

Durkan JA: A new diagnostic test for carpal tunnel syndrome. *J Bone Joint Surg*, 73A:535-538, 1991.

The results of the Tinel percussion test, the Phalen wrist-flexion test, and the new carpal compression test were evaluated in 31 patients (46 hands) in whom the presence of carpal tunnel syndrome had been proved electrodiagnostically, as well as in a control group of 50 subjects. For the diagnosis of carpal tunnel syndrome, the carpal compression test was found to be more sensitive and specific than the Tinel and Phalen tests.

Gellman H, Kan D, et al: Analysis of pinch and grip strength after carpal tunnel release. *J Hand Surg*, 14A:863-864, 1989.

This study evaluated the time required for grip and pinch strength to return to preoperative levels after carpal tunnel release. Grip strength returned to the preoperative level by three months; pinch strength returned sooner, being 96% by six weeks. Their data is useful in predicting when patients may be able to return to their previous work.

Jakab E, Ganos D, et al: Transverse carpal ligament reconstruction in surgery for carpal tunnel syndrome: a new technique. *J Hand Surg* 16A:202-206, 1991.

The authors present a two-year follow-up on 104 hands using a technique to reconstruct the transverse carpal ligament in surgery for carpal tunnel syndrome. Ninety-seven percent of patients returned to work with an average disability of two months. The authors claim that transverse carpal ligament reconstruction stabilizes the transverse carpal arch, provides protection to the median nerve, prevents bowstringing of the flexor tendons, and maximizes postoperative grip strength.

Lowry WEJ, AB Follender: Interfascicular neurolysis in the severe carpal tunnel syndrome: a prospective, randomized, double-blind, controlled study. *Clin Orthop,* 227(February):251-254, 1988.

This is the study to read for those still advocating internal neurolysis in carpal tunnel syndrome. Fifty patients with severe carpal tunnel syndrome (thenar atrophy and/or fixed sensory deficit) were prospectively and consecutively selected and randomized into two groups prior to surgery. Half were treated by standard ligament release alone; the other half also had adjunctive interfascicular neurolysis. All patients had neurologic examination and nerve conduction studies performed by a "blind" examiner at one and three months postoperatively with comparison of these findings with preoperative data. There was no significant difference between the two groups and, therefore, no benefit derived from adjunctive interfascicular neurolysis.

Schuind F, Ventura M, et al: Idiopathic carpal tunnel syndrome: histologic study of flexor tendon synovium. *J Hand Surg,* 15A:497-503, 1990.

Flexor tenosynovium of 21 patients with idiopathic carpal tunnel syndrome histologically were similar and typical of a connective tissue undergoing degeneration under repeated mechanical stresses.

Szabo RM: Carpal tunnel syndrome. *Nerve Compression Syndromes—Diagnosis and Treatment,* p. 101-120, Slack Inc., New Jersey, 1989.

This chapter is a review of the history, physical exam, and treatment options for carpal tunnel syndrome with an in-depth discussion of sensibility testing and the role of electrodiagnosis.

Pronator Syndrome

Fuss FK, Wurzl GH: Median nerve entrapment. Pronator teres syndrome. Surgical anatomy and correlation with symptom patterns. *Surg Radiol Anat,* 12(4): 267-271, 1990.

The surgical anatomy of interest in the pronator teres syndrome is nicely detailed. The patterns of the median nerve, the number of its muscular branches and their branching levels are described as are the location of the fibrous bands that may cause median nerve entrapment.

Johnson RK, Spinner M: Median nerve compression in the forearm: the pronator tunnel syndrome. *Nerve Compression Syndromes—Diagnosis and Treatment,* p. 137-151, Slack Inc., New Jersey, 1989.

The authors present their results of 103 cases of operative decompression of the median nerve for pronator syndrome. Their clinical observations clarify the picture of this clinical syndrome and help differentiate it from other compression neuropathies.

Anterior Interosseous Nerve Syndrome

Chidgey LK, Szabo RM: Anterior interosseous nerve compression syndrome. *Nerve Compression Syndromes— Diagnosis and Treatment,* p. 153-162, Slack Inc., New Jersey, 1989.

The authors describe the anatomy, presentation, etiology, and treatment of this syndrome and clearly present the differential diagnoses that should be considered when evaluating patients.

Miller-Breslow A, Terrono A, et al: Nonoperative treatment of anterior interosseous nerve paralysis. *J Hand Surg,* 15A:493-496, 1990.

The authors present 10 cases of spontaneous partial anterior interosseous nerve paralysis that achieved complete recovery, and draw the conclusion that all anterior interosseous nerve paralysis is a form of neuritis and can safely be treated without operation. All of their patients were seen initially with a history of pain and seven had signs of other nerve involvement either by physical examination or electromyogram analysis. This paper alerts us to a differential diagnostic dilemma: whether to observe patients with anterior interosseous nerve syndrome or to explore and decompress the proximal median nerve.

Cubital Tunnel Syndrome

Dellon AL: Review of treatment results for ulnar nerve entrapment at the elbow. *J Hand Surg,* 14A:688-700, 1989.

This review of 50 published reports between 1898 and 1988, comprising more than 2,000 patients treated for ulnar nerve compression at the elbow, demonstrated that little more than personal bias is available for guidance in selecting treatment. This analysis suggested that for a minimal degree of compression, excellent results can be achieved in 50% of the patients by nonoperative techniques and in almost 100% of patients by any of five surgical techniques. For a moderate degree of compression, the anterior submuscular technique gave the best results with the fewest recurrences. For a severe degree of compression, the anterior intramuscular transposition gave the fewest excellent and the most recurrent results.

Rogers MR, Bergfield TG, et al: The failed ulnar nerve transposition: etiology and treatment. *Clin Orthop,* 269:193-200, 1991.

The authors evaluated 14 patients who had previously undergone surgical treatment for cubital tunnel syndrome and had persistent pain, paresthesia, numbness, and motor weakness. These patients were then treated by neurolysis and submuscular transposition of the ulnar nerve. Revision surgery was successful for relief of pain and paresthesias; however, recovery of motor function and return of sensibility were variable and unpredictable. The causes of continued pain after initial surgery are discussed.

Ulnar Tunnel Syndrome

Gelberman RH: Ulnar tunnel syndrome. *Operative Nerve Repair and Reconstruction,* p. 1131-1143, JB Lippincott, Philadelphia, 1991.

This is a comprehensive description of the etiology and treatment of ulnar nerve compression at the wrist as related to the three distinct anatomical zones.

Radial Nerve Entrapment in the Arm

Nakamichi K, Tachibana S: Radial nerve entrapment by the lateral head of the triceps. *J Hand Surg,* 16A:748-750, 1991.

The authors present a case of compression of the radial nerve by a musculotendinous arch of the lateral head of the triceps, with a good reference list for further study of this unusual compression syndrome.

Posterior Interosseous Nerve Compression Syndrome

Fuss FK, Wurzl GH: Radial nerve entrapment at the elbow: surgical anatomy. *J Hand Surg,* 16(4):742-747, 1991.

The surgical anatomy of interest in the posterior interosseous nerve syndrome is presented, pinpointing the location of the fibrous bands that may cause radial nerve entrapment.

Peimer CA, Wheeler DR: Radial tunnel syndrome/posterior interosseous nerve compression. *Nerve Compression Syndromes—Diagnosis and Treatment,* p. 177-191, Slack Inc., New Jersey, 1989.

This chapter details the diagnosis and treatment of radial nerve compression in the proximal forearm.

Radial Tunnel Syndrome

Lister GD: Radial tunnel syndrome. *Operative Nerve Repair and Reconstruction,* p. 1023-1037, JB Lippincott, Philadelphia, 1991.

The author presents his experience with this syndrome and demonstrates by way of excellent intraoperative photos different surgical approaches to the radial nerve in the forearm.

Ritts GD, Wood MB, et al: Radial tunnel syndrome; a 10-year surgical experience. *Clin Orthop,* 219 (June):201-205, 1987.

The authors followed 34 patients after radial tunnel release for an average of two years and found that the area of maximal tenderness combined with anesthetic nerve block were the best predictors of accurate diagnosis.

Wartenburg's Syndrome

Dellon A, Mackinnon S: Radial sensory nerve entrapment in the forearm. *J Hand Surg,* 11A:199-205, 1986.

By describing the history, physical findings, and treatment of radial sensory nerve entrapment, the authors "rediscovered" Wartenburg's syndrome and brought it to our attention.

Lateral Antebrachial Nerve Compression

Nunley JA II, Howson P: Lateral antebrachial nerve compression. *Nerve Compression Syndromes—Diagnosis and Treatment,* p. 201-208, Slack Inc., New Jersey, 1989.

The largest experience with this rare nerve compression syndrome comes from Duke Medical Center where these authors examine its anatomy, pathomechanics, and management.

Thoracic Outlet Syndrome

Wood VE, Twito R, et al: Thoracic outlet syndrome. *Orthop Clin North Am,* 19(January): 131-146, 1988.

The authors report good and excellent results in 90% of 121 first rib resections in 100 patients with TOS. They conclude that there are no laboratory tests, radiographs, electrical studies, or infallible clinical tests to establish the diagnosis and because there will always be errors in diagnosis, surgery is advised on a basis of exclusion with great reservation.

22

Peripheral Nerve Injuries

Susan E. Mackinnon, MD

Introduction

Peripheral nerve injury is common and frequently disabling. Functional recovery following nerve repair in upper extremity and hand injuries is often the rate-limiting factor in determining ultimate hand function. In spite of the frequency and importance of these nerve injuries, results following nerve repair and grafting are often disappointing. The large volume of traumatic nerve injuries treated during World War II has provided the important foundation for surgeons interested in the management of nerve-injured patients. Although the functional results achieved with these early repairs were generally poor, the clinical material and surgical techniques used provided an important reference point from which our current surgical management has evolved. A unique group of individuals have made contributions that have combined to shape the direction of peripheral nerve surgery. Sunderland's anatomical studies, Millesi's pursuit of tension-free nerve repair and nerve grafting, and Moberg's efforts to quantify sensibility have provided critical cornerstones for patient management. More recently, Dellon has taught the importance of sensory re-education and rehabilitation. Lundborg alerted us to the potential for neurobiology to impact on ultimate function recovery following nerve injury.

Classification of Nerve Injury

There are several patterns of nerve injury which may vary from fascicle to fascicle, and along the longitudinal axis of the nerve. An understanding of the classification of nerve injury is critical in assisting the surgeon in planning appropriate patient management.

In 1943, Seddon described three types of nerve injury: neurapraxia, axonotmesis, and neurotmesis. In 1951, Sunderland expanded this classification to include two degrees of nerve injury which are intermediate between axonotmesis and neurotmesis. Briefly, neurapraxia (Sunderland first-degree injury) involves a localized area of conduction block. If histological changes are noted they are those of segmental demyelination. Because there is no axonal abnormality, a Tinel's sign will not be present and function is restored with correction of the conduction block or remyelination. Axonotmesis (Sunderland second-degree injury) involves an injury to the axons such that Wallerian degeneration occurs distal to the level of the injury. A Tinel's sign progresses distally at the rate of one inch per month, corresponding to axonal regeneration. These axons regenerate along their original endoneurial tubes to their original distal receptors. Recovery should be complete unless the level of the injury is so far from the sensory or motor targets as to

allow time of denervation to become a factor in influencing ultimate end-organ function.

There is no Seddon counterpart for Sunderland's third- and fourth-degree injuries, yet these are common and important injury patterns. Sunderland's third-degree injury yields the most variable degree of ultimate recovery. In this injury, axonal injury is associated with endoneurial scarring. The amount of scar tissue and the type of fascicle involved influence the ultimate recovery. If the fascicle contains both sensory and motor fibers, then a mixing or mismatching of motor and sensory fibers can occur, resulting in a poorer functional result than if the injury involved a "pure" motor or sensory fascicle. Thus, the variation of recovery from a Sunderland third-degree injury can extend from almost complete recovery to almost no recovery depending on how pure or mixed the fascicle is and the degree of endoneurial scarring that is present. This is the type of injury most frequently seen in the medical-legal arena when some, but not complete, recovery occurs following an iatrogenic nerve injury.

In a Sunderland fourth-degree injury, the nerve is in continuity, but at the level of the injury there is complete scarring across the nerve, such that regeneration cannot occur. A Tinel's sign is present at the level of the injury, but does not proceed distally. Neurotmesis (Sunderland's fifth-degree injury) involves complete transection of the nerve with no functional recovery anticipated. Another injury is a neuroma-in-continuity, which combines various injury patterns from fascicle to fascicle and along the longitudinal length of the nerve (Fig. 22-1). This injury provides the greatest surgical challenge in that normal fascicles or those with potential for good recovery must be protected and Sunderland fourth- and fifth-degree injuries reconstructed with repair or grafting techniques (Table 22-1).

How to Examine the Nerve-injured Patient

Preoperative evaluation of neurological function is critical in planning surgical intervention. If the nerve is completely divided then there is no motor or sensory function in the distribution of the nerve involved. Outline 22-1 lists the critical points of a physical examination for each of the three major nerves in the upper extremity. Pinch and grip measurements should be assessed, recognizing that grip strength will be a measurement not only of function in all three major nerves, but also of patient motivation.

Significant effort has been directed towards developing tests to evaluate sensory function in the hand. These tests and the correlation between these tests and fiber/receptor systems are well developed. A simple analogy has been useful to describe and understand the concept between innervation

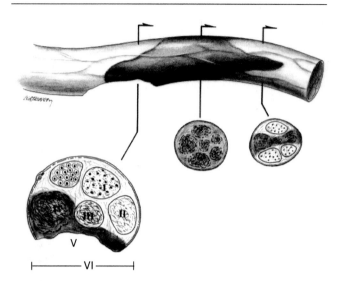

Figure 22-1. A cross section of mixed, neuroma-in-continuity injury. At one o'clock, a first-degree injury (neurapraxia) is noted with segmental demyelination. At three o'clock, a second-degree injury with axonal injury is noted (axonotmesis). In the center of the nerve, a fascicle demonstrates a third-degree injury with a significant amount of scarring in the endoneurium. A fourth-degree injury is noted at nine o'clock with complete scarring of the fascicle noted such that no regeneration can occur. A fourth-degree injury (neurotmesis) with division of the fascicle is noted in the lower portion of the nerve. The diagram demonstrates that the nerve injury can vary in a longitudinal as well as transverse extent. Reproduced with permission from Mackinnon SE, Comparative analysis of nerve injury of the face and hand, implications for surgical treatments, *Oral Maxillofacial Surg Clin North Am,* 4:2, 1992.

Outline 22-1.　Critical Physical Examination Points in Diagnosis of Nerve Injury

I.　Muscles to test for unambiguous diagnosis of motor nerve injury
   A. Radial nerve: extrinsic
      1. Wrist extension
      2. Extension of fingers at metacarpophalangeal joints
      3. Extension of thumb
   B. Median nerve: intrinsic
      1. Thumb-palmar abduction
   C. Median nerve: extrinsic
      1. All flexor sublimi
      2. Flexor profundus to index
      3. Flexor pollicis longus
      4. Flexor carpi radialis
   D. Ulnar nerve: intrinsic
      1. First dorsal interossei
      2. Hypothenar muscles
   E. Ulnar nerve: extrinsic
      1. Flexor profundus to little finger
      2. Flexor carpi ulnaris

II.　Areas to test for unambiguous diagnosis of sensory nerve injury
   A. Radial nerve: dorsal radial aspect of hand toward the first web
   B. Median nerve: pulp of thumb and index finger
   C. Ulnar nerve: pulp of the little finger
   D. Palmar cutaneous branch of median nerve: proximal palm near thenar eminence
   E. Dorsal cutaneous branch of ulnar nerve: dorsal ulnar surface of hand
   F. Digital nerve: not the tip of the finger (overlap), but the proximal third of the distal phalanx and distal third of middle phalanx, adjacent to the distal skin crease

Outline 22-1 reproduced with permission from Mackinnon SE, Dellon AL, *Surgery of the Peripheral Nerve,* Thieme Medical Publishers, New York, 1988.

Table 22-1. Relationship of Injury to Recovery

Degree of injury	Tinel sign present/ progresses disability	Recovery pattern	Rate of recovery	Surgical procedure
I. Neurapraxia	- / -	Complete	Fast, days to 12 weeks	None
II. Axonotmesis	+ / +	Complete	Slow (1" per month)	None
III.	+ / +	Great variation*	Slow (1" per month)	None or neurolysis
IV. Neuroma-in-continuity	+ / -	None	No recovery	Nerve repair or nerve graft
V. Neurotmesis	- / -	None	No repair	Nerve repair or nerve graft

VI. Varies with each fascicle, depending on the combination of injury patterns as noted above.

* Recovery is at least as good as a nerve repair but can vary from excellent to poor depending on the degree of endoneurial scarring and the amount of sensory or motor axonal misdirection that is possible within the injured fascicle.

Table 22-1 reproduced with permission from Mackinnon SE, Dellon AL, *Surgery of the Peripheral Nerve,* Thieme Medical Publishers, New York, 1988.

density and threshold and the various tests currently used to measure sensibility (Fig. 22-2). Two-point discrimination reflects the innervation density and provides an indication of the number of innervated receptors. Static two-point discrimination, which reflects the slowly adapting receptor function, is evaluated by holding two points against the skin for several seconds, at which time the individual indicates whether one or two prongs are felt. The smallest spacing at which the subject is able to identify correctly two of three trials is recorded in millimeters. Moving two-point discrimination is assessed by slowly moving the two prongs longitudinally along the distal portion of the finger pulp with just enough pressure to elicit a response. The subject then indicates whether one or two prongs are felt. The smallest spacing at which the subject is able to identify accurately—on two of three trials is recorded in millimeters.

A more sensitive test of receptor function is the use of a vibrometer to quantify the threshold of the quickly adapting fibers. The vibrating portion of the vibrometer is placed against the skin, and the smallest stimulus perceived is identified as the baseline vibration threshold and recorded in microns of motion. Pressure thresholds are assessed quantitatively using Semmes-Weinstein monofilaments. The nylon monofilaments are applied perpendicularly to the cutaneous surface and the pressure is increased until bending of the monofilament is observed. The probes are sequentially applied to each of the test sites. The number of the probe on the filament represents the logarithm of the force in 0.1 milligrams required to bow the monofilament. The number of the lightest probe that can elicit perception is recorded.

There are several problems with the use of the Semmes-Weinstein filaments. Damaged monofilaments can invalidate the test. The method of testing alters the patient's perception and response in that as the contact time on the fingertip increases, the amount of force required to continue to perceive the presence of filament also increases. The fact that the number on the filament is a logarithm means that the difference between filament numbers is disproportionately discontinuous and as such, measurement cannot be summed and averaged.

Nerve Repair

The use of microneurosurgical technique to reconstruct nerve injury is now generally recognized. Several key points can be emphasized: (1) Microsurgical technique with appropriate magnification, instrumentation, and suture material should be used. (2) A nerve repair must be tension free (Fig. 22-3). (3) When a tension-free repair is not possible, an interposition or interfascicular nerve graft should be used. (4) The proximal and distal extent of the nerve injury must be carefully assessed so that the damaged nerve, which heals with scar tissue, is resected (Fig. 22-4). (5) Extreme postural positioning of the extremity to facilitate an end-to-end repair is discouraged. Both a nerve repair and a nerve graft must be carried out without tension at the repair site. (6) When clinical and surgical conditions per-

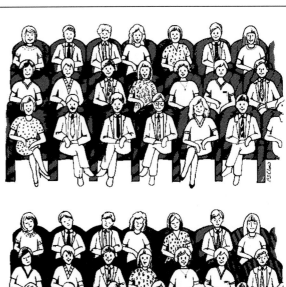
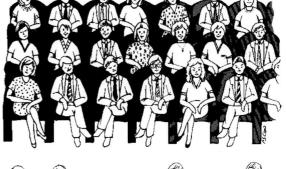
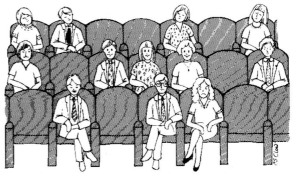

Figure 22-2. A simple analogy helps to describe the relationship between innervation density and threshold. If each person in the audience is considered as a single fiber/sensory receptor unit, then the number of people present in the audience can be considered the innervation density. The "status, health, or well-being" of the individuals can be considered their threshold. **(Top)** If all the seats in the audience are full and the individuals in the audience are "awake and content" then all testing for fiber receptor function will be normal (both innervation density and threshold tests). **(Middle)** The threshold testing will be abnormal (vibration and Semmes-Weinstein monofilaments) if the individuals are not "awake and content" but are "asleep or unhappy." It will take more effort (i.e., greater pressure, larger amplitude) to wake up these sleepy receptors. Moving and static two-point discrimination will be normal because all of the people in the audience are present. **(Bottom)** If individuals in the audience vacate the auditorium, the innervation density test (two-point discrimination) will be abnormal. If the remaining individuals are other than "happy and content," the threshold tests will be abnormal as well. Figure 22-2 (Bottom) reproduced with permission from Mackinnon SE, Peripheral nerve injuries in the hand. In Vistnes LM (ed) *How They Do It: Procedures in Plastic and Reconstructive Surgery,* p. 625, Little, Brown and Company, Boston, 1991.

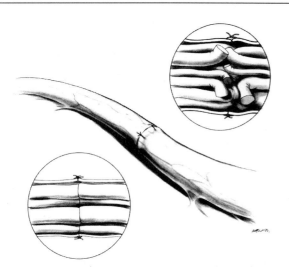

Figure 22-3. The surgeon must take care that the proximal and distal faces of the fascicles are not turned back on themselves (upper circle). A satisfactory appearance on the exterior surface of the nerve can belie poor fascicular alignment.

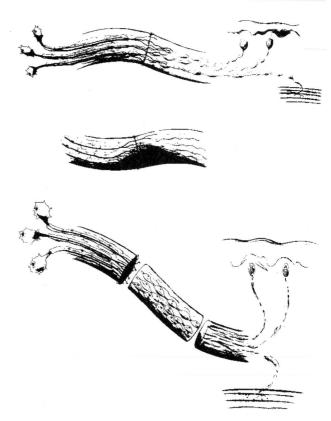

Figure 22-4. **(Top)** Given the use of microneurosurgical instruments and technique, the bottom diagram emphasizes that if the nerve repair is performed between damaged proximal and distal nerve, nerve regeneration will be inhibited. It is often difficult to estimate the proximal and distal extent of the nerve injury. **(Bottom)** A nerve graft serves as a conduit to direct nerve regeneration. Figure 22-4 (Bottom) is reproduced with permission from Mackinnon SE, Upper extremity nerve injuries; primary repair and reconstruction. In Cohen M (ed): *Mastery of Surgery: Plastic Surgery,* Little, Brown and Company, Boston, 1992.

mit, a primary nerve repair should be performed. (7) An epineural repair should be performed unless the intraneural topography of the peripheral nerve dictates a group fascicular repair. (8) Postoperative motor and sensory re-education and rehabilitation may maximize the potential of the surgical result.

The majority of acute nerve injuries can be repaired primarily. The nature of the injury suggests the proximal and distal extent of the nerve injury. If the patient has sustained a relatively clean injury then a primary repair with an end-to-end group fascicular technique is preferred. With a sharp instrument, the surgeon trims back the divided proximal and distal ends of the nerve. For ulnar nerve injuries in the region of the cubital tunnel, primary transposition of the ulnar nerve provides decreased tension on the nerve repair. The surgeon gains approximately 2-3 cm of "length" by this technique. Its usefulness is for ulnar nerve injuries very close to the region of the cubital tunnel. By the time the ulnar nerve is at the level of the proximal to mid forearm, the muscular attachments are such that ulnar nerve transposition is not helpful in gaining any length or decreasing tension.

For injuries at the level of the wrist, the author recommends decompression of the carpal and Guyon's canal distally for median and ulnar injuries respectively. This also confirms motor/sensory orientation in the distal part of the nerve. Appropriate magnification and fine instrumentation is critical in effecting a good nerve repair. When the nerve injury is acute, the fascicular orientation of the proximal and distal surfaces are easily matched. If there is any concern about the motor/sensory orientation on the proximal surface of the nerve, then awake electrical stimulation can be used. This technique finds its greatest use in secondary nerve reconstruction, but occasionally is useful for primary nerve repair. Awake stimulation is a useful technique in determining motor and sensory fascicular grouping in the proximal stump.

Compliance by the patient and support by the anesthetist is critical in the success of this technique. Initial dissection is carried out with neurolept and local regional anesthesia technique. A short-acting anesthetic hypnotic agent must be used when the proximal portion of the nerve is sharply transected, as this is painful. A disposable nerve stimulator usually does not deliver enough stimulus to be reliably perceived by the patient, and more sophisticated electrical equipment that allows the stimulus to be gradually increased is required. Stimulation of sensory fascicles is interpreted by the patient as significant burning or "electrical" pain in a specific cutaneous distribution. By contrast, stimulation of the motor fibers (which contain afferent sensory fibers) is interpreted by the patient as a dull, nonspecific stimulus which is usually localized to the mid portion of the muscle belly of the corresponding motor nerve. Chemical staining of the nerve can also be useful. Several chemical staining techniques have been utilized to identify motor (acetylcholinesterase, cholineacetyltransferase), and sensory (carbonic anhydrase) fibers. The incubation technique for processing tissue has been decreased to one hour; however, the enzyme staining technique requires compliance by a pathologist or a trained technician and is not yet universally available.

At the time of the nerve repair the surgeon moves the digits and extremity and visualizes the amount of movement of the extremity that is acceptable on the nerve repair. The author recommends protecting the nerve repair with a plaster or some type of splint for approximately three weeks, and beginning early protected movement in the early postoperative period; eg, a median nerve repaired at the wrist would be managed with a splint to hold the wrist in neutral and the metacarpal phalangeal joints flexed. The patient is encouraged to begin early active movement of the fingers. This allows the adhesions that form between the median nerve and surrounding tendons and soft tissue to be long adhesions, which facilitates subsequent gliding of the nerve.

Nerve Grafting

When a nerve repair without tension is not possible, a nerve graft should be considered. The ability to align appropriately the motor and sensory fascicles in the proximal and distal stumps is critical to improving results following repair or grafting. If the nerve grafts are placed between the proximal and distal ends of the nerve gap without consideration for both proximal and distal sensory/motor topography, then the mathematical probability of inappropriate sensory motor alignment increases dramatically. Several techniques can be used to aid in identification of sensory and motor fascicles in the proximal nerve stump. These include anatomical clues (surgical identification of fascicles going to specific muscles or cutaneous territories), topography maps, awake stimulation, and enzyme staining. Distally, it is not possible to use awake stimulation or enzyme staining; it is better to rely on anatomical surgical dissection aided by topography maps.

Median nerve injuries at the distal forearm and wrist level requiring nerve grafting are usually performed at a time after injury that would preclude recovery of muscle function (Fig. 22-5). In these cases, the incision is extended into the hand in order to determine anatomically exactly the fascicles destined for specific digits. Proximally, awake stimulation could theoretically be used to separate the majority of the sensory fascicles from the few fascicles that innervate the thenar and lumbrical muscles. From a practical point of view, the distal dissection is used to exclude the motor fascicles to the thenar muscle and accept the "contamination" of the motor fibers from the proximal nerve stump. The nerve grafts coapt the proximal median nerve into the distal median nerve with exclusion of distal motor fascicles. In the distal extremity there is a paucity of plexus formation between fascicles, this orthotopic alignment of the grafts from the proximal stump to the distal stump results in sensibility recovery with good localization (Fig. 22-6).

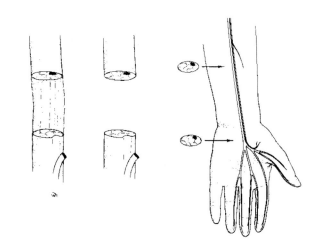

Figure 22-5. Reconstruction of established median nerve injuries in the distal forearm and hand in which recovery of motor function is not anticipated can include exclusion of the distal motor branch, determined by anatomical dissection. Proximally, the motor fascicles could theoretically be identified with awake stimulation, but from a practical point of view satisfactory sensibility will be recovered even if this motor component is not excluded. Reproduced with permission from Mackinnon SE, Upper extremity nerve injuries; primary repair and reconstruction. In Cohen M (ed): *Mastery of Plastic and Reconstructive Surgery*, Little, Brown and Company, Boston, 1994.

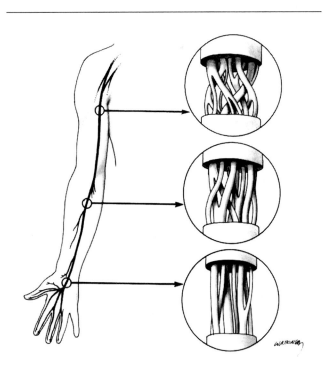

Figure 22-6. A schematic diagram of the internal topography of the median nerve. The degree of plexus formation that occurs between fascicles decreases in the distal portion of the extremity. Reproduced with permission from Mackinnon SE, Dellon AL, *Surgery of the Peripheral Nerve*, Thieme Medical Publishers, New York, 1988.

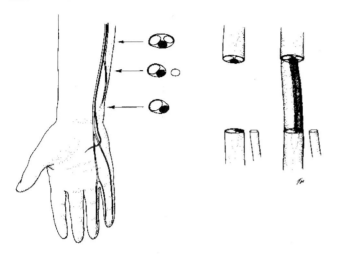

Figure 22-7. Reconstruction of ulnar nerve injuries when the surgeon anticipates both sensory and motor recovery includes identification of the motor (black) and sensory (white) fascicular groups in the hand. Proximally, the motor group is located between the sensory components to the glabrous skin and the dorsal skin of the hand. Awake stimulation and nerve-staining techniques can be used to identify the sensory and motor groups in the proximal portion of the ulnar nerve. The surgeon anticipates the motor group to be slightly smaller than the sensory group and located medial to the main sensory bundle. Reproduced with permission from Mackinnon SE, Upper extremity nerve injuries; primary repair and reconstruction. In Cohen M (ed): *Mastery of Plastic and Reconstructive Surgery,* Little, Brown and Company, Boston, 1994.

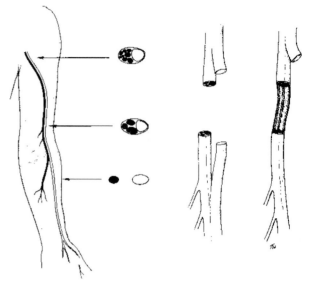

Figure 22-8. Reconstruction of the radial nerve injury is directed at reconstruction of the motor fascicles (black). Distally, the radial sensory nerve (white) should be excluded from the distal nerve repair. Proximally, awake stimulation can be used to separate motor from sensory, which are located in discrete areas of the proximal nerve. Reproduced with permission from Mackinnon SE, Upper extremity nerve injuries; primary repair and reconstruction. In Cohen M (ed): *Mastery of Plastic and Reconstructive Surgery,* Little, Brown and Company, Boston, 1994.

In contrast to the median nerve, the ulnar nerve at the wrist is composed of a significant amount (40%) of motor fibers. The sensory and motor fascicular groups are located in distinct positions in the ulnar nerve; thus, the opportunity exists for excellent functional recovery if the sensory motor/alignment is correct or no functional recovery if the proximal or distal stump is malaligned by 180° (Fig. 22-7). The topography of the ulnar nerve in the forearm has been well described. Proximally, the motor group is located between the sensory groups to the dorsal cutaneous territory and those to the glabrous skin of the hand. After the dorsal cutaneous branch has separated from the main nerve in the mid forearm, the alignment remains such that the motor group is medial and slightly dorsal to the sensory group. This topography is constant until the region of Guyon's canal, where the motor group passes dorsal and radial to the cutaneous group. Orientation of the distal stump in an ulnar nerve graft is determined by extending the incision into the region of Guyon's canal so the surgeon can easily identify the motor and sensory groups. Proximally, awake stimulation and staining have been useful to reassure the surgeon that the motor and sensory fascicular groups have been appropriately determined.

Radial nerve grafting technique can be viewed from a similar perspective (Fig. 22-8). Proximally awake stimulation can be useful in identifying motor and sensory groups. Distally, the radial sensory nerve can be identified and followed proximally to the site of the distal stump. The radial sensory nerve can then be excluded from the distal nerve repair to ensure that no motor fibers regenerate into the sensory nerve distribution. If necessary, the radial sensory nerve can be used as nerve graft material. Motor fibers determined by awake stimulation proximally will be directed into the distal motor branches of the radial nerve. If nerve graft material is at a premium, the branches to the brachioradialis can be excluded, as they do not provide important motor function in isolated radial nerve injuries.

Donor Nerve Grafts

The traditional donor nerve graft is the sural nerve. This will provide 30 cm to 40 cm of useful nerve graft material. The nerve is found adjacent to the lesser saphenous vein just posterior to the lateral malleolus. A longitudinal incision follows the course of the sural nerve. For the hand surgeon, donor nerve grafts in the upper extremity are useful. The lateral antebrachial cutaneous nerve is found adjacent to the cephalic vein in the forearm. This nerve is located on the ulnar border of the brachioradialis muscle. There are usually two branches at this level. A maximum of 8 cm of nerve graft can be harvested. The diameter of the nerve graft is suitable for digital nerve reconstruction and the loss of sensibility is minimal; however, the scar on the forearm is a consideration. The medial antebrachial cutaneous nerve is found adjacent to the basilic vein in the groove just medial to the biceps muscle. There are two branches on either side

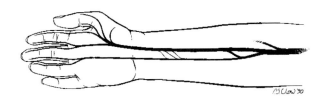

Figure 22-9. Schema of the internal topography of the fascicles to the third digital web space. A microinternal neurolysis of the fascicles to the third web space can be carried out proximally to a level of approximately 145 mm proximal to the radial styloid to meet a large plexus, which precludes further dissection.

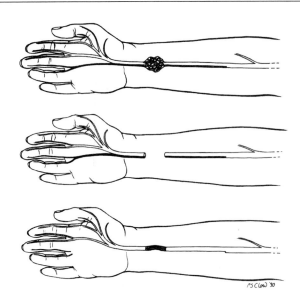

Figure 22-10. In the situation of a fourth-degree injury of the median nerve, the neuroma-in-continuity is resected **(Middle)**, and the fascicles to the third digital web space are dissected both proximal and distal to the injury site to facilitate reconstruction of the nerve injury using the third-web-space fascicles as the donor nerve graft **(Bottom)**. Reproduced with permission from Ross DO, Mackinnon SE, Chang YZ, Interneural topography of the median nerve facilitates nerve sharing procedures. *J Reconst Microsurg*, 8:225-232, 1992.

of the basilic vein. The anterior branch is recommended, as the sensory loss will not be on the important ulnar border of the elbow and forearm. Because of its location in the medial aspect of the arm, the scar from harvesting the medial antebrachial cutaneous nerve is more acceptable than that associated with harvesting the lateral antebrachial nerve. If necessary, 18 cm to 20 cm of nerve-graft material can be harvested from the medial antebrachial cutaneous nerve and on occasion both anterior and posterior branches have been harvested when a contraindication existed to harvesting a sural nerve graft. In a situation of established median and ulnar nerve injuries in which nerve grafting is considered, frequently an expendable portion of the median or ulnar nerve is used to reconstruct more critical components of these nerves. For example, proximal and distal to a median nerve injury, the nerves destined to the third web space can be harvested as donor nerve grafts (Figs. 22-9 and 22-10). Twenty-four centimeters of nerve-graft material can be obtained from this source prior to reaching major plexus formation in the proximal forearm. Thus, the patient who presents with no sensation in the median nerve distribution and the five radial digital nerves is reinnervated using nerve-graft material which would otherwise provide sensation to the two digital nerves to the third web space. Thus, the patient has no added sensory morbidity from harvesting this donor nerve graft. Similarly, the dorsal cutaneous branch of the ulnar nerve in established ulnar nerve injury in which this nerve is not functioning is frequently used as donor nerve material to reconstruct the remainder of the ulnar nerve. Upper extremity nerves have a more favorable neural-to-connective tissue ratio than lower extremity nerves, which may enhance nerve regeneration. Also, securing the donor nerve graft from the same extremity as the nerve injury is of benefit.

Neuroma Incontinuity

Neuroma incontinuity is one of the most challenging of surgical peripheral nerve problems. Careful clinical evaluation using sensory tests that quantify sensibility allows the surgeon to determine preoperatively which fascicular groups are normal or partially or completely injured. The challenge

is to repair the damaged components of the nerve (fourth- and fifth-degree injury) and at the same time not "downgrade" normal fascicles or those with potential for recovery. Recently a simple technique was described for management of the neuroma incontinuity in a situation in which functioning motor fibers must be maintained at the same time as sensory fibers that are either not functioning or are producing disabling pain are identified and reconstructed. The neuroma incontinuity is identified and a simple, disposable nerve stimulator can be used to identify the motor fascicles proximal and distal to the level of injury. These motor fibers are protected and the electrically silent sensory fascicles, both proximal and distal to the neuroma incontinuity, are divided and reconstructed with a nerve graft. In this way, a tedious and potentially dangerous dissection through the neuroma incontinuity itself is avoided (Fig. 22-11). In the reverse situation, when sensory fascicles need to be protected and motor function reconstructed, tendon transfers are frequently appropriate. If reconstruction of the nerve is appropriate, then nerve-to-nerve fascicle recordings are necessary to identify and protect functioning sensory fascicles.

Vascularized Nerve Grafts

Evaluation of both the experimental and clinical studies on vascularized nerve grafting does not demonstrate a superi-

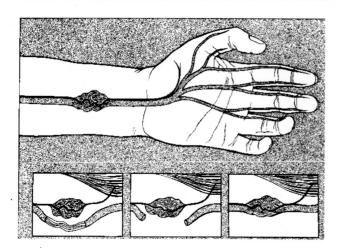

Figure 22-11. Schema of the bypass operation for management of the neuroma-in-continuity of the median nerve in which the motor fascicles (black) are protected and preserved and the sensory component of the median nerve is reconstructed with a nerve graft.

ority of either technique when small-caliber nerves (eg, sural nerve) are used. In the rare instance when a large trunk graft could be considered, (eg, ulnar nerve in brachial plexus reconstruction) then the graft would have to be revascularized to prevent central necrosis.

Results of Nerve Repair and Grafting

In spite of the large number of nerve repairs, there are, in fact, very few publications of results following nerve repair or nerve grafting. Most surgeons who do not actively treat a large number of patients with peripheral nerve problems perceive that the results following nerve surgery are poor. This arises in part from the published results dealing with nerve injuries during World War II. Woodall and Bebee published a five-year follow-up of 3,656 nerve injuries. Nerve grafting was used in only 30 cases. Seddon's report of the war experience demonstrated equally poor results. While these injuries would now be treated differently with microneurosurgical technique and nerve grafting, our attitude towards peripheral nerve surgery has been significantly influenced by this large series of patients with long-term follow-up. In 1988, the published results of nerve repair and grafting in the upper extremity were reviewed. Where possible, reported results were summarized utilizing the MRC classification of motor recovery and a modification of Hyatt's classification of sensory recovery. There have been only a relatively small number of publications of end-stage results. Careful review of these papers will also highlight significant weaknesses in patient evaluation.

In general, the results following nerve repair and grafting are improving. It is interesting to note, however, that nothing has been published since 1980 on the results of high median nerve injuries treated with nerve repair. There have

been five published results of low median nerve repairs. These results were variable, with McManamny reporting 86% of patients recovering as S3+ or greater and Birch and Raji reporting only 11% of patients S3+ and no patients with S4+. Using sensory re-education, the author in 1992 reported 80% of patients recovering as S3+ following median nerve grafting.

Since 1980, there have been only six reports of results of repair of low ulnar nerve injuries. The results of motor recovery varied from only 10% of patients recovering M4 or M5 (McManamny, 1983 and Posch, 1980) to Birch reporting 91% of patients recovering M4 or M5 motor function. Since 1980, only two reports have been published on results of function following high ulnar nerve repair. No patients recovered M5 function and only 9% of patients in one study recovered M4 function.

It is felt that children recover better neurological function following nerve injury than adults. This likely relates to central plasticity rather than significant differences in peripheral nerve regeneration or motor/sensory recovery. It needs to be stressed that the accepted rating scales for both sensory (Hyatt's) and motor (British Medical Research Council) grading can be criticized. At the moment, there is no uniformity among surgeons as to alternative sensory/motor grading systems. Review of published series should provide stimulus for all of us to attempt better follow-up and consider independent evaluation of patient results as well as the possibility of the establishment of a nerve repair and graft patient registry.

Postoperative Rehabilitation

Motor Rehabilitation

In the postoperative period maintenance of range of motion of all joints will be critical in determining potential outcome after motor recovery. There has been long-term interest on the potential effect of electrical stimulation of denervated muscles. It is hypothesized that even in the absence of neurotrophic influence, contractile activity produced by electrical stimulation would ultimately be beneficial to functional motor recovery. Williams laboratory in Montreal has pursued this experimental question in a number of research studies. Implantable electrodes and pulse generators with continuous stimulation would be required if any effect was to be seen.

At the present time, postoperative muscle stimulation is still at the experimental level. Motor re-education, however, will be useful following nerve regeneration especially when a less than perfectly synergistic nerve has been transferred or when significant motor/sensory fiber mixing has occurred. Late-phase motor re-education emphasizes motions or activities that mimic the patient's job activities. Working in a workshop or with a work simulator is useful prior to returning the patient to the workplace.

Sensory Re-education

Following nerve regeneration there is frequently a misdirection of sensory fibers such that aberrant localization of sensation is experienced. Sensory re-education is a method that assists the patient with a sensory impairment to reinterpret the altered profile of neuro impulses. Recent experimental work by Merzenich and Wall in independent laboratories has demonstrated cortical changes following nerve injury and regeneration in adult monkeys. An improvement in cortical mapping is seen when the primates are forced to use their reinnervated digits frequently (a form of sensory re-education).

Patients may be taught the basics of sensory re-education even prior to their surgery so they are familiar with the techniques in the postoperative period. In the very early postoperative period, desensitization is a form of sensory re-education as the patient is trained to perceive altered stimuli as nonpainful. As soon as the patient perceives any touch in the reinnervated area, the early phase of sensory re-education is started. The goals are to re-educate specific perceptions such as movement as distinguished from constant touch and to begin to re-educate incorrect localization. The patient is encouraged to perform the sensory re-education exercises frequently. As the sensibility improves, more challenging sensory tasks are included in the re-education program. It is important not to introduce sensory tasks that are too difficult before the patient is capable of working with them, or frustration develops. Late-phase sensory education includes exercises to identify and recognize objects, beginning with large objects and progressing to smaller ones. Patients can be given Disk-criminators in the late-phase program and encouraged to practice discrimination between one and two points. Late-phase sensory re-education continues until appropriate functional sensibility has returned and the patient is using the hand to perform sensory re-education on a continuing basis.

Annotated Bibliography

Dellon AL: *Evaluation of Sensibility and Re-education of Sensation in the Hand,* Williams & Wilkins, Baltimore, 1981.

A single-authored textbook describing the historical background of sensory evaluation and techniques of sensory re-education.

Gelberman RH: *Operative Nerve Repair and Reconstruction,* J.P. Lippincott, Philadelphia, 1991.

Over one-hundred authors contributed to this textbook presenting various perspectives on surgical management of nerve injuries.

Lundborg G: *Nerve Injury and Repair,* Churchill Livingstone, Edinburgh, 1989.

A single-authored textbook outlining the neurobiology as it would impact on nerve injury and repair.

Mackinnon SE: Comparative analysis of nerve injury of the face and hand, implications for surgical treatments. *Oral and Maxillofacial Surg Clin North Am,* 4(2), 483-502, 1992.

This chapter outlines in detail sensory evaluation in the hand and the classification of nerve injury.

Mackinnon SE, Dellon AL: *Surgery of the Peripheral Nerve,* Thieme, New York, 1988.

Comprehensive textbook outlining the investigation and management of peripheral nerve disorders; surgical techniques are described in detail.

Mackinnon SE: Double and multiple crush and entrapment syndromes in compression nerve syndromes of the upper extremity. *Hand Clin North Am,* ed Rayan GM, WB Saunders, 8(2) 369-390,1992.

This chapter summarizes the concept of double and multiple crush and multiple entrapment neuropathies. This is important in managing problems with compression neuropathy in the upper extremity as it relates to cumulative trauma disorders.

Mackinnon SE: Management of the peripheral nerve gap. *Clinics in Plastic Surgery,* ed Schwarz WM, WB Saunders Co., Philadelphia, July, 16(3) 587-603, 1989.

This chapter outlines the evaluation and management of the neuroma-in-continuity and the management of the peripheral nerve gap.

Mackinnon SE: Peripheral nerve injuries in the hand. *How They Do It: Procedures in Plastic and Reconstructive Surgery,* ed Vistnes LM, Little, Brown & Co., Boston, 621-642, 1991.

Technical details of peripheral nerve repair and reconstruction in the hand are outlined in detail.

Mackinnon SE: Upper extremity nerve injuries: primary repair and reconstruction. *Mastery of Plastic and Reconstructive Surgery,* ed Cohen M, Little, Brown & Co., Boston, 1994.

The techniques of management of nerve injuries in the upper extremity are described including techniques of reconstruction.

Millesi H: The nerve gap-theory and clinical practice, *Hand Clin,* 2:651,1986.

This chapter reviews Dr. Millesi's thoughts on nerve repair and grafting and summarizes his techniques of managing the surgical nerve gap.

23

Brachial Plexus Injuries

Vincent R. Hentz, MD

Introduction

The typical patient with a brachial plexus injury is a young man injured when thrown from a motorcycle. Prior to modern microneurosurgical techniques, there was little enthusiasm for operating on the nerves of such patients. If the palsy was complete, amputation of the arm was recommended. Today, useful function frequently can be restored, even to completely paralyzed limbs.

Pathology of the Lesion

The extent of injury is due primarily to the level of energy and somewhat to the direction of the force relative to the limb and shoulder. Low-energy injuries, such as a fall onto the shoulder, typically cause mostly reversible injuries such as neurapraxia (Sunderland Level I) or various degrees of axonotmesis (Sunderland Levels II–IV). High-energy injuries, for example being thrown from a speeding motorcycle, are associated with more significant injuries, including rupture of plexal segments at any level (Sunderland Level V) or avulsions of nerve roots from the spinal cord. The force of the blow is imparted first to those structures having the most direct or straightest course from spine to arm, in this case the C-8 and T-1 roots and their continuation as the inferior trunk. The energy is imparted last to those structures having the longest anatomic course from fixed points in the neck to fixed points in the shoulder and arm; in this case the sigmoid course of the C-5 and C-6 roots and their superior trunk afford these structures some protection. The C-7 root and associated middle trunk is intermediate in its course. The lower structures of the brachial plexus suffer more significant injuries such as root avulsion, than more proximally located roots, trunks, and cords (Table 23-1). In the same patient, essentially every Sunderland level of injury, and root avulsion can occur (Fig. 23-1).

Table 23-1. Operative findings for each root from a series of 114 patients presenting with total or near-total brachial plexus palsy

Root	Ruptured	Avulsed	Other
C-5	59	14	40
C-6	44	35	35
C-7	39	53	20
C-8	11	67	31
T-1	11	61	37

Evaluation of the Patient

The goal of the examination is to determine as accurately as possible the extent of the nerve injury, and from this, determine whether or not the patient is a candidate for either early surgical reconstruction of the brachial plexus or a period of further observation.

Physical Signs

One important indicator of severity of injury is the presence of a Horner's sign on the affected side. This may be present immediately but occasionally is not readily apparent for

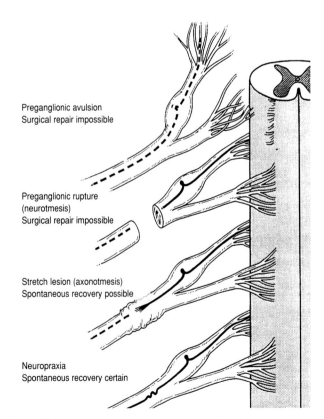

Figure 23-1. In the same patient, a severe traction injury to the brachial plexus may cause nerve injuries of varying severity, including avulsion of the nerve root from the spinal cord (nonreparable), extraforaminal rupture of the root or trunk (surgically reparable), or an intraneural rupture of fascicles (some spontaneous recovery possible).

three to four days following injury. A Horner's sign indicates severe injury to the C-8 and T-l roots and has been correlated with avulsion of one or both of these roots. Severe pain in an anesthetic extremity is also a sign of poor prognosis, indicating some degree of deafferentiation of the limb, again correlated with root avulsion injuries.

Motor and Sensory Examination

A standard motor and sensory examination is performed based on the known metameric levels of innervation. Two important indicators of the level of injury for the patient with near-total palsy are the presence or absence of activity of the rhomboids and serratus anterior muscles. Rapidly accomplished tests such as sharp-dull discrimination, provide sufficient sensory testing.

Radiography

Radiographs of the cervical spine, chest, clavicle, and scapula are necessary. The chest radiograph should include an inspiration and expiration AP view to determine the activity of the diaphragm. A paralyzed diaphragm is an indicator of severe injury to the upper roots of the plexus. The presence of fractures of the transverse processes is also strong evidence of a high-energy injury.

Diagnostic Examinations Including Computerized Tomography, Magnetic Resonance Imaging, and Myelography

Modern imaging techniques have improved the clinician's ability to predict what the microneurosurgeon will find at exploration. Traditional myelography using metrizimide contrast has been largely supplanted by CT or MRI examinations, performed with and without contrast agents (Fig. 23-2). Both CT and MRI may be useful. MRI reformatting provides a better picture of the soft tissues, particularly the T-2 weighted images that highlight the fat content of the cervical spinal cord and nerve roots, but also the T-1 image highlighting the water content associated with a *pseudomeningocoele*. The presence of a pseudomeningocoele has been strongly correlated with avulsion of the corresponding root (Fig. 23-3). When these tests are performed within a few days of injury, especially with contrast, there may be a higher incidence of false positive interpretations because the contrast agent may leak through small tears in the dura, not necessarily associated with avulsion of the root.

Other evidence of significant injury includes empty-appearing root sleeves, or a shift of the cord in one direction or another away from the midline.

Sensory and Motor Evoked Potentials

These tests should be carried out several weeks following injury to allow Wallerian degeneration to proceed. Standard electromyography is not as helpful for severe injuries as are sensory evoked potentials, corticosensory evoked potentials, and spinograms. Stimulation over Erb's point in the supraclavicular fossa and recording from the cortex using scalp electrodes provide evidence that some roots may still be incontinuity with the spinal cord. The spinogram can

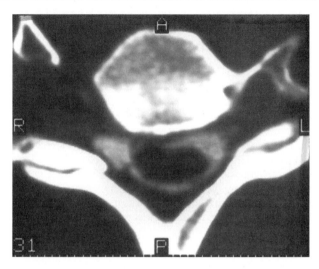

Figure 23-2. Computerized tomography of the cervical spine with contrast demonstrates avulsion of a part of the transverse process and absence of the root shadow at the C-6 level. This appearance suggests that the C-6 root has been avulsed.

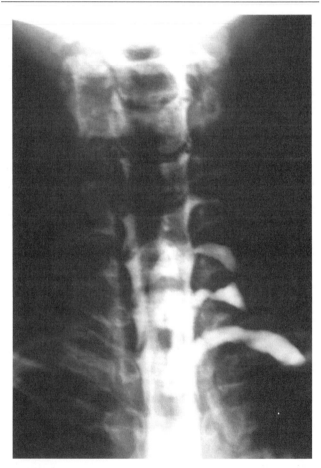

Figure 23-3. Standard cervical myelogram demonstrating multiple large pseudomeningocoeles at several levels. Note the normal root shadows on the contralateral side.

determine information about the level of innervation of the paraspinous muscles. Since these are innervated by the posterior primary rami of the plexus, paralysis of these muscles indicates a very proximal injury but does not tell the examiner whether the injury is associated with avulsion, rupture, or axonotmesis. No one test can be the conclusive basis for surgical decision making. All the information must be assimilated and, most importantly, viewed within the context of the presumed energy of the trauma.

Indications for Surgery

Most of the modern series describing the experience in brachial plexus reconstruction attest to the inverse relationship between time from injury to operation to outcome. In cautious and skilled hands, exploration seldom results in extension of the injury. Even when total palsy exists, less than 20% of patients demonstrate avulsions of all five roots of the plexus, meaning that for the great majority the surgeon will find something to repair or graft and, if this is not possible, reinnervate from another source (nerve transfer). If nerve transfer is included, then virtually all patients might theoretically benefit from microneural reconstruction. These factors imply that when there is a strong suspicion of significant damage to the plexus in the form of root avulsions and nerve ruptures, surgical exploration is warranted.

Timing of Surgery

Immediate Surgery

Immediate surgery is indicated for essentially any patient with a plexus injury of almost any degree of severity secondary to a penetrating injury such as a stab wound or following an iatrogenic injury such as known or suspected injury to the plexus at the time of first rib resection for the treatment of thoracic outlet syndrome. There are many good arguments against immediate reconstruction of the plexus in traction injuries. Most surgeons feel that some period of time must pass to permit delineation of injured from noninjured nerve.

Early Surgery (Three Weeks to Three Months)

Early surgery is indicated for patients who present with total or near-total palsy, or an injury associated with high energy levels. It is also indicated for gunshot wounds to the plexus. For those injuries associated with lower levels of energy and those associated with partial upper-level palsy, it is preferable to follow the course of recovery for three to six months, leaning toward operation if recovery seems to plateau as determined by several successive evaluations carried out at monthly intervals. The presence or absence of an advancing Tinel's sign can be a useful guide. The absence of a Tinel's sign in the supraclavicular fossa in the face of a nearly complete C-5 to C-6 level palsy is a poor prognostic sign for spontaneous recovery and warrants an early exploration with the likelihood that C-5 and C-6

nerve roots may be avulsed. In this case, nerve transfer is necessary.

Controversial Indications

An occasional patient presents with a partial C-8 and complete T-1 lesion, with some finger flexors working but with essentially an intrinsic palsy and anesthesia in the C-8 and/or T-1 distribution. This represents somewhat of a dilemma in decision making because it seems almost impossible to recover intrinsic muscle function in the adult. When injured, the C-8 and T-1 nerve roots are so often avulsed from the spinal cord that it is unlikely that anything reparable (or even worth repairing) will be found at surgery.

Surgical Findings

Unless the injury is clearly limited to one area of the plexus, as for example a stab wound, the entire plexus from neck to axilla may need to be exposed by relatively standard techniques. A variety of presentations may be seen. If the upper roots are avulsed, the rootlets and swollen dorsal root ganglion may be found twisted and lying either behind the clavicle or slightly above it in the region of the C-8 root. If the upper roots or superior trunk and/or the middle trunk have ruptured, the distal ends typically lie behind the clavicle. The avulsed (often) or ruptured (infrequently) C-8 and T-1 structures are usually found much closer to their respective foramina than is the case with C-5 or C-6. Essentially any combination of injuries may occur, including avulsion, rupture, and a neuroma incontinuity. The supraclavicular dissection usually allows this assessment. However, it is critical to complete the remainder of the dissection if the findings above favor some type of reconstruction by nerve grafting because there exist a sufficient number of lesions occurring at two levels, for example, rupture of the superior trunk in combination with avulsion of the axillary nerve from the deltoid, or rupture of the musculocutaneous nerve at the level of the shoulder.

Intraoperative Evoked Potentials

Intraoperative evoked potentials (Fig. 23) are helpful although not foolproof in determining when, for example, an intraforaminal avulsion, which is uncommon, has occurred rather than ruptured. They are also helpful in determining whether there exists only an empty root sleeve, ie, only connective tissue with no axons therein, which is more common. By two to three months after injury, evoked potentials across a neuroma incontinuity are reliable in assisting in decision-making. When stimulating and recording across a neuroma incontinuity, it is unnecessary to average a large number of stimulations. If there exists no easily discernible response above the noise level without averaging, the neuroma and adjacent damaged nerve is resected using the microscope to assist in determining when debridement is adequate, and nerve grafts are placed in the resultant defect. If a clear signal is identified above the noise, then only a neurolysis under magnification is performed.

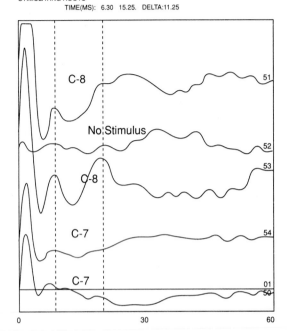

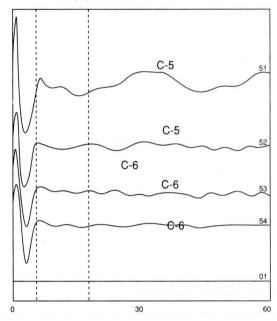

Figure 23-4.   The results of intraoperative corticosensory evoked potential tests are demonstrated in a patient with a C-5, C-6, and C-7 palsy. At exploration, all roots could be found exiting their foramina but the C-5, 6, and 7 roots appeared somewhat firm compared to the C-8 and T-1 roots. The upper three tracings on the left are the result of stimulating (or recording but not stimulating) the C-8 root. With C-8 root stimulation, a large response could be measured with the scalp recording electrodes. Stimulation of the C-5, C-6, and C-7 roots (as indicated on the tracings) resulted in no measurable brain response indicating probable avulsion of these roots proximal to the point of stimulation.

Intraoperative Decisions and Priorities of Repair

When the patient presents with essentially total brachial plexus palsy, the priorities of repair include

- provisions for elbow flexion by biceps/brachialis muscle reinnervation;
- provisions for shoulder stabilization, abduction, and external rotation by suprascapular nerve reinnervation;
- provisions for brachiothoracic pinch (adduction of the arm against the chest) by reinnervation of the pectoralis major muscle;
- sensation below the elbow in the C-6-7 area, by reinnervation of the lateral cord;
- provisions for wrist extension and finger flexion by reinnervation of the lateral and posterior cord.

These priorities have been chosen for three reasons. The first is their functional significance, the second relates to the likelihood of obtaining the chosen function by nerve reconstruction (more proximal muscles are reinnervated more successfullly than very distal muscles), and the third relates to the degree of difficulty in achieving the individual functions listed above by secondary surgery.

Surgical Techniques for Plexoplexal Nerve Reconstruction

The surgeon should take advantage of the knowledge gained by others in internally mapping the plexus (Fig. 23-5). At the root level, the posterior and anterior division bound areas are delineated in an attempt to guide these axons to appropriate target nerves. Next the distal targets are dissected. These usually include the suprascapular nerve, which is frequently difficult to find, the lateral cord and posterior cord. Typically, there are far more targets for nerve grafts than proximal resources.

Choice of Nerve Grafts—Conventional and Vascularized

Both standard fascicular grafts and, for certain cases, vascularized nerve grafts are used. The typical first choice is the two sural nerves. Other donor sites for standard grafts include both medial brachial and medial antebrachial cutaneous nerves. Standard microsuture techniques are typically used, although some surgeons now use autologous-derived fibrinogen as a tissue adhesive to glue together nerve ends more rapidly, apparently with equal success.

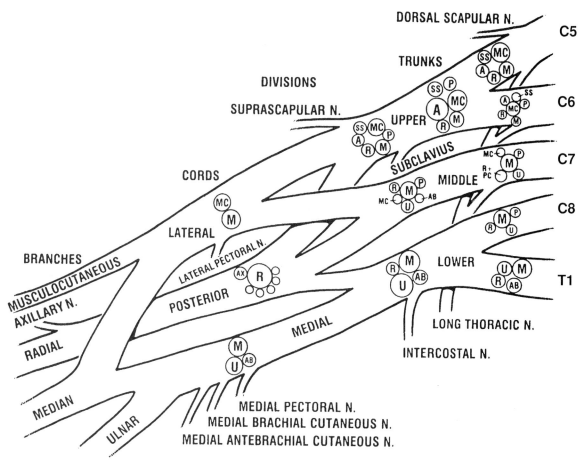

Figure 23-5. The intraneural fascicular architecture of the brachial plexus is depicted. M, median nerve; MC, musculocutaneous nerve; R, radial nerve; U, ulnar nerve; AB, medial brachial and antebrachial nerve; PC, posterior cord; SS, suprascapular nerve. Redrawn with permission from Narakas A: Surgical management of brachial plexus injuries. In *Reconstructive Microsurgery*, Daniels RK, Terzis JK, (eds), p. 451, Little, Brown and Company, Boston, 1977.

Vascularized Nerve Grafts

The principal reason to consider a vascularized nerve graft in plexus reconstruction is to maximize the amount of nerve-graft material for reconstruction. The best indication for a vascularized graft in plexus reconstruction is a case involving proven avulsion of C-8 and T-1 in association with large root stumps of the remaining plexus. In this case, there is no possibility of spontaneous recovery of the ulnar nerve innervated structures or areas, and it makes little sense to waste precious proximal axons to recover some sensibility in the ulnar side of the hand. Intrinsic muscle recovery is essentially never seen in the adult when C-8 and T-1 have been badly injured. In this instance, the best source of a vascularized nerve graft is the ulnar nerve itself, based in the upper arm on one of several branches of the brachial artery, usually the superior ulnar collateral artery.

Surgical Techniques for Nerve Transfer

In the most severe injuries, those with all or most nerve roots avulsed, there are insufficient numbers of proximal axon resources from the remaining parts of the plexus still incontinuity with the spinal cord. In these cases, it has been necessary to turn to extraplexal sources of especially motor and also sensory axons. Many different nerves have been advocated by knowledgeable surgeons; however, the most common sources of extraplexal motor axons have been the spinal accessory nerve and the intercostal nerves from C-3 to C-6. Additionally, motor branches of the cervical rami or even cross chest branches of the contralateral plexus, such as a branch from the lateral pectoral nerve, are used. The most appropriate targets for neurotization are the suprascapular nerve (shoulder abduction and external rotation), the musculocutaneous nerve (elbow flexion), or the lateral pectoral nerve (thoracohumeral pinch).

Neurotization in the Neglected Plexus Injury

It is possible to combine microneural reconstruction with free vascularized functional muscle transfers for neglected cases of total brachial plexus palsy. In these cases the time since injury is too long (in the adult, beyond two years) for successful neurotization or reinnervation of previously denervated muscles. Either the opposite latissimus dorsi, the gracilis, or another muscle is transferred to the shoulder and arm by microvascular free transfer. The motor nerve of the transferred muscle is joined to the donor motor nerve, usually an extraplexal motor nerve such as the spinal accessory or intercostal.

Postoperative Care

At the completion of the operation, a cervical collar is fitted about the neck to restrict neck motion. The shoulder and elbow are immobilized, the shoulder in adduction and the elbow in 90° of flexion for two weeks; range of motion exercises are then renewed without restrictions. After initial healing, the progress of nerve regeneration is assessed about every three months. At least two and perhaps three years are necessary before the results of nerve reconstruction can be assessed.

Results of Nerve Reconstruction by Graft and Neurotization

Analysis of recently published series (Tables 23-2 and 23-3) lead to several conclusions. Repair does improve the prognosis. Infraclavicular injuries have a better prognosis than supraclavicular. Supraclavicular injuries associated with at least two reparable roots have a better prognosis and partial injuries more so than complete. The results of nerve transfer have been more mixed.

Microneural Reconstruction for Obstetrical Palsy

The approach to the infant who has suffered a traction injury of the brachial plexus differs somewhat from the adult, though the mechanism of injury is absolutely similar, ie, excessive direct traction on the brachial plexus associated typically with a difficult delivery or perhaps by compression of the plexus by the first rib. In most cases, a similar set of circumstances prevails, including a high birth weight, usually greater than 4000 grams (frequently associated with maternal diabetes or short, heavy mothers), a difficult presentation (shoulder dystocia), cephalopelvic disproportion, or forceps delivery. Since the first reported attempts at repair in 1903, the role of surgical reconstruction has been far more controversial than for the adult cases and remains so to this day. The principal reason behind the controversy regarding the role of microneural reconstruction lies in the lack of a uniform system of evaluation. Most studies lack reliable data on the initial clinical picture and there is no consensus on what constitutes a good result. For most studies, a good result translates into a well-functioning hand regardless of the condition of the shoulder, which frequently

Table 23-2. Results of Reconstruction with Total Supraclavicular Palsy

Author	Number of patients	Developed useful function
Millesi	20	10/20 *
Sedel	26	22/26#

* Shoulder 5/8, elbow flexion 9/18, wrist/finger 2/18, additional 6 patients explored but nothing repaired.

Grade 3 = 11; grade 4 = 12; grade 5 = 3.

Results of Reconstruction with Partial Palsy

Author	Number of patients	Developed useful function
Millesi	11 supraclav. lesion	9/11
	12 infraclav. lesion	10/12
Sedel/Narakas	23	20/23

Table 23-3. Results of Nerve Transfer for Elbow Flexion

Nerve	Author	Number of patients	Good results	Bad results
Spinal	Allieu	15	3	12
Accessory	Narakas	3	2	
Nerve	Merle	7	3	4
Intercostal	Millesi	22	11	11
Nerve	Narakas	24	9	15
	Nagano	117	80	37

lacks normal external rotation and abduction. However, the hand is frequently spared because a majority of lesions involve C-5 and C-6 (plus or minus the C-7) roots (Fig. 23-6). Most of these cases retain or regain good function of the hand. The recent interest in operating on infants has been stimulated primarily by a better appreciation of the natural history of the spontaneous evolution following injury provided by several longitudinal studies that determined that

- complete recovery seems possible only if the biceps and deltoid have reached the M1 stage by the second month;
- the results, though still good, are nevertheless incomplete if initial contracting of these two muscles requires three to 3.5 months;
- if the biceps is not at stage M3 by five months, the results will be highly unsatisfactory.

Preoperative Evaluation

The posture of the newborn is frequently diagnostic with either a flail limb, indicating complete palsy or an internally rotated, adducted limb with the forearm pronated and the wrist flexed, indicating an upper root problem (Fig. 23-6). A simpler muscle testing scheme is employed where M0 is no contraction, M1 represents contraction without movement, M2 is slight movement, and M3 is complete move-

three months of age will be necessary to determine indications for surgery. At three months of age, the child is retested. If any biceps function is evident, surgery is not recommended. For those without biceps function, an EMG is scheduled although the results of EMG have been difficult to correlate with final outcome. However, total absence of electrical evidence of reinnervation at this time indicates avulsion of the corresponding roots. A final evaluation is cervical myelography. In skilled hands, there is minimal morbidity, and the absence of a pseudomeningocoele essentially confirms the presence of an extraforaminal lesion.

Surgical Approach

The supraclavicular part of the incision alone will usually suffice for C-5, C-6, and C-7 palsies. Otherwise, the dissection is the same as that for the adult.

The operative findings (Table 23-4) differ from the adult in that a neuroma-in-continuity is far more frequently encountered in the infant, typically at the level of the superior trunk. If C-7 is affected, it is usually adherent to this neuroma. The clavicle can be lifted up off the plexus allowing exposure of the divisions and the proximal cords. The suprascapular nerve can frequently be found exiting the neuroma. When all roots have been identified, they are sequentially stimulated and the evoked potentials measured. It is rare to find a root both injured extraforaminally and also avulsed from the cord. Even C-8 and T-1 can be visualized from the supraclavicular approach. In cases of total palsy, if these roots are normal by electrical studies, then an infraclavicular injury must be suspected and the infraclavicular portion of the incision made. If grafting from a supraclavicular to infraclavicular location is to be done, the clavicle is sectioned obliquely. When fibrous scar extends into the subclavicular region, one can expect to find one or two avulsed roots curled within the scar.

Surgical Decision Making

With the presence of a neuroma, it is tempting to perform only a neurolysis. This has led to disappointing results. In most instances, a purposeful decision to resect the neuroma and perform interpositional nerve grafts is made. Frequently, essentially no healthy-appearing nerve fibers are found in the distal neuroma on serial histology. In summary, for subtotal lesions, lesions of C-5, C-6, and C-7 are nearly always extraforaminal ruptures, frequently incontinuity lesions. The lesions are all above the clavicle and may

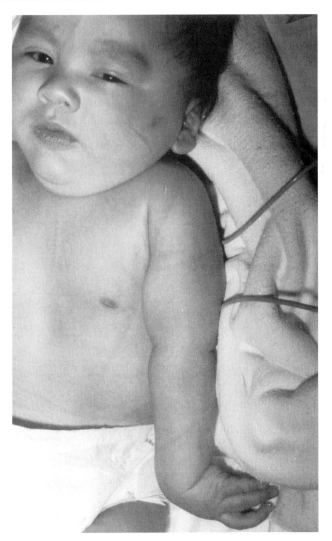

Figure 23-6. A typical presentation of an infant with an upper plexus birth palsy. The arm is held by the side, the elbow extended, the forearm held in pronation and the wrist in flexion. Depending upon the remaining function of the C-7 root, the fingers may either be held in flexion or demonstrate active extension. Wrist and finger flexion are typically strong.

ment. The sensory exam is even less precise; the examiner tests the reaction to pinching the skin only. Other signs to be observed include evidence of trophic changes such as differences in hair growth or color, and the presence of a Horner's sign. EMGs are not obtained until later.

The infant is reexamined at one month of age. Recovery may already be evident and will probably ultimately be complete. For the remaining babies, several presentations are evident: if the palsy is still total and is associated with a Horner's sign, the outlook for spontaneous recovery is poor and early surgery is indicated. If the hand is recovering, but no biceps or shoulder recovery is evident, there is still a chance for spontaneous recovery. A third evaluation prior to

Table 23-4.   Anatomic lesions on upper roots in 75 cases of subtotal obstetrical palsy

Nerve	Rupture	Avulsion	AV + Rupture
C-5, C-6	38	1	1
C-5, C-6, C-7	19	1	5

be repaired through limited incisions. For complete palsy, C-8 and T-1 are almost always avulsed and there is always at least one root available for reconstruction. This justifies systematic surgical intervention. No isolated lower root injuries without injury to the upper roots were found.

Postoperative Care

The postoperative care is essentially that for the adult except that the infant is placed into his clam-shell splint for approximately three weeks. Exercises aimed at maintaining good shoulder external rotation and abduction, elbow extension, and forearm rotation are initiated at three weeks.

Results of Surgery

The results of surgery must be categorized according to the severity of the initial presentation and surgical findings. Table 23-5 outlines the results following reconstruction in subtotal palsy in the largest series published to date. These results indicate that two-thirds of the operated group achieved a more functional shoulder than if they been allowed to evolve spontaneously. Reconstruction of the infant plexus also seems to result in improved growth of the affected limb, but not to normal. Too few cases of total palsy are available for review; however, in contrast to the adult situation, where neurotization of muscles of the hand has almost been abandoned, in the infant it is possible in more than 50% of cases to recover some intrinsic muscle activity and in 90%, some active digital flexion is obtained. When compared to the group allowed to evolve spontaneously, the results of surgery are fundamentally improved. These hands are functional and are used.

Summary

- The typical palsy is a traumatic traction injury caused by forced lowering of the shoulder during delivery.

- While the lesion may affect all roots, the upper roots are usually ruptured while lower roots are frequently avulsed.

Table 23-5. Surgical results in subtotal obstetrical palsy shoulder function

Rupture C-5, G*	two years p.o.	50% Level IV or V
	five years p.o.	70% Level IV or V
Rupture C-5,6,7#	two years p.o.	35% Level IV or V
	five years p.o.	45% Level IV or V

* In contrast, in a control group of babies allowed to evolve spontaneously, all achieved shoulder function at the Grade III level; no patient obtained Grade IV or V shoulder function.

\# In the conservatively treated group, the shoulder achieved Grade II in 30% and Grade III in 70%. No patient achieved shoulder function at the Grade IV level.

- Spontaneous recovery is possible but its quality depends greatly on how early recovery begins.
- Microneural reconstruction is always possible, usually by grafting or by neurotization.
- The results of surgery are better than the results of spontaneous evolution in similar injury patterns.
- Palliative treatment of the sequellae of birth palsies is difficult and the results obtained are rarely totally satisfactory.

For these reasons, the initial surgical intervention should be on the plexus itself in those cases meeting the above criteria. It is important to make this decision as quickly as possible before neuroplasticity is diminished and joint contractures have occurred.

Annotated Bibliography

Akasaka Y, Hara T, Takahashi M: Restoration of elbow flexion and wrist extension in brachial plexus paralysis by means of free muscle transplantation innervated by intercostal nerve. *Ann Hand Surg,* 9:341-350, 1990.

Dual free-muscle transfer using rectus femoris and gracilis muscles and innervated by intercostal nerves has been used to restore elbow flexion and wrist extension. If wrist extension is restored, grasping and pinching may be possible through dynamic tenodesis.

Aziz W, Singer RM, Wolff TW: Transfer of the trapezius for flail shoulder after brachial plexus injury. *J Bone Joint Surg,* 72-B:701-704, 1990.

Twenty-five of 27 patients experienced functional gains. This is a good alternative to shoulder fusion.

Bonnel F: Microscopic anatomy of the adult human brachial plexus: an anatomic and histologic basis for microsurgery. *Microsurgery,* 5:107-117, 1984.

One hundred brachial plexi were dissected to determine angular variations of roots. An additional 21 plexi were serially sectioned to determine fascicular histologic organizations. These studies demonstrate the great differences that exist from individual to individual and call into question the reliability of published maps of the plexus as a guide to reconstruction.

Bonney G, Birch R, Jamieson A, Eames R: Experience with vascularized nerve grafts. *Clin Plast Surg,* 11:137, 1984.

The authors report their experience at the Royal National Orthopaedic Hospital in the use of vascularized nerve grafts to reconstruct long defects in total brachial plexus palsy. They typically used the ulnar nerve when C-8 and T-1 were avulsed, reconstructing the upper plexus. They concluded that regeneration seemed more rapid but could demonstrate no significant gain in ultimate functional recovery.

Dumontier C, Gilbert A: Traumatic brachial plexus injuries in children. *Ann Hand Surg,* 9:351-357, 1990.

Twenty children with traumatic brachial plexus injuries were studied and 16 underwent plexus reconstruction. Elbow flexion was regained in all but one, but shoulder and wrist recovery was unpredictable. The chief goal of surgery was restoration of elbow flexion and hand sensation. Surgery is indicated if there is no recovery within three months.

Gilbert A, Razaboni R: Indications and results of brachial plexus surgery in obstetrical palsy. *Orthop Clin North Am,* 19:91, 1988.

Gilbert has by far the largest experience in the surgical management of obstetrical palsy. The article discusses his philosophy regarding patient selection, timing of surgery, surgical techniques, and preliminary results.

Kanaya F, Gonzalez M, Park C-M, Kutz JE, Kleinert HE, Tsai T-M: *J Hand Surg,* 15A:30-36, 1990.

Fifty-two patients were assessed more than two years following nerve grafting, neurolysis, and nerve transfer. Overall results were good in 58% of cases, fair in 15%, and poor in 27%. Nerve grafting was more successful than nerve transfer. Best results were obtained by operating within three months of injury.

Kline DG: Civilian gunshot wounds to the brachial plexus. *J Neurosurg,* 70:16G-174, 1989.

Many patients with gunshot wounds to the plexus do not improve with time. The major indication for surgery was persistent complete loss of function (on average 17 weeks after injury) in the distribution of one or more elements. Intraoperative electrical testing of neuroma incontinuity was helpful in determining the need for resection and repair or grafting. The best recovery was obtained in upper trunk and lateral and posterior cord injuries.

Leffert RD: Clinical diagnosis, testing, and electromyographic study in brachial plexus traction injuries. *Orthop Clin North Am,* 237:24-31, 1988.

A comprehensive and coordinated plan for evaluating a patient with a traction injury of the plexus is presented.

Millesi H: Surgical management of brachial plexus injuries. *J Hand Surg,* 55:367-379, 1977.

Millesi reports his results in 56 patients with either complete or partial lesions. Examination of the results showed that 38 of 54 (70%) recovered a useful motor function in at least one important area.

Narakas A: Brachial plexus surgery. *Orthop Clin North Am,* 12:303-323,1981

Narakas discusses his clinical experience with 800 cases of brachial palsy. More than 300 patients underwent operation. Indications for early surgery include high-energy injuries, especially with complete palsy. The surgical approach includes a complete exposure of the supraclavicular and infraclavicular plexus. Repair includes nerve grafting, nerve transfer, and neurolysis. In the 100 grafted cases, useful results were obtained in 64% of proximal lesions and 73% of distal lesions.

Sedel L: The results of surgical repair of brachial plexus injuries. *J Bone Joint Surg,* 64-B:54-66, 1982.

Of 139 patients operated on for traumatic brachial plexus injuries, 32 patients with complete palsy had been followed for at least three years and 31 with partial palsies for two years. Repair techniques included nerve grafting, direct repair, nerve transfer, and occasionally, neurolysis. In no case was the lesion made worse by operation. Of the cases with total palsy, 22 of 26 had some improvement but of limited functional value, and four were failures. The results for partial palsy were better. When these groups were compared to 49 cases treated nonoperatively, operation gave more useful results, especially if at least two roots can be used for grafting.

Thomas DGT, Sheehy JPR: Dorsal root entry zone lesions for pain relief following brachial plexus avulsion. *J Neurol Neurosurg Psych,* 46:924-928, 1983.

In 19 patients with severe pain following avulsion injuries of the brachial plexus, 16 experienced some degree of pain relief following DREZ lesions.

Zancolli EA: Classification and management of the shoulder in birth palsy. *Orthop Clin North Am,* 12:433-457, 1981.

Zancolli identifies a larger group of children with post-plexus palsy shoulder joint contractures and a much smaller population with flaccid palsy of the shoulder. He subcategorizes the former group according to the type of contracture, with or without joint deformity or dislocation, and discusses methods to correct the deformity.

24

Painful Upper Extremity

L. Andrew Koman, MD

Physiology of Pain

Pain is defined as an unpleasant sensory and perceptual (emotional) experience associated with actual or incipient (potential) cellular damage. The perception of pain intensity is complex and depends upon the mechanism of the initiating event; the afferent information transmitted; efferent modulation; and central nervous system interpretation of these data. Conscious pain is dependent, in part, on the balance of afferent and efferent mechanisms and individual physiologic capacity to modulate acute and chronic "painful" events. Painful (nociceptive) information is triggered in the periphery by cellular insult or injury. The injury and secondary inflammatory response activate polymodal afferent neurons—pain receptors—which relay information through peripheral nerves to the spinal cord and then to higher centers.

Nociceptors

Terminal polymodal nociceptors may be activated by mechanical, thermal, chemical, or ischemic events. The mechanism of this information exchange (Fig. 24-1) is an incompletely understood physiologic process (transduction) in which painful or noxious stimuli are converted to neural impulses for transmission through peripheral nerves to higher levels. Nociceptive information is transmitted through peripheral nerves primarily in small myelinated (A-Δ) and small unmyelinated (C) afferent peripheral nerve fibers. The response of nociceptor terminal neurons is related

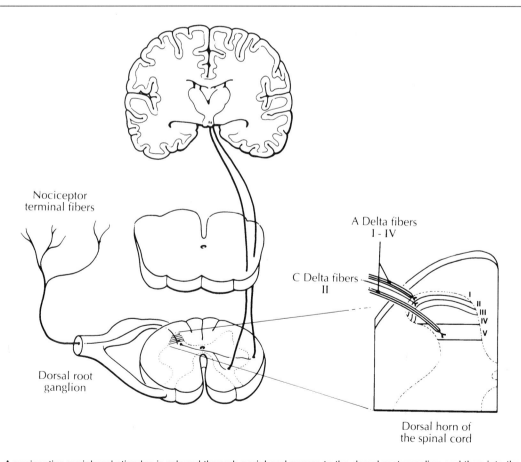

Figure 24-1. A nociceptive peripheral stimulus is relayed through peripheral nerves to the dorsal root ganglion and then into the dorsal horn of the spinal cord.

to the magnitude, duration, and frequency of repetition of the noxious insult. Nociceptors may be sensitized by repetitive stimuli; chemical mediators released by injured cells (eg histamine); or locally synthesized enzyme(s) (eg prostaglandins). Once stimulated, nociceptors may release transmission-enhancing material(s), such as substance P.

Afferent nociceptive information then is relayed through peripheral nerves to the dorsal root ganglia and then into the dorsal horn of the spinal cord, which has five anatomic divisions (I through V). Unmyelinated presynaptic afferent (C) fibers terminate in the substantia gelantinosa (Level II) and myelinated (A-Δ) presynaptic fibers enter Levels I and V. Postsynaptic Level II fibers modulate Levels I and V. From the dorsal horn afferent information crosses to the spinothalamic tract, which ascends in the anterolateral quadrant of the spinal cord to brain stem and thalamic nuclei (Fig. 24-2).

Descending Pathways

Nociceptive pain is modulated by descending pathways from the cerebral cortex, brain stem, and spinal cord. The mechanisms of cortical modulation are not completely understood, but descending pathways include the periaqueductal gray region of the midbrain, the nucleus raphe magnus of the medulla, and the dorsal horn of the spinal cord.

Pain also is modulated by endogenously produced neuropeptides (eg neurotensin), beta endorphins, and dynorphins.

Perception of Pain

Conscious perception of pain is a complex event. Activation of the nociceptive pathways is necessary, but cortical interpretation (nociceptive information) as "pain" is dependent on a complex interplay of individual physiologic events and psychological factors. The cortical (central nervous system) perception of nociceptive information is an important protective mechanism. Polymodal nociceptor activity is important in the inflammatory process through three modes of action. First, evoked pain signals the initiation of injury and simultaneously stimulates endogenous inflammatory mediators. Second, repetitive sensitization initiates these protective responses in an earlier time frame with repetitive injury. Third, nociceptors, by direct release of peptides and neuromodulators, affect the inflammatory process and promote tissue repair.

Chemical and Neurogenic Mediation of Pain

There are both nonneurogenic and neurogenic mediators that, when endogenously released, participate in the transmission of information received consciously as pain (Fig. 24-3).

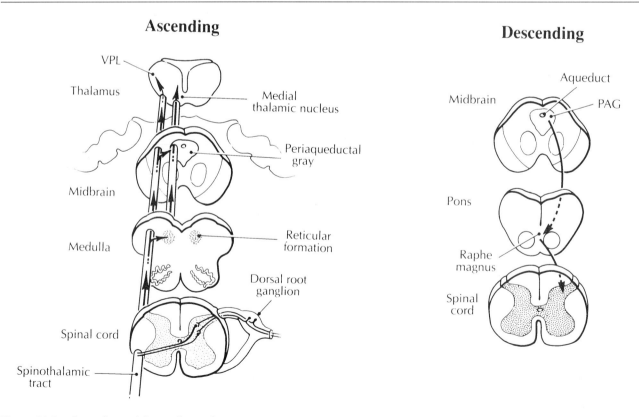

Ascending   ## Descending

Figure 24-2.   Ascending and descending pathways.

Nonneurogenic
  Bradykinin
  Serotonin
  Histamine
  Acetylcholine
  Prostaglandins E_1 and E_2
  Leukotrienes
  Norepinephrine
Neurogenic
  N-methyl-D aspartic acid (NMDA)
  Substance P
  Vasoactive intestinal peptide (VIP)
  Calcitonin gene-related peptide (CGRP)
  Gastrin-releasing peptide
  Dynorphin
  Enkephalin
  Galanin
  Somatostatin
  Cholecystokinin-like substance
Interneural
  Gamma aminobutyric acid (GABA)
  Dopamine
  Glycine

Figure 24-3. Physiologic Mediators of Pain

Nonneurogenic pain mediators include bradykinin, serotonin, histamine, acetylcholine, prostaglandins E1 and E2, and leukotrienes. Neurogenic pain mediators include neuropeptides produced in primary afferent neurons such as substance P, vasoactive intestinal peptide, calcitonin gene-related peptide, gastrin-releasing peptide, dynorphin, enkephalin, galanin, somatostatin, and a cholecystokinin-like substance. In addition, there are mediators in the interneural connections that inhibit sensations, including gamma aminobutyric acid, dopamine, and glycine. These biologically active peptides are produced by primary afferent neurons, and additional factors continue to be discovered.

Gate Theory of Pain

The "gate theory," a dynamic yet unproven theorem developed by Melzack and Wall, is an appropriate aid in the conceptualization of pain. The "gate" is the dorsal horn of the spinal cord, and the volume of peripheral information received at cortical levels is assumed to be finite. Thus, "painful" information either can be displaced or modified by less noxious data or can be modulated at the "gate" level. Although an oversimplification, the gate theory aids in the conceptualization of the pain process.

Pain Syndromes

Pain is a protective mechanism and the complete absence of pain can lead to inadvertent severe tissue damage and destruction, as seen following spinal cord injury or peripheral nerve injury. However, pain that persists after tissue damage has stabilized and/or healed, or pain that is out of proportion to the tissue insult is disruptive and may severely interfere with function.

Acute pain occurs in the presence of tissue damage and its intensity is related to the magnitude and duration of the

Pain—an unpleasant perception associated with actual or potential cellular damage.
Analgesia—absence of pain in response to an insult that should produce pain.
Nociception—response to an unpleasant (noxious) stimulus that would produce pain in a human subject under normal circumstances.
Allodynia—pain associated with light touch to skin of affected area.
Hyperalgesia—an exaggerated painful response to a painful stimulus.
Hyperesthesia—increased sensitivity (pain in response to a mild, nonnoxious stimulus).
Sympathetic—pain in presence of and associated with maintained pain sympathetic dysfunction.

Figure 24-4. Pain Definitions

noxious insult. Chronic pain is pain that persists past an arbitrary three-to-six-month interval and continues in the absence of ongoing tissue damage or threat. Chronic pain can include neuropathic or mechanical components. However, persistent pain secondary to ongoing mechanical damage (eg torn triangular fibrocartilage) generally involves ongoing tissue damage or inflammation. Symptoms of chronic neurotrophic pain include allodynia, hyperalgesia, and hyperesthesia, and may be sympathetically maintained or nonsympathetically maintained (Fig. 24-4). Following injury, it is normal and physiologic to experience pain. It is abnormal to have pain out of proportion to mechanical injury or pain that persists after cellular recovery or repair.

Acute Pain—Pathophysiology

In the normal state, there is an acute and conscious awareness of pain after tissue injury. Normal (physiologic) perception of pain requires sensory discrimination carried by myelinated A-Δ, A-r fibers; and affective-motivational awareness conducted via peripheral unmyelinated C-fibers. The acute pain response after injury may be beneficial or harmful. Beneficial effects include maintenance of blood pressure, cardiac output and intravascular volume, and improved hemostasis; acute pain also immobilizes the injured extremity and thus prevents additional contact or repetition. The persistence of these protective pain responses may be adverse and induce hypertension, tachycardia, hypercoagulable states, hyperglycemia, hypervolemia, anxiety, fear, and chronic pain states. For acute pain to be physiologic, it must be protective; appropriate in intensity; and of reasonable duration. Thus, the intensity and duration of a painful response must reflect the physiologic damage.

Chronic Pain—Pathophysiology

Chronic pain persists in the absence of ongoing tissue destruction or inappropriately reflects ongoing tissue damage in terms of intensity, magnitude, and duration. The pathophysiology is not completely understood and may involve persistent mechanical irritation of peripheral mechanical and/or neural structures, incomplete reinnervation of peripheral nerves (ie neuroma or neuroma-in-continuity), abnormal neural transmitter activity (ie. sympathetically maintained pain), or dystrophic responses.

Neuromas

The formation of a neuroma is a normal peripheral nerve response to interruption of fascicular topography. Following axonal interruption and Wallerian degeneration of a nerve containing sensory fibers, axonal regeneration, stimulated by target-derived neurotrophic factors, is initiated and may result in successful reinnervation if the distal endoneural tissue (nerve stump) is reached. If no distal endoneural tube is available, a disorganized mass of neurons, fibroblasts, connective tissue, etc.—the neuroma—is formed. The proliferative response of the distal stump (the glioma) is less pronounced and rarely painful. The three Sunderland subgroups of neural injury that are most frequently complicated by pain syndromes are neuroma incontinuity, posttransection neuroma, and amputation stump neuroma. Fortunately, the percentage of painful neuromas following injury is small.

The size of a neuroma is multifaceted and depends on the distance from the anterior horn cells, the percentage of connective tissue in the injured nerve, and the age of the patient. The etiology of excessive pain associated with neuromas is poorly understood and unpredictable. However, it is known that neuromas are sensitive to local irritation and mechanical deformation (pressure), and may generate spontaneous action potentials that contribute to nociceptive activity. Thus, neuromas may provide a mechanical and/or chemical trigger of nociceptive pain.

A neuroma incontinuity occurs after an incomplete nerve injury with untransected neurons adjacent to or surrounding the neuroma. Neuromas of completely severed nerves include those of unrepaired and separated peripheral nerve transections and amputation stump neuromas. In both instances, pain and impaired function may be intensified by scarred surroundings and the vulnerable position of the neuroma.

The diagnosis of neuroma is based primarily on history and physical examination. Usually, a history of blunt or open trauma is present. Symptoms include dysesthesia, hyperalgesia, burning pain, and a specific area of point tenderness—often masked by diffuse dystrophic symptoms. Signs include a palpable mass (trigger point), positive percussion test (Tinel's sign), and response to local injection with neural blocking agents (eg lidocaine).

Treatment depends on the location and type of neuroma. If a dystrophic response is present, this should be treated simultaneously with the neuroma. Often, the dystrophy (Outline 24-1) will require management before the extent of pain secondary to the neuroma can be determined fully.

Nonoperative treatments include oral medications, desensitization, transcutaneous nerve stimulation, and local or regional injections. Often, a combination of these techniques is effective. If nonoperative treatment fails, surgical intervention is indicated. Management techniques (Outline 24-1) include alteration of the proximal nerve or neuroma by physical or chemical methods, alteration of the neuroma's environment by rerouting or relocating the neuroma, modification of the environment, nerve repair, nerve wrap, or implanted nerve stimulators. Often, a combination of two or more of these methods is employed. Stump neuromas are not amenable to end-to-end repair or nerve grafting. The management of a neuroma incontinuity requires a patient-oriented approach, which must factor in the specific nerve involved, the extent of the neuroma, the location of the injury, and the functional impairment related to pain as opposed to nerve injury. Painful neuromas incontinuity involving mixed motor-sensory nerves (eg, median nerve in forearm with intact fascicles providing innervation to thenar intrinsics and thumb sensory dermatomes) have a significant risk of functional loss if internal dissection and nerve grafting are performed. The alternative is acceptance of the neural deficit and management of the pain by nonsurgical or surgical means. The choice between nonsurgical pain management and surgical attempts to restore neural function and relieve pain often is difficult, and management of the neuroma incontinuity remains controversial.

Outline 24-1. Management of Painful Neuroma

I. Nonoperative
  A. Oral medications
  B. Desensitization
  C. TENS unit
  D. Local injections
II. Operative
  A. Alteration of proximal nerve
    1. Physical—crush, cauterization
    2. Proximal ligation
    3. Epineural ligation
    4. Capping
  B. Neural rerouting
    1. Neurocampsis
    2. Cross-union
    3. Centrocentral anastomosis
  C. Relocation
    1. Muscle implantation
    2. Bone implantation
  D. Environmental modification
    1. Muscle flap
    2. Skin flap
    3. Vein wrap
  E. Nerve repair
    1. End to end
    2. Nerve graft
    3. Nerve to vein
  F. Nerve wrap
  G. Nerve stimulator-implanted

Reflex Sympathetic Dystrophy

Reflex sympathetic dystrophy is a complex clinical disorder that has undefined pathophysiologic criteria. Therefore, the body of medical literature concerning RSD is confusing and contradictory. The most common synonyms include causalgia, from the Greek for "burning pain" following an unrepaired vascular lesion and a partial injury to a major peripheral nerve; Sudek's atrophy, based on the roentgenographic findings of osteoporosis associated with later-stage dystrophies; and sympathetically mediated (or maintained) pain, reflecting a sympathetic autonomic dysfunction.

Altered extremity physiology after trauma mediated by local neural and/or central factors is a normal response. However, these normal responses may become abnormally prolonged and may involve complex pathophysiologic abnormalities in extremity physiology. Over time, irreversible changes in end-organ anatomy may occur. Thus, RSD is an abnormally severe and prolonged manifestation of a normal postinjury response. Clinical manifestations include pain out of proportion to the identifiable injury, diminished function, stiffness, and trophic changes. Burning pain and restlessness may be the earliest symptoms. Reflex sympathetic dystrophy, as described by the International Association for the Study of Pain Taxonomy, is a descriptive term referring to a complex disorder or group of disorders that may develop as a consequence of trauma affecting an area of the body with or without obvious nerve lesion(s). It consists of pain and related abnormalities of one or more of the following: sensation, blood flow, thermoregulation (sweating), motor systems, extremity anatomy, and/or physiology (trophic changes). All components need not be present.

Reflex sympathetic dystrophy is a dynamic physiologic process that may vary in time, course, and intensity. Due to the variability of extremity adaptation, peripheral and central nervous system modulation, and alterations in natural history secondary to partial treatment, the presentation may be misleading. Furthermore, RSD has no agreed upon objective marker; no single test—including technetium bone scan—is pathognomonic for the process. Thus, the natural history of RSD has been based upon arbitrary staging and grading systems defined by time or clinical signs and/or symptoms.

Following trauma or surgery, a transient period of dystrophic extremity function is normal. Persistence of hyperpathia (increased pain), allodynia (painful response to a normally nonpainful stimulus), vasomotor disturbances, and functional deficits are not normal, and if untreated, may progress to permanent compromise of the extremity. Thus, a normal process becomes a dystrophic cycle produced and/or encouraged by peripheral mechanisms and central abnormalities. Initiation of the process is peripheral and involves local factors and neurovascular responses. Over time, central mechanisms play a more important role. A normal reflex arc may be activated by a painful stimulus and then perpetuated by local factors (eg, substance P), abnormal nociceptor activity by alpha adrenoreceptors (eg, sympathetically maintained component), the formation of ectopic pacemakers, and exaggerated and/or persistent central factors (eg abnormal activity of spinal-cord level, wide dynamic-range neurons, or abnormal higher-level modulation mechanisms).

Reflex sympathetic dystrophy most commonly involves patients between the ages of 30 and 50, but patients of any age may be affected. Women are more frequently affected than men (4:1). Specific mechanical trauma is identifiable in fewer than 50% of cases. The most common associated injury historically is fracture of the distal radius or ulna. In the upper extremity, RSD and dystrophic responses may be seen in conjunction with

- injury of the palmar cutaneous branch of the median nerve (during carpal tunnel release);
- injury of the superficial branch of the radial nerve (during de Quervain's release);
- injury of the dorsal branch of the radial nerve (during resection of the distal ulna); and
- simultaneous carpal tunnel release and resection of palmar fascia from Dupuytren's disease.

Early treatment of RSD is the most important variable in predicting pain relief and functional recovery. Eighty percent of patients treated within one year of injury show significant improvement, while fewer than 50% of those treated after one year will improve significantly. Thus, early diagnosis and prompt, appropriate, therapeutic intervention are the most important prognostic factors for successful recovery.

The diagnosis of RSD is based upon clinical findings of pain, trophic changes, vasomotor or anatomic dysfunction, and functional impairment. Since there are no defined physiologic abnormalities, more than one pathologic entity may be involved. Since irreversible changes in extremity anatomy and/or physiology may occur over time, the objective findings may vary in spite of a constant cause (diagnosis). Objective testing provides important insight into physiologic events and may support clinical impressions. Bone scans have been used and provide a 75% to 98% specificity and a 50% to 90% sensitivity. Objective measurements of vasomotor and thermoregulatory capacity also are useful and allow specific physiologic staging.

Laboratory tests are useful in establishing a diagnosis of RSD and in providing objective baseline measurements of thermoregulatory and vasomotor control. Objective measures that appear to be useful in the evaluation of RSD include

- plain radiographs;
- three-phase bone scans;
- estimation of vasomotor or thermoregulatory capacity;
- endurance testing; and
- evaluation of nutritional flow.

However, it must be remembered that no single existing laboratory test is diagnostic of RSD.

Radiographic evaluation of RSD typically shows diffuse, patchy osteopenia, which is periarticular initially and then becomes diffuse (Sudeck's atrophy). Osteopenia is not a prerequisite for the diagnosis of RSD; 20% of patients with definite RSD have been found to be without bony resorption by radiographs, and similar radiographic findings may be seen after prolonged immobilization, hyperparathyroidism, thyrotoxicosis, and any condition with increased turnover of trabecular bone. Five patterns of resorption have been described by Genant and associates: (1) irregular resorption of trabecular bone in the metaphysis, creating a patchy appearance; (2) subperiosteal bone resorption; (3) intercortical bone resorption; (4) endosteal bone resorption; and

(5) surface erosions in the subchondral and juxtachondral bone.

Three-phase Radionuclide Bone Scan

Three-phase bone scan analysis has assumed an important role in the assessment of RSD, although the positive predictive value of three-phase technetium bone scanning has been questioned because of the variable autonomic activity that occurs during the course of RSD. The suggested requirement that the third-phase bone scan be positive in order to verify RSD does not address a physiologic mechanism, limits the diagnosis, and does not necessarily correlate with clinical symptoms. Current data supports the specificity of the bone scan in the diagnosis of RSD (75% to 98%), but suggests insufficient sensitivity (50% or less) for it to be used as an isolated definitive study. The role of the bone scan in variant forms of RSD has not been evaluated. Overall, bone scans of the upper extremity do not correlate with existing staging criteria for RSD, do not predict recovery, and have no demonstrable prognostic implications.

Quantitative and qualitative evaluation of peripheral autonomic regulation and physiologic estimations of microcirculatory function provide valuable information. The extent of upper extremity microcirculatory abnormalities associated with RSD require evaluation of both thermoregulatory and nutritional components of total flow. In the normal state, total flow is primarily thermoregulatory (80% to 95%) and nutritional (5% to 20%). Evidence suggests significantly abnormal changes in nutritional flow in many patients with clinical RSD, and the ability to monitor quantitative extremity blood flow and differentiate nutritional from thermoregulatory flow has diagnostic significance. Control of extremity flow is a dynamic process and requires stress to be evaluated fully. Static evaluations of microcirculatory function may be misleading and confusing. Any form of stress—heat, psychological, emotional, ischemia—may be employed. Testing involving monitoring by temperature, laser Doppler fluxmetry, and vital capillaroscopy continues to be evaluated and provides objective data for analysis.

Relief of symptoms following interventions that diminish sympathetic activity (eg, stellate ganglion block) provides support for the clinical diagnosis. Diminished pain during an intravenous infusion of phentolamine (an a_1 and a_2 blocking agent) is presumptive evidence of a sympathetically maintained component of RSD. Relief of symptoms after stellate ganglion block is highly supportive of the clinical diagnosis of RSD.

The treatment of RSD is controversial and difficult to evaluate in the absence of a complete understanding of its pathophysiology. In general, a combination of interventions is necessary. Treatment options include physical (occupational) therapy (Fig. 24-5), non-injectable pharmacologic agents (Table 24-1), injectable pharmacologic agents (Table 24-2), surgical or ablative intervention (Fig. 24-6), and physiological interventions (i.e. biofeedback).

Physical (occupational) therapy
Active/passive range of motion
Stress loading
Contrast baths
Continuous passive motion

Figure 24-5. RSD Management Options: Non-pharmacological

Table 24-1. RSD Management Options: Non-injectable Pharmacologic Agents

Medication	Method of Administration
Amitriptyline hydrochloride (Elavil®)	Oral
Phenytoin (Dilantin®)	Oral
Phenoxybenzamine hydrochloride (Dibenzyline®)	Oral
Nifedipine (Procardia®)	Oral
Corticosteroids	Oral
Carbamazepine (Tegretol®)	Oral
Clonidine (Catapres-TTS® -2, -3)	Patch

Table 24-2. RSD Management Options: Injectable Pharmacologic Agents

Medication	Most Common Method of Administration
Guanethidine sulfate	IV regional
Clonidine	Continuous epidural
Phentolamine (Regitine®)	IV injection
Cortisone sulfate (usually with lidocaine)	IV regional
Reserpine	IV regional
Brytilium	IV regional

Neurolytic blockade
  Percutaneous ethanol (alcohol)
Surgical sympathectomy
  Cervicothoracic
Neurosurgical procedures
  Dorsal column stimulators
  Thalamic stimulators
  Periventricular gray matter stimulators
  Cingulotomy
  Peripheral nerve stimulators

Figure 24-6. RSD Management Options: Invasive Procedures

Annotated Bibliography

Genant HK, Kozin F, Bekerman C, McCarty DJ, Sim T: The reflex sympathetic dystrophy syndrome. A comprehensive analysis using fine-detail radiography, photon absorptionmetry, and bone and joint scintigraphy. *Radiology,* 117:21-32, 1975.

Excellent descriptions of the radiographic findings in RSD.

Gould JS: Treatment of the painful injured nerve-in-continuity. In: Gelberman RH, (ed) *Operative Nerve Repair and Reconstruction.* JB Lippincott, pp. 1541-1550, New York, 1991.

An excellent discussion of the management of the painful incomplete nerve injury.

Kozin F, Soin JS, Ryan LM, Carrera GF, Wortmann RL: Bone scintigraphy in the reflex sympathetic dystrophy syndrome. *Radiology,* 138:437-443, 1981.

Problems in specificity and sensitivity of bone scanning are outlined in this classic paper.

Mackinnon SE, Holder LE: The use of three-phase radionuclide bone scanning in the diagnosis of reflex sympathetic dystrophy. *J Hand Surg,* 9A:556-563, 1984.

A retrospective analysis of patients having undergone three-phase bone scan with a diagnosis of reflex sympathetic dystrophy. This study shows a high sensitivity and specificity for three-phase bone scanning.

Melzack R, Wall PD: Pain mechanisms: a new theory. *Science,* 150:971-979, 1965.

The classic article on pain.

Pollock FE Jr, Koman LA, Smith BP, Poehling GG: Patterns of microvascular response associated with reflex sympathetic dystrophy of the hand and wrist. *J Hand Surg,* 18A:847-852, 1993.

This study demonstrates that a positive technetium bone scan does not correlate with vasomotor disturbances in RSD patients.

Tupper JW, Booth DM: Treatment of painful neuromas of sensory nerves in the hand: a comparison of traditional and newer methods. *J Hand Surg,* 1:144-151, 1976.

Comparison of different methods of treating painful neuromas.

Watson HK, Carlson L: Treatment of reflex sympathetic dystrophy of the hand with an active "stress loading" program. *J Hand Surg,* 12A:779-785, 1987.

A report of successful treatment using a stress loading program on patients with early sympathetic dystrophy. Results and long-term follow-up of 41 patients treated with stress loading program.

Wilder RT, Berde CB, Wolohan M, Vieyra MA, Masek BJ, Micheli LJ: Reflex sympathetic dystrophy in children. Clinical characteristics and follow-up of seventy patients. *J Bone Joint Surg,* 76A:910-919, 1992.

Seventy patients under 18 years of age are presented. The differences in the clinical course of RSD in children vs. adults are outlined. The prognosis for complete relief of symptoms, in spite of a multidisciplinary treatment approach, is poor with 38 of 70 manifesting residual pain and dysfunction at follow-up.

VI
Skin and Soft Tissue

25

Physiology of Wound Repair

Elof Eriksson, MD

Introduction

The process of wound repair is the single most important physiologic or pathophysiologic event for a surgeon. Successful surgical procedures are based on predictable and uncomplicated repair. Wound healing has been the target of studies for several thousand years (for review see Brown). Triggered in particular by Stanley Cohen's discovery of epidermal growth factor, and by Howard Green's developments in keratinocyte culturing techniques, there has been a surge of interest in peptide growth factors. A great deal of this interest has been proprietary or commercial, but it has resulted in a renewed research focus on the process of wound repair. Currently, several dozen peptides, other molecules, dressings, and devices are claimed to promote wound repair, based on many experimental and a few clinical studies. In the author's opinion, few of these, if any, have reached a level where they can be recommended for clinical use without reservation. However, many of the suggested treatment modalities are promising, and it is possible and even likely that our wound-treatment practices will change when we have gathered more documentation. Even if nothing is dramatically new in the physiology of the wound-repair process, the understanding of the details has become much more sophisticated.

Wounding

There is little doubt that the degree of systemic reaction to wounding is proportional to the degree of trauma. The best example of this is perhaps a burn; a minor burn has minimal systemic consequences, while a major burn has a catastrophic systemic impact. It appears that similar reasoning can be applied at the local level. Minimal surgical trauma with sharp instruments and delicate technique causes less local necrosis and inflammatory changes. This in turn leads to lesser aberrations in the healing process. It is attractive to speculate that the whole repair process is programmed at the time of wounding. It can be modified by later events, but only to a limited degree. It should also be pointed out that initial trauma from, for instance, a burn or an abrasion, can be increased by letting the wound desiccate. The injury can also be worsened by the use of cytotoxic agents, such as hydrogen peroxide. In a philosophical sense, the wound could be viewed as a tissue culture and the dressing as part of an incubator. It then becomes natural to avoid exposing the wound to any cytotoxic agent. Wounding triggers the subsequent events leading to repair (Fig. 25-1).

Hemostasis

A severed blood vessel constricts and the coagulation cascade is activated. Platelets adhere to the walls of the vessels at the site of injury as well as to themselves, and form a platelet thrombus. The intrinsic and extrinsic coagulation cascades are activated, resulting in the formation of fibrin. Fibronectin, as well as platelets and red cells, are added to the fibrin network to form a clot which prevents the further loss of blood from the severed vessel.

Inflammation

The inflammatory response is initiated by the trauma and starts instantaneously. The local signs are edema, redness, increased tissue temperature, and pain. Neutrophils, lymphocytes, and macrophages are attracted to the area of injury; they adhere to the walls of venules, emigrate through these venules into the tissue where they migrate to phagocytose microorganisms, foreign bodies, and necrotic tissue. In the process they release a number of enzymes and cytokines, which further activate the inflammatory process, as well as the early phases of healing.

There are numerous mediators involved in the inflammatory response. Epinephrine and norepinephrine are secreted in increased amounts immediately after trauma. Free oxygen radicals, histamine, kinins, serotonin, prostaglandin, and complement are released. They appear to be the main cause of edema by means of vasodilation and increased permeability. The amount of edema formed usually peaks in 24 hours. As the same cells and many mediators are involved in both the inflammatory process and the early repair, there is an almost imperceivable evolution from inflammatory changes to changes that make the wound heal.

The inflammatory process has several regulatory pathways and so does early wound repair. The most conspicuous regulatory cell in the early wound-repair process is the macrophage. However, most cells that participate in hemostasis (particularly platelets) and inflammation seem to have some function in initiating and regulating the early wound-repair process. The same is true for fibroblasts and epithelial cells already in the wound. Through the secretion of various peptides that have the ability to work in either an autocrine, paracrine, or endocrine fashion, these cells have the potential to initiate and regulate the wound-healing events.

The Normal Wound Healing Response

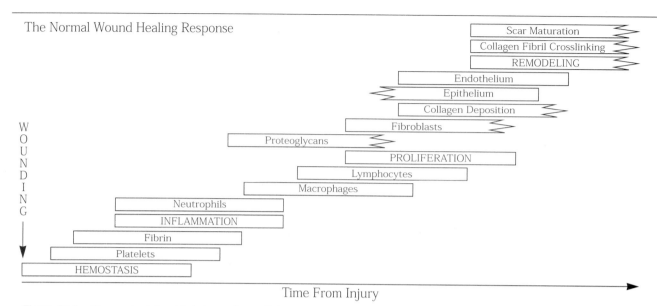

Figure 25-1. Temporal relationship between the multiple processes occurring in dermal wound healing. Reproduced with permission from Mast BA: The skin. In Cohen IK, *Wound Healing—Biochemical and Clinical Aspects*, p. 347, Saunders, Philadelphia, 1992.

Angiogenesis

Effective diffusion distances in the human body rarely exceed 50 microns, and therefore every repair process has to be paralleled by the formation of new blood vessels. Experimental studies have shown that arterioles and venules form solid sprouts into the regenerating wound (Fig. 25-2). These sprouts canalize and connect with other sprouts or vessels. If a graft is revascularized, for instance, it appears that these sprouts connect with existing vascular channels within the graft (inosculation). Many factors seem to stimulate angiogenesis, particularly heparin-binding growth factors such as the ones belonging to the fibroblast growth-factor family. It appears that in favorable circumstances, regenerating vessels can advance by a speed of approximately 1mm per day.

Wound Repair

The discussion deals with epidermal repair and dermal repair. In a partial-thickness wound, re-epithelialization constitutes a major portion of the healing process. In the incisional wound or the full-thickness wound, re-epithelialization becomes a much smaller portion of the changes during repair. In these latter cases, matrix deposition and wound contraction are more prominent events.

Epidermal Repair

Within 24 hours after injury, epithelial repair begins (Fig. 25-3). Epithelial cells from the basal layer of the edge of the wound or from epidermal appendages at the bottom of the wound begin migrating into the area which is denuded of

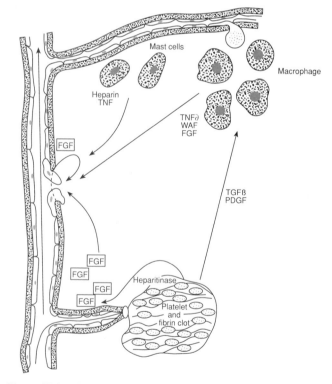

Figure 25-2. Some of the cells that can affect wound healing angiogenesis. TNF∂ = tumor necrosis factor-∂; WAF = wound angiogenesis factor; FGF = fibroblast growth factor; TGFβ = transforming growth factor-β; PDGF = platelet-derived growth factor. Reproduced with permission from Whalen GF, Zetter BR: In Cohen IK, *Wound Healing—Biochemical and Clinical Aspects*, p. 87, Saunders, Philadelphia, 1992.

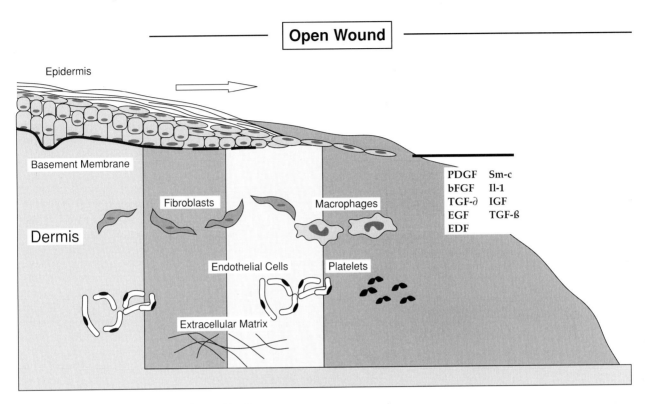

Figure 25-3.   Growth factors in epidermal wound healing.

epithelium. These cells begin dividing and populate the wound surface by epibolic cell migration (as the most proposed mechanism) with a monolayer of cells at the leading edge. This process continues until the entire wound is covered with several layers of epithelial cells. If epithelial cells can migrate on top of an intact basement membrane, regeneration is quicker if this is absent. Without the presence of a basement membrane, epidermal cells migrate on provisional matrix elements, such as Types I, III, or IV collagen, fibronectin, laminin, or vitronectin. During mitosis and migration, epithelial cells also produce the constituents of the new basement membrane (laminin, collagen Type IV). Fibronectin and epibolin also serve as stimulators of epithelial cell migration. When the epithelial cells have repopulated the surface, they differentiate into cell layers that have an appearance similar to the various layers of the intact epidermis.

Several growth factors seem to stimulate epithelialization. Epidermal growth factor, platelet-derived growth factor, and transforming growth factor-alpha, are most commonly mentioned (compare Fig. 25-3).

Dermal Repair

The dermis contains several cell types and a number of matrix components (Fig. 25-3). The most prominent cell is

the fibroblast. Fibroblasts are seen migrating and dividing in the dermal component of the wound. This coincides with angiogenesis in the same area. The migration and mitosis of fibroblasts are stimulated by a number of factors: TGF-beta, EGF, thrombin, PDGF, fibronectin, various lymphokines, complement, several peptide growth factors, and collagen are some of them.

The fibroblasts divide and are the dominating long-term cell type in the wound. Within days after wounding, these fibroblasts begin to produce various proteins and proteoglycans. The most studied protein is collagen (Fig. 25-4), and currently there are at least 13 types of collagen described (Table 25-1). Collagen accounts for the majority of tensile strength in the wound matrix, and it has therefore been studied intensely in relation to the healing of fascia and tendon, where tensile strength is essential. In skin wounds, tensile strength is of lesser importance and early wound strength is usually only important to the degree that it determines when the sutures should be removed. Collagen metabolism is well described in the standard wound healing texts and is therefore not repeated here.

Wound Contraction

All wounds contract to a certain degree, but the phenomenon of contraction is particularly obvious in full-thickness

Collagen Biosynthesis

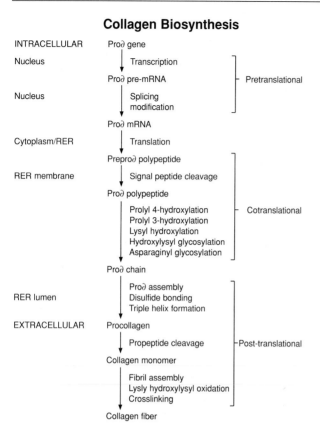

Figure 25-4. Steps in the biosynthesis of a collagen fiber and the location in the cell where they occur. RER = rough endoplasmic reticulum. Reproduced with permission from Wenstrup RJ, Murad S, Pinnell SR: Collagen. In Goldsmith LA (ed): *Biochemistry and Physiology of the Skin,* Second ed, Oxford University Press, New York, in press.

open wounds. The edges are sometimes pulled together at the rate of up to .75mm per day. Usually the process of contraction is only active for approximately two weeks. The degree of contraction is also limited by the tension of the surrounding skin. If surrounding skin tension is high, wound contraction is less pronounced. Wounds in young individuals tend to contract faster than wounds in older individuals.

A popular current theory is that contraction is caused by myofibroblasts. These are cells with a morphology that falls somewhere in between fibroblasts and smooth muscle cells. Myofibroblasts have microfilaments in the cytoplasm and they are most commonly seen in the wound between 10 and 20 days after wounding, which coincides with the maximum speed of wound contraction. They also have the ability to contract *in vitro.* It has not been conclusively shown that myofibroblasts contract *in vivo,* but the theory about their function is still attractive.

Excessive Repair (Scars)

Excessive repair can take place in terms of hypertrophic scars and keloids on the skin surface or as adhesions between deep structures that are not supposed to be connected with the scar. In hand surgery, the most striking example is the healing tendon, which not only forms a scar across the tendon juncture, but also forms scar tissue parallel to the tendon connecting it to the tendon sheath. Attempts to reduce the undesired scarring have included the application of pressure, application or injection of steroids, lathyrogens, and calcium channel blockers.

Up-regulation of Healing

Several factors are necessary for adequate wound healing: adequate circulation, oxygenation, availability of glucose and amino acids, oxygen, various vitamins (particularly vitamin C) and trace elements, particularly zinc. Absence of one or more of these factors will retard wound healing.

Growth factors have been the focus of a large number of studies recently (Table 25-2; Fig. 25-5). Epidermal growth factor, for instance, was found to accelerate epidermal healing. TGF-beta was found to accelerate fibroblast proliferation and collagen secretion. PDGF and TGF-alpha were found to stimulate epithelial healing. Several members of the fibroblast growth factor family have been found to stimulate angiogenesis. Mainly because of the lack of a practical delivery system, the use of growth factors has not reached a level of clinical acceptability yet. For the same reason, it has not been possible to establish *in vivo* dose response curves and a definition of the timing, sequencing, and combination of growth factors in order to achieve optimal results. This area should provide some very interesting results over the years to come.

Growth hormone has been found to speed healing of both incisional wounds and split-thickness skin graft donor sites. Several hormones, particularly the thyroid hormones, have the potential of influencing wound healing. Steroids have significant retarding influence on healing, depending upon the dose and the type of hormone used.

Oxygen has been studied intensively over the past several decades. Attempts have been made to increase rates of healing, both by increasing oxygen concentration and by increasing the atmospheric pressure of oxygen delivered. There is evidence that oxygen suppresses angiogenesis, but stimulates the secretion of collagen.

Several physical modalities have been attempted with a goal of accelerating the healing process, some of the more common being electrical fields, magnetic fields, and ultrasound. In bone, electrical stimulation seems to speed osteogenesis. Typically a low-intensity direct current has been used.

Down-regulation of Healing

In cases of excessive scarring and adhesions, there has been significant interest in trying to down-regulate, or even stop

Table 25-1. Vertebrate Collagen Types

Type	Chain(s)	Locus of Human Gene (Chromosome)*	Major Molecular Species	Distribution	Function
I	α1(I) α2(I)	17 7	[α1(I)$_2$α2(I)]	All connective tissues except hyaline cartilage and basement membranes	Formation of striated supporting elements (fibers) of varying diameter
II	α1(II)	12	[α1(II)]$_3$	Hyaline cartilages and cartilage-like tissues, eg, vitreous humor	Formation of striated supporting elements (fibrils) of generally smaller diameter than type I fibers
III	α1(III)	2	[α1(III)]$_3$	The more distensible connective tissues, eg, blood vessels	Formation of small fibrous elements, similar to type II, but may also form cofibers with type I collagen molecules
IV	α1(IV) α2(IV) α3(IV) α4(IV) α5(IV)	13 13 X	[α1(IV)$_2$α2(IV)]	Basement membranes Glomerular basement membrane	Formation of meshlike scaffold
V	α1(V) α2(V) α3(V)	 2	[α1(V)$_2$α2(V)]	Essentially all tissues	Similar to type III collagen
VI	α1(VI) α2(VI) α3(VI)	21 21 2	[α1(VI),α2(VI),α3(VI)]	Essentially all tissues	Formation of microfibrillar elements
VII	α1(VII)		[α1(VII)]$_3$	Dermal-epidermal junctions	Anchoring fibrils
VIII	α1(VIII) α2(VIII)		Unknown	Descemet's membrane, produced by endothelial cells	Unknown
IX	α1(IX) α2(IX) α3(IX)	6	[α1(IX),α2(IX),α3(IX)]	Hyaline cartilage	Forms coaggregates with type II collagen
X	α1(X)		[α1(X)]$_3$	Hypertrophic cartilage	Unknown
XI	α1(XI) α2(XI) α3(XI)	 6 12	[α1(XI),α2(XI),α1(XI)]	Hyaline cartilage	Unknown, but may form cofibers with type II collagen molecules
XII	α1(XII)		[α1(XII)]$_3$	May be similar to type I collagen	Unknown, but may form coaggregates with type I collagen
XIII	α1(XIII)		Unknown	Synthesized by certain tumor cell lines	Unknown

Reproduced with permission from Miller EJ, Gay S: Collagen Structure and Function. In Cohen IK, *Wound Healing—Biochemical and Clinical Aspects*, p. 132, Saunders, Philadelphia, 1992.

Table 25-2. Molecules of the Wound Environment That May Influence Epidermal Wound Closure

Molecule	Molecular Weight	Source	Action
Basic fibroblast growth factor	18kDa	Keratinocyte, fibroblasts	Stimulates epidural cell growth
Calcium	111 daltons ($CaCl_2$)	Milieux	Stimulates differentiation in high concentration, stimulates proliferation in low concentration
Epidermal growth factor (EGF)	6 kDa Single chain	Salivary gland	Stimulates epidermal cell proliferation
Hypothalamic keratinocyte growth factor	~1.7 kDa	Hypothalamus	Stimulates epidermal cell growth
Interleukin-1	31 kDa	Macrophages, epidermal cells	Stimulates epidermal growth and motility
Platelet-derived growth factor	Dimer of 30-32 kDa and 14-18 kDa	Platelets, endothelium	Stimulates epidermal hyperplasia in combination with EGF
Placental growth factor	Nondialyzable, heat sensitive	Placenta	Enhances keratinocyte growth
Scatter factor	50kDa	Fibroblasts	Stimulates epidermal cell motility
Transforming growth factor-∂	5.6 kDa	Transformed cells, placenta, embryonic tissue	Stimulates epidermal growth
Transforming growth factor-ß	23-25 kDa (two subunits that may combine as TGF-β_1, TGF-β_2, or TGF-$\beta_{1,2}$)	Fibroblasts, platelets	All forms inhibit epidermal cell proliferation but stimulate motility

Reproduced with permission from Stenn KS, Malhorta R: Epithelialization. In Cohen IK, *Wound Healing—Biochemical and Clinical Aspects,* p. 123, Saunders, Philadephia, 1992.

the wound-healing process at a certain stage, usually when adequate tensile strength has been achieved in the structure of interest. Deletions of any of the cells, substrates, enzymes, vitamins, or trace elements that are essential for wound repair result in a reduced rate, or even absence of healing. Smoking, alcoholism, diabetes, connective tissue disease, and conditions with decreased liver and renal function impair the healing process. Therapeutic administration of steroids and chemotherapeutic and immunosuppressive agents also reduce the rate of healing.

Lathyrogens, particularly beta-aminoproprionitrile, are potent inhibitors of collagen cross-linking and have been used to reduce excessive formation of adhesions with some encouraging results. D-penicillamine colchicine, and more recently calcium channel blockers have also recorded some success in reducing the amount of excessive healing.

Possibilities for Improvement of the Repair Process

The old dogma used to be that the repair process can only be optimized and not stimulated beyond the point of optimal healing. In clinical practice this is still true. Nonhealing wounds should be carefully evaluated to identify deficiencies in the wound-healing process. Clean wounds heal faster and with fewer aberrations if covered with a dressing that does not allow desiccation. However, many of the stimulators of the repair process, particularly certain hormones, cytokines, and growth factors, appear to have the potential to stimulate the healing process beyond normal, based on the results from *in vitro* studies and experimental studies in animals. We need to evaluate these modalities carefully in an unbiased fashion. This includes the study of minimizing the use of cautery, as well as cytotoxic agents, such as peroxide. This should be done in carefully designed, prospective randomized studies with defined starting and ending points.

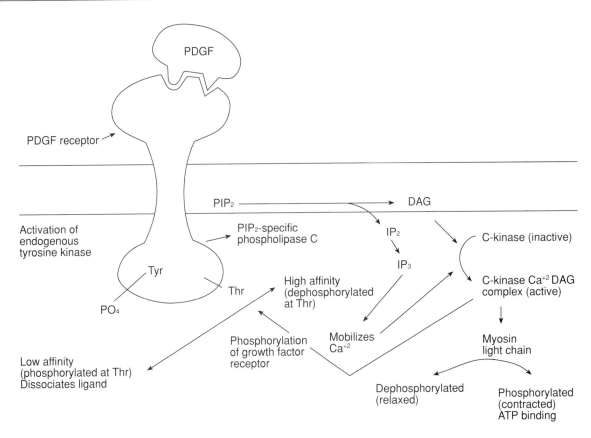

Figure 25-5. Schematic diagram of biochemical events that tranduce the chemotactic signal to the cytoskeleton. C-Kinase = protein kinase-C; DAG = diacylglycerol; IP$_3$ = inositol 1,4,5-trisphosphate; PIP$_2$ = phosphatidylinositol 4,5-bisphosphate; Thr = threonine; Tyr = tyrosine. Reproduced with permission from Grotendorst GR: Chemoattractancts and Growth Factors. In Cohen IK, *Wound Healing—Biochemical and Clinical Aspects,* p. 239, Saunders, Philadelphia, 1992.

Annotated Bibliography

Adzick NS, Longaker MT: *Fetal Wound Healing.* Elsevier, New York, 1992.

A comprehensive up-to-date text on fetal wound healing.

Brueing K, Eriksson E, Liu P, Miller D: Healing of partial-thickness porcine skin wounds in a liquid environment. *J Surg Res,* 52:50-58, 1991.

The feasibility of healing wounds in a liquid environment is demonstrated experimentally in pigs.

Grotendorst GR: Chemoattractants and growth factors. In Cohen IK, *Wound Healing—Biochemical and Clinical Aspects,* Saunders, p. 239; Philadelphia, 1992.

General and specific aspects of the various growth factors are reviewed.

Hunt TK, *et al: Soft and Hard Tissue Repair—Biological and Clinical Aspects.* Praeger, New York, 1984.

Excellent review of wound repair with an emphasis on collagen biochemistry and the importance of oxygen.

Jonkman, MF: *Epidermal Wound Healing Between Moist and Dry.* Thesis, Rijks University, Groningen, 1989.

A comprehensive analysis of the different types of dressings designed to provide a moist wound environment.

Lawrence WT: Wound Healing I: Basic Principles. Foundations of Plastic Surgery Practice: Wound Healing Concepts and Applied, Practical Principles. *PSEF Instructional Courses,* Volume 3, 1991.

An in-depth review of the physiology of wound healing.

Liu PY, Eriksson E, Mustoe TA: Wound Healing—Practical Aspects. In Foundations of Plastic Surgery Practice: Wound Healing—Concepts and Applied, Practical Principles. *PSEF Instructional Courses,* Volume 3, 1991.

This review takes a systematic approach to the clinical diagnosis and treatment of different types of wounds.

Mast BA: The skin. In Cohen IK, *Wound Healing—Biochemical and Clinical Aspects.* p. 347, Saunders, Philadelphia, 1992.

This article provides an up-to-date review of the chronologic events in the healing of the skin.

Miller EJ, Gay S: Collagen structure and function. In Cohen IK, *Wound Healing—Biochemical and Clinical Aspects.* p. 132, Saunders, Philadelphia, 1992.

The biochemistry of the various types of collagen, as well as their molecular genetics, is comprehensively reviewed.

Peacock EE: *Wound Repair.* Saunders, Philadelphia, 1984.

A classic description of the experimental and clinical aspects of wound repair.

Phillips C, Wenstrup RJ: Biosynthetic and genetic disorders of collagen. In Cohen IK, *Wound Healing—Biochemical and Clinical Aspects.* p. 153, Saunders, Philadelphia, 1992.

Excellent review of various collagen disorders.

Stenn KS, Malhotra R: Epithelialization. In Cohen IK, *Wound Healing—Biochemical and Clinical Aspects,* p. 123, Saunders, Philadelphia, 1992.

An in-depth morphological description of the epidermis.

Vogt P, Eriksson E. Aktuelle Aspekte der epidermalen wundheilung. *Handchirurgie, Mikrochirurgie, Plastische Chirurgie,* p. 24, 1992.

This review in German describes the various aspects of epithelialization.

Wise DL: *Burn Wound Coverings*—Volumes I and II, CRC Press Inc., Boca Raton, 1984.

A comprehensive description of various dressings used in burn care.

Whalen GF, Zetter BR: Angiogenesis. In Cohen IK, *Wound Healing—Biochemical and Clinical Aspects,* p. 87, Saunders, Philadelphia, 1992.

An up-to-date review of angiogenesis and various angiogenic factors.

26

Dupuytren's Disease

Lawrence C. Hurst, MD

History

Elliot's recent trilogy on the history of Dupuytren's disease is an extraordinary review of this colorful era of surgical development. Although Dupuytren's disease was studied by many 18th century surgeons, their individual experience was limited. In fact, this disease was a surgical curiosity during a time when life was short, anesthesia did not exist, and death from surgical sepsis was a reality.

Despite these surgical problems, the study of hand anatomy was vigorous. Three centuries before Dupuytren, the anatomist Vesalius (1514-64) had dissected and described the palmar aponeurosis. Bartholinus (1666) and Albinus (1734) also wrote about the palmar aponeurosis. The earliest known description of the diseased palmar aponeurosis was written by Felix Plater of Basel in 1614. In his book *Observations* he described fixed digital contractures, but he believed they were caused by tendon trauma.

The anatomist, surgeon, and father of British surgery, John Hunter, described Dupuytren's disease in 1777. His student Henry Cline lectured on this disease and did the first fasciotomy in Britain. As Elliot aptly points out, Dupuytren was born in 1777. Cline's trainee, Sir Ashley Cooper, also discussed Dupuytren's disease in his 1822 publication, *A Treatise on Dislocations and Fractures.* Cooper used the pointed history to perform subcutaneous fasciotomies of narrow palmar bands.

The first French recognition of Dupuytren's disease was Boyer's 1826 dermatological diagnosis, "Crispatura Tendinum." Despite the work of Boyer and the English surgeons, the eponym for palmar fibromatosis credits Baron Von Dupuytren because of his 1831 lectures and open fasciotomy. Undoubtedly, the very active medical press of Paris facilitated Dupuytren's notoriety. Despite the many derogatory statements about Dupuytren, he was an extraordinary clinician who gave his life to his work. His demanding personality was partially due to the Napoleonic era where every step on the professional ladder was won by participating in "cut-throat" competitive public examinations. The French medical community called this part of the 19th century the "age of Dupuytren."

Dupuytren believed this disease involved only the aponeurosis; he overlooked the fact that the normal aponeurosis did not extend into the finger, which frequently contained pathological cords. He also believed that work and trauma were important etiologic factors and that his open transverse incision was the best technique. In the Academie Royale de Medicine, Dupuytren's competitors like LisFranc, Malgaigne, Goyrand, and Velpeau were eager to argue with him. For example, Goyrand showed in his dissections that the digital cord was new pathological tissue

which was anatomically located in an area that normally contained no aponeurotic fascia. He questioned why the coachman who whipped with only one hand had disease in both. He recommended the longitudinal incision. Meanwhile, LisFranc boldly reminded the French medical audience that Cooper had described palmar fibromatosis in 1822.

Despite controversies, Dupuytren won the eponym while Cooper's closed fasciotomy became the popular operation for the few elective cases of this century. Even after the introduction of general anesthesia in the United States in 1842 and 1846 by Long and Morton, respectively, and the reduction in surgical infections with Lister's antiseptic technique in 1865, Cooper's procedure remained the procedure of choice for most surgeons.

Pathophysiology

Although the clinical features of Dupuytren's disease are well understood, our understanding of the pathobiology has progressed slowly during the last 150 years. A prerequisite for appreciating the pathobiology of Dupuytren's disease is a careful review of the normal fascial anatomy. The fascial components that become involved with Dupuytren's disease are the pretendinous bands, the spiral bands, the natatory ligaments, Grayson's ligaments, Cleland's ligaments, and the lateral digital sheath (Fig. 26-1). An appreciation of the cross-sectional fascial anatomy is also important to the operative treatment of this disease (Fig. 26-2). In the diseased state, these normal ligaments, sheaths, and bands become the pathological cords of Dupuytren's disease. Currently, the named cords are the central cord, the abductor digiti minimi cord, a spiral cord, a lateral cord, a retrovascular cord, a natatory cord, an isolated digital cord, and the first web's intercommissural cords (Fig. 26-3). The abductor digiti minimi cord extends from approximately the abductor digiti minimi's musculotendinous junction or tendon to the ulnar side of the base of the middle phalanx. This cord commonly adheres to the lateral skin. A spiral cord develops from the pretendinous aponeurosis, the spiral bands, the lateral digital sheaths, and Grayson's ligament, and usually connects to the middle phalanx. The web space fascial coalescence is composed of the vertical septa of Legueu and Juvara, the spiral band, the lateral sheath, and the natatory ligaments. The only part of the web space coalescence not involved in the spiral cord is the natatory ligament. The spiral cord's presence is difficult to predict preoperatively but is often associated with more severe proximal interphalangeal joint contractures. A spiral cord always puts the neurovascular bundle at risk because the bundle

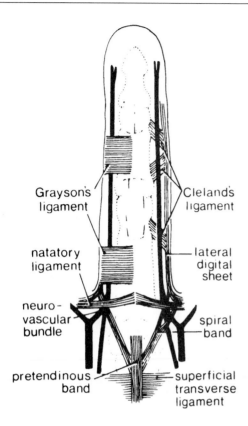

Figure 26-1. Normal fascial structures that can become involved with the pathological cords of Dupuytren's disease. Figure shows the pretendinous bands, the spiral bands, the natatory ligaments, the lateral sheath, Grayson's ligaments, and Cleland's ligaments. Reproduced with permission from McFarlane, RM: Patterns of the diseased fascia in the fingers in Dupuytren's contracture. *Plastic Recon Surg,* 54:31, 1974.

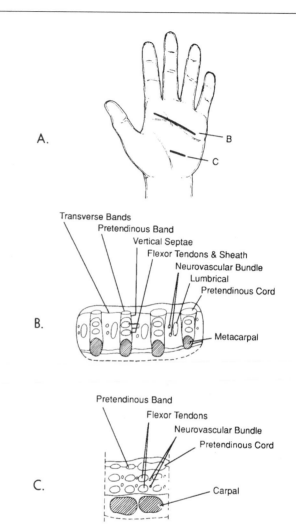

Figure 26-2. **(A)** the locations of the cross sections B and C. **(B)** cross sectional anatomy at the level of the metacarpo-phalangeal joints. Note the small pretendinous bands volar to the index and long metacarpals and the large pretendinous cords volar to the fourth and fifth metacarpals. Note the vertical septae of Legueu and Juvara. These vertical septae divide the hand into nine compartments. Five sections contain nerves, vessels, and muscles. Four sections contain pretendinous bands or cords, flexor tendons, and the metacarpal bones. **(C)** cross sectional anatomy at the level of Kaplan's line (just proximal to the superficial arch). There are no vertical septae separating the tendons into different sections. The normal structures are much more compressed and the pretendinous cords are also confluent at this level.

passes superficial to the cord. Dissection of this cord actually reveals a spiraling neurovascular bundle and a straight "spiral" cord. As the proximal interphalangeal contracture increases, the spiral cord pushes the bundle volarly toward the midline and proximally toward the first flexion crease. A lateral cord starts in the lateral digital sheath. It can involve the spiral band and natatory ligaments. A retrovascular cord involves longitudinal fibers dorsal to the bundle. This cord is commonly seen in combination with other cords. A natatory cord contracts the web by involving those aponeurotic bands that go from midvolar subcutaneous tissue through the web to the adjacent's digit midvolar subcutaneous tissues. The four intercommissural cords of the first web involve pathological changes in the pretendinous band (radial longitudinal fiber), superficial transverse fibers of the palm (proximal transverse commissural ligament), and the first web natatory ligaments (Grapow's ligament).

Histologically, the important cells in the Dupuytren's disease are the myofibroblasts (Fig. 26-4). Myofibroblasts were first described in 1971 by Gabbiani and Majno. The

relationship of the myofibroblasts to Luck's three stages of Dupuytren's contracture has been studied thoroughly. In the first stage (proliferative stage), the typical number of large myofibroblasts increases significantly, the excellular matrix is minimal, and there are numerous cell-to-cell connections (gap junctions). These nodules are vascular with numerous pericytes. In the second (involutional) stage, there is a dense myofibroblast network aligned to the long axis of collagen bundles' so-called stress lines. The ratio of

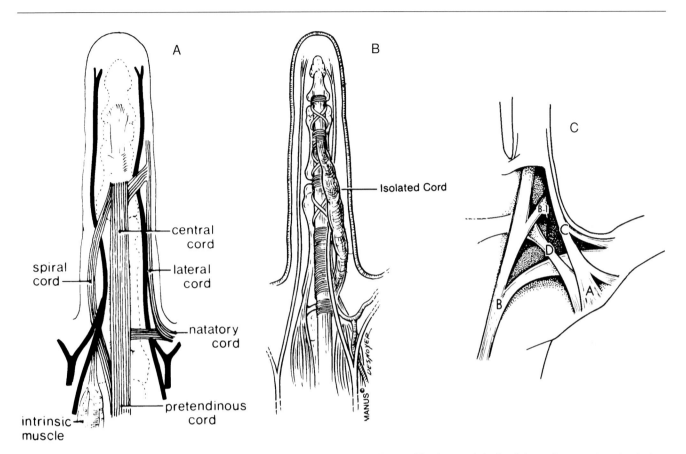

Figure 26-3. (A) the five pathological cords that can develop in Dupuytren's disease. The four cords in the digit are the central cord, spiral cord, lateral cord, and natatory cord. The cord in the palm is the pretendinous cord. Figure 26-3A reproduced with permission from Chiu HF, McFarlane RM: Pathogenesis of Dupuytren's contracture: a correlative clinical-pathological study. *J Hand Surg,* 3A:1-10, 1978. **(B)** the isolated digital cord of Basset and Strickland. Figure 26-3B reproduced with permission from Basset RL, Strickland JW: The isolated digital cord in Dupuytren's contracture: anatomy and clinical significance. *J Hand Surg,* 10A:118-124, 1985. **(C)** the intercommisural cords. Figure 26-3C reproduced with permission from Tubiana R, Simmons B, DeFrenne H: Location of Dupuytren's disease on the radial aspect of the hand. *Clin Orthop,* 168:222-229, 1982.

Type III collagen to Type I collagen is increased. In the third stage (residual stage), the myofibroblasts disappear and a smaller population of fibrocytes are the dominant cell type. With electron microscopy the distinguishing characteristics of a myofibroblast are cytoplasmic myofilament bundles, cell-to-cell and cell-to-stroma connections, dense bodies, and large indented nuclei. Myofibroblasts are also known as transformed fibroblasts, contractile fibroblasts, and specialized contractile fibroblasts. Recently, it has also been shown that the intracellular filaments in myofibroblasts are composed of actin and nonmuscle myosin. The presence of cytoskeletal proteins (intermediate filament proteins) containing the vimentin, desmin, and alpha-smooth muscle actin isomers have been used to define four heterogeneous phenotypes of myofibroblasts in Dupuytren's disease. Some of these phenotypes may actually represent different stages of the development in the myofibroblast. The myofilaments are also associated with a pH-dependent

adenosine triphophatase.

This enzyme is necessary for cellular contraction in muscle. The termini of the myofilaments are connected to the extracellular matrix by a filamentous extracellular material composed primarily of fibronectin. The myofibroblasts are also connected to each other by fibronectin. The cross linking of extra-cellular procollagen molecules during the formation of matrix from fibrin is catalyzed by the enzyme, transglutaminase (Factor XIII), which is found in increased amounts in active Dupuytren's nodules. Other cells recently investigated in conjunction with Dupuytren's nodules are the mobile fibroblasts and the macrophage. Ehrlich reports that a mobile fibroblast contracts the collagen while myofibroblasts orient and fix its position. Meanwhile, Andrew's group found macrophages in numbers proportional to the numbers of myofibroblasts. Phagocytic macrophages are important sources of growth factors, free radicals, and can acquire myofibroblastic ultrastructural characteristics.

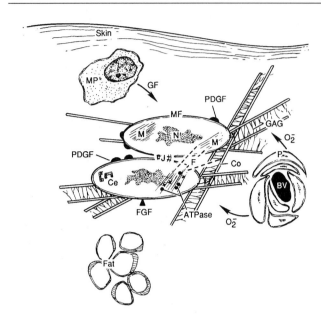

Figure 26-4. The schematic diagram shows the histological and biochemical features of Dupuytren's disease. MF=myofibroblasts; M=myofilaments; N=indented nucleus; CE=centriole; J=gap junctions; AT-Pase=adenosine triphosphatase; CO=collagen; GAG=glycosaminoglycans; F=fibronectin; MP=macrophage; GF=growth factors; PDGF=platelet derived growth factor; FGF=fibroblast growth factor receptor; BV=blood vessels; P=pericytes; °2=oxygen-free radical.

Despite many studies, the cell of origin for the nodular myofibroblast remains obscure. It originates from a fibroblast, a smooth muscle cell, or a pericyte. It is possible that the myofibroblast may develop from several different cells. The disappearance of myofibroblasts in the residual stage is another mystery. The answers to these questions are unknown but the microvascular changes and a secondary relative aponeurotic hypoxia may play a role. Kischer's and Andrew's groups have shown end arteriole narrowing or occlusion by endothelial hyperplasia and associated pericytes proliferation. There are also increased low-chain and volatile fatty acids in the diseased palmar fat, which may be secondary to hypoxia. In addition, Murrell's group has shown a six-fold increase in hypoxanthine in Dupuytren's tissue. This implies a significant potential for greater oxygen-free radical formation in Dupuytren's disease. In tissue culture, low concentrations of oxygen-free radicals can stimulate fibroblast proliferation. Hypoxia is also a known stimulus to angiogenesis and collagen synthesis in wound healing. Murrell's group has hypothesized that oxygen-free radicals are released by the damaged Dupuytren's microvessels, leading to the transformation of the fibroblast to a myofibroblast and possibly to their proliferation.

Other chemicals that may play a role in the pathogenesis of Dupuytren's disease are the recently discovered hormone-like peptides called local growth factors or cytokines. The first fibroblast-related growth factor to be discovered was platelet-derived growth factor. PDGF, a cationic glycoprotein derived from human platelets, may play an important role in the transformation of fibroblasts to myofibroblasts. PDGF is known to increase in peripheral vascular disease. PDGF is a potent fibroblast mitogen (induces mitosis), can stimulate collagen synthesis (especially Type III), binds to matrix components such as acidic glycosaminoglycans, promotes reorganization of cytoskeletal actin filaments, and induces arachidonic acid release with the formation of prostaglandins, particularly E2 and F2 alpha, which are increased in Dupuytren's disease.

Myofibroblast aggregations contract in response to F2 alpha and relax in response to prostaglandin E2. The author's group recently demonstrated PDGF in association with the myofibroblast cell membrane. These growth factors can modulate plasminogen activator levels. Plasminogen levels are increased in aggressive and recurrent cases of Dupuytren's disease. Plasminogen, the zymogen (proenzyme) of plasmin, is responsible for lysing fibrin clot. Finally, Lappi's group recently studied fibroblast growth factor which can stimulate Dupuytren cells to proliferate in a dose-dependent manner in tissue culture. Myofibroblasts can also synthesize FGF, have receptors for FGF, and contain messenger RNA for synthesis of FGF.

The biochemistry of Dupuytren's disease has also been studied extensively. There is an increase in the III/I collagen ratio, increased hexosamine glycosaminoglycan in the matrix, increased amounts of hydroxylysine, increased reducible cross links and the presence of mydroxylysino-hydroxynorleucine. The connection between clinical contractures and these biochemical abnormalities is yet to be explained. Recently, it has been proposed that the collagen changes are not secondary to a genetic defect but are caused by increased cell density. This seems unlikely in that Brickley-Parsons' group found chemical changes in histological normal fascial tissues.

Incidence

The incidence of Dupuytren's contracture appears to be greatest in Northern Europe and in emigrants of Celtic origin from this area. The disease is rare in African countries and only recently have cases been reported in Japan, China, Taiwan, and from the Indian subcontinent. Cases in these groups are rare and the genealogical data is incomplete. The incidence in the United States is unknown. One early study from New York City found an incidence of 2% to 3%. Perhaps the best epidemiological study is Mikkelsen's from Norway (Fig. 26-5). He found Dupuytren's contracture in 9% of males and 3% of females. Age was an important factor with incidence being 7% under age 40 and more than 30% after age 65. Hand dominance does not play a role in the incidence. The reported sex ratio generally indicates the contractures are most common in males but the ratios vary from 2:1 to 10:1. Women have later onset and usually less severe disease. A group of patients in which the prevalence exceeds that of the general population is the HIV-positive population. Patients with HIV also have an increased activity of oxygen-free radicals.

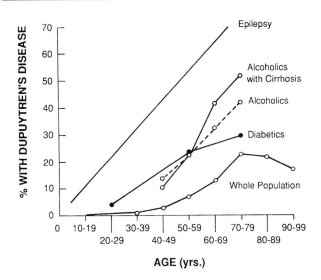

Figure 26-5. The graph shows the relationship of age to the percentage of the population with Dupuytren's disease. These data are from Mikkelsen's Norwegian study. Other superimposed graphs were constructed from data from multiple sources. Epilepsy drugs, alcoholism, and diabetes increase the incidence of this disease.

The connection between diabetes and Dupuytren's contracture has been studied by Noble's group, who recognized that Dupuytren's disease in diabetics is a mild often non-surgical, more radial disease. When the group looked for Dupuytren's disease in a diagnosed diabetic population with the diagnosis of contracture made by hand surgeons, they found 40% of the diabetic patients with evidence of Dupuytren's disease. Other studies have also shown a high incidence of chemical diabetes in patients with Dupuytren's disease. The link between diabetes and Dupuytren's disease may be related to the diabetic microangiopathy, the nonenzymatic glycosylation in diabetes that causes slower collagen turnover, and/or to advanced fibroblast aging.

The studies of Skoog, Lund, and Early have also shown an increased incidence of Dupuytren's disease in epileptic populations. The incidence of contracture increases with the duration of the epilepsy and with the age of the patient. Epileptic Dupuytren's contracture does follow the typical pattern with primarily ulnar involvement; however, these contractures tend to be bilateral, symmetrical, and aggressive. Patients with traumatic epilepsy also have an increased incidence of this hand disorder. However, nonepileptic patients with Dupuytren's contracture do show EEG changes that are not entirely explained by aging. The link between these two disorders is probably the effect the antiepileptic drugs have on collagen metabolism.

Dupuytren's contracture is inherited as an autosomal dominant with variable penetrance. The abnormal gene associated with Dupuytren's disease is probably associated with collagen formation, and homozygous expression may lead to more aggressive disease. To date no specific HLA antigen pattern has been associated with this dominant mode of transmission. However, in cultured myofibroblasts chromosomal karotyping has shown a trisomy abnormality at chromosome number eight. The variable penetrance probably accounts for the fact that only 10% of the patients with Dupuytren's contracture have a positive family history. Patients with a positive family history can also belong to an important subgroup: those with Dupuytren's diathesis. These patients have an aggressive early-onset form of the disease which involves the hands, feet, and penis. Dupuytren's contracture is commonly associated with several diseases including chronic alcoholism, diabetes mellitus, epilepsy, smoking, chronic pulmonary disease and occupational hand trauma (Fig. 26-5). The most controversial of these associations is between Dupuytren's contracture and hand trauma. At this time, the consensus favors the view that heavy manual labor in itself cannot cause Dupuytren's contracture but that a mild form of the disease can be aggravated by traumatizing an early nodule.

An association between alcoholism and Dupuytren's contracture was initially noted by Skoog and Wolfe. Since then, numerous studies both in Dupuytren's populations and in alcoholic populations have tended to support this hypothesis. The connection between Dupuytren's contracture and alcoholism may be related to the effect of alcohol on the microcirculation and its metabolic effect on fat and prostaglandin metabolism.

Clinical Findings

Dupuytren's contracture is typically found in men during the fifth to seventh decades of life and usually begins with one or more mildly painful nodules in the pretendinous bands of the palmar fascia of the ring and little finger rays, often associated with skin dimpling over and around the nodules. The pain is generally short-lived and deserves observation only. The persistence of severe pain, especially night pain in a young patient without classical nodules, should lead to the suspicion of fibrosarcoma, which is extremely rare. As the disease progresses, the digital fascia described above becomes involved, usually producing at first contracture of the metacarpal phalangeal joints. The presence of an isolated nodule over the proximal phalanx should alert the surgeon to an impending PIP joint contracture. Web-space contractures can occur including the thumb-index web space and even rotational contractures in the little finger secondary to contractile cords arising from the abductor digiti quinti and blending with the digital fascia. The true Dupuytren's diathesis is often associated with knuckle pads, plantar (Ledderhose's disease), and penile fibromatosis (Peyronie's disease). One may also encounter trigger fingers and carpal tunnel syndrome in patients with Dupuytren's disease.

Treatment

Conservative treatment with Vitamin E and splinting has proved to be ineffective in the treatment of Dupuytren's contracture. Ketchum has shown that cortisone injection of nodules, which have not formed cords, can suppress the development of these nodules. Current laboratory investigations have led to nonsurgical, untested treatment proposals with compounds such as fibroblast growth factor-saporin, transglutaminase inhibitors, anti-basic fibroblast growth factor, gamma interferon, and more specific collagenases. Currently, surgery is not indicated for static, painless nodules and rarely for knuckle pads. Hueston's table-top test is positive when the palm is placed upon a flat surface and the digits, because of contractures, cannot be simultaneously placed fully upon the same surface. A positive test is an indication for the consideration of surgical intervention. This is not an absolute indication, however because mild metacarpal phalangeal contractures less than 30° may be safely observed, for their correction is almost always complete. However, any degree of PIP joint involvement is an indication for early surgical intervention. Severely contractured PIP joints may not be connected by fasciectomy alone. Additional procedures such as opening the flexor tendon sheath or releasing the check rein ligaments and/or the accessory collateral ligaments may improve the immediate surgical result but ultimately leaves a digit with significant limitations. Only rays involved with disease should be operated upon. Total palmar fasciectomy in the hope of eradication of potential foci of disease is a formidable procedure that in the past often led to multiple complications and did not eliminate recurrence.

Outpatient surgery is appropriate for simple regional fasciectomies. The suction drain is removed before discharge from the ambulatory surgery center or at an early follow-up visit. Older patients with significant medical problems should be hospitalized for 48 hours with the hand elevated and the suction drain in place. A drain is not needed if the palm is left open. During hospitalization prophylactic intravenous antibiotics are given to patients with diabetes, skin grafts, or recurrent Dupuytren's disease.

Technique

The arm should be exsanguinated and an accurate tourniquet should be used. The tourniquet should be released at the end of the procedure and meticulous hemostasis achieved before closing. Loupe magnification is helpful. Current methods utilize various incisions followed by partial or complete regional fasciectomy of the pathological cords. Recently, two series have shown that segmental aponeurectomies are as effective as regional fasciectomies.

Palmar fasciotomy alone may be a temporary method to relieve a severe metacarpal phalangeal joint contracture, but it is not definitive therapy. Closed fasciotomy should never be done in the digits because of the high likelihood of neurovascular injury. Fasciotomy may be useful in patients of limited life expectancy or as a prelude to a definitive partial palmar and digital fasciectomy.

The choice of incisions is elective and depends largely on the degree of contracture and the surgeon's preference. Currently, various zig-zag, z-plasty, and transverse incisions are popular (Fig. 26-6). When the contracture involves

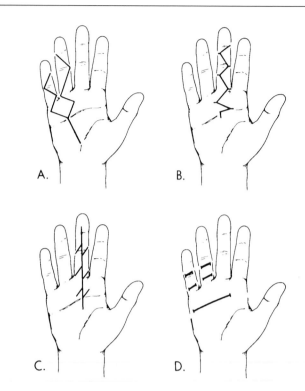

Figure 26-6A-D. The drawing shows four currently used skin incisions for the surgical treatment of Dupuytren's disease. **(A)** is the zig-zag-plasty incision with its linear extension proximal to the palmar flexion crease. **(B)** shows the Littler-Bruner incision with small transverse extensions. Watson uses these for V-Y-plasty closures and Bedeschi leaves them open in the honeycomb technique. **(C)** shows the longitudinal incision which is closed by z-plasties (oblique incision lines). **(D)** demonstrates the transverse incisions of McCash's open-palm technique.

largely the metacarpal phalangeal joint with or without associated PIP joint involvement, a zig-zag-plasty over the pretendinous cord provides excellent exposure. Extreme care must be taken in elevating the flaps. This is a fasciodermal disease and the dissection should remove all involved diseased tissue, yet preserve the uninvolved subcutaneous fat, skin, and vessels. Flaps can be elevated with a scalpel, iris scissors, or blunt dissecting scissors depending on the degree of adherence. Flaps should be retracted gently with small retractors or retention sutures. When dissecting a central cord, exposure of the neurovascular bundles in the palm is facilitated by dividing the transverse bands and cutting the pretendinous cord at the superficial palmar arch level and then pulling it distally. Next, the vertical fibers of Juvara and Legueu are excised. As the dissection approaches the proximal phalanx, the neurovascular bundle may sometimes seem virtually to disappear into a rock-hard Dupuytren's nodule. Slow, meticulous dissection from proximal to distal and vice versa may be needed to free the entrapped neurovascular bundle.

When dissecting the abductor digiti minimi cords, the ulnar neurovascular bundle must be carefully protected because this cord can act like a spiral band. The nerve may spiral dorsal to the abductor digiti minimi cord or spiral through it. Terminal portions of the dorsal ulnar sensory nerve may also be closely applied to the dorsal lateral aspects of this cord. When dissecting spiral cords, the preservation of the neurovascular bundle is challenging. Both the cord and the bundle may have to be dissected bidirectionally. The cord may have to be divided at the point where the bundle twists around it and then dissected. Gentle pulling on the neurovascular bundle with a delicate nerve hook can help locate the neurovascular bundle distal to the point of the spiral. When dissecting natatory cords, which go from one digit to another through the web, the bifurcation of the vessels and nerves has to be carefully localized while preserving the web fat. The natatory cord may have to be dissected from two separate starting points on either side of the web. When dissecting the commissural cords in the first web, special attention must be given to the index radial neurovascular bundle and the digital nerves of the thumb. A first web two- or four-flap z-plasty or skin graft is often needed. A more detailed discussion of the techniques for dissecting these cords and other combination cords can be found in the works of Barton, Hall-Finlay, Landsmeer, McFarlane, McGrouther, Stack, Strickland, Tubiana, and White.

The open technique of McCash may be the approach of choice in older patients who are at risk for postoperative stiffness. This is especially true with multiple ray involvement, severe skin adherence, marked MP joint contractures, and with endomorphic body configurations. The McCash technique allows and encourages early active motion, tends to prevent edema and stiffness, and avoids postoperative immobilization for skin grafts. In the open technique, a transverse incision is made across the palm at the level just proximal to the distal palmar crease and the flaps again are carefully elevated. The digital exposure and dissection is done with zig-zag incisions or digital transverse incisions and, as in the palmar wound, dressed open with nonadherent gauze. In six to eight weeks, the palmar incision with a 3-4 cm gap will heal into a fine linear transverse scar. Leaving the wounds open prevents hematoma formation, pain, and edema, all of which are precursors to reflex sympathetic dystrophy. The disadvantage of this technique vs. primary skin closure is the extra time it takes for wound healing.

The excision of involved skin and its replacement by full-thickness skin grafts is still a matter of controversy. Hueston and Gonzalez are strong advocates of replacing skin densely adherent to diseased cords, because they feel that recurrence is secondary to retained diseased fascia precursor cells in the dermis. This is especially true for patients with recurrent disease, in younger patients, and in those exhibiting Dupuytren's diathesis. Hueston has stated that he has never seen recurrence beneath a graft, but recent studies by Tonkin's group have shown that this may occur. McFarlane disagrees with this premise and contends that

grafting is unnecessary if all diseased fascial cords are excised. Grafts, if utilized, should be thick partial-thickness grafts and should be harvested from a hairless area of the body such as the upper medial arm or from the groin lateral to the inguinal area. It is axiomatic that both the graft and recipient site be so designed that suture lines do not cross flexion creases perpendicularly. The hypothenar area serves as an excellent source for small grafts. Should the flexor tendons be exposed either deliberately or inadvertently in the course of dissection, either a cross finger pedicle flap or local transposition flaps are sometimes used to cover the defect.

Adjunctive Procedures

If trigger fingers are associated even with noncontractile Dupuytren's disease, the local diseased fascia should be excised along with release of the A-1 pulley. Pulley release without local diseased fascial excision may instigate a rapid progression of the Dupuytren's disease.

When carpal tunnel syndrome exists, it should be treated conservatively and not concomitantly with an extensive palmar and digital fasciectomy. Surgical treatment of a persistent carpal tunnel syndrome should be performed at a later date. Prophylactic carpal tunnel release at the time of fasciectomy is not wise, because accelerated scar formation may cause a less-than-optimal result. An exception to this axiom should be made when early proximal palmar Dupuytren's disease coexists with severely symptomatic carpal tunnel syndrome. In this situation a simultaneous carpal tunnel and limited fasciectomy release are usually safe. Upon occasion, particularly in severe recurrent disease especially involving the little finger, PIP arthrodesis or arthroplasty may be necessary. Rarely is amputation performed, but for severely contracted digits, again most frequently the little finger, amputation may be performed, filleting the digit for use as a palmar flap after excising severely involved palmar skin.

Postoperative Care

Whether the skin is to be closed or left open following fasciectomy, it is imperative to release the tourniquet and achieve meticulous hemostasis with a bipolar cautery in order to avoid a palmar hematoma, skin loss, and subsequent infection. A small drain with or without suction, exiting from the proximal palmar wound, is appropriate and should be removed by 48 hours. The dressing itself consists of nonadherent gauze on the wounds and a voluminous fluff dressing supported by a splint or foam rubber. The digital tips are always left visible for neurovascular checks. Markedly contracted joints should not be fully extended in a postoperative dressing for fear of vascular compromise or total digital loss. Postoperatively, the hand is immediately elevated in an arm sling (hand bag) with the elbow on a pillow. There should be little pain; should pain develop requiring increased narcotics for relief, immediate wound inspection is mandatory. If a hematoma has developed, the patient should be returned to the operating room, the wound opened, the hematoma removed, the bleeding vessel coagulated, and the wound reclosed or revision to the open-palm technique.

In five to seven days a light circular dressing is applied and active motion with night extension splinting is begun, supervised by the hand therapist. Sutures are removed at two weeks. Night extension splinting is continued for four months. Continuous passive motion machines have not been shown to improve range of motion or do not reduce residual contractures after fasciectomies. When the open-palm technique is used, daily soaks augment the active motion and splinting.

Complications

Hand edema with finger stiffness is controlled by immediate elevation and early active motion. Skin necrosis secondary to a palmar hematoma is avoided by prompt evacuation of the hematoma and control of the offending bleeding vessel. Hematoma is avoided by meticulous hemostasis with the tourniquet deflated prior to wound closure. Neurovascular damage at the time of dissection should be rare, but severed nerves and vessels should be repaired before the tourniquet is deflated. The development of reflex sympathetic dystrophy is usually related to the pain-edema-stiffness triad and may be more common in women.

Results

Early results of Dupuytren's surgery, regardless of the technique used, are generally good. The patient's function is improved. Those with only metacarpophalangeal contractures are often very pleased with the results. On the other hand, proximal interphalangeal contractures are rarely corrected to a truly normal range of motion, although significant improvement is often achieved initially. The normal postoperative expectation is a full range of flexion and extension in 80% of patients seen primarily. Those with recurrent disease or marked PIP contractures will not fare as well. Return to sports and heavy work is variable and depends upon the severity of the initial involvement and the extent of the dissection, but is seldom less than eight weeks. Patient cooperation and the absence of complications are obvious factors enhancing a rapid return of normal hand function.

Ultimately, recurrence in the original operative area or extension of the disease to previously "normal" parts of the hand are the rule, not the exception. Fortunately, only a small group (i.e. the young patient with a strong diathesis) will need multiple repeat operations. The longer the follow-up the higher the recurrence rate. Long-term studies show recurrent rates ranging from 26% to 80%. The surgeon must always remember to tell the preoperative patient that surgery can not cure Dupuytren's disease.

Annotated Bibliography

Elliot D: The early history of contracture of the palmar fascia (Parts 1-3). 13-B:246-253, 371-378, *J Hand Surg,* 1988; and 14B:25-31, *J Hand Surg,* 1989.

This trilogy of articles is the best recent review of the history of Dupuytren's disease.

Hill N, Hurst L: Dupuytren's contracture. *Hand Clin,* 5(3):349-357, 1989.

This article is a readily available and thorough review with 81 references.

Hueston JT, Tubiana R: *Dupuytren's Disease,* (Second ed.) 1-215, New York: Churchill Livingstone, 1985.

This an excellent collection of papers originally collected and published in France by the Groupe d'Etude de la Main. The monograph contains several classic papers from well-known scholars of Dupuytren's disease.

Hurst L, Badalamente M: Dupuytren's contracture. In: Dee R, Hurst L, Mango E, (eds) *Principles of Orthopaedic Practice,* p. 775-779, vol 1, McGraw Hill, New York, 1989.

A thorough, well referenced, easy-reading summary for those interested in a quick overview.

Hand Surg, (American Volumes) 16A, 1991, and 17A, 1992.

The two latest volumes of the American Journal contain numerous important articles on Dupuytren's disease. Some of the topics covered in these volumes are the relationship of Dupuytren's disease to work and injury, transglutaminase, PDGF, FGF, prognosis in Dupuytren's disease, and lack of effect of continuous passive motion.

J Hand Surg, Br 16A, 1991, and 17A, 1992.

The two latest volumes of the British Journal also contain numerous important articles on Dupuytren's disease. Some of the topics covered in these volumes are collagen in Dupuytren's disease, macrophages in Dupuytren's disease, segmental fasciectomies, day surgery, alcoholism and Dupuytren's disease, and McFarlane's latest overview editorial.

Landsmeer J: Pathoanatomy of Dupuytren's contracture. In *Atlas of Anatomy of the Hand.* Churchill Livingstone, Edinburgh, 1976.

The book on the pathoanatomy of this disease.

McFarlane R, McGrouther D, Flint M: Dupuytren's disease biology and treatment. (First ed.) *Hand and Upper Limb Series,* 5:1-451, Churchill Livingstone, New York, 1990.

This book is currently the best single source on Dupuytren's disease. It contains summaries from many current authors. It has two bibliographies with hundreds of references. The first bibliography is entirely reserved for the historical references.

Sappino A, Schurch W, Gabbiani G: Biology of disease-differentiation repertoire of fibroblastic cells; expression of cytoskeletal proteins as marker of phenotype modulations. *Lab Invest,* 63(2):144-161, 1990.

   An update on myofibroblasts, cytoskeletal proteins, and local growth factors (cytokines).

Seyfer A, Hueston J, ed: Dupuytren's contracture. *Hand Clin,* 7:617-776, 1991.

   The latest complete monograph on Dupuytren's disease with extensive editorial remarks by Hueston.

Stack H: *The Palmar Fascia.* Churchill Livingstone, Edinburgh, 1973.

   The first classic book on the pathoanatomy of Dupuytren's disease.

27

Soft-tissue Coverage of the Upper Extremity

Benjamin E. Cohen, MD

Introduction

Adequate soft-tissue coverage is particularly important in the hand because of its complex form and function. This chapter deals with basic principles and effective and predictable methods of achieving coverage of hand defects. Fingertip injuries and free-flap transfers are considered in other chapters.

The first and foremost principle in the management of acute hand soft-tissue injury is thorough cleansing, irrigation, and conservative debridement of devitalized tissue. Pulsed-jet irrigation by machine or hand-held syringe should be performed with normal saline or a balanced salt solution rather than antimicrobial skin prepping solutions, as they may be harmful to tissues exposed in the wound.

Wound closure may be immediate or delayed. Though many wounds can be dealt with immediately, certain complex wounds, such as electrical burns or those secondary to high-velocity missiles or crush injuries should be cleaned and conservatively debrided initially. Subsequent operative debridements are performed at 24- to 48-hour intervals until the wound is ready for coverage. Repeated debridement often allows for more accurate assessment of tissue damage rather than assessment at initial observation. Similarly, if ischemia develops with initial attempts at advancement (Fig. 27-1), distally based avulsion flaps can be conservatively managed in two stages.

Treatment alternatives for soft-tissue injuries of the hand should be considered in a logical manner. Options range from simple (primary closure or skin graft) to complex (flap or free-tissue transfer). The simplest effective method should be used. Only if primary closure or healing by secondary intention is not appropriate should a skin graft or flap be considered.

Skin Grafts

When nerves, blood vessels, and tendons are not injured or exposed and a healthy recipient bed is present, a skin graft provides excellent coverage. For example, deep partial-thickness burns, full-thickness burns, and skin avulsions are best covered by skin grafts. For avulsion or degloving injuries, the avulsed skin may at times be used after defatting. Using avulsed skin eliminates an additional donor site and minimizes color mismatch.

If a skin graft is indicated, the choice between a split- or full-thickness skin graft is determined by a variety of factors. Some factors to consider are the location, size, and nature of the wound. Most proximal injuries and dorsal hand wounds are best treated with split-thickness skin grafts (Fig. 27-2). Split-thickness skin grafts of intermedi-

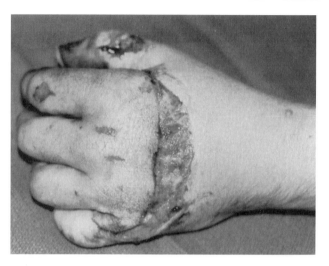

Figure 27-1. Distally based avulsion flaps can be managed in two stages if attempts at initial closure cause ischemia. Nonviable portions should be excised and skin grafting used rather than closure with excessive tension.

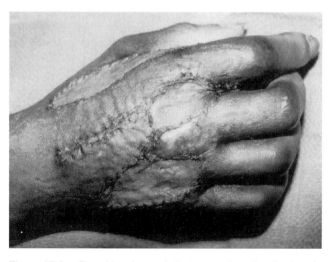

Figure 27-2. Dorsal hand wounds that cannot be primarily closed are often best treated with a split-thickness skin graft. This patient is shown soon after multiple open wounds were grafted.

ate thickness (.012-.015 inches) are usually chosen. Thin (.008-.01 inches) thickness skin grafts can provide excellent temporary coverage as biologic dressings and are also useful following fasciotomies. Following resolution of edema and improvement of the local conditions, grafts in fasciotomies can often be excised and the wound edges advanced and closed. Palm wounds may benefit from the thicker, more durable coverage of a full-thickness skin graft. The size of the full-thickness skin graft is generally limited by the ability to close the donor site primarily. Alternatively, a larger full-thickness graft may be taken and the donor site closed with a split-thickness graft.

The skin graft donor-site location should be chosen carefully. Needs at the recipient site include skin color, texture, and thickness. Donor-site morbidity should also be considered. For split-thickness skin grafts, the lateral buttocks and upper thighs provide ample amounts of skin and relatively inconspicuous donor sites. Good donor sites for full-thickness grafts include the lateral groin crease and gluteal fold. If a relatively small skin graft is needed for the palmar surface of a finger (less than 3 cm square), skin from the ulnar border of the hand is a good option for both split- and full-thickness grafts. An option for larger palmar defects requiring full-thickness coverage is the nonweightbearing plantar skin. Plantar and palmar skin are similar in color and texture. The plantar donor site may require a split-thickness skin graft for closure. To minimize the risk of failure, use of plantar skin is probably best reserved for elective or secondary surgery.

Wound contraction should be considered in the postoperative management of skin grafts. This phenomenon, due to scar tissue maturation, continues for at least 12 months after wound closure. Wound contraction can be reduced somewhat by joint splinting and graft compression (Fig. 27-3). When skin grafts cross joints, prolonged use of splints may be helpful in preventing the development of contractures. Once the wound has healed, these splints should be removed frequently to prevent joint stiffness and to allow range of motion exercises. Hypertrophic scarring can be reduced by the use of compression garments; wearing of the garments begins about two weeks after grafting and continues for six to 18 months.

Flaps

If local tissue is available, a rotation flap often can be designed to cover a small defect (Fig. 27-4). Local flaps yield good results because of tissue similarity. Flaps generally consist of skin and subcutaneous tissues with a donor-site attachment for circulation. Flaps provide durable coverage to areas of the hand with loss of tissue in which bones are without periosteum or cartilage is exposed. Skin grafts will not take over bone without periosteum, tendon, or cartilage. Nerves covered only by skin grafts are frequently hypersensitive. Flaps may also be required when extensive secondary reconstruction is planned.

Specialized flaps can also include fascia, muscle, or nerves. Flaps may have a random pattern blood supply, with nutrition arising from unnamed vessels traveling primarily

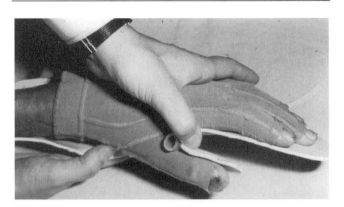

Figure 27-3.   Joint splinting helps to minimize contractures after skin grafting, and compression elastic garments aid in reduction of hypertrophic scarring.

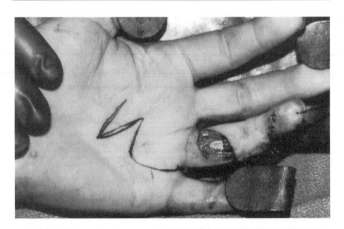

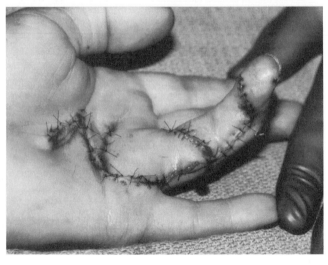

Figure 27-4.   Local rotation flaps can provide durable coverage when a skin graft would be inadequate **(Top)**. A bilobed rotation flap was used to cover this open wound following tenolysis and joint contracture release **(Bottom)**.

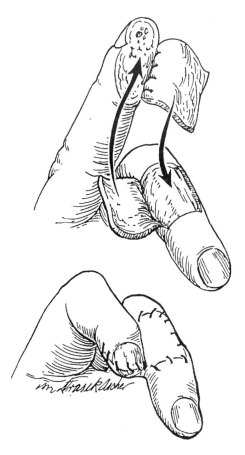

Figure 27-5. Cross-finger flap. A full-thickness skin graft is sutured to the defect on the same side as the donor digit. The flap from the donor finger is elevated leaving paratenon intact. The skin graft and flap are now sutured in place. A flat bolster dressing may be used over the graft. Tape is used to hold the fingers, as well as a bulky protective dressing and splint. Reproduced with permission from Lister GD: Skin Flaps. In Green DP (ed): *Operative Hand Surgery,* 3:1857, Churchill Livingstone, New York, 1988.

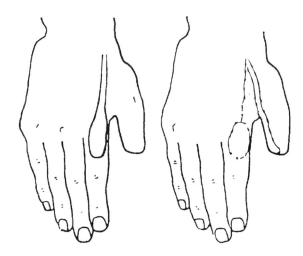

Figure 27-6. The first dorsal metacarpal artery flap has the cutaneous portion donated from the dorsum of the index finger. This can provide sensate coverage for volar thumb injuries. **(Left)** Flap outlined. **(Right)** Flap transferred to thumb with skin graft applied to donor defect. Reproduced with permission from Holevich J: A new method of restoring sensibility to the thumb. *J Bone Joint Surg,* 45B:500, 1963.

in the dermal/subdermal plexus, or they may have an axial pattern blood supply in which the circulation is provided by a named artery and vein. Axial flaps are generally more secure in their circulation than random flaps. Axial flaps can more frequently have a relatively small, mobile pedicle allowing greater flexibility. Axial flaps may be subdivided into peninsula flaps with a skin and vessel pedicle and island flaps, with only a vascular pedicle.

Local Pedicle Flaps from Within the Hand (Smaller Defects)

With the exception of fingertip injuries dealt with elsewhere, three flaps used for defects of the proximal digit and distal palm are the cross-finger, first dorsal metacarpal artery, and flag. The cross-finger flap finds its primary use in covering digital defects (Fig. 27-5). The donor digit is

adjacent to the injured finger. The flap is constructed on the dorsum of the middle or proximal phalanx of the donor finger with the base of the flap adjacent to the injured finger. The flap is elevated, leaving the paratenon intact so that it may receive a full-thickness skin graft. The flap is then tailored and sutured in place. The base is divided two to three weeks later. The main disadvantages are donor site scarring and the possibility of finger stiffness. Due to the possibility of finger stiffness, cross-finger flaps are more satisfactory for younger patients. Hand therapy should be initiated after pedicle transection to reduce the chance of joint stiffness.

Used much less frequently is the first dorsal metacarpal artery flap or Holevich flap. A primary use of the FDMA flap is volar thumb defects (Fig. 27-6). This flap is based upon the first metacarpal artery. The skin paddle is raised from the dorsum of the proximal phalanx of the index finger. A skin bridge from the dorsum of the hand may or may not be included as part of the first dorsal metacarpal artery pedicle. An incision is made from the base of the pedicle to the defect in order to inset the cutaneous portion of the pedicle. Use of a doppler probe makes dissection of this flap quite a bit easier.

Another flap choice, based on a dorsal digital artery branch, is the axial flag flap (Fig. 27-7). This flap can be used to cover defects over the dorsum of an adjacent digit, the volar side of the same digit, or defects on the palm or adjacent web space. The flag flap is taken most reliably from the dorsum of the proximal phalanx of the index or middle fingers. The arterial supply on which this flap is based is less predictable in the other digits. The flap should extend from the distal margin of the web to the most prox-

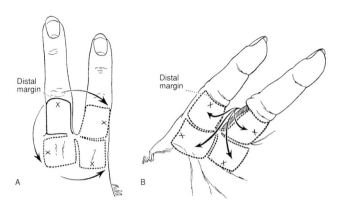

Figure 27-7. **(A)** An axial flag flap raised on the dorsum of the middle finger can be rotated to cover defects on the proximal phalanx of the index finger or over the MP joint of either of those two digits. **(B)** Carrying the flap through the web space allows it to reach defects on the palmar surface of the MP joint of either index or middle fingers. Reproduced with permission from Lister GD: Skin Flaps. In Green DP (ed): *Operative Hand Surgery,* 3:1857, Churchill Livingstone, New York, 1988.

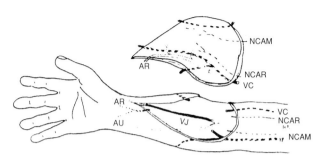

Figure 27-8. Radial forearm flap anatomy. The flap here has been lifted away but can be left attached by the radial artery and cephalic vein to be transposed to the hand as an island flap. The radial artery has been reconstructed with a vein graft. AR, Radial Artery; AU, Ulnar Artery; AB, Brachial Artery; VC, Cephalic Vein; VJ, Vein Graft; NCAM and NCAR, Antebrachial Cutaneous Nerves. Reproduced with permission from *Grabb's Encyclopedia of Flaps,* Strauch B, Vasconez LO, Hall-Findlay EJ (eds): 3:1857, Little, Brown and Co., Boston, 1990.

imal crease over the PIP joint and from midlateral line to midlateral line. The extensor mechanism paratenon should be left intact for grafting. The pedicle is divided in two to three weeks.

Larger hand defects can be managed with the distal-based radial forearm flap. The flap is axial and useful for dorsal hand defects (Fig. 27-8). The flap is based on retrograde flow through the palmar arch and radial artery. The radial artery must be divided at the proximal edge of the skin island. Before using the flap one must check patency of the radial and ulnar arteries with an Allen test as the ulnar artery will be the sole supply to the hand. The radial artery and accompanying *venae comitantes* travel in the lateral intermuscular septum to nourish this fasciocutaneous flap. The flap can be distally or proximally based. For distally based flaps the distance between the defect and the radial styloid is measured. By means of a doppler the radial artery course is marked on the skin. A pattern is made of the defect and then transferred to the forearm reversed proximal to distal, as the flap itself will be reversed due to its distal pedicle. The skin may extend from the wrist to the antecubital crease and from midlateral radius to the volar ulna. Elevation of the flap is begun along its ulnar border and continued until the intermuscular septum is reached. Care is taken to include the deep forearm fascia in the flap. Dissection of the intermuscular septum is continued from distal to proximal, deep to the radial artery. The radial artery and cephalic vein are ligated and divided proximally. The flap is inset and the donor site is closed primarily or with a split-thickness skin graft. Innervation can be achieved by using the lateral antebrachial cutaneous nerve and a segment of radius can be included if bone is needed. The radial forearm flap is predictable and mobile; how-

ever, the donor site tends to be unsightly, and the radial artery is sacrificed unless reconstruction of this vessel is undertaken with a vein graft. If the ulnar artery is normal, reconstruction of the radial artery is not needed.

Muscle flaps are not as useful in the upper limb as in the lower limb. Sacrifice of function is generally unacceptable and aesthetic results can often be wanting.

Occasionally, a distally based forearm flap can be designed which can preserve function. The latissimus dorsi muscle or musculocutaneous flap, either as a pedicle or as an island flap, is useful for large defects from the shoulder to the elbow (Fig. 27-9).

Distant Flaps to the Hand (Larger Defects)

Random Pattern Flaps (Thoracoabdominal Flap)

The majority of large upper limb wounds needing flap coverage will require transfer of distant tissue. A time-honored method is the staged transfer of a random pattern flap. Though these flaps can be designed almost anywhere on the anterior torso, they are usually located on the lower chest or upper abdomen. These locations result in a relatively comfortable upper limb position prior to pedicle division and take advantage of the thinner subcutaneous tissue in this area (Fig. 27-10).

Before surgery, different limb positions are tried in relation to different donor sites to ascertain the most comfortable position. Often, a donor site in the contralateral upper thoracoabdomen is most comfortable, a good source of thin tissue, and maintains some hand elevation. Most of these flaps are superiorly based, particularly for dorsal wounds. Careful planning and use of cloth patterns help assure optimal fit.

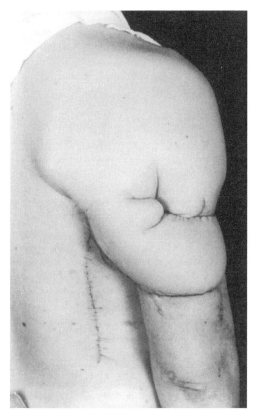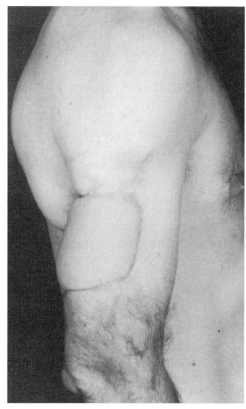

Figure 27-9. **(Left)** The latissimus dorsi as either a pedicle or island flap can be used to cover defects on the upper arm and shoulder. **(Right)** When transferred as a pedicle flap, a second stage to divide the pedicle is required at approximately three weeks after surgery.

In surgery, planning is repeated as final markings are made. Frequently enlarging the defect to conform to more natural anatomical lines is beneficial; a length-to-width ratio of 2:1 is generally reasonable for a random flap. The flap is elevated with about 1 cm of subcutaneous fat. The donor site is closed, or if skin is grafted a bolster (tie over) dressing is applied.

Once the flap is sutured to the margins of the defect, the limb is carefully taped into place to minimize tension on the pedicle. Liberal use of talcum powder and dressing material minimize maceration in the axilla and wherever skin contacts skin. Postoperatively, in bed, the elbow is supported on pillows to help maintain a proper position. The patient can usually be discharged in a day or two and is seen frequently in the office during the two- to three-week interval before pedicle division. Prior to pedicle division, most patients do quite well with minimal tape and elastic bandages. Flap division and inset can be done under general or local anesthesia.

Axial Pattern Flap (Groin Flap)

The axial pattern groin flap is based on the superficial circumflex artery and vein. Advance planning includes the flap's angle of approach to the defect, pedicle length, and the width of the defect. Upper limb joint stiffness may make positioning awkward or uncomfortable. If the patient is unable to tolerate the required position, an alternative flap is chosen.

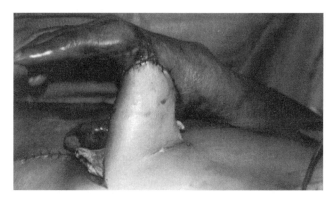

Figure 27-10.   The lower chest/upper abdomen is a good choice for a random pattern pedicle flap for the hand because it allows a comfortable upper-extremity position and has a relatively thin subcutaneous layer. This shows use of such a flap inset into a first-web space defect.

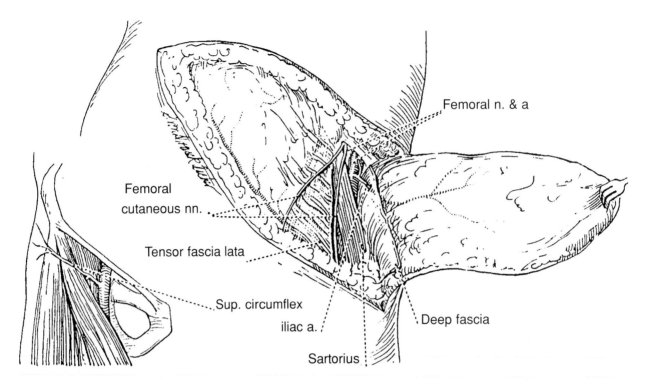

Figure 27-11. Groin flap. The groin flap is based on the superficial circumflex iliac artery, which runs parallel to and approximately one inch inferior to the inguinal liagment. It emerges through the deep fascia as it crosses the sartorious and breaks up into branches at the level of the anterior superior iliac spine. The fascia that is divided at the lateral margin of the sartorious can be seen. Reproduced with permission from Lister GD: Skin Flaps. In Green DP (ed): *Operative Hand Surgery,* 3:1857, Churchill Livingstone, New York, 1988.

Method of Elevation

The superficial circumflex vessels travel two to three centimeters inferior to parallel the inguinal ligament. The vessels' course is traced on the skin, and the flap is centered on the vessels. The width of the base should allow inclusion of the vascular pedicle and tubing of the proximal flap. Distal (superiolateral) to the anterior superior iliac spine, the flap is random and should have a 1:1 or 2:1 length-to-width ratio.

Elevation of the flap begins distally; the depth is at or near the fascia depending upon subcutaneous tissue thickness (Fig. 27-11). As one approaches the anterior superior iliac spine, the dissection should be at the fascial plane and the sartorius muscle is sought. The sartorius muscle fascia is incised along the lateral border and the vessels are visualized on the deep surface of the fascia.

Thigh flexion usually permits primary closure of the donor defect; if not, a split-thickness skin graft is used. The flap may be carefully thinned distally if necessary and the proximal portion is generally tubed prior to flap inset. Elevating the edges of the extremity defect allows an everted closure, especially in the older wound. After inset, limb positioning and taping are used to prevent tension or kinking of the pedicle. Pillow support under the elbow is helpful.

The patient should be transferred directly from the operating table to the hospital bed.

Positioning requirements should be reviewed with the nurses and patient. Flap circulation and arm position should be frequently checked during the first 48 hours after surgery. On the second postoperative day, the patient is allowed out of bed and dressings are changed. Usually the patient can be discharged by the third postoperative day.

Pedicle division is usually done three weeks after flap application. If the tubed portion of the flap is not needed, the pedicle can be divided and inset loosely. If a portion of the pedicle is required to complete the reconstruction, the pedicle is partially divided (delayed) to enhance the flap's vascularity. In seven to 10 days, the pedicle may be completely divided and the flap inset.

Conclusion

Though by no means exhaustive, the above serves as a guide to management of soft-tissue injuries of the hand. Every wound should be carefully assessed and each patient individually evaluated prior to treatment.

Annotated Bibliography

Skin Grafts

Madden JW: On the "contractile fibroblast." *Plast Reconstr Surg,* 52:291-292, 1973.

Myofibroblasts are responsible for wound contraction and possibly for other contracture-type diseases, and this may allow pharmacologic inhibition.

Rogers BO: Historical development of free skin grafting. *Surg Clin North Am,* 39:289-311, 1959.

A concise history of various types of free skin grafts since ancient times.

Sawhney CP, Subbaraju GV, Chakravart RN: Healing of donor sites of split skin grafts. *J Plast Reconstr Surg Br,* 22:359-364, 1969.

A study in pigs which showed that donor-site epithelialization is done by day six and complete epidermal regeneration is accomplished in 21 to 30 days, and no regeneration of dermis occurs. These events are not related to graft thickness.

Local Pedicle Flaps from Within the Hand

Cohen BE: Local muscle flap coverage of the proximal ulna without functional loss. *Plast Reconstr Surg,* 70:745-748, 1982.

A case report of use of the proximal portions of the extensor carpi ulnaris and flexor digitorum profundus to cover an upper-extremity defect with loss of function of the donor muscles.

Cohen BE: Shoulder defect correction with the island latissimus dorsi flap. *Plast Reconstr Surg,* 74:650-656, 1984.

A description of an island flap of the latissimus dorsi based on the thoracodorsal vessels, used to cover shoulder defects.

Holevich J: A new method of restoring sensibility to the thumb. *J Bone Joint Surg,* 45B:496-502, 1963.

A description of restoring sensation to the thumb by using the dorsal branch of the radial nerve with or without a skin paddle.

Iselin F: The flag flap. *Plast Reconstr Surg,* 52:374-377, 1973.

A brief description of types of flag flaps, the anatomic limitations, and operative technique.

Kappel DA, Burech JG: The cross-finger flap: an established reconstructive procedure. *Hand Clin,* 1:677-684, 1985.

A review of the indications and technique of the cross-finger flap reveals functional sensibility in many cases.

Muhlbauer W, Herndl E, Stock W: The forearm flap. *Plast Reconstr Surg,* 70:336-342, 1982.

The author describes the radial forearm free flap using cadaver studies and clinical cases.

Song R, Gao Y, Song Y, Yu Y, Song Y: The forearm flap. *Clin Plast Surg,* 9:21, 1982.

Use and surgical technique of the radial forearm free flap to cover the neck of a patient with burn scar contracture excision.

Soutar DS, Tanner NSB: The radial forearm flap in the management of soft-tissue injuries of the hand. *J Plast Surg Br,* 37:18, 1984.

A good overview of the radial forearm pedicled flap and its use in soft-tissue trauma coverage of the hand.

Timmons MJ: The vascular basis of the radial forearm flap. *Plast Reconstr Surg,* 77:80, 1986.

A complete anatomic cadaver analysis of the arterial supply, perfusion zones, and venous drainage of the radial forearm flap.

Distant Flaps to the Hand

Lister GD, McGregor IA, Jackson IT: The groin flap in hand injuries. *Injury,* 4:229, 1973.

Surgical aspects and use of the groin flap to cover hand defects are shown.

McGregor IA, Jackson IT: The groin flap. *J Plast Surg Br,* 25:3, 1972.

The original description of the groin flap and its multiple uses.

White WL: Flap grafts to the upper rxtremity. *Surg Clin North Am,* 40:389, 1960.

A good overview of pedicled thoracoabdominal flaps to the upper extremity. This classic paper is still relevant today.

General Reference for Flap Coverage of the Hand

Lister GD: Skin flaps. In Green, DP (ed): *Operative Hand Surgery,* vol. 3:1839-1933. Churchill Livingstone, New York, 1988.

A complete review of the use and surgical technique of flap coverage to the hand.

Grabb's Encyclopedia of Flaps, vol. 3, Strauch B, Vasconez LO, Hall-Findlay EJ (eds): Little, Brown and Co., Boston, 1990.

A thorough and detailed description of flaps to the upper extremity.

28

Nail Bed and Fingertip Injuries

Elvin G. Zook, MD

Introduction

Injury of the fingertip and/or nail bed is by far the most common hand injury for the simple reason that when the hand is withdrawn from potential harm, the ends of the fingers are removed last. For the same reason, longer fingers are more commonly injured. Although fingertip and nail-bed injuries rarely cause long-term serious disability, they have significant financial impact on society because of their frequency and time lost from work.

Anatomy

Although the anatomy of the finger and its tip has been described in the past, the possibility of replantation and free-tissue transfer, including the tip and nail along with bone, have encouraged studies of the arterial and venous systems. The common digital artery trifurcates approximately 1 cm distal to the DIP joint, sending one branch to the nail fold, one branch to the paronychial area, and a third major branch into the pulp of the fingertip. The paronychial branch sends two communications to a similar branch from the opposite side: one just distal to the lunula and one near the hyponychium. These two branches have many arborizations. Some venous drainage on the volar surface of the fingertip is primarily associated with the common digital artery, but the majority of the venous drainage is on the dorsum of the finger. There is a series of dorsal venous arches, one over each phalanx, with connections by multiple longitudinal veins. The palmar venous blood flow joins the dorsal system through intercapitular veins. It includes the system of valves present in all veins as far as the pulp, which direct flow from distal to proximal, palmar to dorsal, and radial to ulnar. These veins are the basis of the vein-to-vein transfer of nail from a toe to a finger.

A relatively consistent branching of the terminal digital nerve has been documented to occur at approximately the eponychial level bilaterally. This consists of branches going to the skin proximal to the nail bed, to the lateral border of the nail bed and into the nail bed, and a larger branch going into the pad of the finger. Division of the digital nerve proximal to the distal border of the lunula can be repaired under the microscope, and nerve grafts may be used for reconstruction of nerve.

Fingertip Injuries

Although the fingernail is part of the tip, in this section we will consider only the care of the pad of the finger.

Injuries to the fingertip may involve the skin of the tip, varying amounts of underlying fat, and bone. The angle of the injury is important since volar angulation usually eliminates the use of local finger flaps such as the Kutler or V-Y. If bone is exposed, it is essential to provide padding over the bone by closure with a flap, or shortening of the bone and approximation.

Grafts

When only skin is missing from the fingertip and the fragment is available, it is best replaced as a free full-thickness graft. If fat is present on the amputated part, it may either be replaced intact in a child or defatted and placed as a full-thickness graft in the adult. In the child, a composite fingertip including bone, nail bed, and pad distal to the level of the lunula can be replaced with an excellent chance of take.

When large pieces of composite fingertip amputations are replaced, several techniques have been described that allow overlapping of de-epithelialized skin in an attempt to make more vascularized surface available for rapid vascularization of the tip. Some have advocated techniques that involve de-epithelization of a proximal strip of skin on the amputated part and under lapping the skin of the finger. This increases the raw surface in contact and theoretically hastens the return of blood supply to the fragment.

The controversy continues in regard to permitting healing by secondary intention. Some insist that the tip somehow regenerates, but radiographs of the injured fingertip compared with the opposite finger show that the lost distal phalanx does not regenerate. Some studies comparing spontaneous epithelization (conservative treatment), skin grafting, amputation further back, or flaps have shown, (particularly in children) that conservative treatment gives superior results. If significant skin and fat of the tip are lost, the contracture of secondary healing almost universally causes the nail bed to be pulled over the end of the tip with some degree of resultant curvature of the distal nail. If the tip is not available, but there is fat over the bone, a split-thickness graft from the hypothenar eminence or lateral finger will give durable skin similar to that lost. Grafts can be taken freehand with a Weck blade or Goulian knife under local anesthetic.

Flaps

In some instances the upside-down cross-finger flap will reach a fingertip that cannot be reached by the classic cross-finger flap. With the upside-down cross-finger flap, the epithelium is removed from the flap and the de-epithelialized surface sutured into the defect. A skin graft is then placed over the undersurface (raw surface) of the flap and the donor finger.

Dorsally angled amputations or straight amputations are best covered with either volar V-Y advancement or Kutler flaps. Under certain circumstances, particularly on the thumb, the volar arterialized advancement (Moberg) flap is indicated.

With the volarly angled amputation the cross-finger flap is available, but the resultant disfiguring scar on the dorsum of the adjacent finger is sometimes too high a price to pay. If adjacent fingers are injured they are not available as donor sites.

The thenar crease flap hides the donor scar in the volar MP crease of the thumb and does not require as much flexion of the finger PIP joint to reach the donor site as does the thenar or palm flap. However, from middle age onward, either flap may result in permanent PIP joint stiffness.

The vascularized flag flap from the dorsum of the proximal phalanx of the index finger may be used for amputations of the pad of the thumb and the flap dorsal sensory nerve anastomosed to a common digital nerve of the thumb. This allows at least some normally oriented sensation to the flap. It has been shown that after transfer the ulnar side of the flap is more innervated than is the radial side by the radial nerve. Unfortunately, either with a flap left attached to the index finger or dissected as a neurovascular pedicle, the ulnar border (more sensation) of the flap is on the radial side (least important) of the thumb. If a nerve anastomosis from the flap to the nerve of the thumb is done, the ulnar side of the thumb is best connected.

Nail Bed

The past several years have been a productive time for surgical care of the perionychium. Many authors have made contributions particularly in the area of microvascular composite reconstruction of the perionychium. Little has changed in our knowledge of the anatomy (Fig. 28-1) and physiology of the perionychium, but the application of this knowledge to patient care has progressed.

The most significant recent advances have been the use of free toe pulp, bone, and nail bed to restore the length and shape of the fingertip following amputation. These are usually done as a secondary procedure and the best results have been with dissection of dorsal foot veins and the dorsal pedal artery from the dorsum of the foot. This provides long arteries and veins which may be tunneled under the finger skin and anastomosed to palmar common digital arteries and dorsal hand veins.

Acute Injuries

It is important that the injured nail be treated appropriately at the time of the injury for, as a rule, reconstruction does not give as good a result as proper early care. Accurate approximation of the nail bed with fine chromic suture (7-0 ophthalmic double arm suture on a microspatula needle with magnification) is the preferred method and has been shown to give good or better results in 90% of nail-bed injuries. It is important that fractures of the tuft be accu-

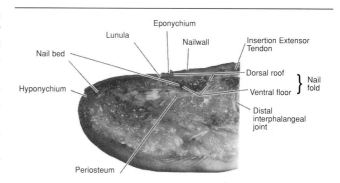

Figure 28-1.   Anatomy of the nail bed.

rately reduced because an offset of the dorsal surface of the bone will cause deformity in the nail as it grows distally. Studies show that the 50% of nail-bed injuries that involve fracture of the distal phalanx do not have as good a result as nail-bed injuries not associated with fracture. After the nail bed has been approximated as accurately as possible, the nail (if available) is the best conformer to shape the nail bed edges between the stitches, maintain the nail fold open, hold bony fractures reduced, and decrease postoperative pain. If the nail is not available, a nail-shaped piece of 0.020" reinforced silicone sheeting or commercially available nails may be used. These maintain the nail fold open and to some degree mold the nail-bed surface. If the substitute is too soft, it is difficult to maintain in the nail fold, and if it is too hard, it may erode the nail fold. When using silicone sheeting, a suture is placed in the lateral recesses of the nail fold and through the silicone sheet to hold it in place for two to three weeks until the injury is healed. If none of these options are available, nonadherent gauze such as adaptic may be placed over the nail bed and into the nail fold to prevent scar adhesions from the dorsal roof to the ventral floor.

The question of nail removal with repair of the underlying nail bed or evacuation of a hematoma remains unanswered. Although it is known that blood under the nail must come from an injury to the nail bed, it is not known how extensive that injury must be to cause subsequent nail deformity. It has been quoted that if more than 50% of the nail is undermined by hematoma the nail should be removed and the nail bed repaired. Although a study advocating removal showed excellent results, another study from the emergency medicine literature reports that subungual hematomas treated by nail trephination, regardless of the size of the subungual hematoma or whether fracture was present, did not affect final result in the patient with an intact nail.

Split-thickness Sterile Matrix Grafts

Approximately 15% of nail-bed injuries involve avulsion of a portion of the sterile and/or germinal matrix. The use of skin graft, dermal, and reversed dermal grafts as coverage

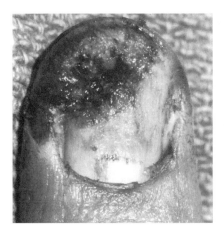
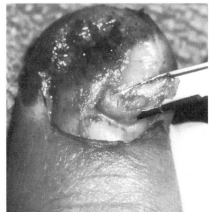
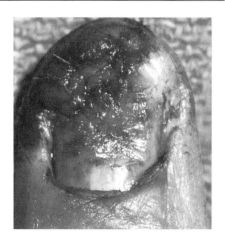
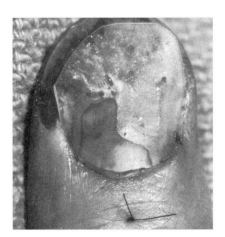
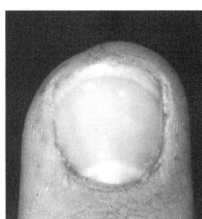

Figure 28-2.

(Top Left) A crushing injury has torn the skin of the tip and avulsed a segment of the sterile matrix.

(Top Middle) A split-thickness sterile matrix graft is removed from the adjacent nail bed with a #15 blade.

(Top Right) The graft is sutured into the defect on the finger.

(Bottom Left) A nail-bed-shaped piece of .020" silicone sheet sutured into the nail fold.

(Bottom Right) The patient one year after trauma.

for avulsion of the sterile matrix has been suggested but does not give a reliably good result. The best treatment is to use the avulsed matrix as replacement. The avulsed fragment or fragments may be found on the undersurface of the nail. Fragments should be carefully removed, replaced in the matrix defects as accurately as possible, and after suturing with fine chromic suture the nail may be replaced to mold the fragments. Nail-bed fragments may be attached to the finger by bits of tissue. They do not provide a blood supply but, rather than being debrided, should be puzzled back into place.

If a small fragment of nail is avulsed with its undersurface covered with matrix, the nail is accurately repositioned and held with stitches in the fingertip and/or steri-strips. Attempts to remove the sterile matrix from a small fragment of nail can cause more injury to the nail bed than leaving it attached and replacing it accurately with the nail as a stent. If the nail avulsion is large, for example more than half of the matrix, the lateral 2 mm of the nail may be freed and removed from the matrix to allow the matrix to be

accurately sutured into place. It is also acceptable, if one feels a more accurate approximation can be achieved, to remove this large fragment of nail bed from the nail, suture it in place, and then replace the nail fragment over it. Also, in some instances, a composite of the perionychium will be avulsed, including sterile matrix, germinal matrix, eponychium, nail fold and/or the paronychium. Again, the best treatment is replacement of the composite avulsed soft tissue as accurately as possible.

If the avulsed composite tissue is not available, but the same area on another finger that is unsalvageable is available, it can be harvested and used as a composite graft. An appropriately sized piece of similar tissue from a toe may also be used. This, of course, will leave a defect of the toe-nail.

A split-thickness sterile matrix graft from a finger or toe nail can be used to replace avulsed sterile matrix and may be placed directly on the cortex of the distal phalanx (Fig. 28-2). Blood supply from the lateral edges will nourish the graft.

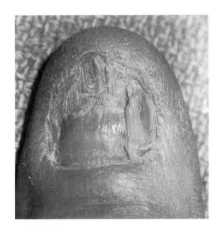
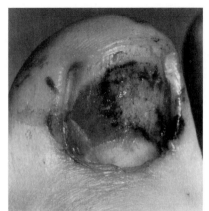
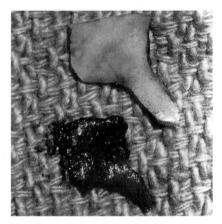

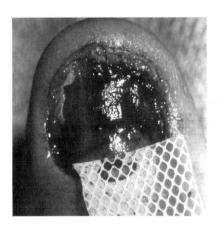
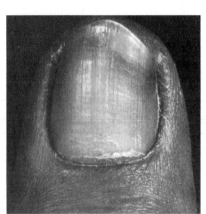

Figure 28-3

(Top Left) A nail deformity of the thumb in a 50-year-old woman following a car door crush.

(Top Middle) The nail remnants have been removed and the area of scarring has been outlined with Methylene Blue.

(Top Right) A pattern made with a piece of rubber glove, placed on the large toe and a split-thickness sterile matrix graft of the same size and shape removed.

(Bottom Left) The split-thickness sterile matrix graft sutured in place on the thumb.

(Bottom Right) The patient one year after injury.

A split-thickness sterile matrix graft may also be used in reconstruction of the sterile matrix when the nail is split or nonadherent (Fig. 28-3). As a rule with either trauma or reconstruction, if the area of split-thickness sterile matrix loss is large enough that adequate sterile matrix cannot be harvested from the adjacent sterile matrix of the nail bed, one must use a sterile matrix graft from the large toe to obtain the necessary volume. The nonadherent or split nail should be removed and the sterile matrix explored. This is best done with loupes, or preferably, 10-X power of the operating microscope. The area of scarring is outlined and resected. A pattern is made with a piece of rubber glove or suture package and transferred to the toe. One must be careful not to reverse the pattern since it will not fit when it is brought back to the nail bed defect. The skin graft may be taken with the tip or the side of a #15 blade by moving it back and forth like a dermatome. The edge of the blade should always be visible through the nail bed to prevent the graft being taken too thick and causing deformity of the donor nail. *Alert: split-thickness sterile matrix graft will work as a replacement for sterile matrix only.* If the germinal matrix is avulsed, neither a split-thickness graft of sterile matrix or germinal matrix will be satisfactory as a replacement. For germinal matrix replacement, the basilar layer of germinal cells must be retained. This layer is not included in a split-thickness graft but only in a full-thickness graft.

Germinal Matrix Grafts

Free nonvascularized germinal matrix grafts have been thought successful in reverse proportion to the age of the patient and have not been recommended for older adults. As more experience has been gained in their use, the results have not been found as discouraging as previously thought (at least into middle age). Germinal matrix grafts are most commonly taken from a toe, but may be from another finger which cannot be replanted. The second toe is recommended, especially in women, since they usually are reluctant to have the disfigurement of the large toenail that occurs with use of the germinal matrix. The germinal matrix of a second toe will usually supply adequate germinal matrix for reconstruction of a finger, but may not be of adequate size for the thumb. The patient must be told of the resultant deformity.

Composite Grafts

Composite grafts of nail fold, germinal, and sterile matrix, as well as paronychium as a nonvascularized replacement for avulsed segments of nail work well in acute injuries as a rule. This is probably true because there is a more adequate blood supply soon after injury than after scar has formed when most reconstruction is attempted.

Eponychium

Free composite grafts of the dorsal roof (eponychium) of a toe to correct a deformity of the finger eponychium work well in that they contour the eponychium and improve the surface of the nail that grows from beneath it. The second toe may provide adequate replacement for the finger but usually for a thumb the eponychium from the large toe is

necessary. The volume of toe eponychium needed is excised after the edges of the finger defect are freshened and measured. The donor site on the toe is covered with ointment, nonadherent gauze and is allowed to heal by secondary intention. This gives some widening of the lunula, but rarely nail deformity since the surface of toenails are usually not as smooth as a fingernail.

The Hooked Nail

Attempts at correction of the hooked nail have eluded the hand surgeon throughout history. The cause of the hooked nail is either loss of the bony support of the distal phalanx allowing the nail bed to fall over the tip, or the surgeon's pulling the nail bed to cover a tip defect. If the nail bed curves around the tip of the finger, the nail will follow its course and become hooked. The best treatment to date is to reestablish the defect, allow the nail to return to the dorsum of the distal phalanx, and replace the tip soft tissue with a cross-finger or thenar flap. This, in most cases, improves the deformity, but does not correct it completely and leaves a shortened nail. In view of the contributions of several authors, the solution to this problem appears to be transfer of a composite vascularized toe tissue transfer of distal phalanx, nail bed, and toenail soft tissue to replace the defect of the fingertip.

Annotated Bibliography

Ashbell TS, Kleinert HK, Putcha S, Kutz JE: The deformed fingernail, a frequent result of failure to repair nail bed injuries. *J Trauma,* 7:177190, 1967.

Classic early article on care of nail injuries and deformities.

Ketchum LD, (Ed): Skin and soft-tissue coverage of the upper extremity. *Hand Clin,* 1:4, WB Saunders, 1985.

A good discussion of management of acute injuries and chronic problems of the fingertip.

Shephard GH: Treatment of nail bed avulsions with split-thickness nail bed grafts. *J Hand Surg,* 8:49-54, 1983.

First description of the use of split-thickness nail-bed grafts for nail-bed avulsion secondary to trauma.

Shibata M, Seki T, Yoshizu T, Saito H, Tajima T: Microsurgical toenail transfer to the hand. *J Plast Reconstr Surg,* 88;102-109, l991.

Demonstrates use of vascularized toe tissue to reconstruct fingertip deformities.

Zook EG (Ed.): Hand Clinics. Vol 6, #1. *The Perionychium,* WB Saunders, 1990.

Multiple contributions from leaders in perionychium problems.

Zook EG, Van Beek AL, Russell RC, Beatty ME: Anatomy and physiology of the perionychium: a review of the literature and anatomic study. *J Hand Surg,* 5:528-536, 1980.

Basic anatomy and physiology of growth of nails.

VII

Vascular

29

Vascular Disorders of the Hand

E. F. Shaw Wilgis, MD

Introduction

Several significant articles dealing with vascular disorders of the upper extremity have been published during the last ten years. They can be grouped into three categories: evaluation techniques, occlusive disease, and vasospastic disorders.

Evaluation Techniques

Maurer reviewed the use of three-phase bone scans to evaluate various disorders of the hand and wrist. Modern three-phase studies are carried out by an intravenous injection of the gamma-emitting radionuclide 99MTC coupled to methylene diphosphate. The phosphate complex produces high skeletal binding resulting in excellent bone images two to three hours after injection (Phase III). Pictures taken during the first two minutes after injection, while the nuclide is within the vascular tree, produce an extremity arteriogram (Phase I). Pictures taken five to 10 minutes following injection create soft-tissue images as the radionuclide diffuses into the soft-tissue spaces (Phase II).

The vascular images obtained in Phase I can be used to diagnose vascular occlusion of the radial or ulnar artery, but cannot image the individual vessels of the palmar arch or digits, which are usually seen as an early blush. Vasospastic disorders such as Raynaud's phenomenon are identified by decreased perfusion in two or more digits which usually persists into Phase II. Arteriovenous malformations show as early Phase I areas of increased perfusion while hemangiomas produce increased activity in Phase I that persists into Phase II. Radionuclide imaging is useful in diagnosing reflex sympathetic dystrophy, producing a diffusely positive Phase III study, which does not always correlate with increased blood flow and hyperemia in Phases I and II. The authors noted that, with disuse, some patients may show decreased blood flow with a positive Phase III study.

Osteomyelitis produces a positive Phase III image while cellulitis, or other inflammation of synovium or joints, produces positive Phase I and II images. To rule out increased uptake of bone adjacent to an area of infection, delayed 24-hour films (Phase IV) are useful to differentiate osteomyelitis with increased bone turnover and uptake from adjacent cellulitis, which will not cause increased bone activity and radionuclide uptake. Radionuclide imaging is a painless, minimally invasive technique that does not cause vasospasm and may be useful in select cases when other imaging techniques are not possible.

Baxter and associates reviewed their use of available upper extremity vascular studies including digital brachial indicis, segmental plethysmography, Doppler studies, duplex scanning, and stress tests to diagnose the extent and location of acquired or congenital vascular disorders. Segmental limb pressures are easily obtained using proximal blood pressure cuffs at least 1.2 x the diameter of the extremity and a unidirectional 10 MHz Doppler flow probe. Pressures are recorded at various levels along the extremity by the return of an audible Doppler signal as the proximal tourniquet is deflated below arterial pressure. There is normally no difference within or between arm pressures in a healthy individual. A difference of 20 mm or more of mercury indicates a significant obstruction. Normal digital pressure should not differ more than 1 mm of mercury from each other. The authors caution that this method may not be accurate in patients with bilateral disease or in identifying lesions in patients who are hemodynamically normal at rest. Such patients may require exercise or reactive hyperemia to enhance SLPs sensitivity. The authors also show how Doppler wave form analysis can be used to help locate and determine the degree of arterial vascular disease.

The use of photoplethysmography and strain gauge volume recordings to localize arterial disease by analyzing wave forms at different levels in the extremity was also discussed. Changes in wave forms, such as loss of the dicrotic notch or the rate of rise in the systolic peak, are the earliest signs of proximal arterial obstruction that can be seen using photoplethysmography. Duplex scanning can be used to diagnose suspected arterial intimal lesions causing digital embolization, true and false aneurysms, arteriovenous fistulae, and for surveillance of venous bypass grafts. Cold sensitivity testing was used to distinguish Raynaud disease, which is characterized by episodes of digital ischemia secondary to vasospasm, from Raynaud phenomenon, which includes partial arterial occlusive disease. Patients with arterial disease require more than 20 minutes to return to pre-exposure temperatures when submersed for 20 seconds in ice water, while controls reached this temperature within 10 minutes. Photoplethysmography can also be used to aid in the diagnosis of thoracic outlet syndrome by recording changes in the wave form of a sitting patient when moving their shoulder girdle into various positions. Impedance plethysmography can also be a valuable method for assessing upper extremity venous outflow obstruction as can the use of a bidirectional Doppler examination. Bidirectional venous flow is usually found in patients with chronic venous insufficiency. Venous duplex scanning is also a good method to identify axillary and subclavian vein thrombosis. This is an excellent review of the available noninvasive techniques.

Hosokawa and associates presented a retrospective analysis of routine Allen's tests performed on 1,470 surgical patients (2,490 arms) by their anesthesiology department over a one-year period. A positive test was defined as return of color to the digits more than five seconds after release of the ulnar artery alone. An abnormal Allen's test was found in 85 patients (5.8%) and 105 arms (3.5%). There was no difference between men and women or right and left arms. The incidence increased from 2.2% in the first decade to 6.9% in patients 80 or older. Surprisingly, there was no correlation in patients with diabetes or cardiac disease. The authors suggest that patients who have had a forearm artery divided, as when elevating a radial forearm flap, might be at increased risk of developing future vascular compromise as they age. This retrospective study, however, could not analyze the hemodynamic changes which occur routinely to redistribute blood flow into the extremity following occlusion or transection of the radial artery.

Stein and associates evaluated the measurement of transcutaneous Po_2 ($Ptco_2$) as a noninvasive method for assessing whether limb salvage should be attempted. Using a complex statistical analysis based on the generalizability study analysis of 36 measurements from each individual, they suggest $Ptco_2$ determination is useful in evaluating patients with peripheral vascular disease as candidates for limb salvage. The technique is not reliable for screening normal patients for peripheral vascular disease.

Goodman and associates studied the use of upper limb exercise testing in combination with myocardial scintigraphy and oxygen consumption determinations to evaluate the cardiac status of patients with peripheral vascular disease. The authors compared their results from a comprehensive evaluation of upper limb exercise tolerance to those obtained by standard treadmill performance in normal individuals and in 33 patients with known peripheral vascular disease.

They showed that upper limb exercise testing is a reliable method to evaluate the cardiac status of patients with peripheral vascular disease. Twenty-five of 33 patients with peripheral vascular disease who were asymptomatic for cardiac problems developed positive thallium scans during upper limb testing, suggesting latent myocardial disease. Thirteen of 25 exhibited abnormal exercise EKG's during upper limb testing. This study showed that arm exercise testing with myocardial scintigraphy may be able to detect occult cardiac ischemia in patients with peripheral vascular disease.

Occlusive Disease

Sotta reviewed vascular problems seen in the proximal upper extremity of athletes. He reviewed the pertinent anatomy of the proximal upper extremity vascular tree and discussed individual cases with arterial and/or venous problems. The author concluded that proximal vascular injury can be diagnosed clinically by changes in the pulse, temperature, and the presence of pain or swelling in the upper extremity. The most common presenting symptom in athletes with proximal upper limb vascular problems is easy fatigability and paresthesias. Suspicious lesions were confirmed in most cases by angiography. The etiology for the majority of proximal upper extremity vascular problems

was thought to be repetitive or acute trauma with subsequent clot formation. Aggressive treatment with thrombectomy and the use of interpositional grafts was recommended in the majority of cases involving young individuals.

Bollinger reviewed vascular conditions that cause upper extremity pain, including arterial stenosis and occlusions, vasospastic disorders, and venous thrombosis. The primary value of this paper is to alert the physician to the symptoms of vascular problems when treating a patient with vague upper extremity symptoms.

Vasospastic Disease

Treatment of hand vasospastic disorders was discussed by Kaarela who used rabbits as the experimental model. Perivascular sympathectomy by adventitia stripping was performed on one forepaw metacarpal artery using the other forepaw metacarpal artery as a control. Vessels were then harvested and analyzed utilizing catecholamine histofluorescence at one and three weeks after surgery. Their studies showed that although the material stripped from vessels did contain adrenergic nerve fibers, vessels distal to the stripped areas also showed evidence of adventitial nerve fibers. This paper implies perivascular sympathectomy fails to remove distal adrenergic innervation. Catecholamine histofluorescence studies show that some sympathetic tissues travel with peripheral nerves rather than with the vessels. It is important to realize these comments do run counter to previous literature on rabbits indicating that perivascular sympathectomy does control adrenergic innervation. Comments involving the success or failure of perivascular sympathectomy for relief of vasospastic hand disorders should be reserved because this study contained no clinical correlates such as measurements of temperature or vascular flow differences between forepaws.

Freedman and associates investigated the effect of digital nerve block on preventing vasospastic attacks in patients with Raynaud disease. Vasospastic attacks were initiated in symptomatic patients with Raynaud phenomenon or scleroderma by a combination of environmental and local cooling. The incidence of vasospastic episodes was documented by alternatively blocking and unblocking patients' digits using 2% Lidocaine. The results clearly show that the incidence of vasospastic attacks in Raynaud's patients is no different in blocked or unblocked fingers. These data argue in favor of the Lewis' "local fault" hypothesis (in which precapillary resistance vessels are hypersensitive to local cooling, resulting in classic vasospastic symptoms) and against the hypothesis of sympathetic hyperactivity.

Bodelsson and associates studied the effect of cooling on vasoconstriction in human hand veins. The complicated study utilizing alpha 1 and 2 agonists and antagonists in combination with cooling showed that cooling has a significant effect on augmenting vasoconstriction of human hand veins. The increased vasoconstriction induced by cooling appears to be secondary to an increased response of alpha 2 adrenoreceptors. Agonist-antagonist studies in the same paper show that as temperature decreases, the effect of alpha 2 adrenoreceptor mediated vasoconstriction in human hand veins increases relative to other receptors. This study suggests that an alpha 2 antagonist such as Yohimbine might be of therapeutic value in patients with cold-induced vasoconstriction.

Engelhardt and associates investigated the effect of temperature on patients exhibiting vasospastic characteristics such as primary Raynaud phenomenon, systemic sclerosis, and undifferentiated connective tissue disease. The findings reveal that a transient vasoconstrictor response of both arterial and venous microvascular beds can be evoked in all patient groups. However, they note that while additional central cooling has no influence on arterial flow, the systemic sclerosis patient subgroups manifest a failure to maintain nutritive perfusion at finger temperatures associated with Raynaud phenomenon. This may be the reason for the propensity of systemic sclerosis patients to develop finger ulceration, and appears to separate these patients physiologically from other forms of Raynaud phenomenon.

Pelmear and associates reviewed the current international, British, and American standards dose response criteria for various vibrating tools which propose safety limits for their use. The current International Standards Organization uses a weighted average in which higher frequencies appear to be less damaging than lower frequencies. The authors reviewed data collected since 1983 by the Ontario government to measure the hand vibration levels of various tools. Their study concluded that current ISO threshold limits are questionably low for almost all tools tested. Vibrations of 150-250 Hz tend to be isolated to the hands and fingers that are directly in contact with the tool while vibrations less than 100 Hz are transmitted directly to the forearms. The most dangerous frequencies for blood vessels in their study were from 30-200 Hz and at 480 Hz. Those most dangerous for nerves ranged from 60-700 Hz with the most sensitive range between 250 and 350 Hz. The authors believe that all frequencies from as low as 6 Hz to as high as 5 kHz should be evaluated and that frequency weighting should be discontinued in favor of unweighted measurements.

Other articles by Nagata, Stark, and Hedlund discuss the role of vibration and/or cold exposure in the production of vasospastic disorders relating to various occupations and/or tool use. They suggest there is an increased incidence of vasospastic disorders in workers exposed to vibration. Cherniack provides an extensive literature of Raynaud phenomenon of occupational origin.

Annotated Bibliography

Evaluation Techniques

Baxter BT, Blackburn D, Payne K, et al: Noninvasive evaluation of the upper extremity. *Surg Clin N Am,* 70(1):87-97, 1990.

An overview of noninvasive tests that can be used in the diagnosis of upper extremity vascular problems. These tests are chosen on the basis of the history and physical exam.

Goodman S, Rubler S, Byrk H, et al: Arm exercise testing with myocardial scintigraphy in asymptomatic patients with peripheral vascular disease. *Chest,* 95(4):70-6, 1989.

A study involving the use of arm exercises along with myocardial scintigraphy and oxygen consumption is presented. This is seen as an effective method of detecting occult ischemia in patients with peripheral vascular diseases.

Hosokawa K, Hata Y, Yano K, et al: Results of the Allen test on 2,940 arms. *Anls Plast Surg,* 24(2):149-52, 1990.

Two thousand nine hundred forty adult hands (683 men and 787 women) were assessed with bilateral Allen radial artery compression tests. Abnormalities were found in 105 (3.6%). Incidence increased with age. Circulatory failure in the hand develops after several decades when the radial artery is removed during youth.

Maurer A: Nuclear medicine in evaluation of the hand and wrist. *Hand Clin,* 7(1):183-200, 1991.

Skeletal scintigraphy (bone scan) has developed into a widely used tool for early detection and staging of metastatic diseases to the evaluation of many skeletal disorders. This article reviews the technique of three-phase scintigraphy and application to the study of the hand and wrist.

Stein M, Provan JL, Prosser R, et al: A statistical assessment of the dependability of transcutaneous tissue oxygen tension measurements. *J Surg Research,* 46(1):70-5, 1989.

A study comparing transcutaneous oxygen tension measurements is reviewed in a group of peripheral vascular patients and a central group with readings from the arm, knee, and foot. The dependability of these values and a study analysis are included.

Occlusive Disease

Bollinger A: Arm pain due to vascular causes. *Therpapeutische Umschau,* 45(11):794-800, 1988.

Sotta RP: Vascular problems in the proximal upper extremity. *Clin Sports Med,* 9(2):279-88, 1990.

Vascular problems of the proximal upper extremity present with signs of venous and arterial occlusion. The treating physician must be aware of these and ready to treat vascular occlusion.

Vasospastic Disease

Bodelsson M, Arenklo-Nobin B, Nobin A, et al: Cooling enhances alpha 2 adrenoceptor-mediated vasoconstriction in human hand veins. *Acta Physiologica Scandinavica*, 138(3):283-91, 1990.

The contribution of different receptor subtypes in the contractile response during cooling in human hand vessels is of interest in the understanding of cold-induced peripheral vasospasm as it appears in Raynaud phenomenon.

Cherinak MG: Raynaud phenomenon of occupational origin. *Arch Int Med*, 150(3)519-22, 1990.

Vibration to the hand and arm by industrial power tools can cause vascular and neurovascular problems including cold-induced vascular spasm and peripheral neuropathies with paresthesis, dysesthesis, and sensory abnormalities. It can be difficult for the clinician to differentiate these from Raynaud phenomenon.

Engelhart M, Sibold JR: The effect of local temperature versus sympathetic tone on digital perfusion in Raynaud phenomenon. *Angiology*, 41(9pt1):715-23, 1990.

A study involving patients with peripheral vascular diseases suggests that finger temperature is the principal determinant of arterial flow in systemic sclerosis and that arterial flow is the principal determinant of microvascular perfusion.

Freedman RR, Mayes MD, Sabharwal SC: Induction of vasospastic attacks despite digital nerve block in Raynaud disease and phenomenon. *Circulation*, 80(40):859-62, 1989.

Vasospastic attacks were introduced to 21 patients with Raynaud or scleraderma. Two fingers on the hand were anesthetized with Lidocaine. There was no significant difference in the fingers' response.

Hedlund U: Raynaud phenomenon of fingers and toes of miners exposed to local and whole-body vibration and cold. *Int Arch Occup & Environ Hlth*, 61(70):457-61, 1989.

A study was done with 27 miners and a control group. They were both exposed to cold or other vasoconstrictive environmental factors and the miners also to hand or whole-body vibration. Those exposed to vibration had more Raynaud-like phenomenon.

Kaarela IO: Perivascular sympathectomy of the metacarpal artery of the rabbit paw fails to remove distal adrenergic innervation. *Scandinavian J Plast Recon Surg & Hand Surg*, 25(2):121-4, 1991.

Vasospastic disorders of the hand are commonly treated by perivascular sympathectomy, which is believed to remove distal adrenergic innervation. This experiment using rabbit forepaws failed to support this belief.

Nagata C, Yoshida H, Mirbod MS, et al: Raynaud phenomenon and cutaneous changes due to hand-arm vibration. *Sangyo Igaku-Japanese J Ind Hlth*, 32(5):366-70, 1990.

This paper describes the findings obtained from the observation of the skin of the hands exposed to vibration and evaluates the relation between Raynaud phenomenon and cutaneous changes.

Pelmear PL, Leong D, Taylor W, et al: Measurement of vibration of hand-held tools: weighted or unweighted? *J Occup Med*, 31(11):902-8, 1989.

The standards for hand-arm vibration used today were developed in the 1960s and were based on discomfort and tolerance levels. The recent epidemic of vascular and neurologic components of hand-arm vibration suggests the need to update these standards.

Savin E, Kedra AW, Oliva I, et al: Comparison of humeral blood flow during rewarming and recooling of the hand in normal subjects or presenting Raynaud phenomenon. *J Des Maladies Vasculaires*, 14(4):312-9, 1989.

A study comparing the effects that blood cooling and warming have on the circulation system in normal subjects versus those with Raynaud phenomenon. Subjects with Raynaud had limited vasodilation but vasoconstriction capacity was not disturbed.

Stark G, Pilger E, Klein GE, et al: White fingers after excessive motorcycle driving: a case report. *Vasa*, 19(3):257-9, 1990.

A case study of an 18-year-old male with Raynaud phenomenon who had arterial lesions in both hands much like those found in patients with vibration-induced white fingers. The only likely cause was in exposure to vibration due to excessive off-street motorcycle driving.

30

Replantation Surgery

Richard D. Goldner, MD

Introduction

Replantation is the treatment of choice for many amputations occurring in the upper extremity. Factors that must be considered in deciding whether to replant an amputated part are the predicted morbidity to the patient, the expected chance of survival and functional outcome of the replanted part, and the total cost incurred by the patient or third-party payer. For replantation to be selected as the treatment method, the anticipated function should be equal to or better than that achieved with amputation revision or prosthetic replacement, although cosmesis should not be ignored.

Factors that influence the decision to attempt replantation include the level of amputation; the type of injury, such as guillotine, crush, or avulsion; the presence of segmental injuries; the length of warm or cold ischemia; the age, general health, and occupation of the patient; and the potential for rehabilitation.

Indications and Contraindications for Replantation

Replantation should be considered in most cases of thumb amputation. Even avulsion injuries requiring thumb shortening, metacarpophalangeal joint fusion, or vein and/or nerve grafting are often functionally and cosmetically superior if successfully replanted when compared to alternative methods of reconstruction.

Individuals with multiple digit amputations are candidates for replantation. In some instances, only the least damaged digits can be replanted, and these digits are often shifted either to the most functional positions or to the least injured parts of the hand.

Successful replantation at the level of the palm, wrist, or distal forearm generally results in better function than would be achieved with a prosthesis. Sensibility, although decreased, is usually adequate and extrinsic muscles provide sufficient grasp and release, although intrinsic function is often poor.

In some individuals, replantation at the humeral level provides useful hand function while in others it may permit conversion of an above-elbow amputation to a more functional below-elbow level. Muscle necrosis and subsequent infection can complicate replantation through the humerus, and the surgeon must be selective in deciding to attempt replantation at this level.

Replanted digits distal to the superficialis insertion function well, although often the distal interphalangeal joint must be fused. Proximal interphalangeal and metacarpophalangeal joint motion is excellent, sensibility is good, the cosmetic results are pleasing, and operative time is usually less than four hours.

Replantation of nearly all amputated parts should be attempted in healthy children. Epiphyseal growth continues after replantation, sensibility is usually good, and useful function can be anticipated although the range of motion is often decreased.

Some types of injuries are not suitable for replantation. Amputations with severely crushed or mangled parts, or those with a prolonged warm ischemia time, especially when at the humeral or forearm level, or amputations with injuries at multiple levels are poor candidates for replantation. Additional contraindications include amputations that occur in patients with other serious injuries or systemic disease, in individuals with severely atherosclerotic vessels, in mentally unstable patients, or in those who cannot withstand anesthesia safely.

Replantation of a single digit proximal to the flexor superficialis insertion generally does not improve hand function and seldom is indicated, particularly if it involves the index finger. One review of 59 single digit amputations reported an average PIP joint motion of only 35° after replantation proximal to the flexor digitorum superficialis insertion. However, special consideration is given to certain musicians who must have 10 digits, and to individuals whose major concern is the appearance.

Care of the Amputated Part

Replantation is usually not recommended if the warm ischemic time is greater than six hours for an amputation proximal to the carpus, or greater than 12 hours for an amputated digit. Cooling the amputated part to 4° to 10°C can prolong the ischemic time to 10 to 12 hours for an amputation proximal to the carpus and to 24 hours or longer for a digit that has no muscle.

The amputated part should not be placed directly on ice and should not be frozen. Digits should be placed in a sterile, plastic specimen container filled with ringers lactate solution and the entire container placed on ice. An amputated hand or arm can be wrapped in sterile gauze or in a sterile towel moistened with ringers lactate solution, and placed in a plastic bag which is then placed on ice.

Assessment of Arterial Injury

A distal, sharp amputation with little or no crush or avulsion, and a short ischemic time, in a young, healthy patient is most likely to survive and function after replantation. Unfortunately, many amputations have crush and/or avulsion components that require the amputated parts and adjacent tissues to be inspected carefully and debrided meticulously. The "red line sign" is caused by traction on the neurovascular bundles, which tears branches along the course of the vessel, producing hemorrhage and a visible "red line" on the side of the finger. The "ribbon sign" describes an artery that is tortuous and twisted from traction injury, which distorts the adventitia and separates the media and intima. This is caused by a longitudinal traction force and the elastic recoil of the artery. Either of these signs is usually a contraindication to replantation due to injury to long segments of the digital vessels. Replantation may still be accomplished in selected cases by resecting the injured segment of artery or vein and spanning the defect with an interpositional vein graft between healthy vessel ends, without tension.

Operative Sequence — Digital Replantations

Slightly dorsal midlateral incisions are used to elevate dorsal and palmar skin flaps to locate volar digital arteries and nerves and dorsal veins. The proximal and distal wound edges are debrided to avoid infection, which is the most common complication after replantation. Bone shortening of 0.5 to 1 cm in digits often enables primary repair of digital arteries and veins without tension and allows primary closure.

Skeletal fixation in the digits can be achieved by longitudinal or crossed K-wires, intraosseous wires, intramedullary fixation, or plates. Although K-wires have been the most widely used method for fixation of replanted digits, problems include a lack of rigid fixation, difficulty with accurate bone opposition, and possible transfixion of soft tissues. Intraosseous wires placed perpendicular to each other have been shown to have the lowest angulation and nonunion rates. A single K-wire with an intraosseous wire can also yield good results. Although most methods produce "adequate" fixation for replantation, one study documented a 21% nonunion rate when using crossed K-wires, 8% with K-wire and intraosseous wire, and no known nonunions when using perpendicular intraosseous wires. It is notable that one-third of the patients in that series who demonstrated a nonunion at four months, healed with prolonged splinting.

After bone stability is achieved, the flexor and extensor tendons are repaired using a Tajima or modified Kessler stitch, and the lateral bands are repaired. Digital arteries and nerves are repaired or grafted, as are dorsal veins. At least one artery and two veins are anastomosed in each digit and both arteries and three veins are repaired when possible. Soft-tissue coverage is achieved using split- or full-thickness skin grafts or local rotation flaps as necessary.

If there is a skin and vein defect, a venous flap can be used to provide both skin coverage and venous repair. The flap can be based on a proximal venous pedicle from an adjacent digit or can be harvested as a free-tissue transfer from the volar wrist or dorsal hand. If skin coverage is needed over an arterial defect, a venous flap can be harvested, reversed, and the flap vein used to reconstruct the digital artery. Unfortunately, neither of these methods is completely reliable.

Techniques in Replantation of Distal Digital Amputations

Amputations distal to the interphalangeal joint of the thumb or the DIP joint of the fingers can be replanted successfully if digital arteries and dorsal veins can be located in the amputated part. Approximately 4 mm of dorsal skin proximal to the nail plate must be present on an amputated digit for dorsal veins to be located. A volar vein may be used if dorsal veins cannot be identified in the amputated tip.

If a vein in the amputated tip cannot be identified, an arteriovenous shunt can be established. One digital artery is repaired first while the contralateral unrepaired distal digital artery is anastomosed to a proximal vein allowing retrograde flow through an arteriovenous shunt.

If no venous return can be established by any method, the nail plate can be removed, and a heparin-soaked cotton pledget applied to the raw nail matrix. Every hour the nail matrix is rubbed with a sterile cotton applicator to stimulate bleeding. It may be necessary to heparinize the patient, but care must be taken to monitor PTT, platelet count, and hematocrit as this technique can result in substantial blood loss.

Use of Leeches

Medical grade leeches are available and can be placed on a fingertip if venous congestion occurs. The leeches become engorged in 15 to 30 minutes and then detach from the digit. However, they secrete a local anticoagulant, Hirudin, which allows the incision to bleed for eight to 12 hours preventing congestion. When the bleeding stops a leech is applied again to the fingertip. In one study that included four digits with no vein repairs and three digits with postoperative venous congestion, six of seven digits survived after being treated with leeches for an average of 4.7 days.

Leeches will not remain on avascular tissue and can infect the patient with aeromonas hydrophilia, identified as a gram negative anaerobic rod. This bacteria is endosymbiotic within the leech, inhibiting growth of other bacteria and producing digestive enzymes including amylase, lipase, and proteolytic hemolysin, essential to the breakdown of red cells and hemoglobin. Treatment of aeromoneas infection consists of early surgical debridement, and antibiotic treatment with aminoglycosides, Tetracycline, Chloramphenicol, Septra, third generation Cephalosporins, or Azthreonam.

Postoperative Management

Protective dressings and plaster splints are applied after surgery. The extremity is either elevated or placed at heart level depending on the arterial and venous status of the replanted part. Initially, the patient remains at bed rest in a quiet, warm room. Adequate peripheral blood flow is maintained by eliminating products with nicotine or caffeine and by keeping the patient well hydrated. Anticoagulants are used, depending on the degree of crush or avulsion, the appearance of the vessels before and after anastomosis, and whether or not vein grafts were used. Options include various combinations of aspirin, Persantine, low molecular weight Dextran, and heparin.

The digit is monitored hourly with attention to color, capillary refill, turgor, and surface temperature. Although various monitors have been used, skin surface temperature is reliable, noninvasive, reproducible, and safe. A temperature drop of greater than 2°C in one hour, or a temperature below 30°C indicates decreased digital perfusion, which may require re-exploration of the vessel repairs.

Results of Thumb Replantation

Early reports indicated approximately 75% of replanted thumbs survived, although avulsion injuries succeeded in only 40% to 45% of cases. More recently, aggressive debridement of injured tissue and the use of vein grafts have improved thumb replantation survival to greater than 90% of cases. One recent study reported an 82% survival rate in 19 of 23 patients who at 20.5 months follow-up had an average grip strength of 95% and a key pinch 77% of the unaffected side. Twenty percent of the patients achieved a two-point discrimination of less than 5 mm.

In another series, replantation was attempted for 42 complete thumb amputations regardless of the mechanism or severity of injury. Sixteen thumbs or 38% of cases failed intraoperatively or postoperatively. Thumbs with a narrow zone of injury had a significantly higher survival rate of 76% than those with a wide zone of injury of only 41%, while 46% of avulsed thumbs survived. The total active motion of the MCP and IP joints averaged 68°. Grip strength averaged 77%, key pinch 44%, and pulp pinch 60% of the uninjured side. Two-point discrimination averaged 11 mm and cold intolerance was not a problem after one year. The authors recommend attempted replantation of all thumb amputations but note that three patients with primary amputations had stronger grip strength, pulp pinch, and key pinch than their normal contralateral side.

Other authors reviewed results of thumb amputations that were not replanted including 13 at the distal phalanx and 12 at a more proximal level. The final outcome was good in eight patients, fair in 12 and poor in five. Only patients with amputations at or distal to the IP joint had normal key and pinch grip. Six patients never returned to work and two carpenters worked at a lower capacity. The median time off work was 114 days. The most frequent complaints were hypersensitivity, difficulty in picking up small objects, cold intolerance, and pain when using the remaining part of the digit. These problems were not related to thumb length.

Another study divided patients with complete thumb amputations into those replanted and those who underwent revision amputations. Twenty-five of the patients with replanted thumbs and 18 of those with revision amputations underwent testing that consisted of interview and physical examination, test of activities of daily living, Jebsen test of hand function, and both static and dynamic testing on the BTE work simulator. Ninety percent of replantations were between the MCP joint and the proximal third of the distal phalanx. Shortening averaged 11 mm and range of motion was 42% ± 28% that of the uninjured thumb.

Twenty-one percent had 7 mm or less two-point discrimination and 38% had between 8 mm and 20 mm. Eighty percent of patients in both groups were able to perform activities of daily living at 80% of their uninjured side. Grip strength was approximately 84% that of the uninjured hand in each group. Lateral pinch averaged 68% ± 25% that of the normal side in the replant group and 91% ± 9% in the amputation group. BTE work simulator assessment of lateral and three point pinch was better in the amputation revision group. Scores on Jebsen testing were slightly better for those with replanted thumbs, but in general neither replant nor revision-amputation patients functioned as well as did Jebsen's normal patients. Median time for return to work for patients with replanted thumbs was 11 weeks compared to eight weeks for those with amputations, but the range was large in these groups. Eighty-seven percent of patients in the replant group (26/30) returned to their pre-injury job, compared with 70% (12/17) in the amputation revision group.

It was not possible in this group of patients to demonstrate a uniform superiority of replantation over amputation revision. Patients with an isolated thumb amputation distal to the MCP joint, whether replanted or revised, had some degree of functional impairment. Function decreased in both groups of patients with injuries proximal to the proximal third of the proximal phalanx, especially if final sensibility was poor. Function of thumbs amputated through the IP joint or proximal phalanx depended on the extent of injury and the patient's motivation. Good results were seen in certain individuals in both the replant and amputation groups. The most frequent patient complaint was poor sensibility. Those with replanted thumbs and good sensibility tended to perform better in tasks requiring fine dexterity than did those with amputations. Patients with isolated thumb loss usually had stronger pinch than did those with a replantation although they had more difficulty holding certain objects. Most patients with isolated thumb amputation distal to the MCP joint, whether replanted or revised, adapted to their injury and resumed activities of daily living and their jobs.

Classifications of Ring-avulsion Injuries and Results of Treatment

There are several classifications of ring-avulsion injury but that described by Urbaniak is used most commonly.

Class 1: Circulation is adequate. Standard bone and soft-tissue treatment is sufficient.

Class 2: Circulation is inadequate. Vessel repair preserves viability. (Other authors have subdivided Class 2 injuries to distinguish between those in which digital arteries are compromised but bones, tendons, nerves, and veins are intact; those in which circulation is inadequate and bone, tendon, or nerve injury exists; and those in which only venous compromise exists.)

Class 3: Complete degloving or complete amputation.

Complete amputations, especially those proximal to the flexor digitorum superficialis insertion, or with complete degloving of the ring finger, have the worst prognosis for replantation and often are best managed by surgical amputation of the digit. However, one review of seven patients with Urbaniak Class 3 avulsions revealed there was an average 85% replantation success rate leading to a useful digit. MCP joint motion ranged from 0° to 85°, with PIP motion from 15° to 90° and DIP motion from 0° to 15°. Protective sensation was present in all patients and sensation was good in three. If the amputation was distal to the superficialis insertion and if vein and nerve grafts were used, these authors felt the results justified the procedure. When the PIP joint was damaged or the proximal phalanx was fractured, amputation was recommended. Another series demonstrated excellent functional results if only venous compromise was present.

One of the largest series of ring-avulsion injuries reviewed 55 cases. Three patients with Class 1 injuries were all successful. Replantation was successful in 86% of patients with Class 2 injuries and in 73% of those with Class 3 injuries. Seventy-five percent of 12 successful patients with Class 2 and 69% of 13 successful Class 3 patients had 90⁰ or more PIP and DIP motion.

Sensory Recovery after Replantation

One review summarized the results of 12 previously published reports including 367 fingers and 87 thumbs replanted successfully. The mean patient age was 32.5 years and mean follow-up was 33.5 months. Mean static two-point discrimination was 9.3 mm in cleanly amputated thumbs and 12.1 mm in crush/avulsion thumb injuries. The mean overall was 11 mm in thumb and 12 mm in finger replantation.

Return of sensibility was better after replantation of sharply amputated fingers, which averaged 8 mm while those with crush-avulsion injuries averaged 15 mm. Sixty-one percent of replanted thumbs and 54% of replanted fingers regained two-point discrimination of 15 mm or less. Recovery of sensibility appears to be better in children and in patients with distal replantations.

Cold intolerance can be the most disabling symptom after digital replantation. It is present in most replanted digits and usually improves after two years. One study showed cold intolerance and a normal thermoregulatory response to return as sensibility recovered. That is, if one to two years following replantation, a static two-point discrimination of S3 or greater is achieved, symptoms of cold intolerance are minimal and vasoregulation approaches normal.

Control of thermoregulation after replantation appears to be a combination of vascular and neural mechanisms. Controversy remains as to the relationship between cold intolerance, the number of digital vessels repaired, digital pulse pressure, and the recovery of sensibility.

Flexor Tendolysis after Replantation

Other authors reviewed data on patients with 37 amputated fingers and four replanted thumbs requiring flexor tendolysis at an average of 10 months after replantation. These cases represented 13% of the authors' total series. The indication for digital tendolysis was a significant discrepancy between passive and active flexion after four to six months in the presence of demonstrable return of sensibility. The total active motion increased from a mean of 72° to 130° after tendolysis. There were 13 excellent, 11 good, 6 fair, and 11 poor results. The thumbs had two fair and two poor results. The poor results were also seen in crush or avulsion injuries, hands with more than two digits amputated, and those requiring PIP joint capsulotomy. Complications included tendon ruptures and infections but no digits were lost. Despite the absence of major complications, 25% still had poor results. The study supports flexor tendolysis after replantation of fingers but not thumbs. Digits sustaining avulsion amputation, in close proximity to the MCP joint, with significant PIP joint stiffness, or associated with multiple digit amputations, are less likely to have a good functional result.

Techniques in Major Limb Replantation

The problems associated with major limb replantation proximal to the wrist are different from those associated with digital replantation. Prolonged ischemia prior to a hand replantation, for example, can lead to intrinsic muscle fibrosis and contracture, while excessive ischemia in a more proximal amputation can result in forearm or arm muscle necrosis. Skeletal muscle is very sensitive to ischemia and must be protected by cooling during transfer and/or by rapid revascularization to prevent cell death; therefore a synthetic shunt is inserted initially during hand or arm replantation cases to provide arterial inflow to muscles as quickly as possible. Unhealthy tissue is debrided extensively to prevent subsequent myonecrosis and infection. Fasciotomy is performed routinely to prevent developing a compartment syndrome after surgery. Inadequate debridement that leads to infection, and inadequate decompression of muscle compartments, are the two most common causes of failure in major limb replantation cases. The bone is stabilized, usually with plates and screws while the synthetic shunt is in place. Two to four centimeters of bone shortening is usually necessary in the forearm while the humerus can be shortened up to 8 cm to permit soft-tissue closure. We routinely insert an arterial shunt for replantation cases proximal to the wrist, or perform arterial anastomosis before the veins are repaired. This sequence provides a physiologic washout of lactic acid and toxic breakdown products of anaerobic metabolism to prevent them from being transported systemically as occurs when veins are repaired prior to arteries. Intravenous sodium bicarbonate may also be given to the patient prior to completing the venous repairs. If venous reconstruction is performed first, the return of toxic catabolites through the system microcirculation can cause myofobinoria, renal failure, systemic acidosis, and hypercalcemia. The disadvantage of re-establishing arterial flow first is that blood loss is increased. However, if a pneumatic tourniquet is used intermittently, and if the surgeon and anesthesiologist are cognizant of the amount of blood being lost during the procedure, the patient's blood volume can be maintained adequately with blood transfusions.

Heparin is not used after forearm or arm replantation because the lacerated muscle associated with these amputations can cause excessive bleeding if the patient is anticoagulated. Patients with forearm or arm replantation are returned to the operating room 48 to 72 hours later for wound inspection and further soft-tissue debridement if necessary.

Results of Transhumeral Replantation

One series reviewed seven patients with complete transhumeral amputations. The mechanism of injury was avulsion in all cases, and the average ischemic time was 12 hours. Seventy percent of replanted arms (5/7) survived, yielding useful elbow flexion of 90° or more and adequate strength. Two patients with surviving arms had useful distal function in the wrist and hand. Most patients required multiple additional procedures averaging 2.8 per patient, including the following: corrective osteotomies; release of muscle, joint, and skin contractures; nerve grafting; tendon or muscle transfers; tendolysis; sequestrectomy; free muscle transfer, or below-elbow amputation.

It was concluded that replantation is indicated in selected patients with a transhumeral amputation. The patients most suitable for consideration are those who are medically and psychologically stable and who have relatively isolated injuries. Patients must understand the limited expectations of the procedure. Hand function equal to or better than a prosthesis is achieved in some patients while in others, later below-elbow amputation may be indicated.

Annotated Bibliography

Urbaniak JR: Replantation, pp. 1085-1102, in Green DP (ed): *Operative Hand Surgery,* Churchill Livingstone, New York, 1993.

This comprehensive review of replantation covers patient selection, instruments, preparation of the amputated part for transportation, technique and sequence of surgery, postoperative care, major limb replantation, and expectations following replantation. The references are thorough and current.

Weiland AJ, Raskin KB: Philosophy of replantation. *Microsurg,* 11:223-228, 1990.

This article reviews current concepts of replantation including patient selection, transportation, indications and contraindications for replantation, technique, and postoperative management.

Indications and Contraindications

Axelrod TS, Buchler U: Severe complex injuries to the upper extremity: Revascularization and replantation. *J Hand Surg,* 16A:574-584, 1991.

Twenty-nine patients were reviewed with incomplete (26) or complete (three) amputations of the upper extremity proximal to the wrist with revascularization or replantation. Limb survival rates were 95%. Bone shortening osteotomies helped to reduce the soft-tissue defect size. In this series, all patients with surviving limbs achieved distal limb function superior to that offered by a prosthesis.

Goldner RD, Stevanovic MV, Nunley JA, Urbaniak JR: Digital replantation at the level of the distal interphalangeal joint and the distal phalanx. *J Hand Surg,* 14A:214-220, 1989.

Forty-two complete, single digit amputations at the distal interphalangeal joint or distal phalanx were reviewed. Success rate, return of sensibility, range of motion, time lost from work, and average total cost of treatment are discussed in comparing replantation with conventional procedures.

Meyer VE: Hand amputations proximal but close to the wrist joint: prime candidates for reattachment (long-term functional results). *J Hand Surg,* 10A:989-991, 1985.

One hundred twenty-nine patients (from Shanghai, Louisville, and Zurich) with upper limb replantations were reviewed. Results of the 49 cases of amputation proximal to the wrist but close to the joint (distal forearm) are discussed specifically.

Russell RC, O'Brien BM, Morrison WA, Pamamull G, MacLeod A: The late functional results of upper limb revascularization and replantation. *J Hand Surg,* 9A:623-633, 1984.

The functional results in 25 of 30 patients after successful upper limb revascularization or replantation were evaluated by subjective patient survey and objective measurements. Young patients with complete, sharply amputated extremities at the wrist level or those with incomplete injuries and uninjured peripheral nerves had the best functional results. Multiple-level, diffuse crush or avulsion injuries, even if the injuries were incomplete, and patients with high-level nerve injury had less return of function.

Taras JS, Nunley JA, Urbaniak JR, Goldner RD, Fitch RD: Replantation in children. *Microsurg,* 12:216-220, 1991.

The authors reviewed results of replantation of 162 parts in 120 children over the past 15 years. They suggest that unlike an adult, any child suffering a traumatic amputation should be considered for a replantation. Survival rate for complete replantation in children under 16 years of age was 77%. Long-term studies showed that continued skeletal growth occurred and the digit attained 81% of normal longitudinal length at maturity. Recovery of sensibility in the replanted digit is nearly as good as for isolated digital nerve repair.

Urbaniak JR, Roth JH, Nunley JA, Goldner RD, Koman LA: The results of replantation after amputation of a single finger. *J Bone Joint Surg,* 67A:611-619, 1985.

These authors studied 59 consecutive patients who had replantation of a single finger after traumatic amputation. Fifty-one (86%) of the replanted fingers survived. The functional results were most dependent on the level of amputation. The PIP joint in amputated fingers that were replanted distal to the insertion of the flexor superficialis tendon had an average range of motion of 82° after replantation, while those amputated proximal to the insertion had an average range of motion of only 35° after replantation. Based on this experience, it was the authors' opinion that replantation of a single finger that was amputated distal to the insertion of the flexor superficialis tendon is justified, but that replantation of a single finger that was amputated proximal to this insertion is seldom indicated.

Operative Sequence—Digital Replantations

Brown ML, Wood MB; Techniques of bone fixation in replantation surgery. *Microsurg,* 11:255-260, 1990.

These authors review methods of osteosynthesis in replantation surgery at the level of the phalanges, metacarpals, wrist, forearm, elbow, and humerus.

Whitney TM, Lineaweaver WC, Buncke HJ, Nugent K: Clinical results of bony fixation methods in digital replantation, *J Hand Surg,* 15A: 328-334, 1990.

Phalangeal replants over a five-year period were analyzed retrospectively to assess the outcome of different fixation methods with regard to frequency of angulation, fracture instability, nonunion, and the need for corrective osteotomy. Initial results show similar early angulation deformities in all groups. Intraosseous wires alone were found to have the lowest nonunion and complication rates. Overall, bony problems were seen in nearly 50% of replants in this series.

Techniques in Replantation of Distal Digital Amputations

Fukui A, Maeda M, Inada Y, Tamai S, Sempuku T: Arteriovenous shunt in digit replantation. *J Hand Surg,* 15A:160-165, 1990.

Use of the arteriovenous shunt in digital replantation is described in four cases. Two replantations were successful; necrosis developed in the other two patients.

Koshima I, Soeda S, Moriguchi T, Higaki H, Miyakawa S, Yamasaki M: The use of arteriovenous anastomosis for replantation of the distal phalanx of the fingers. *Plastic Recon Surg,* 89:710-714, 1992.

Arteriovenous anastomosis was used to reestablish either the arterial or the venous drainage system in 33 digits in 23 patients. The success rate was 91%.

Use of Leeches

Brody GA, Maloney WJ, Hentz VR: Digit replantation applying the leech Hirudo Medicinalis. *Clin Orthop,* 24S:133-137, 1989.

This series comprises the authors' first seven patients treated with Hirudo Medicinalis. These conclude that the use of medicinal leeches shows promise as a safe and effective method of providing temporary venous drainage in replanted digits.

Lowen RM, Rodgers CM, Ketch LL, Phelps DB: Aeromonas hydrophilia infection complicating digital replantation and revascularization. *J Hand Surg,* 14A:714-718, 1989.

Two cases of thumb replantation and one finger revascularization complicated by aeromonas hydrophilia infection are reported. Two digits were lost because of infection in the soft tissue and osteomyelitis. One thumb had extensive necrosis. In all cases, the infection was difficult to eradicate, probably because of ischemia. All three patients sustained their injuries while cutting meat or fish. Note is made of aeromonas hydrophilia in medicinal leeches that are used in microvascular surgery and the potential for iatrogenic infection.

Postoperative Management

Goldner RD: Postoperative Management. *Hand Clin,* 1:205-215, 1985.

This article reviews postoperative management of replantation patients including postoperative orders, medications, postoperative examination, monitoring, early complications, and treatment of the compromised replant. Postoperative physical therapy and secondary procedures in replantation patients are discussed briefly.

Results of Thumb Replantation

Bowen CVA, Beveridge J, Milliken RG, Johnston GHP: Rotating shaft avulsion amputations of the thumb. *J Hand Surg,* 16A:117-121, 1991.

Twenty-three of 29 patients with rotating shaft avulsion of the thumb were considered suitable for replantation. Survival was achieved in 19 of 23 replantations. Grip, pinch, and sensibility were good enough to encourage an aggressive microsurgical approach to these injuries.

Goldner RD, Howson MP, Nunley JA, Fitch RD, Belding NR, Urbaniak JR: One hundred eleven thumb amputations: replantation vs. revision. *Microsurg,* 11:243-250, 1990.

Of patients sustaining isolated complete thumb amputations, 25 who underwent replantation and 18 who underwent revision of amputation had testing that consisted of interview and physical examination, test of activities of daily living, Jebsen test of hand function, and both static and dynamic testing on the BTE work simulator.

Hovgaard C, Dalsgaard S, Gebuhr P: The social and economic consequences of failure to replant amputated thumbs. *J Hand Surg,* 14B:307-308, 1989.

Because replantation of the amputated thumb is not always possible, the effect of complete amputation at various levels was examined in 32 patients.

Ward WA, Tsai TM, Breidenbach W: *Per primam* thumb replantation for all patients with traumatic amputations. *Clin Orthop Related Res,* 266:90-95, May 1991.

These authors reviewed 42 patients with complete thumb amputations replanted between 1980 and 1984. Success rate, factors affecting survival, range of motion, sensibility, and results of reexploration are discussed.

Kay S, Werntz J, Wolff TW: Ring-avulsion injuries; classification and prognosis. *J Hand Surg,* 14A:204-213, 1989.

Fifty-five cases of ring-avulsion injuries were reviewed to examine how the extent of injury and the surgical management correlated with results. These authors felt that completely amputated digits (Urbaniak Class 3) are salvageable and have comparable results to ring-avulsion injuries with skeletal injury (Class 2). They propose a revised classification system including new classes for injuries with and without skeletal injury.

Nissenbaum M: Class IIA ring-avulsion injuries: an absolute indication for microvascular repair. *J Hand Surg,* 9A: 810-815, 1984.

The Urbaniak Class 2 ring-avulsion category includes incomplete amputations with inadequate circulation. These authors proposed Class 2A to indicate digits with arterial compromise only and 2B to indicate inadequate circulation with bone, tendon, or nerve injury. They indicated that replantation of a Class 2A ring-avulsion injury results in as close to a normal digit as possible.

Tsai TM, Mansteln C, DuBou R, Wolff TW, Kutz JE, Kleinert HE: Primary microsurgical repair of ring-avulsion amputation injuries. *J Hand Surg,* 9A:68-72, 1984.

Seven patients with ring-avulsion amputation injuries that were reconstructed by use of microsurgical reanastomoses are reported. All were classified as Urbaniak Class 3 avulsions. Six patients (85%) had a successful replantation leading to a useful finger. These authors indicate that if the amputation is distal to the PIP joint, with a functional superficialis tendon, primary microsurgical repair is the treatment of choice in complex ring-avulsion injuries.

Urbaniak JR, Evans JP, Bright DS; Microvascular management of ring-avulsion injuries. *J Hand Surg,* 6:25-30, 1981.

Nine ring fingers were successfully revascularized of 24 acute ring-avulsion injuries reviewed. The classification system is outlined. Complete amputations, especially proximal to the superficial insertion, and complete degloving injuries of the ring finger were best managed by surgical amputation of the digit.

Weil DJ, Wood VE, Frykman GK: A new class of ring-avulsion injuries. *J Hand Surg,* 14A:662-664, 1989.

Sixteen patients with ring-avulsion injuries were reviewed. Follow-up functional measurements showed that the average grip strength of Urbaniak Class 2 patients was no better than that of the Class 3 patients, even though all of the Class 3 patients had amputation revisions. Five Class 2 patients required only venous microvascular repair. The authors proposed to modify Urbaniak's classification to include ring-avulsion injuries with only venous compromise (Class 2C). These patients had excellent functional results, with an average total active motion of 224°.

Sensory Recovery After Replantation

Glickman L, Mackinnon S: Sensory recovery following digital replantation. *Microsurg,* 11:236-242, l990.

These authors reviewed 12 series of digital replantations between 1977 and l989. Three hundred sixty-seven fingers and 87 thumbs were included. Factors that influenced digital sensibility following replantation included the patient's age, level and mechanism of injury, digital blood flow, cold intolerance, and postoperative sensory reeducation. Recovery of sensibility in the replanted digit is comparable to simple nerve repair and to nerve-grafting techniques.

Koman LA, Nunley JA: Thermoregulatory control after upper extremity replantation. *J Hand Surg,* 11A: 548-552, 1986.

Four patients with complete forearm amputations between the wrist and elbow were analyzed prospectively to determine the interrelationships of thermoregulation to pain, cold intolerance, arterial integrity, venous competence, motor nerve recovery, sensory nerve recovery, and time. Cold intolerance and normal thermoregulatory response, as indicated by cold-stress test performances, were temporarily related to attainment of two-point sensory discrimination, or to motor-nerve recovery, or to both.

Flexor Tendolysis After Replantation

Jupiter JB, Pess GM, Bour CJ: Results of flexor tendon tenolysis after replantation in the hand. *J Hand Surg,* 14A:35-44, 1989.

Thirty-seven replanted digital units and four thumb replantations had a flexor tendolysis at an average of l0 months after replantation. The results of this study support flexor tendolysis after replantation of fingers but not after thumb replantation.

Techniques in Major Limb Replantation

Goldner RD, Nunley JA: Replantation proximal to the wrist. pp. 413-425, in Wood MD (ed) *Hand Clinics: Microsurgery,* W.B. Saunders Co., Philadelphia, 1992.

This is a detailed review of techniques used in replantation proximal to the wrist.

Kleinert JM, Graham B: Macroreplantation: an overview. *Microsurg,* 11:229-233, 1990.

These authors review the literature on replantation and summarize pertinent results.

Wood MB, Cooney WP: Above-elbow limb replantation: functional results. *J Hand Surg,* 11A:682-687, 1986.

Seven patients with a complete transhumeral limb amputation had their limb replanted. In all seven limbs, the mechanism of injury was avulsion, and the ischemic time was relatively prolonged. Five patients with surviving limbs achieved useful elbow control. Out of these patients, two achieved useful function distal to the wrist and hand and one had a below-elbow amputation. They suggested limb replantation at the transhumeral levels may be of value for recovery of elbow function in most of these patients. In some instances, this may permit conversion of an above-elbow amputation to a functional below-elbow level. In a few patients, recovery of useful hand function may be achieved.

31

Microsurgical Soft-tissue Coverage

William M. Swartz, MD

Introduction

Reconstruction of soft-tissue defects of the hand by microsurgical techniques has provided solutions to some of the most difficult and challenging hand reconstructive problems. The principal benefit of microsurgical procedures over conventional techniques lies in the ability to select the most ideal tissues for restoration of soft-tissue loss. Examples include specialized tissues for a sensory restoration of the fingertips and the hand, gliding tissue for restoration of a proper bed for tendon and nerve reconstruction, and unique tissues to include combined soft tissue, vascular or bone structures. A second major benefit of these techniques is that the donor site can be distant from the injured hand, thus eliminating the need for increasing trauma to the already compromised extremity.

Recent advances in microsurgical reconstruction over the past five years to be emphasized in this update include: (1) refinement in fingertip reconstruction including sensory restoration and nail restoration with vascularized partial toe transfers from the great toe and second toe; (2) the introduction of venous flaps for restoration of small soft-tissue and vascular loss in the digits; and (3) refinement in free-tissue donor sites for specific reconstructive requirements, notably small muscle flaps such as the serratus muscle for hypothenar reconstruction, the temporoparietal fascia free flap for resurfacing the dorsum of the hand and digits, and the lateral arm flap for reconstruction of substantial soft-tissue loss. Additional nonmicrosurgical methods of providing distally based pedicled forearm tissue from the radial artery-based flaps, the ulnar artery-based flaps and the posterior interosseous flap will be discussed as an alternative to free-tissue transfers.

The applications of microsurgical free-tissue transfer in the upper extremity have become widespread and well accepted. They include the use of emergency free flaps for trauma reconstruction, free-tissue transfers for one-stage reconstruction following limb-sparing tumor surgery, and delayed reconstruction for complex wound problems.

Digital Restoration Using Toe Pulp Flaps

Since the original description of the use of the first web space and toe pulp for digital resurfacing by Strauch and associates in 1984, refinements of this concept have provided the reconstructive surgeon with a number of options in restoring the digital pulp. The advantages of using these tissues over such procedures as thenar and cross-finger flaps are that the pulp volume is restored and the opportunity for providing sensory rehabilitation is maximized. The initial description of the first and second toe web space used

the blood supply from the first dorsal metatarsal artery, a branch of the dorsalis pedis artery. This dorsal dissection, which included the terminal branches of the deep peroneal nerve, did not provide maximum sensory restoration. Additionally, patients who were reticent to have the great toe operated upon stimulated other authors to expand the potential donor sites. Consequently, the second toe was developed as a donor site. Wei and associates described a second toe wrap-around similar to the great toe wrap-around but based on the dorsal circulation from the dorsalis pedis artery. The plantar digital nerves, however, were included in the dissection and these nerves were then used to restore sensibility to an injured digit. The second toe skeleton was amputated leaving a four-toed foot. The two-point discrimination measured in these flaps ranged from 8 mm to greater than 15 mm. Seeking ever greater refinements to this technique, Eadie and associates transferred the web space between the second and third toes using the plantar vascular and neural systems. They demonstrated an improved moving two-point discrimination of 10 mm to 12 mm. This smaller flap was closed with a full-thickness skin graft from the groin (Fig. 31-1). The authors report that an additional advantage for this flap is the avoidance of hypertrophic scars in the first web space, a common problem for people who wear thongs.

Additional indications for these partial toe transfers are for nail bed restoration in traumatized digits. The thin ony-

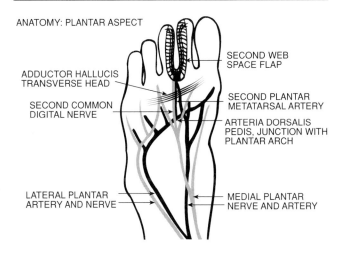

ANATOMY: PLANTAR ASPECT

SECOND WEB SPACE FLAP

ADDUCTOR HALLUCIS TRANSVERSE HEAD

SECOND COMMON DIGITAL NERVE

SECOND PLANTAR METATARSAL ARTERY

ARTERIA DORSALIS PEDIS, JUNCTION WITH PLANTAR ARCH

LATERAL PLANTAR ARTERY AND NERVE

MEDIAL PLANTAR NERVE AND ARTERY

Figure 31-1. The anatomy of the second metatarsal flap illustrating the neurovascular supply from the second metatarsal artery and the second common digital nerve. Reproduced with permission from Eadie et al: Clinical experience with the second metatarsal artery neurovascular flap. *J Plast Surg Br*, 45:136, 1992.

chocutaneous flaps from one-half of the great toe, based on the dorsalis pedis circulation were used by Roshima and associates for reconstruction of distal phalangeal losses of the fingers. The donor-site defects in these cases were also covered with split-thickness skin grafts and the results showed a small but adequate nail remaining in these patients. The flap also included the medial aspect of the big toe, but the distal phalanx was left intact, unlike the wrap-around flap of Morrison. The main advantage of this technique over the wrap-around flap is that it leaves the donor digit of the toe intact with a functioning nail.

The overall impact of these techniques is to restore digital pulp and nail loss with like tissue, which has led to an improved aesthetic and functional result over traditional methods of amputation or soft-tissue coverage only.

Venous Free Flaps

The concept that tissue could be transferred on a vascular pedicle consisting only of venous tissue was first put forth by Takiyama and associates in 1981. Over the past five years several clinical series have been developed utilizing these concepts. Tsai and associates studied a series of 15 patients who underwent replantation or revascularization of a single digit with a substantial dorsal defect. They utilized the dorsal tissues of nonreplantable tissues as a free flap to bridge the venous gap on the dorsum of the finger. The veins were repaired, both proximally and distally, and no arterial inflow was provided. Small skin flaps transferred with this venous tissue survived completely. However, when this concept was utilized to design free-flap donor sites from the forearm or dorsum of the foot, it was unsuccessful. The findings, however, supported the clinical feasibility of venous flaps, and the investigators postulated that a high venous flow was necessary to support skin-flap survival in this system. Iwasawa and others used this concept to reconstruct a fingertip, using a flap from the dorsum of the toe which included part of the nail bed. The nail flap, which included the dorsal veins, was transplanted to the thumb, and vascular anastomoses were performed between the dorsal veins and the digital artery. Thus, this flap was an arterialized venous flap unlike the previous flap described. More recently, Roshima has improved on the concept of arterialized venous flaps and performed extremity reconstruction utilizing flaps overlying the saphenous vein in the medial aspect of the leg. An artery was hooked up to the distal flap vein and the proximal flap vein hooked to a recipient vein, providing sufficient nutrient flow for uniform flap survival.

The size of venous flaps that have been successfully raised in the forearm are 8 cm by 3 cm and up to 11 cm by 7 cm in the medial aspect of the leg. The hemodynamics of these flaps remains controversial. It is thought that vasoparalysis after surgical denervation may account for the failure of venous valves and the opening of arteriovenous shunts, thereby permitting reverse flow against intact venous valves for arterial blood to reach the arterioles.

The conceptual advantage of this technique over conventional free-flap donor sites is obvious. Flaps can be designed with only cutaneous venous circulation in mind and these flaps are more numerous and available than flaps that depend on segmental or septocutaneous arteries. While this concept is still in its infancy, these developments will have significant impact on future flap design.

Refinement of Free-flap Donor Sites

With a wide variety of free-flap donor sites available, a consensus has developed over the past five years as to the most effective donor sites for soft-tissue coverage in the upper extremity. In general, reconstructive surgeons today choose between free-flap donor sites to include the lateral arm flap, the temporoparietal fascia flap, and the scapular flap. Pedicled tissue donor sites from the forearm require microsurgical dissection, and include the reverse radial forearm flap, ulnar artery-based flaps, and the posterior interosseous pedicle flap. The choice between these donor sites depends on the individual tissue requirements, the patient's body habitus, and the extent of the injury. For example, in a hand injury where arterial compromise is present, a pedicled radial artery-based flap or ulnar artery-based flap would not be appropriate. In these circumstances the posterior interosseous flap might be chosen.

The Lateral Arm Flap

First described by Ratsaros and associates, this flap has gained significant popularity and widespread usage due to its versatility. The skin flap is relatively thin and is based over the lateral intermuscular septum of the upper arm, extending from the deltoid grove to the lateral epicondyle. The skin flap can measure up to 6 cm in width and 9 cm to 11 cm in length, still permitting primary donor-site closure. The vascular pedicle of up to 8 cm consists of the posterior radial collateral artery and its vena comitantes (Fig. 31-2). When the flap is centered over the lateral epicondyle, branches of the posterior humeral cutaneous nerve will provide sensory innervation to this flap with the ability to provide protective sensation only. The principal advantage of this flap over other donor sites is that the flap can be elevated from the same extremity that is injured with little, if any, additional trauma. The posterior radial collateral artery sacrifice does not compromise the remainder of the extremity and additional dissection sites and patient repositioning need not be considered. The donor defect is a linear scar that is well tolerated. The only drawback, in this author's opinion, is sensory deprivation to the dorsum of the proximal forearm. In heavy patients, this flap can be bulky, requiring secondary thinning as any flap would require other than the temporoparietal fascia. The experience of Ratsaros, published in 1991, of 20 patients undergoing upper-extremity reconstruction outlines the advantages of this flap.

The Temporoparietal Fascia Flap

The temporoparietal fascia flap, first described by Robert Allan Smith in 1980, has subsequently enjoyed increasing popularity for the resurfacing of hand defects. The flap is

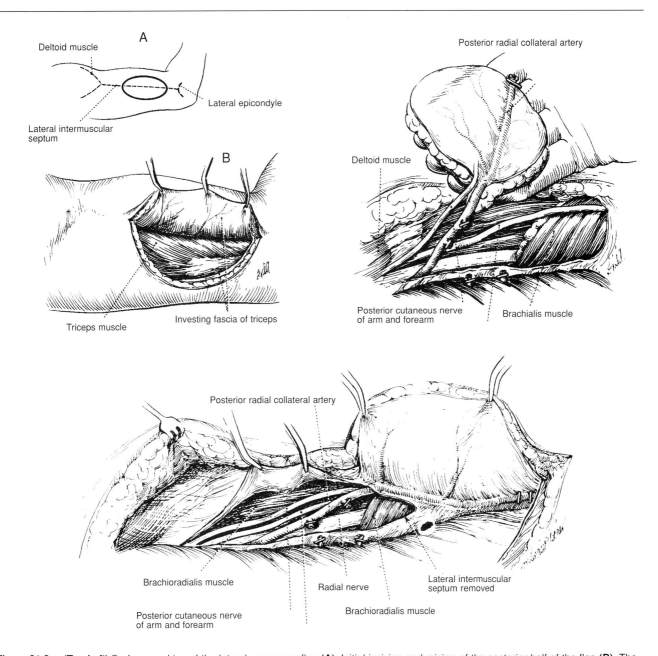

A

Deltoid muscle

Lateral epicondyle

Lateral intermuscular septum

B

Triceps muscle

Investing fascia of triceps

Posterior radial collateral artery

Deltoid muscle

Posterior cutaneous nerve of arm and forearm

Brachialis muscle

Posterior radial collateral artery

Brachioradialis muscle

Radial nerve

Lateral intermuscular septum removed

Brachioradialis muscle

Posterior cutaneous nerve of arm and forearm

Figure 31-2.   **(Top Left)** Surface marking of the lateral upper arm flap **(A)**. Initial incision and raising of the posterior half of the flap **(B)**. The cutaneous branches of the PRCA are readily seen as they arise in the lateral intermuscular septum. Note that deep fascia is included with the flap. **(Top Right)** The flap raise. The posterior cutaneous nerve of the arm has been included in the flap. **(Bottom)** Exposure of the pedicle, showing its relationship to the radial nerve. For clarity of illustration, a window has been cut out of the lateral intermuscular septum and the venae comitantes of the PRCA, which regularly accompany the artery, are omitted. Reproduced with permission from Katsaros et al: The lateral upper arm flap: anatomy and clinical applications. *Ann Plast Surg*, 12:489-499, 1984.

indicated when a thin flap of gliding tissue is required. The dorsum of the hand where the extensor tendons must glide beneath skin and over bone is an ideal indication for the use of this flap. Additionally, a thin coverage for the dorsum of the fingers using this flap has been reported with excellent outcome. The flap itself consists of the temporoparietal fas-

cia, which is the external fascia of the scalp. It is supplied by the superficial temporal artery and vein and provides a flap of up to 10 cm by 12 cm with a pedicle length of 4 cm to 5 cm. The donor site is well tolerated, not painful, and the scars are hidden by the patient's hair. The scalp is elevated just beneath the hair follicles and the flap is lifted off the

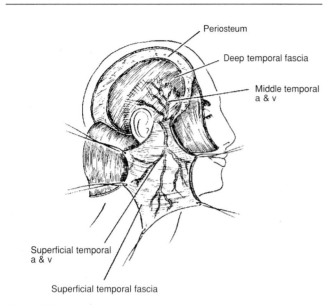

Periosteum

Deep temporal fascia

Middle temporal
a & v

Superficial temporal
a & v

Superficial temporal fascia

Figure 31-3.

pericranium superiorly and the deep temporal fascia inferiorly. Closure of this donor site is by direct approximation of the scalp. This flap provides the thinnest of all tissues and supports a skin graft for final wound closure. An ingenious use of the flap has been described whereby the flap is dissected to include the deep temporal fascia as a separate layer, and in this manner provides thin tissue in which to sandwich tendon reconstructions (Fig. 31-3). In this author's experience, use of the temporoparietal fascia flap has been without donor-site complication, and the results for dorsal hand coverage and extensor tendon gliding have been excellent.

Small Muscle Flaps

The use of free muscle flaps for lower extremity coverage is well appreciated. In the upper extremity, however, its use has not been as popular as cutaneous flaps or fascial flaps described above. Recent use of the serratus muscle for closure of small wounds in the hand and for the provision of dynamic motion of the thumb provide an exciting new application for these procedures. Logan and associates reported use of the serratus anterior muscle for resurfacing complex wounds of the hand where dead space management or wound contamination was consideration. In their series of 18 patients, they describe techniques for both dorsal and palmar hand coverage. It is especially effective, in their experience, for opening the thumb-index web space. As in other free muscle flaps, these tissues have effectively controlled osteomyelitis and chronic wound infections once adequate debridement and antibiotic coverage have been provided. The flap is based on the serratus branch of the thoracodorsal artery vascularizing the distal three slips of the

serratus muscle. The vascular pedicle is up to 10 cm in length and the donor site deformity is minimal. The innervation to this muscle is the long thoracic nerve and the distal portion of this nerve can be anastomosed to the motor branch of the thumb to provide active thumb motion. In Logan's series of patients, three underwent innervated muscle transfers and were provided dynamic restoration for the loss of thenar muscle tissues.

The gracilis muscle has been described for dynamic reconstruction of Volkmann's ischemic contractures in the forearm. Manktelow and others have separated the anterior and posterior divisions of this muscle to provide isolated flexion of the digits and the thumb, based on the fascicular separation of these muscle segments. Early success with these free muscle transfers for dynamic restoration of hand function clearly points the way to the future. Using a combination of electrical stimulation and free muscle transfers it is possible to contemplate the restoration of functional motion in patients with previously unreconstructable extremities.

Distally-based Upper Extremity Pedicle Flaps— New Alternatives to Free-tissue Transfers

The Radial Forearm Flap

The radial forearm flap, first described by Song and associates and known as the "Chinese flap," has enjoyed popularity as a free-flap donor site. Its principal characteristics are that the flap is generally thin, often hairless, and has the potential for sensory reinnervation. Based on the radial artery proximally, this flap has been used for reconstruction of head and neck defects and transferred to the opposite extremity for specific reconstructive purposes. Costa and associates reported the use of a flow-through flap using the radial artery, in which the artery was used to restore circulation to a devascularized hand and the soft tissues of the forearm used to resurface the soft-tissue loss. Additionally, the forearm tissues can be elevated to include segments of tendon (the palmaris longus tendon for example) and the distal radius, to satisfy a wide variety of complex tissue requirements. The radial forearm flap, however, has additional versatility for hand reconstruction. If the injury to the hand is an isolated one, particularly on the dorsum, the flap can be based on its distal blood supply with the venous return through venae comitantes in a retrograde direction. Using this flap design, volar forearm skin can be transferred to the dorsum of the hand without the need for microsurgical anastomoses. Dissection, however, requires the same care and expertise as elevating the flap for microsurgical transfer. Contraindications for the use of this flap would be in the extremity with vascular compromise where dividing the radial artery proximally would deprive the hand of this arterial inflow. Additionally, the ulnar artery must be demonstrated to provide circulation across the palmar arch to the radial side of the hand; a negative Allen's test is a prerequisite for transferring this flap. By including the medial antebrachial cutaneous nerve in the flap design, sensory restoration to the hand can be provided using this flap as a distally based flap (Fig. 31-4). As reported by

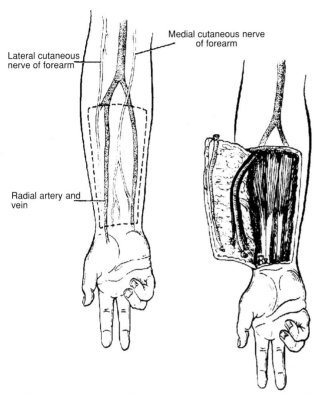

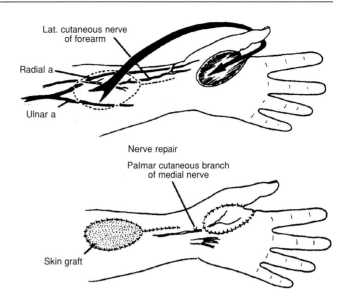

Figure 31-4. **(Left)** Anatomy of the radial forearm flap. This fascia cutaneous flap from the volar forearm is based on the radial artery and venae comitantes. This flap may be innervated using the medial or lateral cutaneous nerves of the forearm, which enter the flap at its proximal border. Swartz WM, Banis JC: *Head and Neck Microsurgery.* Baltimore, MD, Williams & Wilkins, 1992. **(Right)** Distally based radial forearm flap used for palmar restoration. The skin island is located proximal in the forearm and based on the distal blood supply from the radial artery and its venae comitantes. For sensory reinnervation, the flap should be routed over the dorsum of the hand to permit proximal nerve repairs to appropriate sensory nerves. Reproduced with permission from Swartz, WM: Restoration of sensibility in mutilating hand injuries. *Clin Plast Surg,* 16: 515-529, 1989.

Brown and associates, sensory recovery for this tissue is 14 mm moving two-point discrimination.

A variation of the distally based volar pedicle tissue flap is the ulnar artery, distally based forearm flap. Guimberteau and associates reported using this flap in 54 cases. The flap is centered over the ulnar artery in the distal forearm and may be as large as 10 cm x 6 cm. Similar to the radial forearm flap, this flap can be innervated by using a branch of the medial antebrachial nerve. This flap is drained by the venae comitantes of the ulnar artery as well as by a superficial venous system. The authors cite the advantages of this flap over the radial forearm flap to include a more rapid dissection and increased mobility of the flap, allowing it to reach the entire skin surface of the hand. Additionally, the flexi carpi ulnaris muscle and tendon can be included with the flap, or the flexor superficialis to the fourth and fifth fingers can be used to replace lost extensor tendons. These authors admonish potential users of this flap to consider arterial reconstruction should vascular compromise be present upon sacrificing the ulnar artery. It is apparent from these reports that the skin of the volar forearm has a rich subdermal plexus that can be transferred by either of these overlapping arterial systems.

The Posterior Interosseous Flap

Unlike the previously mentioned distally based radial fore-

arm and ulnar forearm flaps, the posterior interosseous island flap does not require the sacrifice of a major inflow vessel to the extremity. Costa and associates, in an extensive series of cadaver dissections and clinical experience, have demonstrated the role of the posterior interosseous vessels in providing blood supply to the fascia on the dorsal forearm. A distally based flap can be devised, utilizing skin from the proximal forearm over the intermuscular septum between the extensor carpi ulnaris and the extensor digiti minimi. The posterior interosseous artery enters the intermuscular septum between the supinator and the abductor pollicis longus and then sends septocutaneous branches to the overlying fascial plexus. In the lower third of the posterior forearm, septoperiosteal branches to the ulna are also present, permitting the transfer of an osteocutaneous flap for thumb reconstruction (Fig. 31-5). This flap was found to be totally reliable with skin flaps elevated as large as 12.5 cm by 8.5 cm (in a series of 21 patients). The principal advantages of using this flap over the radial and ulnar artery-based flaps include the ability to raise larger skin flaps with primary donor site closure. For larger flaps, skin grafts may be placed over muscle without the associated problems of tendon exposure seen in radial or ulnar artery-based flaps. These authors also cite the reduced possibility of iatrogenic fracture using the posterior interosseous compared with the radial artery osteocutaneous flap, since bone

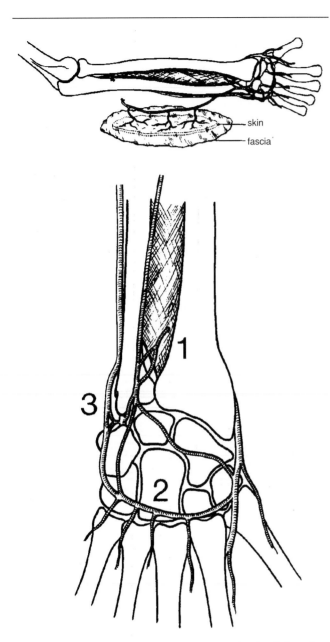

Figure 31-5. Sources of the vascular supply to the distally based posterior interosseous island flap at the level of the distal ulnar head. The following three main patterns of anastomosis are depicted: (1) the anterior interosseous artery, (2) the dorsal carpal arch, (3) the ulnar artery, by the branches that surround the ulnar head. Reproduced with permission from Landi et al: The distally-based posterior interosseous island flap for the coverage of skin loss of the hand. *Ann Plast Surg*, 27:527-536, 1991.

is taken from a region of the ulna that is broad and triangular rather than a narrow tubular section of the radius. The authors warn, however, that the technique of this dissection is more demanding than that of the radial artery flap.

From the foregoing descriptions, it is apparent that a variety of flaps can be designed from both volar and dorsal forearm tissue to satisfy soft-tissue requirements in the hand.

These flaps are included in the discussion of free-tissue transfers since the dissection of these flaps requires considerable expertise with the same care given in the dissection as would be required for free-tissue transfer.

Emergency Free-tissue Transfers

Since the work of Godina and associates, considerable interest has developed in the treatment of complex hand injuries with emergency free-tissue transfers. Godina showed that the use of emergency flaps in the lower extremities significantly improved the flap success rate and decreased the problem of long-term complications such as osteomyelitis. In the upper extremity, however, the use of emergency free flaps must be weighed against the potential of errors in decision making. Proponents for the use of this technique include Ratsaros and associates, who compared 18 free-flap reconstructions for acute hand trauma with 12 groin flaps as historical controls. They showed the rate of complication was the same in both groups but patients covered with an emergency free flap required fewer secondary procedures. The average operating time was the same for both groups, which included two operations for patients with pedicled groin flaps. The average hospitalization time for patients with free flaps, however, was half of that for those with groin flaps. Lister described 31 emergency free flaps applied to the upper extremity with two flaps lost and a severe infection found in one of the 31 patients. Both of these authors stress the need for adequate debridement of these wounds, turning a contaminated, traumatized wound into a cleanly excised wound. In this author's opinion, the advantages to be gained by early wound coverage by emergency free-tissue transfers must be weighed against the potential of delayed tissue necrosis due to inadequate debridement. Despite the best judgment, additional tissue necrosis will change the reconstructive plan or alter the design of the proposed flap. Certainly the exposure of essential longitudinal structures such as arteries and nerves should be treated in this time frame, however.

Conclusion

Microsurgical free-tissue transfer for coverage of soft-tissue defects in the upper extremity has reached increasing levels of sophistication over the past five years. The operations described above require considerable expertise in execution and more thought in their planning. Patients should be assessed for their long-term reconstructive needs and a logical, well thought out reconstructive plan developed before choosing a method of soft-tissue coverage. Tissue requirements such as vascularized nerves, vascularized tendons and vascularized bone can all be incorporated into many of the flaps already described. The thoughtful use of these composite tissue transfers by microsurgical techniques can substantially shorten the time for effective rehabilitation. By combining conventional reconstructive techniques with microvascular free-tissue transfer coverage, a substantial improvement over the traditional, multi-staged reconstructions has been realized.

Annotated Bibliography

Partial Toe Flaps

Eadie PA, Jenner DA, Sakai K: Clinical experience with the second metatarsal artery neurovascular flap. *J Plast Surg Br*, 45:136-140, 1992.

Three cases of innervated web space flaps from the foot based on the second metatarsal artery and the second common digital nerve are described. This flap is used to provide glabrous skin for digital reconstruction with sensory reinnervation and minimal donor site morbidity.

Koshima I, Moriguchi T, Soeda S, *et al:* Free thin osteoonychocutaneous flaps from the big toe for reconstruction of the distal phalanx of the fingers. *J Plast Surg Br*, 45:1-5, 1992.

Free flaps consisting of the nail bed and hemipulp of the big toe are designed as an improvement over the wrap-around flap for restoring digital soft tissues including the nail. This technique eliminates the need for a cross-toe flap, preserving part of the toenail as well.

Strauch T, Tsur H: Restoration of sensation to the hand by a free neurovascular flap from the first web space of the foot. *Plast Reconstr Surg*, 62:361, 1978.

This is the classic description of toe web space innervated free flaps.

Wei FC, Chen HC, Chuang D, *et al:* Second toe wrap-around flap. *Plast Reconst Surg*, 88:837-843, 1991.

This paper describes the use of the second toe wrap-around technique for reconstructing digital loss including a nail bed. Thirteen flaps and 10 patients are presented showing improvement in aesthetic and functional recovery for digital restoration.

Venous Flaps

Chavoin JP, Rouge D, Vachaud M, *et al:* Island flaps with an exclusively venous pedicle. A report of eleven cases and a preliminary haemodynamic study. *Br J Plast Surg*, 40:149-154, 1987.

Eleven cases of island flaps surviving on a venous pedicle only are presented. This paper discusses the theoretical reasons why the flaps survive.

Iwasawa M, Furuta S, Noguchi M, Hirose T: Reconstruction of fingertip deformities of the thumb using a venous flap. *Ann Plast Surg*, 28:187-189, 1992.

A fingertip deformity reconstruction was performed using a venous nail flap. In this case, the dorsal vein was anastomosed to a digital artery and an outflow vein to a digital vein.

Roshima I, Soeda S, Nakayama Y, Fukuda H, Tanaka J: An arterialised venous flap using the long saphenous vein. *J Plast Surg Br*, 44:23-26, 1991.

Elective reconstruction of upper extremity defects using a venous flap designed over the saphenous vein of the medial thigh is presented. The inflow to the flap is an artery and the outflow is a vein. All tissues survived completely with flaps as large as 11 cm x 7 cm.

Tsai T, Matiko JD, Breidenbach W, Rutz J: Venous flaps in digital revascularization and replantation. *J Reconstr Microsurg*, 3:113-119, 1987.

Fifteen patients are presented who underwent restoration of the dorsum of a replanted digit with a free skin flap using venous anastomoses proximally and distally as a flow-through system. The skin was shown to survive with only venous flow present. Attempts at designing venous flaps from the dorsum of the foot and from the forearm were uniformly unsuccessful, suggesting the need for greater blood flow to provide nourishment to the overlying skin.

Free-flap Donor Sites

Brody GA, Buncke JH, Alpert BS, Hing DN: Serratus anterior muscle transplantation for treatment of soft-tissue defects in the hand. *J Hand Surg*, 15A:322-327, 1990.

This paper elaborates upon the use of the serratus anterior muscle for soft-tissue restoration for complex defects involving both the dorsum and palmar aspects of the hand.

Hirase Y, Rojima T, Bang H: Double-layered free temporal fascia flap as a two-layered tendon-gliding surface. *Plast Reconst Surg*, 88:707-712, 1991.

The techniques of using the temporoparietal fascia flap are presented, including a two-layered design that incorporates the deep temporal fascia as well as the superficial fascia. This idea permits the use of the flap to restore tendon grafts for extensor tendon restoration in complex dorsal hand wounds.

Logan SE, Alpert BS, Buncke JH: Free serratus anterior muscle transplantation for hand reconstruction. *J Plast Surg Br*, 41:639-643, 1988.

This paper discusses the use of the serratus anterior muscle for restoring soft-tissue loss in 15 patients, three of whom required dynamic muscle transfer for thumb opposition. Technique and rationale for use of free muscle flaps in hand reconstruction are delineated.

Manktelow RT and Zuker RM: The principles of functioning muscle transplantation: applications to the upper arm. *Ann Plast Surg*, 22:275-282, 1989.

This paper discusses the use of innervated free gracilis muscles to restore elbow function in patients with traumatic injuries and injuries secondary to paraplegia. Principles of muscle transfers are outlined. The paper is an extension of a previous report of restoration of finger flexion using free muscle transplantation.

Upton J, Rogers C, Durham-Smith G, Swartz WM: Clinical applications of free temporoparietal flaps in hand reconstruction. *J Hand Surg*, 11A:475, 1986.

This paper describes the use of the temporoparietal fascia flap for a variety of hand surgical reconstructions. The technique for flap elevation is clearly presented along with the advantages of this flap.

Lateral Arm Flap

Katsaros J, Schusterman M, Beppu M, Banis JC Jr, Acland RD: The lateral upper arm flap: anatomy and clinical applications. *Ann Plast Surg*, 12:489-499, 1984.

This paper describes the lateral arm flap with a series of vascular injections and cadaver dissections. Twenty-three clinical cases are presented.

Katsaros J, Tan E, Zoltie N: The use of the lateral arm flap in upper limb surgery. *J Hand Surg,* 16:598-604, 1991.

An additional 20 patients for upper extremity reconstruction are presented and the advantages of using this flap for upper extremity reconstruction are described.

Distally based Pedicle Flaps

Costa H, Guimaraes I, Cardoso A, et al: One-staged coverage and revascularization of traumatized limbs by a flow-through radial mid-forearm free flap. *J Plast Surg Br,* 533-537, 1991.

The radial forearm free flap was used in two clinical cases to restore both arterial inflow and venous outflow to severely traumatized extremities. Soft-tissue coverage was provided by the volar forearm skin and the arterial reconstruction by the radial artery.

Guimberteau JC, Goin JL, Panconi B, Schuhmacher B: The reverse ulnar artery forearm island flap in hand surgery: 54 cases. *Plast Reconstr Surg,* 81:925-932, 1988.

The authors present their experience with the reverse ulnar artery forearm flap in 54 cases and describe its advantages over the previously described radial forearm flap.

Lin S, Lai C, Chiu C. Venous drainage in the reverse forearm flap. *Plast Reconstr Surg,* 74:508, 1984.

This paper describes the use of the distally-based radial forearm flap and outlines the physiologic reasons that reverse venous flow can occur.

Soutar DS, Tanner NSB: The radial forearm flap in the management of soft-tissue injuries of the hand. *J Plast Surg Br,* 37:1826, 1984.

This paper amplifies the previously described radial forearm flap and its use for soft-tissue reconstructions of hand injuries. In this paper a distally-based radial forearm flap was used; however, venous congestion required anastomosis of a subcutaneous vein to improve venous drainage.

Swanson E, Boyd JB, Manktelow RT: The radial forearm flap: reconstructive applications and donor site defects in 35 consecutive patients. *Plast Reconstr Surg,* 85:258-266, 1990.

Use of the radial forearm flap for a variety of reconstructive problems including nine patients is presented for upper extremity reconstruction. The complications of this flap are outlined and methods are presented to deal with them.

Posterior Interosseous Flap

Costa H, Soutar DS: The distally-based island posterior interosseous flap. *J Plast Surg Br,* 41:221-227, 1988.

This paper describes the anatomic basis for the posterior interosseous flap of the forearm with 22 cadaver dissections and three clinical cases.

Costa H, Comba S, Martins A, et al: Further experience with the posterior interosseous flap. *J Plast Surg Br,* 44:449-455, 1991 .

This paper extends the information previously presented with 50 anatomic dissections and 21 clinical cases.

Landi A, Luchetti R, Soragni O: The distally-based posterior interosseous island flap for the coverage of skin loss of the hand. *Ann Plast Surg,* 27:527-536, 1991.

This paper discusses the use of the Doppler for identifying the presence and size of the posterior interosseous vessel and discusses eight cases where the flap was used on both the volar and dorsal surfaces of the hand.

Free-flap Coverage for Acute Hand Injuries

Lister G, Scheker L: Emergency free flaps to the upper extremity. *J Hand Surg,* 13A:22-28, 1988.

Thirty-one emergency free flaps are presented with an overall flap success rate of 93.5%. The average hospital stay was 11.8 days and only one severe infection occurred. The rationale for use of definitive early free-flap coverage for upper extremity injuries is documented.

Katsaros J, Tan E, Zoltie N: Free-flap cover of acute hand injuries. *Injury,* 20:96-97, 1989.

This paper compares 18 emergency free-flap reconstructions of acute hand trauma with 12 historical controls utilizing the pedicled groin flap. They document approximately half the hospital time for free-tissue transfers, but the total operating time and complications were approximately equal.

Sensory Restoration

Brown CJ, Mackinnon SE, Dellon AL, et al: The sensory potential of free flap donor sites. *Ann Plast Surg,* 33:135-140, 1989.

The potential for sensory reinnervation was studied for a variety of free flap donor sites including the volar wrist, dorsal hand, dorsal foot, and great toe. The paper describes improvement in sensation with sensory reeducation.

Hausman M: Microvascular applications in limb-sparing tumor surgery. *Orthopaed Clin N Am,* 20:427-437, 1989.

The principles of tumor resection and limb-sparing surgery and the contributions of a variety of microsurgical free-tissue transfers in limb restoration are presented.

Lahteenmaki T, Waris T, Asko-Seljavaara S, Sundell B: Recovery of sensation in free flaps. *J Plast Reconstr Surg Scand,* 23:217-222, 1989.

This paper studies recovery of sensibility in 27 free flaps with a variety of donor sites. They conclude that cutaneous nerves freely reinnervate skin transferred to a tissue bed with intact cutaneous nerves whether or not cutaneous nerves are reconnected.

Swartz WM: Restoration of sensibility in mutilating hand injuries. *Clin Plast Surg,* 16:515-529, 1989.

This paper outlines the strategy for providing the sensory restoration for a wide variety of hand injuries utilizing neurovascular free flaps from the toe as well as radial forearm and lateral arm flaps.

32

Elective Microsurgery

Michael B. Wood, MD

Introduction

The initial applications of microsurgery in hand surgery focused chiefly on replantation, revascularization, nerve repair, and nerve grafting. Over the last two decades, however, microsurgical technique has permitted revascularized transfer of a variety of tissues for sophisticated reconstructive procedures in the upper limb. Elective free-tissue transfer procedures to the hand and arm have in many centers become the major application for microsurgery and in future years will likely find even wider application. This chapter concentrates on the current application of elective microsurgical procedures for upper limb reconstruction.

Digit and Partial Digit Transfer

Digit or partial digit transfer permits replacement of some or all components of a missing thumb or finger including skin, nail, nerve, bone, joint, and tendons. Thus, this procedure may provide, with a single compound tissue transfer, a replacement part with the appearance of a thumb or finger and with the functional necessities of stability, sensibility, mobility, and motor control.

Donor Sites

Great Toe

The first described human free microvascular digit transfer was for thumb replacement using the great toe. The great toe remains an excellent choice for thumb replacement although in most patients it is distinctly larger than the thumb and retains a toe-like appearance. An advantage is its single interphalangeal joint which in most patients is quite stable. The vascular pedicle of the great toe may simply be the proper digital arteries and dorsal veins; however, in most cases the arterial pedicle is based on the dorsalis pedis artery, which distally gives rise to the first dorsal metatarsal artery (Fig. 32-1) and/or the first plantar metatarsal arterial arch. The venous pedicle is the saphenous system originating over the dorsum of the foot.

Second Toe

The second toe may be useful for either thumb or finger reconstruction. As a thumb replacement it is considerably more slender than the normal pollex but nonetheless in terms of function seems comparable to the great toe. Its two interphalangeal joints are less stable than the great toe interphalangeal joint; however, in contrast to the great toe, considerable metatarsal length can be harvested with the second toe without adversely affecting foot function. The second

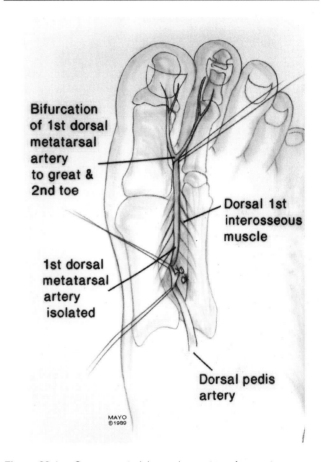

Figure 32-1. Common arterial vascular anatomy for great or second toe isolations. Dorsal view: note dorsalis pedis artery giving origin to first dorsal metatarsal artery which in turn bifurcates to supply great toe and second toe. (Artist's representation.)

toe almost always is the donor toe of choice for finger reconstruction. The vascular pedicle for the second toe is virtually identical to that of the great toe using in most cases the dorsalis pedis and first dorsal metatarsal parent arteries (Fig. 32-1) and saphenous venous system (Fig. 32-2).

Two Toes

The second and third toe may be isolated together as a single composite tissue for replacement of two fingers. This procedure has been used chiefly to reconstruct a hand capable of "three jaw chuck" pinch in a patient missing all fingers but with an intact thumb. The resultant hand function from this procedure may be gratifying, but the donor site

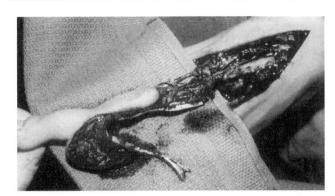

Figure 32-2. Isolated second toe with attached vascular pedicle. Intraoperative photography.

cleft in the foot is often objectionable. Most contemporary authors therefore recommend transfer of two second toes in preference to a second and third double-toe unit. The anatomical basis of the vascular pedicle is essentially the same as for the second toe with the exception that in all cases the medial plantar metatarsal artery and the associated plantar metatarsal arch to the second and third toe should be preserved.

Other Toes

Occasionally there is a need to select other toes, such as unavailability of either the great or second toe. The author (for example) has transferred a fifth toe for thumb reconstruction in a patient with bilateral upper limb adactyly and congenital absence of all remaining toes.

Wrap-around Procedure

The wrap-around procedure is a modified toe transfer technique utilizing a filleted composite tissue flap of skin with digital neurovascular bundles, nail, and in most cases, a portion of the distal phalanx with or without a free bone graft for thumb reconstruction. The advantage of this technique is that it allows reconstruction of a thumb which approximates the normal thumb cross-sectional dimensions. Because it does not include joint or tendons and does not permit growth potential, it is useful chiefly for replacement of thumb loss distal to a mobile metacarpophalangeal joint in the adult. The vascular pedicle anatomy is exactly the same as for great toe transfer.

Fingers

Occasionally free finger or thumb transfer may be indicated for digit reconstruction to the same or opposite hand. The major application would be the free transfer of an already damaged digit which is of little or no use to hand function in its orthotopic location, to a more useful position elsewhere (for example using a partially amputated finger stump for thumb reconstruction either to the same or the opposite hand). This procedure has also been described as a free transfer from a traumatically amputated contralateral limb or from a contralateral flail anesthetic limb resulting from prior peripheral nerve injury. The anatomical basis of such free finger or thumb transfers of course depends upon the specific digit being transferred and coincides with the normal vascular anatomy based on either the radial artery for the thumb or the superficial palmar arch and common digital arteries for fingers.

Indications

The major indication for digit or partial digit transfer is for thumb reconstruction after traumatic loss and less frequently for congenital absence. The selection of great toe or second toe for thumb reconstruction can be interchangeable. It is often based on the particular size dimensions of the great or second toe as it correlates with the patient's opposite normal thumb and other factors including surgeon and patient preference. In terms of function, some studies have demonstrated no appreciable difference in function between the great versus the second toe, while others believe the great toe transfer results in a greater grip strength. Unquestionably, the wrap-around procedure provides the best aesthetic thumb reconstruction because it approximates the normal thumb size.

Less often, digit transfer is used for replacement of missing fingers. Although there are no rigid rules, the author's opinion is that digit transfer should be considered in cases of loss or absence of three or more fingers. Replacement of a single finger loss by digit transfer may be of aesthetic benefit but for most patients is of doubtful functional value. The second toe is the preferred donor site (for finger reconstruction). As previously mentioned, a compound flap of the second and third toe may be useful in cases of total finger loss in the presence of a functioning thumb for reconstruction of "three jaw chuck" grasp. However, the donor site morbidity associated with this transfer often precludes its utility. In selected patients, portions of the second toe may be utilized for fingertip reconstruction involving the nail or hemipulp. The overall effect of such distal digital reconstruction on hand function should be carefully weighed and assessed prior to recommending an exotic procedure of this sort.

Technical Refinements

Toe or partial toe transfer is a complex and technically demanding procedure. However, the challenges of this procedure may be minimized, and the technical results improved, by attention to certain technical refinements.

Primary Skin Supplementation at the Recipient Site

Experience has demonstrated that a surplus of skin at the hand recipient site is a useful requisite prior to toe transfer. Although authors have described the transfer of a major skin flap along with the toe from the foot, such procedures markedly contribute to foot donor site morbidity and attendant problems. Therefore, if the skin status at the hand recipient site is marginal, a first-stage procedure augmenting skin preferably by a pedicle groin flap procedure is recommended. Although alternate means of supplementing skin, including a retrograde-based radial forearm flap or a retrograde-based posterior interosseous flap are possible, the vascular dissection associated with either of these procedures might complicate the second stage toe transfers. For this reason the author prefers using a staged conventional groin flap before considering microvascular digit transfer to the hand. Of course, if a surplus of skin already exists at the recipient site the preliminary step of skin supplementation is not required.

Reduction of Great Toe

The size and dimension of the great toe for thumb reconstruction may be minimized by modifications at the time of toe-to-hand transfer. This procedure offers some of the cosmetic advantages of a wrap-around procedure but with the additional benefits of a great toe transfer procedure. Such a reduction requires bilateral contouring of the condylar flairs of the great toe interphalangeal joint with debulking of the tuft portion of the great toe at the time of transfer. It should be recognized, however, that this modification at the time of primary toe transfer may add to the complexity of the procedure and could jeopardize the vascular integrity of the great toe. Therefore, in most cases, surgical contouring of the great toe to more closely mimic the size of the thumb is more safely and preferably carried out as a secondary procedure.

"Twisted-two-toe" Procedure

The "twisted-two-toe" procedure has been described as a means to allow contouring of the toe transfer as a form of modified wrap-around procedure at the recipient site and yet minimize donor site problems by reconstruction of the great toe portion of the transfer. This procedure is probably best indicated in the patient with aesthetic concerns such that a wrap-around procedure for thumb reconstruction and a concomitant procedure to replace the great toe at the foot is of great importance. In all patients considered for this procedure, the requisites for wrap-around procedure in the hand (in regards to level of amputation of the thumb) require scrutiny. As far as the foot donor site is concerned, most patients can tolerate the loss of the great toe quite well with or without "twisted-two-toe" reconstruction provided the skin cover and integrity of the metatarsal head of the first ray is preserved.

Primary "Fingerization" Toe-to-Hand Transfer

The second toe and to a lesser extent the great toe has a rather bulbous tip with a drum-stick type appearance. Primary or secondary contouring of this drum-stick shape by transverse wedge resection of the tuft portion and defatting of the tuft results in an appearance that more closely mimics the normal fingertip. A transverse elliptical incision is made a few millimeters palmar to the hyponychium of the second toe and through this a modest defatting with primary closure is carried out. Although there may be a higher degree of safety in carrying this out as a secondary procedure, the author has done this as a primary procedure with no untoward problems to date. Provided the defatting is limited and kept well away from the palmar portion of the toe, no impairment of sensibility recovery has been noted in such cases.

Management of Claw Deformity

A claw deformity following toe-to-hand transfer is most characteristic for the second toe and particularly in those transfers which include the metatarsophalangeal joint. In such cases, a three-joint system involving metatarsophalangeal joint, proximal interphalangeal joint, and distal interphalangeal joint may result in a zig-zag or concertina type collapse related to tendon imbalance. This problem may be further accentuated by lateral instability of either interphalangeal joint but especially the distal joint. In such patients, secondary arthrodesis or fibrous ankylosis of proximal or distal or both interphalangeal joints may be warranted. If at the time of transfer there is considerable lateral instability of the distal interphalangeal joint, the author recommends stabilization be carried out primarily. This is safely done by removal of the articular surfaces and transfixion with a Kirschner wire of the distal interphalangeal joint through a linear dorsal incision.

Results

In general, the reported results for tissue survival following toe-to-hand transfer have been high, ranging between 95% and 100%. Most of these procedures are carried out under ideal circumstances as elective operative procedures. Objective data regarding the functional value of toe-to-hand transfer is more variable, but in general, most series report excellent results. The functional outcome (for the thumb) has been particularly gratifying since full range of motion is not necessary and much of the range of motion for function is from the intact carpometacarpal joint. Most series report that protective sensibility predictably recovers and in most instances two-point discrimination ranging between 5 mm and 10 mm has been reported. The results of finger reconstruction have been more modest perhaps because of increased range of motion demands. However, recovery of sensibility has been comparable to that of the thumb. In the author's experience secondary procedures following toe-to-hand transfer are often required for optimal function. The secondary procedures may include chiefly capsulotomy, tenolysis, first web space contracture release, interphalangeal joint fusion or ankylosis for instability, and corrective osteotomy. Patient acceptance in successful cases is gratifying.

Complications

Recipient Site

Complications at the recipient site may be grouped into early and late categories. The most common early complication is vascular thrombosis of either the arterial or venous pedicle, necessitating early reoperation and revision. Authors of most series suggest that a reoperation rate of approximately 10% may be expected but that successful salvage with reoperation is frequent. Usually such instances are related to thrombosis at the anastomosis site related to technical factors or exogenous compression from associated wound hematoma or excessively tight dressings. Additional early complications may include tissue slough or wound sepsis. Late complications are chiefly related to limited range of motion, contracture, or malalignment. In such instances, secondary corrective procedures as mentioned above may be required. Additional late complications include recipient or donor site cold intolerance. Most patients, however, adjust to this problem by appropriate protective garments.

Donor Site

Although variable, the chief reason for secondary foot problems related to toe-to-hand transfer is an overly aggressive toe harvest associated with an attached dorsalis pedis skin flap or excessive resection of the first metatarsal. Harvest of the distal portion of the first metatarsal with the great toe should be avoided. Usually, if metatarsal and metatarsophalangeal joint resection is required, then the second toe should be selected as the donor, since the second metacarpal can be resected to the proximal portion of its shaft. If the second toe with metacarpal is utilized, the void left in the second ray should be closed by approximation of the first to third metatarsal and reconstruction of the transverse intermetatarsal ligament. If a diastasis results between the first and third rays following second toe resection, a progressive hallux valgus deformity is possible. The use of composite second and third toes transfers consistently results in a cleft foot deformity with a secondary hallux valgus deformity of the great toe. Although gait disturbances following this procedure have not been emphasized, donor site problem may occur with complaints of forefoot metatarsalgia. Normally these complaints can be managed by appropriate molded inlays and orthoses.

Bone Segment Transfer

Vascularized bone graft transfer for reconstruction of a long bone defect was first reported in 1975 by Taylor and associates. The procedure has now become an accepted technique in the clinical armamentarium for reconstruction of extensive long bone defects resulting from trauma, tumor resection or osteomyelitis debridement, reconstruction of difficult congenital pseudarthrosis or fibrous dysplasia, the repair of certain resistent nonunions, particularly those associated with radiation-induced osteonecrosis, and bony avascular necrosis. A variety of donor sites have been described, but for most cases of upper limb reconstruction either the fibula or anterior iliac crest is preferred. The indications for microvascular bone transfer in the upper limb are often determined by the availability or lack of simpler alternative procedures including nonvascularized cancellous or cortical autografting and some forms of segmental or osteoarticular allograft reconstruction. Moreover, the utility of palliative procedures such as construction of a one-bone forearm or resection arthroplasties may be appropriate in certain patients.

Donor Sites

Virtually any expendable bone with an identifiable vascular pedicle may be appropriate for transfer. The fibula based on its peroneal vascular pedicle or the anterior iliac crest based on the deep circumflex iliac vessels, are most commonly used for reconstructive procedures in the upper limb.

Fibula

The fibula is especially suited for long bone reconstruction because of its size and linear configuration. Its cortical structure is well suited to stable internal fixation with compression plates for the forearm or intramedullary placement and transcortical screw fixation for the humerus. The diameter of the fibula approximates that of the radius and ulna but is considerably less than the humerus. Nonetheless, clinical series have demonstrated a capacity for hypertrophy of the fibula to approximate the diameter of the humerus over time, provided sufficient mechanical protection of the construct can be ensured for the first six to 12 postoperative months. The fibula is an expendable bone (in the lower limb) with a low incidence of donor site problems. However, in a growing child stabilization of the distal tibiofibular syndesmosis by arthrodesis is recommended to avoid progressive valgus deformity of the ankle. This risk does not exist in the adult or in children with closure of the epiphyseal growth plate. The fibula is based on its specific nutrient artery as well as multiple periosteal perforators originating from the peroneal artery and accompanying *venae comitantes*. Typically the nutrient artery enters the central third of the bone. The technique of fibula harvest is well described in numerous reports. A lateral approach carried out in an extraperiosteal manner is utilized by most authors. A bone graft length of up to 28 cm has been reported.

Anterior Iliac Crest

The anterior iliac crest may provide a length of corticocancellous bone of up to 14 cm. The structure of the iliac crest is less well suited for long bone reconstruction because of its flat cancellous nature. It may, however, be quite useful for metaphyseal bony reconstruction and about the wrist and carpus for the purpose of ensuring wrist arthrodesis. The anterior iliac crest is based on the deep circumflex iliac vessels which are isolated through a transinguinal approach. The advantage of the anterior iliac crest is that it can be isolated in association with a rather large skin flap when concomitant soft-tissue coverage is required or helpful.

Indications

The chief indication for microvascular bone transfer is for reconstruction of bone defects when standard cancellous bone grafting is not applicable or is unlikely to succeed.

Extensive Bone Defects Resulting From Trauma

There is no established lower limit for the length of a bony defect appropriate for a vascularized bone transfer. Most authors recommend consideration of this procedure for bone gaps exceeding 6 cm. However, it is important to recognize that bone defects as great as 12 cm can be managed by nonvascularized grafts provided surrounding soft tissues are healthy, sufficient bone autograft material to completely fill the bone defect can be obtained, and the bone graft construct can be supported over a long period of time. Shorter defects may merit consideration for vascularized bone transfer if the soft-tissue environment is scarred or of poor vascularity, bone autograft material is sparse, or if there is a record of failure with conventional bone grafting.

Bone Defects Resulting From Tumor Resection

Typically bone tumor resection results in bony defects exceeding 10 cm to 12 cm. Moreover, if adjuvant or neoadjuvant chemotherapy or radiation therapy is utilized, nonvascularized bone grafts may be put at a disadvantage for healing. Thus, microvascular bone reconstruction is often required for limb salvage following resection of malignant or locally aggressive bone tumors.

Management of Osteomyelitis

Osteomyelitis involving extensive areas of sclerotic and poorly vascularized bone may require aggressive bony resection for management of local sepsis. Reconstruction of such large bone defects is particularly facilitated by the use of microvascular bone compound tissue transfer resulting in the ability to reconstruct the osseous defect with vascularized bone and if necessary, provide sufficient accompanying soft tissue to obliterate dead space and permit wound closure.

Congenital Defects

A variety of congenital long bone deficiencies may be suited to reconstruction by vascularized bone transfer. Most well known among these indications is congenital pseudarthrosis involving chiefly the tibia or ulna. Additional congenital deficiencies that may benefit from such transfers include fibrous dysplasia and certain forms of fibromatosis or desmoids. Vascularized bone transfer with concomitant epiphyseal growth plate has been suggested for certain bone deficiencies associated with growth arrest or hypoplasia, i.e. radial hemimelia. The results of vascularized epiphyseal transfer have been less predictable and gratifying; the status of this procedure is still under review. At least one major problem for transfer of bone with growth potential is identification of a donor site with a sufficiently consistent and defined blood supply about the epiphysis to minimize the risk of ischemic-induced epiphyseal plate premature closure.

Resistant Nonunions

There may be a variety of instances when a bony nonunion without a substantial defect may be a candidate for repair or reconstruction by vascularized bone transfer. Chief among these categories are the following subgroups.

Failed Prior Bone Graft

Selected patients who have previously undergone (unsuccessful) bone grafting procedures may warrant consideration for a further attempt at repair of a recalcitrant nonunion site by vascularized bone transfer. An effort should be made in all such cases to identify a shortcoming of the initial procedure that can be rectified by a second operative attempt, such as failure to use an adequate amount of cancellous or corticocancellous autograft, inadequate internal fixation, or inadequate postoperative immobilization. If no specific problem can be identified as a probable cause of failure for a prior bone grafting attempt, then local or regional factors about the nonunion site should be considered, such as osteonecrosis of the bone ends or a poor soft-tissue environment that could plausibly explain inadequate incorporation of a conventional bone autograft. Microvascular bone transfer may be an appropriate management (in such cases) but always in conjunction with established principles of nonunion management, including the use of stable internal fixation and adequate postoperative immobilization.

Post-irradiation Fractures

Spontaneous or induced fractures following radiation present a particularly difficult problem to the reconstructive surgeon. Such fractures are associated with avascular bony necrosis, impaired blood supply to the periosteum, and a deficiency of vascularity of the surrounding soft tissues. The extent of external beam radiation damage is dose-dependent. Bone and soft-tissue radiation changes may be seen with radiation doses as low as 3,000 rads and is virtually assured with radiation doses up to 5,000 rads. Frequently the onset of radiation changes in bone and soft tissue are progressive and do not become fully obvious for several years after exposure. Because of multiple problems associated with radiation, conventional onlay bone grafting is generally unsuccessful; therefore, resection of the fracture site and adjacent bone to a level outside of the radiated field with reconstruction by microvascular bone transfer is a useful procedure in such cases.

Allograft Nonunion

In recent years the use of massive segmental or osteoarticular allografts has become well accepted particularly for limb reconstruction following tumor resection. Although many such patients proceed to union and a successful clinical result, allograft nonunion may represent a significant challenge. Onlay bone grafting about the osteosynthesis site may be beneficial in some patients. However, if this fails, totally bridging the segmental allograft by a vascularized bone segment extending from host bone proximally to host bone distally is a rational and successful form of management. Unfortunately, this same concept cannot be applied to osteoarticular allografts. In the latter case, either onlay bone grafting or vascularized bone grafting over the maximal length of osteoarticular allograft may warrant consideration.

Avascular Necrosis

The use of microvascular bone transfer for the management of avascular necrosis is predicated on the principle that such bone grafts may act as a structural support to prevent bony collapse while at the same time serve as a vehicle for revascularization to the avascular bone. This procedure has been used chiefly for the management of osteonecrosis of the femoral head, the management of avascular necrosis of the lunate (Kienböck's disease), and scaphoid nonunion associated with avascular necrosis of the proximal fragment. The role of vascularized bone transfer for the management of hip avascular necrosis is under evaluation. The preliminary data from several centers suggest that this procedure may be useful in those patients who have no preoperative evidence of femoral head collapse. The value of this procedure for the management of Kienböck's disease is not well established but currently is under evaluation by several centers.

Technique Refinements

Isolation of Fibula or Iliac Crest

The standard techniques of isolation of the fibula or iliac crest are described in several available textbooks and publications. Most authors prefer the lateral approach to the fibula as originally described by Gilbert (Fig. 32-3). The iliac crest is best harvested using a transinguinal approach to the deep circumflex iliac vessels (Fig. 32-4).

Stabilization of Bone

The following factor should be considered in order to select the ideal technique of vascularized bone graft stabilization. The specific technique of stabilization and bone insertion will depend upon the peculiarities of the construct needs.

Bone Graft Placement Relationship to the Axis of Load

Intramedullary placement of the fibula (or other vascularized bone graft) into a long bone, i.e., tibia, femur, or humerus, positions the fibula in the long axis of the reconstructed bone and therefore improves the conditions for bone union and subsequent hypertrophy. Although several authors have suggested that bone graft placement in line with the applied load is advantageous, to this author's knowledge there is no experimental work that confirms this point. However, there are many cases in which the transferred vascularized bone segment may best be placed eccentrically because of other factors chiefly related to internal fixation. With the use of an intramedullary rod the vascularized bone must be placed eccentrically either as a single or double strut.

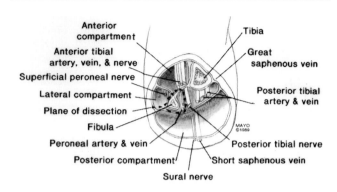

Figure 32-3. Cross-sectional view—course of dissection for isolation of vascularized fibula segment. (Artist's representation.)

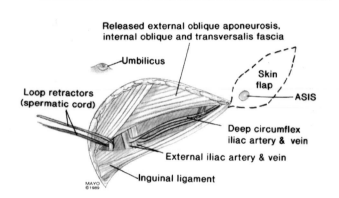

Figure 32-4. Vascular anatomy as viewed by transinguinal approach, anterior iliac crest based on deep circumflex iliac vessels. (Artist's representation.)

Load Bypass of the Bone Graft by Internal Fixation Hardware

Vascularized bone grafts require some form of remodeling or hypertrophy to meet the mechanical needs of the recipient site. This is particularly relevant in the lower extremity where weightbearing is required. Care should be taken in patients to select a form of internal fixation that allows a controlled loading of the transferred bone segment following union at either end (Fig. 32-5). For this reason the use of a long side plate which spans the length of the bone graft construct and hence may load bypass the graft should be avoided. The use of a compression plate at either end of the bone, an external fixator, or an intramedullary rod that may permit dynamization for weightbearing are all appropriate means of internal fixation in such patients.

Adequacy and Stability of Fixation

Consistent with any means of osteosynthesis, rigid internal fixation enhances the likelihood of bony union. The same

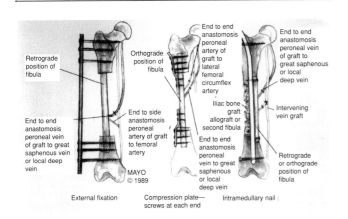

Figure 32-5. Techniques of graft placement and fixation for femur reconstruction by vascularized fibula transfer. (Artist's representation.)

applies for transferred vascularized bone segments where stable internal fixation of both the proximal and distal osteosynthesis sites should be carried out. Prior work has suggested that stable internal fixation is associated with a significantly higher union rate than is unstable or marginal fixation.

Supplemental Bone Grafting

The use of supplemental cancellous autograft material about both the proximal and distal osteosynthesis sites is associated with a significantly higher union rate.

Vascular Monitoring

The most specific and direct technique for determining the vascular status of the transferred bone after surgery is to perform the procedure as an osteocutaneous flap with constant monitoring of the associated skin flap. However, the inclusion of a skin flap with the bone when otherwise not required adds to the complexity of the procedure especially in deeply situated recipient locations like the femur or humerus. The accompanying skin flap may lie awkwardly deep to the normal skin surface of the thigh or upper arm. In patients without a cutaneous flap for monitoring, some authors have recommended the use of bone scanning in the first postoperative week using Technetium-99 EHDP. A positive bone scan has been correlated with a vascularized bone graft and an improved postoperative result. The drawback of this technique, however, is that a negative scan does not provide a sufficiently timely assessment of the vascular status of the transferred bone graft to permit reexploration or revision of a thrombosed vascular anastomosis. A simple, dynamic, and minimally invasive technique for vascularized bone graft monitoring would be useful. At the present time, however, available monitoring devices involve more invasive techniques, including implanted flow meters at the vascular anastomosis sites and bone surface Doppler probes.

Early Reoperation for Delayed Union or Nonunion

Most large series of vascularized bone transfer procedures report a substantial rate of delayed union or nonunion at one or both osteosynthesis sites. This rate approaches 30% of patients in some series. If the transferred bone segment is not united by six months, some authors recommend reoperation with onlay iliac bone autografting to the nonunion site and usually with revision of the internal fixation hardware. In the author's opinion, attempts to obtain union by noninvasive means beyond six months after surgery has been unrewarding and may contribute to prolonging the period of disability and recovery.

Results

Bone union with adequate hypertrophy leading to a successful clinical result has been reported in 81% to 88% of cases for larger series involving all recipient sites in all areas of the body. The failure rate from this procedure is reported to average 13%. The most favorable results for salvage or reconstruction of a bony defect using a vascularized bone transfer has been reported for nonseptic defects. Reconstruction for posttraumatic or congenital pseudarthrosis appears to have a slightly higher success rate than for tumor reconstruction. This is presumably due to the deleterious effects on bone healing of adjuvant and nonadjuvant chemotherapy or radiation therapy in the latter group. An average time to union for major long bone reconstruction is approximately six months. Adequate hypertrophy of the bone segment sufficient to allow unrestricted use or weightbearing in the humerus, tibia, or femur will require an additional 6 to 12 months. Hypertrophy appears to be a gradual process related to controlled loading of the bone segment following union and is chiefly noted in weightbearing bones of the lower extremity.

Complications

As with any major reconstructive procedure, complications are frequent with vascularized bone transfer. Nonunion or delayed union may occur in as many as 39% of patients following the bone transfer procedure. Secondary intervention to the nonunion site involving revision of the internal fixation and/or iliac bone autografting may be required in 20% to 30% of patients for final union. Patients should be advised of this possibility with the expectation that absence of union at one or both osteosynthesis sites by six months should merit consideration of reoperation. The causes of nonunion may be related to inadequate fixation, inadequate bone coaptation, inadequate bone mass, sepsis, or vascular thrombosis of the graft. No series have addressed the relative frequencies of these various causes of nonunion.

Stress fractures are frequently seen in those patients who appear to go on to early union and early weightbearing. In DeBoer's series, it was noted in 27% of patients at an average of eight months after surgery. Often the diagnosis of stress fracture is made retrospectively by the incidental finding of periosteal new bone formation about some point in the transferred bone segment. Stress fracture is almost completely confined to the lower extremity weightbearing bone reconstruction sites.

Donor Sites

Fibula

A number of series to date have evaluated the fibula donor site when used as a vascularized bone transfer with the resultant conclusion that donor-site complications are minimal in the adult. Typically, weightbearing is permitted in the first few days after surgery and recovery of strength is a gradual process although subjectively the patient may perceive minimal problems. Goniometric and gait analysis studies have documented donor-site limb gait disturbances in a minority of patients undergoing vascularized fibula transfer. Peroneal palsy as a transient event has been reported in numerous series but typically is a traction phenomenon with a high likelihood of spontaneous recovery. In the author's reported series of 132 fibula transfers, there were five transient peroneal palsies but all recovered completely. Tenodesis or weakness of the flexor hallucis longus tendon may occur in a small number of patients and be related to a form of otherwise unrecognized compartment syndrome or postoperative peritendinous adhesions of the flexor hallucis longus tendon. Passive stretching of the great toe in extension during the postoperative period is recommended to avoid this complication. In a growing child with open epiphyses, a progressive valgus deformity of the ankle may be seen if failure to stabilize the distal fibular segment following resection is not accomplished. Therefore, in the child with open physes, fusion between the distal fibular segment and the adjacent tibia is recommended. Other complications may occur but are unusual and include compartment syndrome, wound dehiscence, or deep wound infection.

Iliac Crest

Complications related to harvest of the anterior iliac crest based on the deep circumflex iliac vessel chiefly relate to secondary incisional hernia. This is especially true in the obese patient. A careful layered closure is recommended to minimize the risk of this complication. Additional complications associated with an anterior iliac crest graft include neuropathy of the lateral femoral cutaneous, pudendal, or ilioinguinal nerves.

Microvascular Joint Transfer

The role of microvascular joint transfer for reconstruction in the hand is at this point somewhat controversial. Although laboratory data suggest that a vascularized joint transfer preserves articular cartilage and nearly normal joint morphology, the clinical results of this procedure may at times be disappointing with a poor range of motion. The ultimate range of motion achieved may be more dependent on periarticular structures, which include the integrity of the extensor and flexor tendon apparatus. Most vascular-ized joint transfer series report maintenance of a limited range of motion with adequate joint stability and long-term maintenance of joint integrity. Although suggested as theoretical concern, neuropathic progressive joint destruction has not been reported.

Donor Sites

The chief donor site for vascularized joint transfer is the metatarsophalangeal or proximal interphalangeal joint of the second toe. Other toe joints and finger joints harvested from previously damaged fingers are also utilized. The recipient sites most typically have been the proximal interphalangeal joint and less often the metacarpophalangeal joint.

Indications

The chief indication for this procedure is for reconstruction of a destroyed proximal interphalangeal or metacarpophalangeal joint in a young child with associated epiphyseal plate injury. Vascularized joint transfer restores longitudinal growth as well as joint integrity. The second major indication is for restoration of joint function in the adult patient for whom endoprosthetic arthroplasty or joint arthrodesis is not warranted. The latter indications are limited.

Results

Although clinical series vary, a recent summary of the available English literature on vascularized joint transfer has suggested that "a limited but useful range of motion with good lateral stability" can be expected. In the adult patient an average range of motion of 32° and in the child an average range of motion of 37° with vascularized joint transfer have been reported. The range of motion realized demonstrates little difference when utilized for metacarpophalangeal or proximal interphalangeal joint. Secondary procedures involving tendolysis or capsulotomy are frequent. In Tsai's series, nearly one-half the patients required a secondary procedure.

Complications

The major drawback or complication of a vascularized joint transfer is limited range of motion, which is clearly suboptimal compared with the donor joint. This factor should be carefully considered when recommending the procedure to a patient. The role of joint arthrodesis or endoprosthetic versus perichondral arthroplasty should be considered prior to vascularized joint transfer.

Functioning Free Muscle Transfer

Functioning free muscle transfer is indicated for restoration of active muscle function in patients who lack alternative options of tendon or muscle repair, nerve reconstruction, or tendon transfer.

Donor Muscles

The gracilis muscle is preferred for restoration of finger flexion. This muscle is expendable and is well suited because it has a well defined proximal and distal tendon. It is at times excessive in length for restoration of finger flexion across the forearm; however, the tendon of insertion can be shortened as required. The motor nerve of the gracilis, the anterior division of obturator, is quite robust and easily identified. The primary vascular pedicle originating from the medial circumflex femoral vessels, however, is often short and small in caliber. Nonetheless, in most instances gracilis is the muscle of choice for forearm reconstruction either involving restoration of extrinsic finger flexion, wrist extension, or finger extension. Alternative muscles that have been reported with successful outcomes include latissimus dorsi, pectoralis major, rectus femoris, semitendinosis, and medial gastrocnemius.

Indications

A free-functioning muscle transfer is most indicated for restoration of active digital flexion. The clinical outcome is best in a patient who has preserved intrinsic hand muscle function but lacks extrinsic digital flexors. Wrist stability by means of active wrist extension or wrist stabilization is essential. Restoration of full passive finger range of motion must be obtained before surgery. An identifiable healthy donor nerve is required in all cases. Other less common indications for free-functioning muscle transfer are for restoration of active wrist or active elbow flexion. The recipient site motor nerve (for wrist or finger extension) is the posterior interosseous if available. Restoration of active elbow flexion is typically most needed in a patient with late brachial plexus injury lacking alternative means of reanimating elbow flexion combined with a neurotization procedure to the free muscle transfer.

Results

The results of free muscle transfer depend upon the clinical application. The results when used to restore finger flexion are highly dependent upon the presence or absence of a sustained intrinsic motor function and normal finger sensibility. Manktelow reported grip strength following gracilis transfer to be nearly 50% normal. On the other hand, if intrinsics are lacking the results are much less predictable. Nonetheless if there are no other options this is a reasonable procedure to consider. Those cases reported for restoration of elbow flexion have as their chief limitation not the muscle transferred but rather the available donor nerve for neurotization. If reliable donor nerves are available, results comparable to restoration of finger flexion can be expected.

Complications

The major complication of free-functioning muscle transfer is either ischemic necrosis of the muscle or failure of neurotization. A comprehensive review of the available case reports suggests that 83% of free-functioning muscle transfers were "successful," which is indicative that in this group some degree of useful recovery occurred.

Free-tissue Transfer of Useless or Spare Parts

The concept of free-tissue transfer of spare useless parts is particularly attractive because it obviates concerns related to donor-site problems. Although such cases are not frequent, in every patient requiring reconstruction for free-tissue transfer an inventory of possible donor sites that currently are a liability rather than asset to function is warranted. This may suggest the use of innovative free-tissue transfers to accomplish reconstructive goals, such as free-tissue transfer of a useless finger amputation stump for restoration of length in another digit on the same or opposite hand; the vascularized transfer of a joint residing within a useless or nonfunctional digit for reconstruction of an adjacent digit; or the use of vascularized bone transfer from a part either traumatically amputated or one that may be electively amputated without an adverse effect on patient function. The literature contains many examples of this approach. Specific guidelines regarding the transfer of useless parts are not possible; however, the concept of considering this option in any patient undergoing reconstruction is worthwhile and merits emphasis.

Annotated Bibliography

Bourne MH, Wood MB, Cooney WP: Reconstruction by free tissue transfer of electively amputated parts. *Surg Rounds for Orthopaedics*, 56-61, Sep 1988.

Buncke HG: *Microsurgery: Transplantation-Replantation, An Atlas Text*. Lea and Febiger, Philadelphia, 756-758, 1991.

Cobbett JR: Free digital transfer. Report of a case of transfer of a great toe to replace an amputated thumb. *J Bone Joint Surg*, 51B:677-679, 1969.

A case report is presented in which the great toe is transferred in one stage to replace an amputated thumb using microvascular techniques to anastomose the appropriate vessels.

DeBoer HH, Wood MB: Bone changes in the vascularized fibular graft. *J Bone Joint Surg*, 71B:374-378, 1989.

A retrospective study of 64 patients who had vascularized fibular transfer for the reconstruction of large skeletal defects at the Mayo Clinic. Conclusions reached include the need to protect the vascularized graft from stress fractures and that mechanical loading should be gradually increased to enhance remodeling and hypertrophy.

Foucher G, Van de Kar T: Twisted two-toes technique in thumb reconstruction. In Landi E, (ed) *Reconstruction of the Thumb*, Paris, Chapman, 275-279, 1989.

Foucher G, Sammut D, Citron N: Free vascularized toe joint transfer in hand reconstruction: a series of 25 patients. *J Reconstr Microsurg*, 6:201-207, 1990.

A review of 28 vascularized toe-joint transfers in 25 patients is presented noting that various techniques are useful in this procedure. The vascularized joint transfer allows for a one-stage composite transfer and provides rapid bone healing. Potential growth in the young, good long-term cartilage preservation, normal lateral stability in pinch, and limited but useful ROM.

Gerwin M, Weiland AJ: Vascularized bone grafts to the upper extremity: indications and technique. *Hand Clin*, 8:509-523, 1992.

The indications for and techniques of vascularized bone grafting are presented along with three case studies. A good outcome is achievable for the patient with large bony defects that defy the use of conventional graft methods if proper patient selection, evaluation, and techniques are followed.

Han C, Wood MB, Bishop AT, Cooney WP: Vascularized bone transfer. *J Bone Joint Surg*, 74A:1441-1449, 1992.

An overview of the results of 160 patients from 1979-1989 who had reconstruction of a skeletal defect with use of a vascularized bone graft from the illiac crest or fibula. The procedure was found to be of value on appropriate selected patients.

Ishida O, Tsai T: Free vascularized whole joint transfer in children. *Microsurg*, 12:196-206, 1991.

Indications for the reconstruction of the traumatized finger joint with epiphyseal distraction in children and techniques to improve postoperative range of motion are discussed in this review of 19 joint transfers. Almost normal growth was observed in all transferred joints except two that showed premature epiphyseal closure.

Koshima I, Soeda S, Takase T, Yamasaki M: Free vascularized nail grafts. *J Hand Surg*, 13A:29-32, 1988.

A report of two clinical cases in which a free vascularized nail graft and a double onychocutaneous flap were used successfully. It is suggested that the free vascularized nail graft is a superior method in reconstruction to treat fingernail loss or deformity.

Lipton HA, May JW, Simon SR: Preoperative and postoperative gait analysis of patients undergoing great toe-to-thumb transfer. *J Hand Surg*, 12A:66-69, 1987.

The consequences of elective amputations of the great toe for toe-to-thumb microvascular transfer are evaluated with a preoperative and postoperative gait analysis of 12 patients. It is concluded that this procedure results in no major objective disturbance of foot function in gait and that fear of such problems should not discourage the use of this method of thumb reconstruction.

Manktelow RT: Functioning microsurgical muscle transfer. *Hand Clin*, 4:289-296, 1988.

This article emphasizes the use of muscle transfer along with a nerve repair for the reconstruction of finger flexion. The operative technique for muscle transplantation to the flexor and extensor forearm and for the upper arm is also discussed.

Morrison WA: Thumb and fingertip reconstruction by composite microvascular tissue from the toes. *Hand Clin*, 8:537-550, 1992.

The advantages of using toe pull web flaps in reconstructive procedures for deficits of the thumb and fingers are discussed along with the ability to include the toenail in the transfer. This flap can replicate the missing tissues of the thumb and fingers thus giving an optimal result.

Pho RWH, Patterson MH, Kour AK, et al: Free vascularized epiphyseal transplantation in upper extremity reconstruction. *J Hand Surg*, 13B:440-447, 1988.

A review is done of three patients who have had free vascularized transfer grafts to proximal fibular epiphysis in replacement of proximal humeral head or distal radial epiphysis. A discussion of both successes and problems is included in this early analysis of the results.

Salibian AH, Anzel SH, Salyer WA: Transfer of vascularized grafts of iliac bone to the extremities. *J Bone Joint Surg*, 69A:1319-1327, 1987.

Sixteen patients had a large segmental defect of bone in an extremity treated with a vascularized graft of the iliac crest. Technique and indications are reviewed; it is concluded that a vascularized graft of iliac crest is suitable for patients with an open segmental defect that is 6 cm to 9 cm long. Defects 10 cm or longer should be treated with a fibular graft and those 5 cm or shorter with a cancelloid bone graft.

Singer KI, O'Brien BM, McLeod AM, et al: Long term follow-up of free vascularized joint transfer to the hand in children. *J Hand Surg*, 13A:776-783, 1988.

A six-to-eight year postoperative review of four cases involving toe-to-hand vascularized joint transfers in children. NITP to MCP vascularized joint transfers can provide painless, functional, stable motion with near-normal growth potential. Toe PIP to hand PIP joint transfers are limited by the inability to achieve good active extension and have limited growth potential.

Taylor GI, Miller GDH, Ham FG: The free vascularized bone graft: a clinical extension of microvascular techniques. *Plast Reconstr Surg,* 55:533-544, 1975.

A case presentation of two patients in whom extensive bone and soft-tissue loss was restored by free vascularized bone grafts after appropriate flap repairs for skin coverage.

Tsai T, Ludwig L, Tonkin M: Vascularized fibular epiphyseal transfer. *Clin Orthop,* 210:228-234, 1986.

A review of eight patients with free vascularized fibular epiphyseal transfers suggests that an open epiphysis offers some potential for growth in either congenital abnormalities or epiphyseal arrests secondary to trauma and infection.

Tsai T, Wang W: Vascularized joint transfer: indications and results. *Hand Clin,* 8:525-536, 1992.

The indications for vascularized joint transfers are reviewed along with the benefit of doing this procedure. The surgical procedure is described and postoperative management along with results and a discussion are provided.

Uhm KI, Shin KS, Lee YH, Lew JD: Restoration of finger extension and forearm contour utilizing a neurovascular latissimus dorsi free flap. *Ann Plast Surg,* 21:74-76, 1988.

A case history of a burn patient in which a free neurovascular latissimus dorsi flap was used for restoration of wrist and finger extension and forearm contour. This is a rare patient in whom restoration of finger extension was achieved after the nearly total loss of the extensor forearm muscles.

Valauri FA, Buncke HJ: Thumb and finger reconstruction by toe-to-hand transfer. *Hand Clin,* 8:551-574, 1992.

Toe transplantation provides a means of restoring a thumb or finger in a single microsurgical procedure with tissues anatomically similar to those lost or absent. A successful procedure: of 188 toe transplants there was a success rate of 97% and because they are anatomically analogous, the toe transplant affords a reconstruction with many unique attributes of the missing thumb or finger.

Wei FC, Chen HC, Chuang CC, et al: Simultaneous multiple toe transfers in hand reconstruction. *Plast Reconstr Surg,* 81:366-377, 1988.

A presentation of 46 toes from 38 feet transferred to reconstruct 19 hands in 19 patients. Seven transfers were combined second and third toe units and 32 were single toes. It is concluded that simultaneous multiple toe transfers in hand reconstruction is feasible without increased complications both in primary and secondary wound conditions.

Wei FC, Chen HC, Chuang CC, et al: Thumb reconstruction with trimmed toe transfer. *Plast Reconstr Surg,* 82:506-515.

The trimmed-toe transfer is a new modification of the existing great toe transfer for thumb reconstruction. This technique involves reduction of both bony and soft-tissue elements along the medial aspect of the transferred great toe in order to produce a more normal sized thumb. Overall, appearance and usefulness of the reconstructed thumb have been excellent.

Wood MB: *Atlas of Reconstructive Microsurgery.* Aspen Publ, Rockville, 1990.

An atlas providing a basis for and continuation of the process of microsurgery including its potential applications, expectations, and limitations.

Youdas JW, Wood MB, Cahalan TD, et al: A quantitative analysis of donor site morbidity after vascularized fibula transfer. *J Orthop Res,* 6:621-629, 1988.

Eleven patients with free vascularized fibular graft transplants to the upper extermity were studied for donor-site morbidity effects. Donor-site morbidity does not appear to be caused exclusively by surgical soft-tissue trauma. No statistical difference was found between donor and normal control sites in gait factors regardless of follow-up length. Other findings regarding knee and ankle foot motion changes and muscle strength are reviewed.

VIII
Tumors

33

Soft-tissue Tumors: Benign and Malignant

Earl J. Fleegler, MD

Introduction

The evolution of our understanding of and ability to treat tumors of the upper extremity, although slow, continues. The relative scarcity of hand tumors compared to other anatomic regions has required the publication of many case reports and small series as well as information from other specialties, eg, radiology and radiotherapy, oncology, and dermatology. According to McFarland, the following make up approximately 95% of all masses of the hand: reactive lesions; ganglia; giant-cell tumor of tendon sheath; epidermoid inclusion cyst; pyogenic granulomas; foreign body reactions; and fungal infections.

Benign solar (actinic) keratosis of the skin (these are frequently premalignant) should be added to this list.

This section considers other benign and malignant tumors that are less frequent. Their relative scarcity requires study in order to recognize and adequately evaluate and treat them. The list of malignant tumors is large and difficult to present with regard to relative frequency.

Since it is impossible to be knowledgeable about all disciplines required to diagnose and treat tumors of the upper extremity, it is important to involve other specialists including pathologists, oncologists, radiotherapists, and psychiatrists in the evaluation and treatment of these patients.

Once the type and extent of the tumor is determined, adequate removal with sufficient margins of barrier tissues to control the primary tumor is required. Simultaneously, if metastasis has occurred every effort must be made to stage this development and treat involved sites. The following outlines the primary goals of tumor treatment to save the patient's life: (1) The tumor should be staged. (2) A biopsy should be carried out after the staging procedures by the surgeon who is responsible for management of the patient. This surgeon, or team, should consider the subsequent alternative treatment procedures required, plan the biopsy incision (often longitudinal) and carry out the procedure in such a way as to avoid contamination of adjacent areas. (3) Investigative studies of the biopsy tissue should be conducted. (4) A definitive surgical procedure to achieve local tumor control should be performed. The secondary goals include reconstruction and maintenance or recovery of function.

Mankin has reminded us that when evaluating soft-tissue tumors of the hand that are deeply placed and which are not ganglia, giant-cell tumors of tendon sheath, inclusion cysts, or lipomas, the surgeon must be concerned about the lesion's being malignant.

The following tumors are also of relative importance but encountered less frequently than those noted above: lipoma; glomus tumor; fibroma; enchondroma; osteochondroma;

and keratoacanthoma. It is difficult to assign a relative frequency to this group.

Malignant tumors of the hand and upper extremity are less common than those listed above but are of great significance to the patient, posing a threat to limb and/or life. They include squamous cell carcinoma, the most common malignant tumor found involving the skin primarily. Other tumors, all of them rare, include
- Basal cell carcinoma
- Malignant fibrous histiocytoma
- Epithelioid sarcoma
- Synovial sarcoma
- Fibrosarcoma
- Malignant melanoma
- Clear-cell sarcoma
- Osteosarcoma
- Malignant schwannoma
- Kaposi's sarcoma

Of the deep-seated soft-tissue malignancies, epithelioid sarcoma, synovial sarcoma, and clear-cell sarcoma are among the relatively common sarcomas that may involve the hand. All of these may metastasize to regional lymph nodes as well as by the methods that sarcomas are usually thought to metastasize, ie by extension along soft-tissue planes and by hematogenous routes. This list is now recognized to include rhabdomyosarcoma (especially in younger patients) and malignant fibrous histiocytoma, both of which can metastasize by similar methods to the first three described. Clear-cell sarcoma is also known as melanoma of soft parts. By careful preoperative work-up and appropriate biopsy, staging systems have been developed for many of these lesions, including melanoma, which have provided insight into the required surgical resections. This information also may provide an idea about outlook. Biopsies are best carried out through longitudinally oriented incisions, except in special circumstances. Change of gloves, gowns, drapes, and instruments after biopsy is usually required if additional operative procedures are carried out at that time. Copious irrigation after tumor ablation is another principle.

Ongoing research into such basic processes as progression of malignant tumors may shed light on invasion and spread of neoplasms and perhaps treatment. One such area of study focuses on the process of proteolysis and malignant tumors. The growth and invasion as well as metastatic potential of such tumors is thought to be related to their destruction of extracellular matrix.

In order to provide the best treatment, one must have knowledge of the anatomy, biologic characteristics, and natural behavior of these tumors as well as being grounded in the principles of tumor surgery. An institution that has the facilities to provide all of this and colleagues who will be part of the tumor team are a necessity. Such a team should include the hand surgeon, oncologist, radiotherapist, members from radiology, psychiatrists, social workers, and other specialists as needed. References are included that also discuss important anatomic areas.

Basic requirements in the evaluation of the patient with a tumor of the upper extremity necessitate taking a history and a search for exposure to carcinogens, including radiation and chemicals. This is important to document and may have a bearing on future health considerations for the patient. Family history may be positive for syndromes such as the basal cell nevus syndrome or B.K. Mole syndrome.

Past history may reveal underlying problems such as immunosuppression for organ transplantation or human immunodeficiency virus. It appears that other viruses may play a role in the development of neoplasms, for example, the human papilloma virus. Examination of these patients should carefully describe the specific lesion but also consider metastatic disease and other conditions that may affect treatment. One must evaluate regional nodes such as the epitrochlear and axillary areas.

The pattern of tumor growth and type may have significant differences in various age groups. For example, almost 40% of the tumors found in the pediatric study by Azouz and coworkers were vascular tissue tumors. Understanding syndromes that these young patients may have will lead the physician to look for other problems in addition to the vascular tumor, such as is found with the Klippel-Trenaunay syndrome and with the Maffucci syndrome. In the first case there may be absent deep veins and superficial varicosities. Multiple enchondromas in addition to hemangiomas should raise the specter of Maffucci syndrome.

When necessary, CT scan and MRI as well as occasionally angiography are also important in the evaluation of tumor patients.

Benign Tumors

Differential diagnosis of tumors of the hand and upper extremity must be considered any time a mass, ulceration, infection, color change, or even pain needs explanation. Ganglia are the most common mass encountered in the hand and wrist, followed by inclusion cysts and giant-cell tumor of tendon sheath. Ganglia, giant cell tumors of tendon sheath, inclusion cyst, and lipoma, as well as other tumors are reviewed in a recent discussion of common tumors by Diao and Moy.

Ganglia

Presentation may occur in a variety of areas: the typical dorsoradial wrist ganglion; volar radial wrist ganglion; mucous cyst; occult (this form may be found only after careful investigation into the cause of difficult-to-diagnose wrist pain.)

MRI studies have become useful in this evaluation; however, the anterior or volar wrist ganglion has not received similar attention. The recurrence rate appears to be much higher for anterior wrist ganglia in this study compared to dorsal wrist ganglia that have undergone adequate excision. Greendyke, Wilson, and Shepler point out that the anterior variety may account for up to 20% of ganglia, seem to have a higher recurrence rate than the dorsal lesion, and, although it may be seen when it is quite small, the patient often presents with discomfort. Adequate exposure is required to completely remove the lesion and appropriately delineate the joint of origin.

Warts can be difficult lesions to differentiate from sweat gland tumors and other tumors and to treat. Warts, related to human papilloma virus, raise the possibility of the human papilloma virus being involved in the production of squamous cell carcinomas.

Fibrous Tumors

A partial list includes digital fibroma; digital fibrokeratoma; fibroma of tendon sheath; extra abdominal desmoid; fibrous hamartoma; fibromatosis, aggressive; and aponeurotic fibroma.

This is a large group of tumors, which appear to behave differently in different age groups. Excepting Dupuytren's disease, experience of a given surgeon with these lesions is often limited. Aggressive fibromatosis, a rare fibroproliferative neoplasm, is known for its local invasiveness and tendency to recur. Although it may occur in many sites, it may also be seen in the hand. Its evolution is not well understood, treatment requires careful delineation of the tumor, and surgical treatment may necessitate a wide ablation; however, this is still difficult to define.

Lipomas

Many authors have emphasized the difficulty in treating lipomas involving the hand, especially because of the method by which the tumor advances into tight spaces creating an intimate relationship with nerves, vessels, and other structures. These lesions are hazardous to extirpate because of the potential for associated damage. Lipofibromatous hamartoma remains a difficult lesion to treat because of the involvement of peripheral nerves. Incomplete removal and pain are two problems associated with this tumor.

Glomus tumor

Glomus tumor is the classic example of a mass entering into the differential diagnosis of a painful condition. These are most prevalent in the distal finger area, especially in the subungual region. These tumors most frequently occur in middle-aged adults and present as red to purplish discolorations (when they can be seen at all) distorting the overlying nail plate. Recognition and complete excision are usually curative.

Nail-area tumors include an extensive list. A recent review considered 25 neoplasms (both benign and malignant) in a partial listing of tumors in this area. In addition to deformity and/or formation of a mass, subtle presentation, for example infection, may herald an underlying neoplasm. This somewhat unusual presentation of a tumor, when recognized, may at least help resolve an underlying cause for chronic infection. Therefore, even rare tumors must be understood.

Nodular fasciitis should be considered in the differential diagnosis of forearm and even hand tumors because of its presentation as a firm, round-to-ovoid mass that may be fixed to the surrounding tissues. Although careful preoperative work-up is necessary, CT and MRI scans may help visualize the lesion, yet not yield information that allows differentiating it from other neoplasms. This tumor may be easily confused with more serious lesions.

Sweat Gland Tumors

In addition to being rare, these tumors have treatment requirements that are not well understood. They may recur locally, produce deformity and pain, and in some cases, evolve into malignancies.

Syringomas are among the more common sweat gland tumors arising from the eccrine ducts; however, they are unusual in the distal parts of the extremities. They may be multiple and papular. The actual tumors are often small, skin colored to yellowish. It is important to differentiate them from other tumors such as basal cell carcinoma or other sweat gland tumors. These are more frequently found in locations other than the hand (especially about the face).

Malignant sweat gland tumors do occur in the upper extremity. Some appear as asymptomatic masses. In the still-benign aggressive digital papillary adenoma, high recurrence is usual. This, as well as its malignant counterpart, tends to invade the deeper tissues. Once the lesion is frankly malignant, a significant number of patients are at risk for developing metastases.

Eccrine acrospiroma (clear-cell hidradenoma) is a relatively common eccrine sweat gland tumor. Its histologically malignant counterpart is rare. The malignant variety may develop in a benign lesion and has the potential to metastasize and kill. They may enter into the differential diagnosis of squamous cell carcinoma of the skin and may require aggressive surgical treatment.

Malignant Tumors

Malignant tumors of the hand and upper extremity run the gamut of neoplasms encountered virtually anywhere in the body other than those specific for viscera. Basal cell carcinoma is much less common in the hand and upper extremity than in other sun-exposed areas. Yet basal cell carcinoma still is seen at advanced stages, having either been missed by examining physicians, or neglected by patients. This can lead to the perplexing situation described by Craig and coauthors with regard to an advanced basal cell carcinoma of the shoulder. The approach to such lesions should consider a spectrum of surgical procedures from wide excision and skin grafting to the complex reconstruction mentioned in that report.

Squamous cell carcinoma is the most frequently encountered, primary malignant tumor involving the hand. However, some authors report it as a rare tumor. Keratoacanthoma (KA) still causes difficulty in the differential diagnosis between it and squamous cell carcinoma. Keratoacanthomas are thought to arise in hair-bearing skin, frequently from hair follicles; however, there is an increasing body of literature studying subungual keratoacanthomas which have arisen from non-hair-bearing skin. KAs appear to behave locally aggressively yet may be cured by curettage. Those that recur after curettage are treated by limited amputation by some surgeons. However, this author has followed at least one patient with a recurrent subungual keratoacanthoma that seems to be successfully treated by curettage with follow-up exceeding five years postcurettage. Unfortunately, there are inadequate statistics to guide us at the present time. Differentiation between the probably nonmalignant true keratoacanthoma and malignant squamous cell carcinoma is being made by experienced dermatopathologists with what appears to be a high degree of accuracy.

Various agents and conditions have been associated with the development of both keratoacanthomas and squamous cell carcinomas, some of which are common to both of these. Human papilloma virus infection and exposure to certain organic chemicals are mentioned in the recent literature. Conditions such as chronic burn wounds and skin disorders such as epidermolysis bullosa may be associated with more aggressive skin cancers. Reports are now accumulating in literature that have studied significant groups of patients with squamous cell carcinoma of the hand. Some consider this anatomic area to be involved by a squamous cell carcinoma that behaves in a more aggressive fashion than in other areas.

Although spreading through lymphatics to regional nodes is the most common metastatic route for squamous cell carcinoma of the skin of the hand, metastatic tumors may present in a variety of unusual anatomic patterns including perineural and even skeletal metastases. Implantation of squamous cell carcinoma in skin graft donor sites is possible. An apparent relationship between certain types of the human papilloma virus and squamous cell carcinoma in the hand, as well as other areas, is now being reported by multiple workers. Pigmented skin and nail area tumors continue to tax our diagnostic acumen, and it is important not to be tardy in biopsy of such lesions.

Melanoma

Surgeons still try to understand the factors that help decide whether regional node dissections are advisable when dealing with Stage one melanoma. It is possible that methods for detection of occult melanoma cells in elective lymph node dissection specimens have not been adequate. The presence of "regression" and prognosis of melanoma has also been studied.

Efforts at understanding the prognosis for melanoma have led to many papers dealing with thickness and staging. Physicians have also looked at the association of vascular invasion with tumor thickness in trying to understand prognosis. Efforts at determining prognosis for patients have also evaluated those with Stage two (Clark's staging or Stage III AJCC staging; American Joint Committee on Cancer: Manual for Staging of Cancer (ed. 3), Philadelphia, PA, Lippincott, 139-144, 1988) regional node involvement. The most difficult melanoma patient to treat is a patient with recurrence and metastasis. In the experience of some, perfusion of limbs with chemotherapy by isolated regional techniques may produce palliation.

Sarcomas

A variety of masses needs to be considered in the differential diagnosis of soft-tissue sarcomas of the upper extremity. Tumors ranging from desmoid tumors to nodular fasciitis, Dupuytren's disease, erythema nodosum, fibromas of various locations, dermatofibroma, metastatic tumors to the hand and upper extremity, and even masses produced by various microorganisms enter into this consideration.

Epithelioid sarcoma, a tumor that is easily confused with many benign and malignant processes, is one of the more frequent sarcomas seen in the upper extremity. It may initially appear to involve the superficial soft tissues and even ulcerate through the skin. This is a tumor of young adults that requires early and aggressive surgical treatment.

Dermatofibrosarcoma protuberans is another malignant tumor that is seen occasionally involving the subcutaneous tissues as well as skin, and later involving the deeper tissues in young adults. Metastases from this tumor are not as common as with other sarcomas. Minimal treatment is considered to be a wide resection containing good margins of normal tissue barriers including deeper tissues such as fascia and muscle. However, recurrences are common.

A partial list of sarcomas encountered in the upper extremity includes epithelioid sarcoma, dermatofibrosarcoma protuberans, fibrosarcoma, malignant fibrous histiocytoma, rhabdomyosarcoma, and synovial sarcoma. In addition to the usual routes of spread along tissue planes and hematogenously, one should be concerned about lymphatic spread with these tumors.

Treatment of upper extremity sarcoma is obviously still in a state of evolution. Appropriate margins around these tumors, the concept of limb-sparing surgery and complications of that surgery as well as appropriate utilization of radiotherapy and chemotherapy, are still intensely studied. Factors involved in understanding prognosis are coming to light. Efforts at detecting early metastases and their treatment are some of the new developments in this area.

Kaposi's sarcoma, a tumor known to have an association with HIV and AIDS, has now been reported masquerading as infection in the area of the nail fold, in addition to producing its more characteristic red or purple soft-tissue masses. Unusual presentation of this tumor may involve the palmar surface of the hand. See reference to Ozbek and Kutlu in the differential diagnosis section of the annotated bibliography.

Annotated Bibliography

Principles

Adani R, Calo M, Toricelli P, Squarzina PB, Caroli A: The value of computed tomography in the diagnosis of soft-tissue swellings of the hand. *J Hand Surg,* 158:229-232, 1990.

The authors point out the importance of CT as well as MRI and angiography.

Azouz EM, Kozlowski K, Masel J: Soft-tissue tumors of the hand and wrist of children. *J Canadian Assn Radiol,* 40:251-255, 1989.

These authors reported on 23 children with soft-tissue tumors about the hand. The greatest number involved blood and lymph vessels. In this review they found only one malignancy (rhabdomyosarcoma). They discuss imaging techniques, emphasizing that plain radiography is the primary technique. This may be helpful in adults who have calcified phleboliths, commonly associated with cavernous hemangioma. They point out that bony erosion may be produced by a number of tumors that are benign including glomus tumors, vascular tumors, giant-cell tumor of tendon sheath, and some fibromatoses. Keratoacanthoma can also rapidly destroy bone in the subungual area.

Mack GR: Superficial anatomy and cutaneous surgery of the hand. *Advances in Dermatology,* Mosby-Year Book, Inc. 7:315-352, 1992.

This is an extensive review of the skin anatomy as it relates to surgical procedures. One must keep in mind that surgery of this subdivision of the hand requires thorough knowledge of the entire hand, its response to wounding, and the care of the patient postoperatively.

Mankin HJ: Principles of diagnosis and management of tumors of the hand. *Hand Clin,* Vol 3:185-195, 1987.

Dr. Mankin carefully reviews the approach one should consider to a hand mass. He points out the relative rarity of a mass in the hand representing a metastatic focus (although this has been found by this reviewer to include, not only lung, but in rare instances, other tumors including lymphoma). He points out the significant percentage of bone tumors that are benign, especially composed of enchondromas and osteocartilaginous masses but warns about not underestimating large, deeply placed soft-tissue tumors. Rules such as these are laid down throughout this paper. An overview of staging of soft-tissue and bone tumors, grading, and the approach to them is detailed. Advice as to biopsy and principles of management of the tumor are provided. The actual tumor ablation is considered in terms of intralesional, marginal, wide, and radical approaches. These procedures are matched to the staging of the tumor.

Rayner CR: Soft-tissue tumors of the hand. *J Hand Surg,* 16B:125-126, 1991.

Fundamentals are briefly reviewed in this article. Special areas of concern are keratoacanthoma, nail area melanoma, and fibrous tumors. Diagnostic studies that have been shown in recent years to be extremely helpful include the CT and MRI scan.

Schlagenhauff B, Klessen C, Teichmann-dorr S, Breuninger H, Rassner G: Demonstration of proteases in basal cell carcinomas. *Cancer,* 1133-1140, 1992.

These authors considered that the high activity of proteases that they demonstrated in the connective tissue about the basal cell carcinoma, "may be related to the proliferation and invasive growth of basal cell carcinoma."

Zook EG: Anatomy and physiology of the perionychium. *Hand Clin,* Vol 6:1-7, 1990

This article defines the anatomy of the nail area including its lymphatic, arterial, and venous supply.

Differential Diagnosis

Diao E, Moy OJ: Common tumors. *Orthop Clin North Am,* 23:187-196, 1992.

These authors provide a concise review of benign tumors including enchondroma, osteochondroma, osteoblastoma, and bone cysts, as well as soft-tissue lesions. The authors review the ganglion cyst, pointing out that they are most common in the "periscaphoid" areas. Ganglia are also divided into the usual dorsal wrist ganglion, occult dorsal wrist ganglion, and those occurring in the flexor retinaculum and distal interphalangeal joint areas. The authors point out the difficulty in adequate treatment and in choosing the best treatment. Lipomas are also reviewed from the perspective of their difficulty in treatment. Squamous cell carcinoma is emphasized as being the most common malignant hand tumor. References cited list this malignancy as representing 70% to 90% of all hand malignancies. Also a brief review of nerve and vascular tumors is presented.

Ozbek MR, Kutlu N: A rare case of Kaposi's sarcoma: hand localization. *Handchir Mikrochir Plast Chir,* 22:107-109, 1990 .

Common benign tumors of the skin and of the hand and nail area, include ganglia and inclusion cysts, dermatofibroma, fibroma, and fibromatoses, foreign body reactions, infections, for example, related to acid-fast organisms, sporotrichosis, and chronic wounds may confuse this issue. Keratoses, keratoacanthoma, glomus tumors, nevi, sweat gland tumors, and warts are part of the differential diagnosis.

Smith KA, MacKinnon SE, Macauley RJB, Malis A: Glomus tumor originating in the radial nerve: a case report. *J Hand Surg,* 17A:665-667, 1992.

These authors point out that one is always looking for a glomus tumor when dealing with an ungual area, painful lesion. However, these tumors may occur in other sites such as peripheral nerves. In other positions they can also produce pain. Diagnostic methods such as ultrasonography and MRI are discussed.

Virus and Tumors

Guitart J, Bergfeld WF, Tuthill R, Tubbs RR, Zienowicz R, Fleegler EJ: Squamous cell carcinoma of the nail bed: a clinicopathological study of 12 cases. *J American Academy Dermatology,* 123:215-220, 1990.

These articles are but a few of those appearing on this interesting subject that may clarify the role of HPV in certain squamous cell carcinomas.

Moy RL, Quan MB: The presence of human papilloma virus Type 16 in squamous cell carcinoma of the proximal finger and reconstruction with a bilobed transposition flap. *J Dermatologic Surg Oncol,* 17:171-175, 1991.

This is a documented case presentation in which the difficulty in diagnosis of keratoacanthoma versus squamous cell carcinoma is emphasized. Human papilloma virus, type 16 DNA was found in the tumor.

Benign Lesions

Alman BA, Goldberg MJ, Nabers P, Galanopoulous T, Antoniades HN, Wolfe HJ: Aggressive fibromatosis. *J Ped Orthop,* 12:1-10, 1992.

These authors point out that aggressive fibromatosis, which is known by many names, is a difficult disease to control. They had a high recurrence rate and emphasize using IV contrast material to enhance the tumor during the evaluation. They conclude that wide surgical margins decrease the rate of recurrence.

Amadio PC, Reiman HM, Dobyns JH: Lipofibromatous hamartoma of nerves. *J Hand Surg,* 13A:67-75, 1988.

Some of the significant problems in treating lipofibromatous hamartoma are discussed. A high percentage of these conditions was found in association with enlargement of the anatomic part. Complications are emphasized not only by this review but the experience of many working with patients who suffer from this unfortunate condition.

Fleegler EJ: A Surgical Approach to Melanonychia Striata. *J Dermatologic Surg Oncol,* 18:8,708-714, 1992.

This recent review attempts to provide guide lines for the approach to subungual pigmented lesions. Longitudinal pigmented lesions of the nail area are presented as a difficult diagnostic problem. The major differentiation in evaluating these is from melanoma. Differences in racial groups and technical approaches to the problem are covered. The difficulty and danger in this area is emphasized by patient presentations that include young patients exhibiting a spectrum of lesions from completely benign pigmentation to premalignant or early melanoma to melanoma which has been delayed in diagnosis. The importance of follow-up for what are thought to be benign lesions is stressed. Certainly no one would argue with very careful follow-up after treatment of malignancies. For a broader review of these subjects see: *Tumors of the Hand and Upper Limb,* Eds. Bogumill, G. and Fleegler, E.J., Churchill Livingstone. Published in 1993.

Fleegler EJ, Zienowicz RJ: Tumors of the perionychium. *Hand Clin,* 6:113-133, 1990.

This paper points out the frequent delay in diagnosis and/or misdiagnosis of nail bed tumors and which tumors are more frequent. In addition to providing lists of tumors encountered in the nail area, a discussion of biopsy in this difficult site is presented. The authors emphasize that biopsy usually requires some form of nail removal and reconstruction of the nail bed and/or matrix. Listening to the patient's description of the lesion is emphasized. Difficulties in approaching these patients, especially those with pigmented lesions, are discussed.

Gabrielsen TO, Elgjo K, Sommerschild H: Eccrine angiomatous hamartoma of the finger leading to amputation. *Clin and Exp Derm,* 16:44-45, 1991.

In this report a 34-year-old pregnant woman underwent amputation in order to treat a painful eccrine angiomatous hamartoma. This tumor is histologically described as one of a group combining "eccrine, pilar and vascular structures in the same tumor...." This report emphasizes the need to remove such tumors completely. In addition to pain these tumors may present with hyperhidrosis.

Greendyke SD, Wilson M, Shepler TR: Anterior wrist ganglia from the scaphotrapezial joint. *J Hand Surg,* 17A:487-490, 1992.

These authors point out that volar wrist ganglia more frequently arise from the radioscaphoid or scapholunate area. Thoughts on why this happens, the anatomy of the area, and some of the problems that may predispose to recurrence are discussed. They employ an incision (Bruner) that provides adequate exposure, emphasize not rupturing the cyst, and carefully dissect the pedicle in order to identify the joint from which the lesion originates. Anterior wrist ganglia are divided into two groups: the radio-scaphoid/scapholunate group which was approximately 65% and the scaphotrapezial, which accounted for 34% of their series.

Hays SD, Brittenden J, Atkinson P, Eremin O: Glomus tumour: an analysis of 43 patients and review of the literature. *Br J Hand Surg,* 79:345-347, 1992.

Although described as uncommon, a computer search revealed 43 patients in this study with glomus tumors that were treated by the Aberdeen group of hospitals from 1972 to 1990. Males were involved more frequently than females. The history of glomus tumor as well as its histologic classification is reviewed. Pain was the most commonly encountered symptom and a high percentage of the patients had a lesion that could be grossly identified as reddish-purple. Surgical treatment uniformly lessened the pain. Differential diagnosis was considered to include, "pigmented naevi, melanoma, neuroma, and skin nodule."

Marty-Double C, Balmes P, Mary H, Alliu Y, Pignodel C, Targhetta R, Lesbros D, Metge L: Juvenile fibromatosis resembling aponeurotic fibroma and congenital multiple fibromatosis. *Cancer,* 61:146-152, 1988.

A seven-year-old boy with a tumor of the palm of the right hand is presented. Since the development of this tumor at age four, the patient developed discomfort when he began drawing. There followed multiple excisions leading to amputation of the hand. Ultimately lung involvement occurred following involvement of the ipsilateral axillary lymph nodes. The authors review this type of lesion pointing out that classically juvenile aponeurotic fibroma is described as a slow-growing mass that is poorly circumscribed and painless. The two main sites are the hands and feet. The pathology is discussed in detail. They emphasize the uncertain prognosis.

Metze D, Jurecka W, Gephart W: Disseminated syringomas of the upper extremities. *Dermatologica,* 180:228-235, 1990.

Disseminated syringomas in a 66-year-old man are reviewed. Multiple tumors involve the hands and forearms. Considerable information is presented concerning the histology of this tumor.

Meyer CA, Kransdorf MJ, Jelinek GS, Moser RP: MR and CT appearance of nodular fasciitis. *J Comput Assist Tomogr,* 15:276-279, 1991.

The importance of being able to differentiate nodular fasciitis from a sarcoma is reviewed. This lesion of young adults is relatively common in the upper extremity. It can present in many anatomic locations ranging from subcutaneous to deeply situated masses. A variety of radiologic techniques is described for application to the work-up of these patients.

Patel NR, Desai SS: Subungual Keratoacanthoma of the Hand. *J Hand Surg,* 14A:139-142, 1989.

The authors have considered that amputation of the distal phalanx was required in a thumb subungual keratoacanthoma that recurred. They reviewed the available literature pointing out that subungual keratoacanthoma, although benign, grows rapidly and may destroy the distal phalanx quickly. The clinical findings are described, including those of a rapidly growing subungual mass which may produce a soft, white material under the nail plate.

Rankin G, Kuschner SH, Gellman H: Nodular fasciitis: a rapidly growing tumor of the hand. *J Hand Surg,* 16A:791-795, 1991.

Because nodular fasciitis is somewhat uncommon in the upper extremity, it may be difficult to differentiate it from other lesions including sarcoma. Studies have been presented in which the tumor has been mistaken for a fibrosarcoma as well as other types of malignant neoplasms.

Malignant Tumors

Ceballos PI, Penneys NS, Acosta R: Aggressive digital papillary adenocarcinoma. *J American Academy of Derm,* 23:331-334, 1990.

Subtle findings include an asymptomatic mass occurring on the palmar aspects of digits that may be associated with this group of tumors. There is a high recurrence rate. Metastases occur most commonly to the lung and also to "lymph nodes, brain, skin, bone, and kidney." The histologic differentiation of this tumor is described in this report. The authors recommend aggressive therapeutic treatment with either wide or local excision or amputation of the digit.

Cochran AJ, Duan-Ren W, Morton DL: Occult tumor cells in the lymph nodes of patients with pathological stage one malignant melanoma. *Am J Surg Path,* 12:612-618, 1988.

Although the authors found no evidence for microscopic melanoma in the lymph nodes of 100 patients being treated for Stage one cutaneous melanoma by H and E sections, they considered that melanoma was detectible in 16 nodes from 14 of these patients using an "antiserum to S-100 protein in a peroxidase-antiperoxidase." This was confirmed by a reaction of these cells with, "melanoma-directed monoclonal antibody NK 1/C3." The deeply invasive, thicker primary tumors have the highest incidence of nodal involvement. Therefore, these workers considered early melanoma metastasis in stage one "is greater than has previously been appreciated on the basis of assessment of routine hematoxylin-and-eosin-stained sections."

Cochran AJ, Lana AMA, Duan-Ren W: Histomorphometry in the assessment of prognosis in stage II malignant melanoma. *Am J Surg Path,* 13:600-604, 1989.

This paper presents an interesting study of stage two patients' lymphadenectomy specimens. The authors found that a "combination of a number of positive nodes with aggregate tumor diameter was the most accurate..." manner of predicting survival in Stage two patients. They believe that those patients who die of their disease despite relatively favorable lymph-node findings do so because of rapid or extensive hematogenous spread.

Craig DM, Sullivan PK, Herndon JH, Edstrom LE: One-stage arm-preserving shoulder resection with latissimus dorsi flap for basal cell carcinoma. *Ann of Plast Surg,* 20:158-162, 1988.

The Tikhoff-Linberg procedure is presented as a radical resection of the shoulder girdle that spares the patient a forequarter amputation. An alternative approach to what is probably a less aggressive lesion is presented for a more anterior shoulder-chest and neck area tumor in the review of tumors of the skin of the upper extremity in Hand Clinics, 1987.

Mandell L, Ghavimi F, LaQuaglia M, Exelby P: Prognostic significance of regional lymph-node involvement in childhood rhabdomyosarcoma. *Med Ped Oncol*, 18:466-471, 1990.

Rhabdomyosarcomas are reviewed in this paper from Memorial Sloan-Kettering Cancer Center. Regional lymph-node involvement was histologically studied in 28 patients; the primary tumor was found in the upper extremity in 11. Embryonal rhabdomyosarcoma was present in 13 patients and alveolar rhabdomyosarcoma involved 14 patients. The minimum follow-up time from diagnosis was 5.3 years. Overall survival for the group was 48%. This study found that the presence of regional lymph-node involvement, at the time of diagnosis of the rhabdomyosarcoma seemed to be associated with a poor outcome. Multi-agent chemotherapy is reviewed as is a discussion of cell type, clinical and diagnostic evaluation, and staging. Treatment modalities included surgery, radiotherapy, and chemotherapy.

Rooser B, Willen H, Hugoson A, Rydholm A: Prognostic factors in synovial sarcoma. *Cancer*, 63:2182-2185, 1989.

The high-grade nature of this malignancy is emphasized. Other factors that are evaluated in attempting to discern prognosis included mitotic rate, tumor necrosis, and vascular invasion. It was found that sex, age, presence or absence of vascular invasion, type that is monophasic or biphasic, as well as amputation versus limb-sparing surgery did not seem to significantly affect outcome. The factors that did appear to affect outcome included "more than 15 mitoses/10 HPF, tumor size four centimeters or larger, tumor necrosis larger than four millimeters, and a local recurrence..."

Schiavon M, Mazzoleni F, Chiarelli A, Matano P: Squamous cell carcinoma of the hand: 55 case reports. *J Hand Surg*, 13A:401-404, 1988.

These authors have reviewed a large number of patients treated at the plastic surgery institute at the University of Padua, Italy for squamous cell carcinoma of the skin between 1971 and 1983. Of this large group there were 55 cases or 11% where the tumor was primary in the hand. Even with the significant margins of resection they outline, recurrence rate was 22% and metastasis, most often to regional lymph nodes, epitrochlear and axillary, 28%. Mortality at five years after surgery left 82.5% of the patients alive without signs of disease, while only 67% were alive, in good health, at eight-year follow up. In addition to early patient deaths from metastatic disease, they reported three patients who had died from metastasis in their sixth, seventh, and eighth year of follow-up. That is, there was a 10% five-year mortality rate, and 17.5% eight-year mortality rate. A high percentage of the patients who had local recurrence (67%) were noted to have metastatic spread. However, regional lymphadenectomy was associated with survival in 54% of those patients with local recurrence at five years after regional lymph node resection.

Serpell JW, Ball ABS, Robinson MH, Fryatt I, Fisher C, Thomas JM: Factors influencing local recurrence and

survival in patients with soft-tissue sarcoma of the upper limb. *Br J Surg*, 78:1368-1372, 1991.

This paper includes a broad spectrum of the tumors encountered, including MFH, synovial sarcoma, epithelioid sarcoma, clear cell sarcoma, liposarcoma, rhabdomyosarcoma, and others. The synovial sarcoma was the most common encountered by this study. Seventy-five percent of the patients had local recurrences following treatment elsewhere prior to being treated in this soft-tissue sarcoma unit. "The overall five-year survival rate of 80% (95% confidence interval 61% to 90%) supports a policy of conservative surgery."

Stagnone GJ, Kucan JO, Gross K, Mann JL, Zook EG: Malignant acrospiroma. *J Hand Surgery*, 15A:987-990, 1990.

Reviews individual cases, one a man, the other a woman, who were found to have malignant acrospiromas involving their fingers. The malignant, aggressive nature and potential for metastasis leading to death are emphasized. Of these two patients one had a local recurrence eight months postoperatively despite a ray amputation and axillary lymph node dissection. The original resection appeared to have good margins and negative lymph nodes.

Steinberg PD, Gelberman RH, Mankin HJ, Rosenberg AE: Epithelioid sarcoma in the upper extremity.
J Bone Joint Surg, 74A:28-35, 1992.

This series reviews 18 patients retrospectively who have been treated for epithelioid sarcoma in the upper extremity. The authors emphasize the frequency of local recurrence, extension along tendons as well as spread both through lymphatics and hematogenously. The lack of correlation between the grade of the tumor and patient outcome is described. One patient who had positive axillary nodes when seen at the seven-month follow-up, was followed up for a subsequent nine years after an above-elbow amputation plus axillary excision for the positive nodes and found to be free of tumor. Another patient was free of disease 11 years after what was described as "wide axillary excision..." These authors found that a marginal excision was not adequate for tumor control. Late recurrence is always of concern with regard to this tumor. A second group of six patients who had initial wide or radical tumor resection had a survival rate of 100% at the mean duration of follow-up of seven years. Considering patients who had other initial forms of treatment and subsequent wide or radical excision revealed that this form of treatment was successful in nine out of 13 operations. This study also makes recommendations with regard to the work-up of the patient for sarcoma.

Wilson KM, Jubert AV, Joseph JI: Sweat gland carcinoma of the hand (malignant acrospiroma). *J Hand Surg*, 14A:531-535, 1989.

The poor prognosis associated with malignant acrospiroma is reviewed in association with a case presentation. The frequency of local recurrence after what appeared to be adequate surgery for sweat gland carcinomas is discussed. This has led to the opinion of some that the histologic type of the tumor must be heavily weighed in trying to understand the survival. Treatment with hyperthermic isolation chemotherapeutic perfusion is suggested for consideration. Please see the articles discussing this mode of treatment for melanoma in this chapter.

34

Benign and Malignant Tumors of Bone

Clayton A. Peimer, MD

Introduction

The majority of neoplasms common to the hand—whether of bone or soft tissue—are benign. In addition to true neoplasms, there are reactive lesions, nodules, sequelae of systemic connective tissue proliferations and diseases, calcifications, bone spurs, and foreign body reactions. Bone tumors of the hand and upper limb are far less common than in the lower extremities; the literature tends to reflect this, with smaller series and case reports predominating. Some bone tumors in the hand are encountered more frequently, can present challenging diagnostic problems, and result in functional deficits when located. This chapter first presents the common, benign tumors, and then progresses to the troublesome, locally aggressive lesions, and finally to malignant neoplasms.

Because there are no reliable published data of large series of these tumors, it is difficult to determine what *exactly* constitutes a safe margin of extirpation or how much (anatomy and function) must be sacrificed in order to save the life of a patient with a skeletal malignancy. The goal is to eliminate the tumor. Whatever combination of surgery and adjunctive measures are employed, they should be used so as to avoid either annoying or lethal recurrence. Even a benign tumor of bone that recurs presents a problem for the patient who must undergo another operation and disability. The message that tumor control requires local control is repeated in all published articles; the literature remains very clear on this issue if nothing else.

Cartilage Tumors

Chondroma-solitary

Endosteal (enchondromatous) and extraosseous cartilage tumors are some of the most common primary neoplasms of the hand skeleton. Solitary enchondroma is frequently found in the hands of young adults, but virtually only in the phalanges and metacarpals. Carpal bone enchondromas are essentially unknown. Most lesions present as pathological fractures, although they are rarely diagnosed on radiographs taken for other reasons. In situations in which the lesions are very small, they may only require periodic observation. The larger tumors, and those presenting as fractures, should be treated. The literature is not clear on *when* bones are *likely* to break with a benign, albeit quiescent or growing, osteolytic lesion.

With incidental discoveries, the surgeon should carefully assess whether the patient has history of symptoms or local findings of tenderness. A bone scan should be part of the routine work-up to assess the tumor, and to exclude the possibility of other sites. If the patient has findings, complaints, and/or a hot scan, the tumor is presumed to be active and the patient advised about the risks of extirpation versus the problems of pathologic fracture in weakened bone and later treatment.

The occurrence of a fracture through an enchondroma does not assure that the lesion itself will spontaneously resolve as the fracture heals. Accordingly, there is controversy as to whether to treat these tumors and the pathologic fracture at the time of presentation, or to allow the fracture to heal first and then later perform surgery to treat the enchondroma. By treating the tumor and fracture simultaneously there is only one rather than two disability intervals.

These tumors are slow growing, locally destructive, and can be handled by curettage. Autogenous bone graft is added to increase the rate of bone reconstitution if the tumor is relatively large. Bone graft is not required, but may be helpful to assist with stabilization of a curetted "pathologic infraction." The addition of internal fixation—such as Kirschner wires or screws—is appropriate with most pathologic fractures to optimize stability and enhance the start of remobilization. With or without use of bone graft, recurrences are unusual. In the rare circumstance that the tumor proves to be other than an enchondroma, treatment of a pathologic fracture at the time of presentation speeds both the diagnosis and shortens the disability.

Curettage can generally be accomplished through a dorsal or dorsolateral incision in the fingers or metacarpals. It is important to take the time to curette the tumor cavity *thoroughly* to lessen the chance of recurrence. Since many are approached through a "cortical window," the underside edge of the fenestration becomes a "blind area" that needs careful attention—generally with a curved curette—before completing the operation. With recurrences, some cellular atypia is expected, although numerous mitoses per high-powered field should *not* be seen.

Chondroma-multiple

Multiple enchondromatosis (Ollier's) are less frequent than solitary lesions. These tumors tend to be associated with deformities of the axial skeleton and are often larger than the solitary variety. With multiple lesions, there is a considerably greater risk of degeneration into chondrosarcoma, perhaps because of the increased number of tumors, but perhaps also because this problem is a systemic one, with lesions present at a much earlier age.

The possibility of malignant degeneration has to be entertained if known tumors become painful, enlarged, or are associated with a precipitous change in size or other symptoms. In these circumstances, a proper tumor work-up followed by incisional biopsy is recommended. Definitive treatment is best deferred until the pathology is clear by permanent sections. Enchondromas of the large tubular bones should be considered probable chondrosarcomas (they tend to develop symptoms late) whereas low-grade "possible chondrosarcomas," or the more frequent "atypical enchondroma" of phalanges and metacarpals are likely to have a completely benign course. In all events, it is more than prudent to begin any chondroma work-up with a bone scan both for the lesion in question as well as others that may not be easily diagnosable by other methods.

Osteochondromas

Solitary and multiple exostoses are known widely to be well represented in hand bones, often, but not always, on a hereditary basis. There may also be significant skeletal deformities associated with this problem of aberrant bone production via excessive or ectopic enchondral ossification, including limited motion (periarticular), nail deformities, and clinodactyly. In children, the base of the lesion is bony and the top, or cap, is made of cartilage, which continues to increase in size during growth. Most patients present with symptoms caused by the presence of the actual bony mass. This tumor is more frequent in the radius and ulna than in the hand.

The goal of care is to remove the tumor and effect decompression of the normal skeleton and soft tissues. The surgical problem most frequently encountered is the need for reconstructive operation to restore or preserve functional alignment of bones, joints, and other parts. Although virtually uniformly benign, these tumors can be therefore quite troubling if they are not watched carefully, so that a deformity occurs where treatment is delayed. Frequent examinations and radiographs, as well as careful assessment of alignment and mobility, must be pursued if surgery is not elected for whatever reason. Treatment delay until physeal closure is complete is not feasible when neoplastic proliferation causes dysfunctional and unaesthetic angulation, rotation, or limits the range of joint motion.

Chondromyxoid Fibroma

This is an unusual tumor that is rare in the hand but may be more likely to occur more in the forearm. It has a population incidence similar to giant cell tumors of bone (discussed below) and may actually be confused radiographically with that more common bone tumor. Unlike giant cell tumors of bone, chondromyxoid fibromas rarely recur after curettage. The defects are usually large enough to need bone grafting following intralesional removal.

Chondrosarcoma

Chondrosarcomas are uncommon in the hand, especially in patients who have not yet reached their fifth decade. Actually, chondrosarcomas are rare in the hands of other than the elderly where there has *not* been previous exposure to ionizing radiation, *and* multiple enchondromas are absent. The most frequent site in the hand bones is the proximal phalanx, but metacarpal and other phalangeal sites common to benign enchondromas are not surprising. While the presentation is similar to enchondroma, this tumor should be larger, and have a longer history of neglect and associated deformity.

Chondral tumors with histologic findings of mild cellular atypia are not necessarily worrisome. As explained earlier, such is not rare when chondral tumors recur. Because chondrosarcomas generally grow slowly, they can be treated by *en bloc* (marginal) excision when purely intraosseous, or by amputation/ray resection where needed. In certain circumstances, the surgeon may wish to consider allograft replacement of a bone (especially a larger one) and associated osteoarticular reconstruction or (better) fusion. Because this is not a highly aggressive malignancy, the role of radiation and chemotherapy is extremely limited. In all circumstances, the prognosis is typically excellent with adequate surgical treatment.

Bone Tumors

Solitary (Unicameral) Bone Cysts

Solitary bone cysts are benign lytic lesions, which are rare in the hand. They are more common in the humerus or distal radius when they do present in the upper extremity. On radiograph, they appear most often in eccentric metaphyseal sites which are radiolucent (not speckled as with chondral tumors). These cysts may often first present following pathological fracture through the previously weakened bone. Solitary bone cysts have no known potential for malignant deterioration.

These tumors sometimes present the greatest problem because of their juxtaphyseal location, but may be treated semisurgically by the injection of steroids. Injection treatment requires radiographic control, a (#15) Craig needle with stylette and an 18-gauge hypodermic needle, each attached to 5 cc syringes. Both needles are introduced into the cyst, and the fluid aspirated and sent for laboratory analysis. After aspiration, about 40 mg to 80 mg of methylprednisolone (or similar steroid) is injected through the Craig needle. Some large cysts in the long bones have been injected with up to 200 mg of steroids. Fluid extravasation is not unexpected; therefore, a compression dressing is applied. Follow-up radiographs are needed about every six weeks. Healing should occur after eight to 12 weeks, or the technique may be repeated up to two or three times, as indicated. If injection treatment fails and if the tumor is repeatedly recurrent, or otherwise unsuitable, surgery must include thorough and meticulous curettage to remove the entire cyst wall (lining). Bone grafting can be appropriate and helpful to speed osseous reconstitution following curettage. Radiation therapy is contraindicated. As some of these lesions heal spontaneously without treatment, the smaller ones may be observed, understanding the risk issues of pathologic fracture.

Osteoid Osteoma

The osteoid osteoma is a benign bone-forming neoplasm which most often presents as a painful but obscure problem in the young individual. The area in question may appear radiographically benign, or may show only cortical enlargement/thickening. This tumor is found most commonly in the first and second decades. Osteoid osteomas have been reported both in the diaphyses and metaphyses of the tubular bones of the hands as well as the flat carpal bones and the large bones of the axial skeleton. Although the "textbook history" includes nocturnal pain and pain relief from aspirin, this is actually a rather variable phenomenon. When located by X-ray, the tumor has the appearance of an eccentric area of cortical sclerosis which surrounds a small radiolucent zone in which is contained a dense bony nidus. The lesion rarely exceeds a diameter of 1 cm and more often is so small in the hand bones as to be easily *missed* on routine radiographs. It often may require a combination of suspicion plus tomography, bone scan and/or CT scan for proper diagnostic visualization.

The most difficult part of treating an osteoid osteoma is the diagnosis. Cure without recurrence is typical after local excision of the nidus via cortical window. However, it is critical that the entire nidus is removed, otherwise symptoms will not improve or may rapidly recur. Radiographic and/or histologic confirmation of complete excision of the nidus is important, although the former method may be difficult with small lesions of the phalanges that have been imaged only on computerized tomography or similar sophisticated studies.

Osteoblastoma

The osteoblastoma consists of smaller islands of mature bone in osteoid tissue. There are no true, clear histologic criteria to distinguish it from osteoid osteoma. Osteoblastomas tend to be larger but may also occur in the tubular bones of the hand. They are classically represented on radiograph as an expanding radiolucent zone with sometimes irregular areas of opacification. Treatment should be curettage, with the addition of bone grafting as required.

In rare circumstances, in which such a tumor has recurred or has been neglected and allowed to become locally destructive, cure may require more extensive bony resection and reconstruction by autogenous or allograft bone tissues. It is unusual, however, for extensively destructive lesions to be located other than in the axial skeleton.

Aneurysmal Bone Cyst

Aneurysmal bone cysts are uncommon tumors in the hand although they are not rare in larger, more proximal long bones and the spine. They arise most frequently in patients during the second and third decades as benign but rapidly expansile cystic/hemorrhagic (osteolytic) bone tumors. Unless removed completely, this neoplasm has a significant tendency to recur locally and invade its region of origin.

Once diagnosed by appropriate tumor work-up and confirmed histologically, surgical resection is the treatment of choice. Intralesional excision, or curettage, is unlikely to result in cure; *en bloc* excision of involved bone is necessary to minimize the chance of recurrence. Appropriate bone reconstruction by corticocancellous or allograft methods may be necessary. Ray resection should be performed only in those circumstances in which the tumor is large or recurrent and not amenable to a less destructive removal.

Giant Cell Tumor of Bone

Although relatively infrequent in the bones of the hand, a giant cell tumor of bone is more likely to occur in young adults. Generally, patients present with swelling and pain, and often the radiographic findings include pathologic fracture. Typically this is a solitary bone lesion, but the *multifocal variant* of this neoplasm (whether metachronous or synchronous) seems to involve the bones of the hand in many cases. It is important that a bone scan be obtained as part of the routine work-up for these patients in order to assess the possibility of multicentric lesions.

On radiograph, the giant cell tumor of bone is often an expansile, somewhat eccentric, radiolucent defect of the epiphyseal region of tubular bones. It is actually uncommon for a lytic lesion to involve and invade the subchondral region of a small tubular bone, so these radiographic findings should make the physician suspect that the lesion is a giant cell tumor.

The GCT is reported to have an high tendency to recur in and about the bones of the hand and wrist—up to 95% in some series. Accordingly, while curettage of this tumor— with or without bone grafting—may be appropriate in locations other than the hand, it cannot be recommended unhesitatingly here. *En bloc* excision with replacement by autogenous bone graft, vascularized bone, or allograft (or ray resection, for appropriate digital locations) must be regarded as the definitive method of treatment. Based on available literature, it is not evident that intralesional surgical methods will produce a cure in the bones of the hand. In addition, use of the 1940s (Jaffe) "histologic grading criteria" is no longer justified because there is no relationship between clinical behavior and the historical microscopic findings. Distant metastases from single and multiply operated lesions are uncommon but certainly have been reported (most often from origins in larger bones, however).

Osteogenic Sarcoma

Osteogenic sarcoma is a potentially lethal malignancy but an unusual tumor in the hand. When present, it tends to be found in the first and second decades of life, with locations in the proximal phalanges and metacarpals. The tumor usually presents as an increasingly painful and progressively swollen site whose course is ominously rapid. Plain radiographs often reveal a sclerotic and expanding, destructive bone tumor. After a full work-up, the surgical biopsy will have a differential which must still include osteoblastoma, a distinction that may sometimes be difficult. Treatment requires aggressive surgery in the context of appropriate adjuvant therapies. Adjuvant chemotherapy, including use of preoperative systemic or regional medications, should be strongly encouraged, potentially improving ultimate survival and allowing a definitive yet limb-sparing procedure. The value of radiation therapy has not been consistently defined in the literature.

Ewing's Sarcoma

Ewing's sarcoma is very rare in the hand skeleton. This round cell tumor is more common in young patients, usually those in their first decade, and has been reported in the phalanges and metacarpals, most often with a soft-tissue component. While any neoplastic process may present as an inflammatory problem, this neoplasm is often characterized by associated erythema, swelling, and discomfort in the presence of a systemic response which includes fever and an elevated erythrocyte sedimentation rate. Radiographs usually show an osteolytic destructive lesion with soft-tissue swelling.

After appropriate tumor work-up, incisional biopsy may be performed in preparation for wide *en bloc* resection or amputation. Ewing's sarcoma is radiosensitive; adjuvant chemotherapy is also widely recommended. Surgery is actually a more practical treatment method, where therapeutic radiation includes tissues that may be sensitive to fibrosis, such as nerve plexuses, and especially in children. Survival following presentation with a lesion in the hand may be better, possibly due to earlier recognition when the tumor is still small and more likely to be limited.

Metastatic Tumors

Skeletal metastases are not frequently found below the elbow but may arise in patients with primary malignancies of breast, colon, kidney, and lung. These may be the most common malignant bone tumors in the hand. The distal phalanx is the most frequent location when hand bones are involved; the carpals are unusual sites.

The clinical course may suggest an infection, especially if the primary tumor is still unknown; symptoms will often include erythema, induration and discomfort. Radiographs often show a destructive bony process. Diagnosis is confirmed by biopsy which may be done via needle aspiration if a primary lesion has already been diagnosed. Standard infection and tumor protocols should prevail where distant primary sites are unknown.

Treatment choices depend on the status of the primary tumor and health of the patient. Commonly, local palliative *en bloc* excision, amputation, or radiotherapy will be recommended. Radiation to prevent impending pathologic fractures is not generally appropriate for the hand; in patients without a high chance for survival, and in whom there is a special need to preserve body parts, curettage and filling with methylmethacrylate may be considered. In any event, metastatic bone tumors of the hand carry a poor prognosis in that the majority of patients will *not* have a significant chance of one-year survival.

Summary

While generalizations and specific tumor information are important, it is critical to remember that each patient and each tumor is somewhat different. The problem must be handled in a way likely to produce a cure and yet salvage maximum function where that secondary goal is also possible. The surgeon who biopsies a tumor should be prepared to treat. Hand surgeons need to be part of a team including knowledgeable radiologists, pathologists, and oncologists to jointly envision a plan for diagnosis, resection, reconstruction, and adjuvant therapy to assure the best possible outcome.

Annotated Bibliography

Amadio PC, Lombardi RM: Metastatic tumors of the hand. *J Hand Surg,* 12A:311, 1987.

Data from 18 patients with 22 metastatic hand lesions are reviewed. Guidelines are provided for the evaluation and management of such lesions.

Ambrosia JM, Wold LE, Amadio PC: Osteoid osteoma of the hand and wrist. *J Hand Surg,* 12A,5:794-800, 1987.

A retrospective study of 19 patients with osteoid osteoma of the hand or wrist. Diagnosis of this condition is frequently delayed due to lack of clinical findings. The signs, symptoms, distribution, and results of treatment are reviewed.

Averill RM, Smith RJ, Campbell CJ: Giant cell tumor of the bones of the hand. *J Hand Surg,* 5:39-50, 1980.

Giant cell tumors are uncommon to the hand. When treated with curettage alone or with bone grafting the recurrence rate is over 90%. Resection or amputation is recommended.

Bacci G, Dallar D, DiScioscio M, Caldora P, Picci P, Ferrari S, Malaguti C, Avella M, Prasad R: Importance of dose intensity in neoadjuvant chemotherapy or osteosarcoma. *J Chemotherapy,* 2:127-135, 1990.

A retrospective study was done involving 125 patients with osteosarcoma of an extremity analyzing the relationship between dose-intensity (amount of drug given per unit time) and outcome. Dose-intensity was found to be determinant of treatment outcome; therefore, every effort should be made to avoid reduction of doses and delays of cycles of chemotherapy.

Bauer RD, Lewis MM, Posner MA: Treatment of enchondromas of the hand with allograft bone. *J Hand Surg,* 13A,6:908-916, 1988.

After comparing 12 patients with 19 endochondromas of the hand treated with corticocancellous allograft to 16 patients with similar background treated with autogenous iliac crest bone graft, it was concluded that allograft corticocancellous bone graft is effective in treating this tumor.

Bickerstaff DR, Harris SC, Kay NR: Osteosarcoma of the carpus. *J Hand Surg,* 133:303-305, 1988.

A case report and literature review of a case of osteosarcoma of the carpus. Osteosarcoma should be considered in the differential diagnosis of a painful wrist.

Campanacci M, Capanna R, Picci PL: Unicameral and aneurysmal bone cysts. *Clin Orthop,* 204:25, 1986.

The authors provide a retrospective review of 319 unicameral bone cysts, of which 178 were treated with curettage and bone grafting and 141 were treated with cortisone injection, along with a review of the surgical treatment of choice of aneurysmal bone cysts. The authors analyze the outcome of treatment in relation to radiographic features and type of therapy.

Creighton JJ, Peimer CA, Mindell ER, Boone DC, Karakonis CP, Douglass HO: Primary malignant tumors of the upper extremity: retrospective analysis of one hundred twenty-six cases. *J Hand Surg,* 10A:805-813, 1985.

Primary malignancies of the upper extremity are rare. This is a retrospective study of 126 patients with upper extremity malignant tumors to evaluate the Musculoskeletal Tumor Society staging system. The system was found still to be valid and its use is recommended.

Diao ED, Moy OJ: Common tumors. *Clin Orthop,* 23:187-196, 1992.

Any tumor that appears anywhere in the body can appear in the hand or wrist, although the most common tumors of the hand are benign conditions. This paper reviews common bone tumors.

Dick HM, Angelides AC: Malignant bone tumors of the hand. *Hand Clin,* 5:373-381, 1989.

Although rare, primary malignant tumors can occur in the hand. The authors propose the use of the Musculoskeletal Tumor Society Grading System to standardize reports, thus leading to more meaningful statistics, diagnosis and treatments.

Doyle LK, Ruby LK, Nalebuff EA, Belsky MR: Osteoid osteoma of the hand. *J Hand Surg,* 10A:408-410, 1985.

Seven cases of osteoid osteoma of the wrist and hand are described. Delay from presenting symptoms to definitive diagnosis and treatment averaged 13.5 months with a range of seven to 30 months. Although unusual, osteoid osteoma should be considered as a cause of pain in the wrist and hand.

Finci R, Gultekin N, Gunhan O, Demiriz M, Somuncu I: Primary osteosarcoma of a phalanx. *J Hand Surg,* 16B:204-207, 1991.

A case report is discussed describing a rare case of osteosarcoma arising from a phalanx of the hand without any known predisposing factor.

Fleegler EJ, Marks KE, Sebek BA, Groppe CW, Belhobek G: Osteosarcoma of the hand. *Hand,* 12:316-322, 1980.

Osteogenic sarcoma, a rare malignant tumor in the hand, is reviewed in two case reports and the literature on this tumor is discussed.

Frassica FJ, Amadio PC, Wold LE, Beabout JW: Aneurysmal bone cyst: Clinicopathologic features and treatment of 10 cases involving the hand. *J Hand Surg,* 13A,5:676-683, 1988.

A study of 10 aneurysmal bone cysts in the hand which examines treatment and outcome. It was concluded that aneurysmal bone cysts of the small bones of the hand require either thorough exteriorization, curettage, and bone grafting or excision and bone grafting for effective treatment.

Frassica FJ, Amadio PC, Wold LE, Dobyns JH, Linscheid RL: Primary malignant bone tumors of the hand. *J Hand Surg,* 14A:1022, 1989.

Primary malignant lesions located in the small bones of the hand are rare but still must be considered in the differential diagnosis of tumors, as surgical control of these lesions requires careful preoperative planning and wide-spread surgical margins.

Healy JH, Turnbull ADM, Miedema B, Lane JM: Acrometastases: a study of twenty-nine patients with osseous involvement of the hands and feet. *J Bone Joint Surg,* 68A:743, 1986.

A retrospective study of 29 patients with 41 metastatic lesions of the hand or foot is reviewed to describe the experience with the diagnosis and treatment of the acrometastases. Two case histories are presented.

Johnston AD: Aneurysmal bone cysts of the hand. *Hand Clin,* 3:299-310, 1987.

A review of aneurysmal bone cysts and the wide range of precursors, many of which raise problems in differential diagnosis.

Kuur E, Hansen SL, Lindequist S: Treatment of solitary enchondromas in fingers. *J Hand Surg,* 14B:109-112, 1989.

This paper presents the results of 21 solitary endochondromas of finger bones. The symptoms prior to diagnosis, radiographic findings and groupings, and treatments are discussed.

Link MP, Goorin AM, Horowitz M, Meyer WH, Belasco J, Baker A, Ayala A, Shuster J: Adjuvant chemotherapy of high grade osteosarcoma of the extremity: updated results of the multi-institutional osteosarcoma study. *Clin Ortho Rel Res,* 270:8-15, 1991.

An update of the results of the Multi-Institutional Osteosarcoma Study, this recommends that the administration of immediate adjuvant chemotherapy has significant favorable impact on event-free survival for patients with nonmetastatic, high-grade osteosarcoma of the extremity.

Peimer CA, Moy OJ, Dick HM: Tumors of bone and soft tissue. In Green DP (Ed) *Operative Hand Surgery,* Third ed., Churchill Livingstone, 1993, in press.

Peimer CA, Schiller AL, Mankin HJ, Smith RJ: Multicentric giant-cell tumor of bone. *J Bone Joint Surg,* 62A:652, 1980.

Five patients with primary multicentric giant cell tumors of bone (18 lesions) were followed for four to 14 1/2 years. Eleven of the 18 lesions were in small bones of the hand. The methods and infection rate are discussed. There was no metastases.

Tordai P, Hoglund M, Lugnegard H: Is the treatment of enchondroma in the hand by simple curettage a rewarding method? *J Hand Surg,* 15B:331-334, 1990.

Forty-six hand enchondromas were reviewed, all treated by simple curettage without bone. Eighty-two percent healed, 16% were left with small bone defects, and one patient required reoperation due to recurrence.

Trias A, Basora J, Sanchez G, Madarnas P: Chondro-sarcoma of the hand. *Clin Orthop,* 134:297-300, 1978.

A case report of a hand chondrosarcoma; this case has the longest following of any hand chondrosarcoma reported. Due to the rare occurrence of these tumors, it is important to report such cases and document their characteristics, behavior, and prognosis.

35

Aggressive Tumors of the Hand and Forearm

Richard R. McCormack, Jr., MD

Introduction

In the last 10 years, the treatment of aggressive tumors of the musculoskeletal system has benefited from the advent of improved techniques of histologic identification, improved preoperative imaging to evaluate extent of disease and assist surgical planning, the use of limb-sparing surgery and microvascular free-tissue transfer to avoid amputation when possible, and the use of adjuvant chemotherapy and radiation therapy to control micrometastases and allow closer surgical margins. Although the term "aggressive" most often refers to malignant lesions of the hand and forearm, there are some benign but locally aggressive tumors such as giant cell tumor of bone, desmoplastic fibroma, or aneurysmal bone cyst that may also be considered in this category.

The treatment of such lesions begins with a classification system adopted by the Musculoskeletal Tumor Society to stage tumors of bone and soft-tissue origin excluding skin and hematopoetic malignancies. From such a grading system, decisions about prognosis and proper treatment can be made. In addition, because the stage of the tumor has so much to do with prognosis, results of different treatment protocols for a given stage of tumor can be compared from one institution to another, assuming that the application of the staging system is uniform.

Grading of Musculoskeletal Tumors

Tumors of musculoskeletal origin are divided into three grades: benign, low grade malignant (G1), and high grade, fully malignant (G2). Determination of grade is based on the histologic appearance of the tissue obtained at the time of biopsy. Because of the anaplastic nature of these sarcomas, precise identification by morphologic criteria alone can be difficult. In some cases, even the distinction between sarcoma and carcinoma can be equivocal. The use of special immunochemical staining techniques (vimentin, desmin, muscle specific antigen, keratin, S-100 protein, and immunoperoxidase) to confirm the presence or absence of characteristic intracellular identifying components is most helpful in this regard. The histologic grading is critical in the staging of the tumor. An outline of the most common malignant sarcomas, divided into low- and high-grade forms, is shown in Table 35-1.

Surgical Site

The location of the tumor can be described as A—intracompartmental, or B—extracompartmental, based on pre-

Table 35-1. Surgical Grade (G)

Low (G1)	High (G2)
Parosteal osteosarcoma	Classic osteosarcoma
Endosteal osteosarcoma	Radiation sarcoma
	Paget's sarcoma
Secondary chondrosarcoma	Primary chondrosarcoma
Fibrosarcoma,	Fibrosarcoma
Kaposi's sarcoma	Malignant fibrous
Atypical malignant	histiocytoma
fibrous histiocytoma	Undifferentiated primary
	sarcoma
Giant cell tumor, bone	Giant cell sarcoma, bone
Hemangioendothelioma	Angiosarcoma
Hemangiopericytoma	Hemangiopericytoma
Parosteal osteosarcoma	Classic osteosarcoma
Myxoid liposarcoma	Pleomorphic liposarcoma
	Neurofibrosarcoma
Clear-cell sarcoma	Rhabdomyosarcoma
tendon sheath	Synovial sarcoma
Epithelioid sarcoma	
Chordoma	
Adamantinoma	
Alveolar cell sarcoma	Alveolar cell sarcoma
Other and undifferentiated	Other and undifferentiated

Reproduced with permission from Enneking W, Spanier S, Goodman M. *Clin Orthop Rel Res,* 153: 106-120, 1980.

operative studies to evaluate the extent of disease. These studies include the physical examination, routine plane radiographs, bone scan, CT scan, MRI, and regional angiography. From these studies, a determination is made as to whether or not the tumor is still confined to the compartment in which it arose. A classification of surgical sites as compartments is given in Table 35-2. Tumors confined to the tissue in which they arose (bone, joint, muscle, or fascial envelope) are considered to be intracompartmental. Note that for purposes of this system a ray of the hand, and volar (flexor) and dorsal (extensor) compartments of the forearm are considered to be separate compartments. Those tumors that have extended to the mid-hand or antecubital fossa are deemed to be extracompartmental. Any involvement of regional lymph nodes or distant metastases indicates spread of the tumor from its original compartment with systemic involvement implying a dismal prognosis.

Based on these studies, tumors arising in bone are determined to be still within the bone (intracompartmental) or to have outgrown the confines of the bone into the surrounding muscles and soft tissues (extracompartmental). Likewise, tumors arising in muscles are said to be extracompartmental when they have outgrown their fascial envelope. Proximity to adjacent important nerves, blood vessels, and tendons can be determined from preoperative imaging studies. This

Table 35-2.   Surgical Sites (T)

Intracompartmental (TI)	Extracompartmental (T2)
Intraosseous	Soft-tissue extension
Intra-articular	Soft-tissue extension
Superficial to deep fascia	Deep fascial extension
Paraosseous	Intraosseous or extrafascial
Intrafascial compartments	Extrafascial planes or spaces
Ray of hand or foot	Mid and hind foot
Posterior calf	Popliteal space
Anterolateral leg	Groin-femoral triangle
Anterior thigh	Intrapelvi
Medial thigh	Mid-hand
Posterior thigh	Antecubital fossa
Buttocks	Axilla
Volar forearm	Periclavicular
Dorsal forearm	Paraspinal
Anterior arm	Head and neck
Posterior arm	
Periscapular	

Reproduced with permission from Enneking W, Spanier S, Goodman M. *Clin Orthop Rel Res,* 153: 106-120, 1980.

Table 35-3.   Surgical Stages

Stage	Grade	Site
IA	Low (G1)	Intracompartmental (TI)
IB	Low (G1)	Extracompartmental (T2)
IIA	High (G2)	Intracompartmental (TI)
IIB	High (G2)	Extracompartmental (T2)
III	Any (G) Regional or distant metastases	Any (T)

Reproduced with permission from Enneking W, Spanier S, Goodman M. *Clin Orthop Rel Res,* 153: 106-120, 1980.

Table 35-4.   Surgical Margins

Type	Plane of Dissection	Result
Intralesional	Piecemeal debulking or curettage	Leaves macroscopic disease
Marginal	Shell out *en bloc* through pseudocapsule or reactive zone	May leave either "satellite"or "skip" lesions
Wide	Intracompartmental *en bloc* with cuff of normal tissue	May leave "skip" lesions
Radical	Extracompartmental *en bloc* entire compartment	No residual

Reproduced with permission from Enneking W, Spanier S, Goodman M. *Clin Orthop Rel Res,* 153: 106-120, 1980.

Table 35-5.   Surgical Procedures

Margin	Local	Amputation
Intralesional	Curettage or debulking	Debulking amputation
Marginal	Marginal excision	Marginal amputation
Wide	Wide local excision	Wide through bone amputation
Radical	Radical local excision	Radical disarticulation

Reproduced with permission from Enneking W, Spanier S, Goodman M. *Clin Orthop Rel Res,* 153: 106-120, 1980.

information is of utmost importance in planning the surgical approach and margins of resection.

The hand and forearm represent a special case in this regard. The ray of a hand is considered a separate compartment for a tumor growing in a finger. However, a tumor arising in the mid-palm is considered already to be extracompartmental because of the possibility of proximal and distal extension afforded by flexor tendon sheaths. Thus, a fully malignant tumor arising in the mid-palm (extracompartmental) may require a mid-forearm amputation for control of local disease.

Staging

Based on histologic grade, location (whether intra- or extracompartmental) and the presence or absence of metastasis, each tumor can be staged as outlined in Table 35-3. Based on such a staging system, appropriate surgical and adjuvant treatment can be prescribed for these sarcomas. Surgical margins of resection and their consequences with regard to residual tumor are defined in Table 35-4.

Types of Surgical Procedures

Surgical procedures for the treatment of musculoskeletal sarcomas are divided into four types based on surgical margin as outlined in Table 35-5. Intralesional procedures, such as curettage and marginal excision, leave portions of the tumor behind. Wide excision and radical excision are the best procedures for complete control of local tumor. In some cases, the efficacy of wide excision can be enhanced with adjuvant chemotherapy or radiation therapy depending on the tumor type. Lesions unresponsive to adjuvant treatment are better dealt with by radical surgical excision.

The primary goal of the surgeon is to eradicate the tumor and the secondary goal is to preserve as much function as possible without jeopardizing the cure rate. Such radical surgery can be conceptually difficult for the hand surgeon who is trained to preserve function wherever possible. There are many cases in which amputation is the treatment of choice and no reconstructive possibilities exist.

Although we will be considering the surgical and adjuvant treatment of Stage IIA or Stage IIB lesions and to a lesser degree Stage III tumors, it should be remembered that some Stage I lesions, such as giant cell tumor of bone, may behave aggressively and warrant treatment normally reserved for Stage II lesions to achieve adequate control.

Preoperative Evaluation

As discussed above, the determination of staging is based not only on histologic grade, but also on the location of the tumor with respect to musculoskeletal compartments. Often, many of the staging procedures are carried out prior to the actual biopsy when a tumor is suspected. In many cases, this sequence is preferred as the trauma and reaction to the biopsy can artificially extend a Stage IIA lesion to Stage IIB on imaging studies. This is particularly true with MRI, which is becoming the preferred technique for evaluation of tumor extent. Plane radiographs and CT scans are excellent for bony lesions but do not show marrow extension (skip lesions) and soft-tissue involvement as well as MRI.

Angiography remains the diagnostic study of choice to evaluate for involvement of major vascular structures as well as origin of abnormal tumor vessels. This information is most helpful in planning limb-sparing procedures. Recently described techniques using MRI angiography (MRA) have revealed remarkably good vascular detail without the invasive intervention of arteriography. Bone scan is helpful in determining bone involvement in soft-tissue tumors without apparent bone changes on routine plane films. This may be the only sign of extracompartmental involvement for a soft-tissue lesion, and resection of bone would also be required as part of a wide or radical excision.

Routine chest radiograph and CT scans are helpful in evaluation for pulmonary metastases. MRI is probably more helpful for determination of regional lymph-node involvement.

Biopsy

The biopsy of a potentially malignant tumor in the hand, as elsewhere, is of critical importance in the planning and execution of limb-sparing definitive surgery. A poorly placed biopsy incision (eg transverse) can convert a potentially limb-sparing procedure into an amputation. If the nature of the tumor is unknown, then it is safest to assume that it is malignant, rather than benign, and the incisions can be planned accordingly. The biopsy should be placed within an incision, which can be used for the definitive tumor resection. The biopsy incision is then ellipsed at the time of the resection, leaving the biopsy scar with the tumor as part of the *en bloc* resection. In almost all cases this will result in a longitudinal incision, often less cosmetically acceptable than a transverse scar. However, one would rather have the cosmetically objectionable scar and a benign tumor than use a transverse, cosmetic incision and jeopardize a limb-sparing procedure if the tumor is malignant. Because it is the skin coverage that may be a limiting factor, the use of free-tissue transfer in the form of fasciocutaneous, myocutaneous and composite flaps can be used to salvage difficult situations.

Resection of Aggressive Lesions

Although the concept of removal of the entire compartment or compartments involved by tumor is a sound one, it is often impractical. Surgical treatment depends on the type of malignant tumor and the stage. In fact, most lesions are treated by wide *en bloc* resection with at least a 2-cm margin of surrounding normal tissue, the extent of involvement having been determined by the preoperative work-up. For

those tumors arising in long bones, 4 cm of bony margin is recommended to avoid missing skip lesions. The MRI is helpful in picking up these skip lesions preoperatively. In the hand, a tumor arising in a metacarpal, for instance, requires resection of at least that metacarpal and usually the entire ray.

Recent advances in the techniques of radiation therapy to the extremities have made it possible to deliver adequate ionizing radiation doses to the involved area without circumferential coverage. Treatment portals are customized with shrinking exposure fields allowing different doses to be given to the tumor bed (60-65 Gy) and the surrounding area at risk for micrometastases (50-56 Gy). Custom limb immobilization devices are mandatory for consistent reproduction of dose fields with fractionated treatment schedules. With such techniques, the combination of conservative surgery and moderate dose radiation therapy have been reported to rival radical surgery or amputation for control of local disease, with preservation of limb function. For those cases in which circumferential limb doses are deemed necessary based on preoperative evaluation, amputation is the treatment of choice because of the severe disability rendered by circumferential radiation. In reported series, many of the circumferentially irradiated limbs required amputation for dysfunctional extremities.

The primary goal is to completely control all tumor. The secondary goal is to preserve function. Although the hand surgeon is trained to preserve function, this goal should never interfere with the primary goal of complete tumor excision. If the neurovascular structures to an extremity can be preserved, bone, skin, and even active muscle can be transferred by microvascular technique to reconstruct the defect. Tendon transfers may be performed primarily or staged after free-tissue transfer for adequate coverage. These techniques are reviewed in Chapters 15 and 32.

The use of distant pedicle flaps for coverage in the treatment of malignant disease is contraindicated because of the risk of disseminating tumor to the donor site. Local flaps, skin grafts and free-tissue transfer have a definite role in the coverage and reconstruction of defects created at the time of tumor surgery.

For most lesions arising distally in the upper extremity, the treatment of choice will be amputation. For tumors arising in the distal phalanx, amputation through the middle phalanx with local flap coverage is usually adequate. Tumors arising more proximally in the middle or proximal phalanx are probably best treated with ray amputation, both from the basis of tumor control as well as functional and cosmetic result.

Tumors arising in the metacarpals are also best treated with ray resection, assuming that the lesion is confined to the bone (Stage IIA). This is particularly true of the border digits, index and little finger. The alternative option involves complete excision of the metacarpal with autograft or allograft reconstruction. Arthrodesis proximally and ligament reconstruction with or without implant arthroplasty at the MP joint can be used, but may not give as good functional results as ray amputation. For lesions extending beyond the bone (Stage IIB) or soft-tissue sarcomas arising in the intermetacarpal areas, resection of multiple rays may be required.

For tumors arising in the thumb metacarpal, the surgical options include ray amputation with secondary reconstruction using pollicized index, or excision of the thumb metacarpal and reconstruction with bone graft for Stage IIA lesions. Every effort should be made to preserve the thumb without sacrificing the principles of tumor surgery. Even for those tumors in which all four metacarpals must be resected, there is a functional and aesthetic benefit to preserving the thumb.

Aggressive soft-tissue tumors of the palm often require amputation rather than local or wide excision. The ability to adequately resect the tumor with a cuff of normal tissue and preserve function is related mostly to the size of the tumor. Because of the close proximity of structures from all the fingers in the palm, it is often difficult to spare function and amputation is required. Failure to appreciate this fact and attempts at local excision of large tumors lead to a high local recurrence rate and probable distant metastases.

For malignant tumors arising in the volar aspect of the wrist, *en bloc* limb-sparing tumor resection is often impractical because of the proximity of the median nerve, ulnar nerve, and radial and ulnar arteries. Flexor tendons may also be involved. Whether the malignant tumor arises in bone or soft tissue, in this area mid-forearm amputation is often required. Tumors of the dorsum of the hand and wrist can often be resected by wide local excision without resorting to amputation. With preservation of the flexors and the volar neurovascular structures, reconstruction of dorsal tendons by transfers or grafts can be performed as a primary or secondary procedures. Local axial patterned flaps or free flaps may be required for skin coverage and provide a superior bed for tendon reconstruction when compared to skin grafts.

As with all cases, the ability to resect the tumor with adequate normal tissue margins depends on the size and location of the tumor with respect to important neurovascular structures. Preoperative evaluation is critical in making these decisions. Assuming that these structures can be preserved with adequate tumor resection, limb-sparing reconstruction following resection of portions of the radius and ulna can be carried out with allograft or vascularized fibular autograft depending on the size of the defect (Fig. 35-1). Tendon transfer or tendon grafts can be used to restore function once skeletal stability has been achieved. Tumors confined to the distal half of the ulna alone can be resected without the need for skeletal reconstruction.

Contraindications to Limb Salvage Procedures

Recently, the trend in tumor surgery has been toward limb-sparing or limb-salvage procedures made possible by better preoperative staging and microsurgical reconstructive techniques; however, there are some cases in which limb salvage procedures should not be attempted. When an adequate tumor resection fails to achieve a functional result that is superior to amputation with an appropriate prosthesis, amputation should be performed. When pathologic fracture has occurred and has disseminated tumor cells throughout the fracture hematoma, amputation is the treatment of choice and should include the entire anatomic compartment of what is a Stage IIB lesion (radical resection). Certainly for cases in the lower extremity, skeletal immaturity with resultant limb length inequality from resection of a growth center is a contraindication. In the upper extremity, where limb length inequality is better tolerated and preservation of hand function is more important than limb length, skeletal immaturity is a relative contraindication.

Examples of Aggressive Tumors

Although the frequency, histology, and behavior of these aggressive tumors of the hand and forearm are all different, certain trends regarding their treatment can be realized which are based on the principles of treatment outlined above. At the outset, it must be realized that malignant tumors of the hand and forearm are rare. Most of what is known about the biology of malignant skeletal and soft-tissue tumors is derived from experience in treating the same tumors in other skeletal sites. Because the tumor may be detected at an earlier time and at a smaller size in the hand and forearm, the prognosis may be slightly better in those locations.

As alluded to earlier, some lesions that are considered benign or low-grade malignancies, such as giant cell tumor of bone or desmoplastic fibroma, behave in such an aggressive fashion locally in the hand and forearm, and have such a high local recurrence rate, that a more aggressive surgical approach is warranted for initial treatment.

Bone Tumors

Giant Cell Tumor of Bone

This benign but locally aggressive bone tumor has a propensity to arise in the distal portion of the radius, metacarpals, and phalanges. As in other bones, it is characterized by its lytic, expansile appearance in the epiphyseal-metaphyseal portion of long bones. It is common for the lesion to extend to the subchondral plate and involve the distal articular surface of the radius. The articular cartilage, however, appears to represent a barrier to extension into the joint in cases in which there has been no fracture or prior surgery. The paucity of periosteal reaction belies the rapid growth of this tumor. There is a spectrum of histology for giant cell tumor of bone with 2% to 16% of cases in reported series being fully malignant. There are also sporadic case reports of histologically "benign" pulmonary metastases with giant cell tumor, which have been adequately treated by pulmonary resection without chemotherapy.

Results following curettage with or without bone grafting (intralesional resection) reveal recurrence rates on the order of 60% to 85%. Curettage and cryosurgery with liquid nitrogen or application of phenol decrease the recurrence rate to 11% to 36% in published series. The complications related to cryosurgery such as skin necrosis, nerve dysfunction, and fracture of remaining bone have dimin-

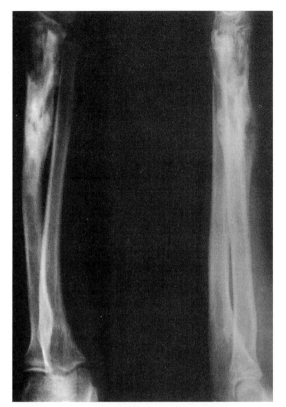

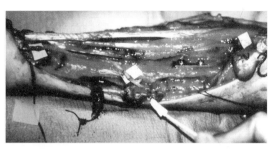

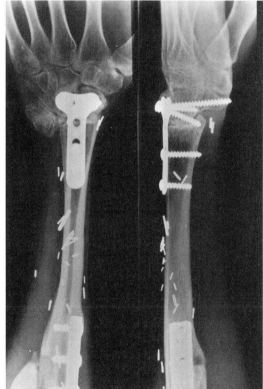

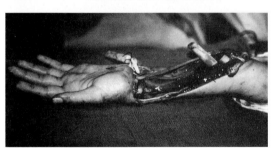

Figure 35-1.   (Top Left) Radiographs of a Stage IIB osteosarcoma of the distal radial metaphysis in a 16-year-old male. The lesion extends along the interosseous membrane toward the ulna. **(Top Right)** After reconstruction with vascularized fibular autograft. The radial artery was reconstituted by anastomosis with the peroneal artery of the flap in both the proximal and distal aspects of the wound. Arthrodesis of the carpus to the fibula was performed. **(Bottom Left)** Appearance of the hand and forearm after *en bloc* resection of three-fourths of the distal radius and one-half of the distal ulna. Median and ulnar nerves as well as finger flexor and extensor tendons were preserved; the radial artery, flexor carpi radialis, palmaris longus, and pronator quadratus were sacrificed with the tumor. **(Bottom Right)** Radiographic appearance three months postoperatively.

ished enthusiasm for this technique despite good local tumor control. The use of a small Cryospray unit has made the application of liquid nitrogen more controlled and precise than the previous reported pour method (Fig. 35-2).

Based on several authors' experience with this tumor, the treatment of choice is *en bloc* excision of the involved distal radius and reconstruction with osteoarticular allograft or free vascularized fibular autograft. Attempts to preserve wrist motion have not met with great success and wrist arthrodesis is preferred by many authors. Because of the

benign nature of most of these tumors, chemotherapy and radiation treatment are not indicated. In fact, malignant transformation has been noted in benign giant cell tumor exposed to radiation therapy.

Osteosarcoma

Osteosarcoma in the hand is rare, with less than one percent hand and forearm involvement in large reported series.

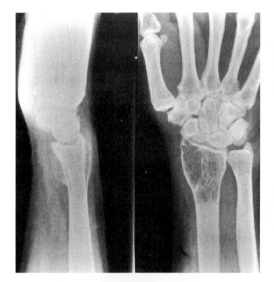
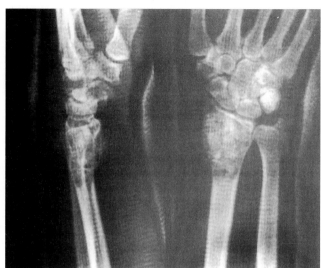
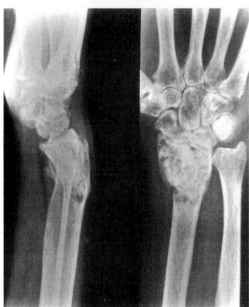

Figure 35-2. **(Top Left)** AP and lateral radiographs of a Stage IA giant cell tumor of the distal radius in a 48-year-old nurse, treated with curettage and cryosurgery with liquid nitrogen using a Cryospray unit. Three freeze-thaw cycles were performed prior to autogenous bone grafting. **(Top Right)** Appearance at nine weeks indicating pathologic fracture of frozen bone. With prolonged immobilization, this fracture went on to heal and the bone graft incorporated. Although wrist motion was limited, a functional, pain-free ROM was achieved and the patient returned to work. **(Bottom)** Radiographic appearance in cast immobilization after bone graft.

Although with better imaging and preoperative staging, more limb-sparing procedures can be done (Fig. 35-1), in many cases of osteosarcoma of the hand and forearm, amputation is the best surgical treatment. The greatest advances in treatment of osteosarcoma involve the use of adjuvant chemotherapy to control the dissemination of subclinical micrometastases prior to and after definitive tumor resection. The addition of chemotherapeutic regimens for osteosarcoma has increased the five-year disease-free survival rate to as high as 70% from what was previously about 20% with surgery alone. The advantages of chemotherapy include not only cytotoxic effects against micrometastases, but also shrinkage of local tumor, perineoplastic vascularity and edema, making wide local excision possible in cases where previously amputation would have been necessary. Frank tumor necrosis has been reported to a varying degree in those specimens resected after preoperative chemotherapy. The most successful regimens include high-dose methotrexate with citrovorum rescue factor, cis-platinum, and adriamycin. When given preoperatively, the efficacy of the chemotherapeutic regimen can be evaluated and postoperative chemotherapy continued with the same agent if effective, or changed to another agent if a poor response is noted. It is also probably true that because of the lack of muscle bellies in the hand and forearm, osteosarcomas arising in this area get noticed earlier and at a smaller tumor size than those in the lower extremity. Aggressive surveillance and excision of pulmonary metastases may also play a role in improved long-term survival in osteosarcoma.

Ewing's Sarcoma

Ewing's sarcoma is a fully malignant round cell tumor of childhood which, when it appears in the hand, represents less than one percent of reported cases for this rare tumor. The inflammatory nature of this tumor leads to frequent confusion with infection, certainly a more common finding for this age group and location. Preoperative staging and biopsy are performed as for other sarcomas. Ewing's sarcoma is quite radiosensitive and the mainstay of treatment has been radiotherapy and chemotherapy. Reports of functional evaluation of patients surviving more than two years revealed that, in this skeletally immature population, radiation was better suited to lesions of the upper extremity, and amputation for sarcomas of the lower extremity, depending on location. Because of recent reports of late local recurrence, many after five years, and radiation-induced osteosarcoma, many surgeons are also adding wide local excision to their treatment protocols. Principles of surgical ablation are no different than those for osteosarcoma.

Chondrosarcoma

Chondrosarcoma arising in the hand or distal forearm is uncommon. Compared to other primary malignant tumors or other locations for chondrosarcoma, in each case the frequency is less than one percent. The incidence is somewhat higher in syndromes of multiple lesions such as Ollier's disease or Maffucci's syndrome. The most common location, as for benign enchondroma, is the proximal phalanx, and there are a number of well documented cases of chondrosarcoma arising in histologically proven enchondroma (Fig. 35-3). When compared to enchondroma, the radiographic appearance is one of increased bone destruction with a soft-tissue mass beyond the confines of the original cortex. The histologic appearance is one of increased cellularity with binucleate forms.

For cases arising in the proximal phalanx, ray amputation is the treatment of choice. Most cases are low-grade malignant tumors and chemotherapy is not indicated. Radiation therapy is of no value.

Malignant Fibrous Histiocytoma

Malignant fibrous histiocytoma is a fully malignant sarcoma of mesothelial origin which can be found arising in bone or soft tissues. It usually presents as a painful mass or pathologic fracture, and in the upper extremity has a predilection for the proximal humeral shaft. Elsewhere in the upper extremity it presents as a soft-tissue mass and is clinically indistinguishable from those tumors discussed below. In most series, males predominate and the average age of onset is 36 years (17 years in females). The radiographic appearance is that of a lytic lesion in the metaphysis of a long tubular bone, often with cortical destruction and pathologic fracture.

The histologic appearance is a pleomorphic mix of fibrous and histiocytic elements with a characteristic "storiform" or woven mat pattern. Bizarre, ana-plastic forms are seen and giant cells are often present. The differential diagnosis includes osteolytic osteosarcoma, medullary fibrosarcoma, and metastatic renal cell carcinoma in bone.

Treatment is by radical resection or wide *en bloc* excision. There may be some benefit to radiation treatment and chemotherapy with a multi-drug protocol similar to that for osteosarcoma. The five-year survival was 67%.

Soft-tissue Tumors

Synoviosarcoma

Synoviosarcoma (synovial sarcoma, synovioma, tendosynovial sarcoma) is an uncommon malignant tumor of mesenchymal origin that histologically resembles the synovial lining of joints, bursae, and tendon sheaths. It appears as two histologic types: monophasic (spindle cell) with a poorer prognosis and biphasic (epithelioid and spindle components) with a better prognosis. Although these tumors arise more commonly in the lower extremity, in the upper extremity they tend to concentrate about the hand and forearm, and commonly present as a tender mass adjacent to but usually not involving a joint. Often the patient will report the presence of an asymptomatic mass for a long period of time prior to the onset of symptoms or change in size.

On plane radiography, synoviosarcoma appears as soft-tissue density with a 30% incidence of calcification. Bone involvement with cortical erosion is reported in about 20% of cases but is less likely in the upper extremity. Metastases to regional lymph nodes have been reported in 16% to 25% of cases, but pulmonary metastases are far more common. Probably the most sensitive predictor of outcome is the size of the tumor, with 74% five-year survival for patients with small tumors (5 cm or less) compared to 26% for tumors larger than 5 cm for the general group of "tendosynovial sarcomas." Those tumors arising in nonfleshy areas of the upper extremity such as in the finger, hand, wrist, and elbow have a better prognosis, presumably because of the likelihood of earlier detection at a smaller tumor size. It should be noted that the staging system adopted by the Musculoskeletal Tumor Society does not take into consideration the size of the tumor, and this has been a major criticism of this grading system. However, larger tumors are more likely to extend out of their original compartment and, in this sense, tumor size is represented in the grading system.

Although some controversy exists regarding the treatment of synoviosarcoma, on one point all studies agree: intralesional or marginal surgical treatment is ineffective, leading to a 90% local recurrence rate. For the "tendosynovial sarcoma" group, even wide, local, *en bloc,* excision may not be adequate because of satellite lesions and the propensity of the sarcoma to extend along fascial planes and tendon sheaths, producing gross or microscopic tumor. The recommended surgical intervention is radical excision or amputation which lowers the local recurrence rate to 2% (Fig. 35-4). High-dose radiation treatment of the local area and regional lymph nodes, chemotherapy, either systemic or intra-arterial with hyperthermic limb perfusion, and

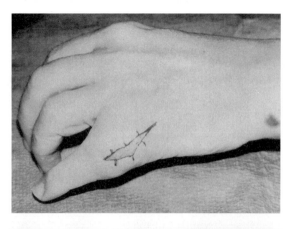

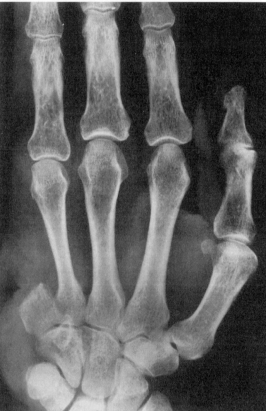

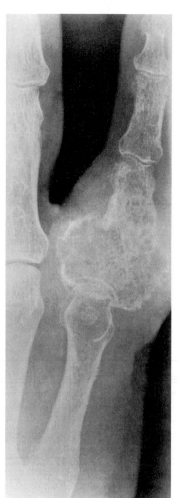

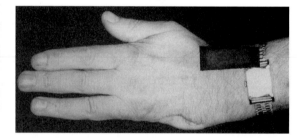

Figure 35-3. **(Top Left)** Clinical appearance at time of biopsy of a Stage IIB chondrosarcoma arising in documented, previously treated, enchondroma of the proximal phalanx. **(Top Right)** Radiographic appearance, with pathologic fracture. **(Bottom Left)** Radiographic appearance after ray amputation. **(Bottom Right)** Clinical appearance after ray amputation.

immunotherapy have all been used with modest improvement in survival. The best treatment remains initial aggressive surgical resection at an early stage of the disease (less than 5 cm tumor size).

Epithelioid Sarcoma

Epithelioid sarcoma presents as a small, painless mass in the hand or forearm, most commonly on the volar surface.

All ages can be affected by this tumor comprised of histologically anaplastic cells with epithelioid, spindle cell, or mixed morphology. The distal part of the upper extremity is more commonly involved with extension along tendon sheaths and invasion of the walls of local vessels. Metastases to regional lymph nodes are not uncommon, especially in cases of recurrence. The prognosis for survival with regional lymph node metastases or pulmonary metastases is dismal. The propensity to invade tendon

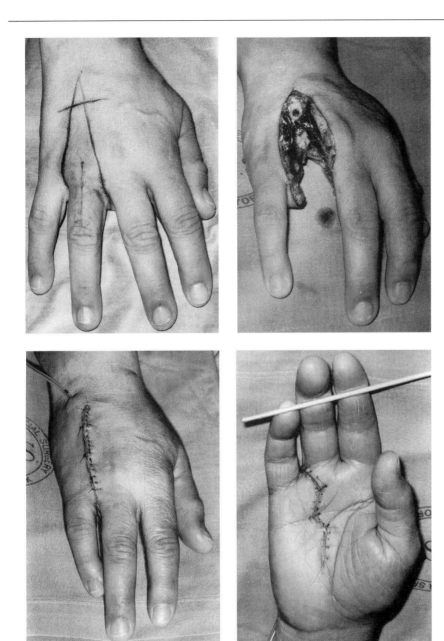

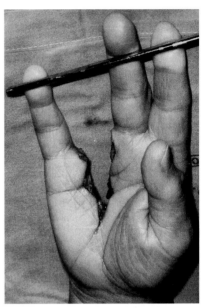

Figure 35-4.   (Top Left) Synoviosarcoma, Stage IIA, arising on the dorsum of the ring finger in a 58-year-old woman. Note longitudinal biospy incision scar. **(Top Center)** Immediate appearance after ray resection. **(Top Right)** Immediate appearance after ray resection. **(Bottom Left)** Immediate appearance after ray resection without transposition. **(Bottom Right)** Immediate appearance after ray resection without transposition.

sheaths and blood and lymph vessels makes it difficult to cure this tumor without radical surgical treatment. The initial small size of the tumor and benign presentation give a false sense of security that an adequate margin of resection has been achieved. Although T2 weighted images using MRI can be helpful in showing the local extent of disease including tendon sheath involvement, axillary node involvement may not be adequately assessed. Axillary lymph node biopsy should be performed as part of the staging procedure as well as chest CT scan. Although both radiation therapy and chemotherapy have been used as adjunctive treatment for epithelioid sarcoma, the one factor significantly affecting long-term survival is the adequacy of the surgical margin of resection. Wide or radical margins of resection yield on the order of 60% five-year survival compared to less than 10% with marginal surgery. Secondary wide or radical resection can also be effective for local recurrence without distant metastases.

Annotated Bibliography

Averill R, Smith R, Campbell C: Giant-cell tumors of the bones of the hand. *J Hand Surg,* 5A:39-50, 1980.

A retrospective study of 28 giant cell tumors in 21 patients with five cases of multicentric lesions. Thirteen of 15 treated with curettage with or without bone graft recurred, whereas three of seven treated with resection and zero of six treated with amputation or ray resection recurred. There were two cases of pulmonary metastases. Bone scan or skeletal survey is recommended to detect multicentric lesions. Resection or amputation is recommended as treatment.

Bickerstaff D, Harris S, Kay N: Osteosarcoma of the carpus. *J Bone Joint Surg,* 18B:303-305, 1988.

A case report of a low-grade osteosarcoma arising in the trapezium of a 66-year-old female presenting initially as basal joint arthritis, treated by wide excision of the thumb, index, trapezium, trapezoid and radial styloid, including median nerve.

Creighton J, Peimer C, Mindell E, *et al:* Primary malignant tumors of the upper extremity: retrospective analysis of one hundred twenty-six cases. *J Hand Surg,* 10A:808-814, 1985.

A multicenter study of 45 sarcomas of bone and 61 of soft tissue to evaluate the effectiveness of the Musculoskeletal Tumor Society staging system to predict outcome. Statistically significant differences between bony and soft-tissue tumors were noted with regard to location (above/below elbow), surgical stage, type of tumor resection and incidence of local recurrence. There was no difference with regard to metastases and survival.

Enneking W, Spanier S, Goodman M: A system for the surgical staging of musculoskeletal sarcoma. *CORR* 153:106-120, 1980.

The classical article for staging of tumors of the musculoskeletal system. A retrospective report of survival by stage of tumor for 258 cases treated at the University of Florida.

Frassica F, Amadio P, Wold L, Dobyns J, Linscheid R: Primary malignant bone tumors of the hand. *J Hand Surg,* 14A:1022-1028, 1989.

Eighteen cases of primary sarcomas of the hand are reviewed retrospectively with a 50% local recurrence rate (85% for intralesional treatment). Careful preoperative planning, wide surgical margins, and comprehensive postoperative follow up were recommended.

Hajdu S, Shiu M, Fortner J: Tendosynovial sarcoma: A clinicopathological study of 136 cases. *Cancer,* 39:1201-1217, 1977.

A retrospective study of tendosynovial sarcoma including synoviosarcoma, epithelioid sarcoma, clear cell sarcoma, and choroid sarcoma, all of which are felt by the authors to originate from a common mesenchymal precursor. The overall five-year survival rate was 40% regardless of treatment, with a 60% recurrence rate with wide local excision. Size was the best predictor of outcome with 74% five-year survival for tumors 5 cm or less. Location distally in an extremity and biphasic histologic type also had slightly better prognosis.

Huston J, Ehman R: Comparison of time-of-flight and phase-contrast MR neuroangiographic techniques. *RadioGraphics,* 13:5-19, 1993.

A discussion of MR neuroangiographic techniques demonstrating the detailed imaging that can be achieved by this noninvasive method, which is also applicable in the hand and forearm.

Lewis R, Marcove R, Rosen J: Ewing's sarcoma – functional effects of radiation therapy. *J Bone Joint Surg,* 59A:325-331, 1977.

A review of 55 patients with greater than two-year survival treated with surgical ablation or radiation, and in most cases, chemotherapy (T2 protocol). Upper extremity cases did better than lower extremity cases with radiation because skeletal growth disturbances were better tolerated. Two patients died of radiation-induced osteosarcoma.

Mankin H, Lange T, Spanier S: The hazards of biopsy in patients with malignant primary bone and soft tissue tumors. *J Bone Joint Surg,* 64A:1121-1127, 1982.

A multicenter study of biopsies of 329 cases with respect to accuracy of diagnosis, complications, and technical aspects. Guidelines for performing the biopsy are offered, including the recommendation that it be performed at the same institution where the definitive procedure is performed.

Marcove R, Weis L, Vaghaiwalla M, Pearson R: Cryosurgery in the treatment of giant cell tumors of bone. *Clin Orthop Rel Res,* 134:275-289, 1978.

A retrospective review of 52 consecutive cases (25 of which previously reported) of GCT of bone treated with cryosurgery. Technique and results of treatment including management of complications. There were six cases in the upper extremity; five in the distal radius.

Murray J: Synovial sarcoma. *Orthop Clin North Am,* 8:963-972, 1977.

A review of the literature and report of 15 cases (eight upper extremity) treated by local excision and high-dose radiation therapy, with one local recurrence in the upper extremity and three of eight dead of distant metastases at two years follow up.

Nelson D, Abdul-Karim F, Carter J, et al: Chondro-sarcoma of the small bones of the hand arising from enchondroma. *J Hand Surg,* 15A:655-659, 1990.

Two cases of chondrosarcoma arising in enchondroma are reported along with a review of 18 cases from the literature.

Okunieff P, Suit H, Proppe K: Extremity preservation by combined modality treatment of sarcomas of the hand. *Int J Radiation Oncology Biol Phys,* 12:1923-1929, 1986.

The authors report on 16 cases of soft-tissue sarcomas of the hand and wrist treated with "conservative" surgery and postoperative shrinking field technique radiation therapy. Local tumor control was achieved in 87% at one to 12-year follow up. Limb function was evaluated and found to be determined by the extent of surgical resection rather than radiation treatment. There were four cases of distant metastases.

Peimer CP, Smith R, Sirota R, Cohen B: Epithelioid sarcoma of the hand and wrist: patterns of extension. *J Hand Surg,* 2:275-282, 1977.

Six cases were evaluated for local and remote extension of tumor. Tumor was found to spread by local extension, fascial planes, tendon sheaths, lymphatic channels, and by the hematogenous route with no preferred pattern noted. Preoperative imaging studies were unreliable in predicting the extent of disease. Wide *en bloc* excision or amputation was recommended as primary treatment along with axillary lymph-node dissection.

Pho R: Malignant giant-cell tumor of the distal end of the radius treated by a free vascularized fibular transplant. *J Bone Joint Surg,* 63A:877-884, 1981.

The author presents a series of five cases of malignant giant cell tumor of the distal radius treated with wide *en bloc* resection and reconstruction with a vascularized fibular graft. The details of the surgical procedure are outlined.

Rock M, Pritchard D, Unni K: Metastases from histologically benign giant-cell tumor of bone. *J Bone Joint Surg,* 64A:269-274, 1984.

A report of eight cases from the Mayo Clinic and a review of the literature (31 cases) of benign pulmonary metastases from GCT with a 25% mortality. A case for aggressive treatment of both the primary and pulmonary lesions is made. Four of the eight cases were in the radius.

Simon M: Biopsy of musculoskeletal tumors (current concepts review). *J Bone Joint Surg,* 64A: 1253-1257, 1982.

A review of the important aspects of biopsy of tumors of musculoskeletal origin including preoperative planning, staging, technique, and timing.

Simon M, Enneking W: The management of soft-tissue sarcomas of the extremities. *J Bone Joint Surg,* 58A:317-327, 1976.

A retrospective report of 54 cases of soft tissue sarcomas of various diagnoses (one-third upper extremity) treated with "adequate" radical local resection or amputation. The study reports a 16.7% local recurrence rate and 62% five-year survival, without adjuvant radiation or chemotherapy.

Smith R, Floyd W: Surgical treatment of aggressive lesions of the hand and forearm. In Green DP (ed), *Operative Hand Surgery,* 62:2363-2390, Churchill Livingstone, New York, 1990.

The authors discuss principles of tumor surgery in the hand and forearm as well as surgical management of aggressive lesions in various locations in the upper extremity. Several illustrative cases are shown.

Steinberg B, Gelberman R, Mankin H, Rosenberg A: Epithelioid sarcoma in the upper extremity. *J Bone Joint Surg,* 74A:28-35, 1992.

A retrospective analysis of 18 cases divided into two treatment groups: marginal versus wide or radical resection with or without adjuvant therapy. Outcome with marginal resection was dismal when compared to those treated by radical or wide (>3 cm cuff of normal tissue) excision. Wide or radical resection for those cases treated initially with marginal excision which recurred locally without metastases was also found to be effective.

36

Pediatric Hand Tumors

Joseph Upton III, MD

Introduction

Few in-depth studies of pediatric hand and wrist tumors exist. Ganglion cysts, epidermal (inclusion) cysts, and vascular tumors predominate. Other soft-tissue and skeletal masses are so unusual that the differential diagnosis may be difficult. A thorough history and physical examination will usually make the diagnosis and a plain radiograph is often the only test needed.

Ultrasonography is helpful in identifying tendon ruptures, foreign bodies, synovitis, cystic, and solid masses. With computed tomography scans, fat and calcium components of masses and normal tissues are clearly delineated. Magnetic resonance scans are particularly good for the differentiation of tissues with varying densities. Enhancement with technetium-labeled red blood cells or gadolineum demonstrates vascular lesions well. With this technology, as well as invasive techniques such as selective angiography, the hand surgeon of the 90s has an abundance of information about a mass before biopsy or excision. Diagnosis is rarely in doubt and there are few surprises.

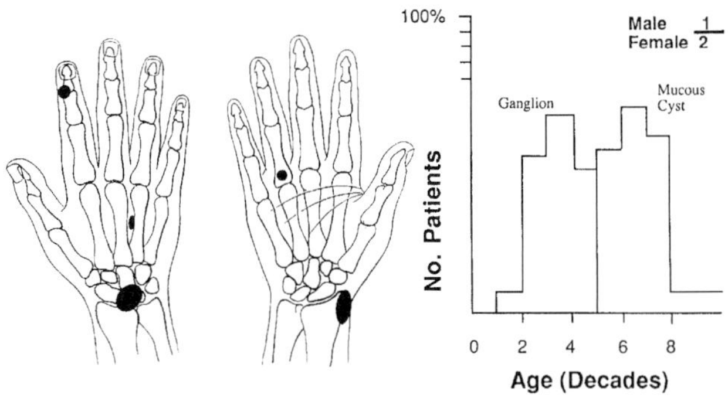

Figure 36-1. Ganglion cysts. The common dorsal and volar wrist locations are pictured. Retinacular cysts are located over the volar surface of the proximal phalanx and synovial cysts over the dorsal metacarpal location. Children do not present with mucous cysts at the DIP joints.

Ganglion Cysts

Ganglion cysts comprise 50% to 70% of soft-tissue tumors of the hand and wrist in both children and adults. There is a female prevalence by a two to one ratio. The incidence in children is probably underestimated. Most pediatric patients do not seek medical treatment because there is little pain or functional impairment. Large reported series do not contain more than a 10% occurrence in the pediatric age group.

These synovial cysts appear in four locations: the dorsum of the wrist with origin from the scapholunate ligament region (approximately 70%); the volar wrist arising from the radiocarpal or an intercarpal joint (approximately 20%); the volar digit (long and ring predominate) with origin from the retinacular sheath (approximately 10%); and the dorsum of the hand in the metacarpal region with origin from an extensor tendon (approximately 2%). (Fig. 36-1) The retinacular cysts are commonly seen in young children and the synovial cysts attached to extensor tendons in teenagers. Cysts in more unusual locations such as the metacarpal, dorsal portion of the digital proximal interphalangeal joint, and first dorsal compartment are uncommon in children. Mucous cysts associated with degenerative arthritis of the distal interphalangeal joint are common in adults and are virtually not seen in children.

Most ganglion cysts are hard and immobile and those originating from the wrist joint characteristically fluctuate in size. Young children are usually brought in by concerned parents and normally do not complain of pain associated

with a palpable mass. Teenagers complain of the appearance. Symptoms are directly proportional to the size of the mass. Occult dorsal ganglia should be considered in older children presenting with wrist pain. Since the diagnosis is evident on physical exam, radiographs, ultrasonography, and arthrography are not routinely necessary but may be helpful with small lesions. The etiology of these synovial cysts has been covered in the section on adult tumors. Examination of the cyst fluid reveals gelatinous material more viscous than joint fluid and with high concentrations of hyaluronic acid, albumin, globulin, and glycosamines.

Treatment of children consists of reassurance for asymptomatic masses. Ineffective modalities include rest, immobilization, and traumatic rupture (Bible treatment). Simple needle aspiration has been reported as effective in 85% of patients; failures with this method are evident within six to 10 months. Excision of pediatric ganglion cysts is recommended for symptomatic patients and should include a small portion of the capsule and evacuation of all intra-articular daughter cysts. In dissections of dorsal wrist ganglia the scapholunate ligament should be preserved. All volar wrist dissections should preserve the often displaced radial artery and superficial branches of the radial nerve. The thumb CMC joint may often be the site of origin in young children with large volar lesions. Retinacular sheath ganglia are most successfully treated by aspiration without steroid infiltration. Excision of flexor sheath lesions in children is seldom necessary.

Recurrence rate is less than 10% with proper excision under controlled operating conditions and may range as high as 40% in other settings. No large series with follow up and recurrence rates in children is available in the medical literature.

Vascular Anomalies

No discussion of pediatric tumors would be complete without the inclusion of vascular lesions, which represent either the third or fourth most common mass lesion of the upper extremity. Although only 10% of all vascular lesions in the body are found in the upper extremity, they still represent significant numbers. Classification is difficult because our understanding of the natural history, biology, and pathogenesis of the many vascular anomalies is incomplete. One conceptual system of classification based on biological characteristics has practical importance for the hand surgeon. Mulliken and Glowacki have divided vascular anomalies into two main groups: hemangiomas, which grow rapidly and spontaneously involute, and malformations, which grow commensurately with the child and do not involute. (Tables 36-1 and 36-2) Two pediatric vascular lesions that are not included in this system are the glomus tumor, a proliferation of specialized perivascular cells, and the pyogenic granuloma, a reactive lesion.

Table 36-1.   Biological Classification of Vascular Birthmarks.

Hemangioma	Malformation
Proliferating phase	Grow with child
Involutional phase	Cellular types: Capillary Lymphatic Venous Arterial Combined

Hemangioma

A hemangioma may be present at birth or may exist initially as a small red spot. Within several months these lesions undergo rapid growth and proliferation and usually reach maximal size by two to three years of age. (Figs. 36-2 and 36-3) Lesions within the hand and wrist are usually circumscribed and have no predominant location. Isolated fingertip lesions are unusual. Hemangiomas are characterized by endothelial hyperplasia and elevated mast cells during the proliferative phase. Fibroblasts, macrophages, and diminishing endothelial turnover are seen during the involuting phase. By age five spontaneous involution is underway. This process is heralded by gray areas of lighter pigmentation called "herald spots." Most of these lesions have the appearance of a "strawberry" if dermis is involved, but many deeper lesions will show few skin changes. The size or shape of a lesion has little effect upon involution (Table 36-2).

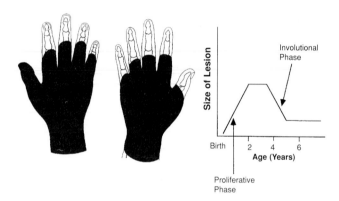

Figure 36-2. Hemangioma. The location of these tumors may be virtually anywhere in the hand.

Table 36-2.   Differences Between Hemangiomas and Vascular Malformations.

Hemangioma	Malformation
Clinical	
Plump endothelium, increased turnover	Flat endothelium, slow turnover
Increased mast cells	Normal mast cell count
Multilaminated basement membrane	Thin basement membrane
Capillary tubule formation *in vitro*	Poor endothelial growth *in vitro*
Radiological	
Circumscribed, lobular parenchymal staining	Diffuse, no parenchyma Slow flow: phleboliths, ectasia Fast flow: tortuous arteries, arteriovenous shunting
Hematological	
Primary platelet trapping (Kassabach Merritt phenomenon)	Primary venous stasis (localized consumptive coagulopathy)
Skeletal	
Infrequent "mass effect" on adjacent bone, hypertrophy rare	Slow flow: distortion, hypertrophy, or hyperplasia
	Fast flow: destruction, distortion or hypertrophy

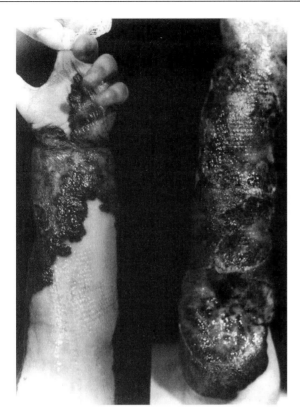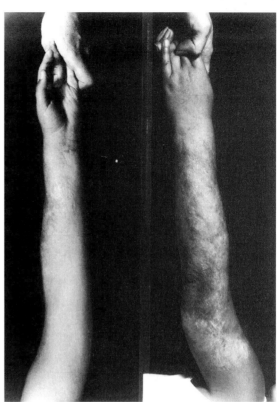

Figure 36-3.   Hemangiomas undergo rapid growth and proliferation and usually reach maximal size by three years of age. Spontaneous involution is underway by age five.

Treatment is conservative. Compression garments for large lesions and reassurance of parents remains the treatment of choice. Ulceration is treated with appropriate dressings and antibiotics if needed. Central scarred areas will contract with time. Areas of redundant fibrofatty tissue can be excised after involution is complete. Earlier surgery is reserved for serious obstructions of the aerodigestive tract, obstruction of vision, gastrointestinal bleeding, and other life-threatening conditions. Early surgery is rarely indicated in the upper extremity. Tunable dye lasers, sclerotherapy, and radiation may add to tissue death during involution and are not needed. Approximately 15% of large, extensive hemangiomas may respond to systemic prednisone. Recent clinical trials with alpha-2a interferon therapy for life-threatening hemangiomas of infancy demonstrate enhanced regression of extensive lesions.

Malformation

Lesions that do not involute and whose endothelial cells show no signs of cellular turnover are called malformations. They exhibit a normal imperceptible endothelial cell cycle. It is clinically useful to subclassify malformations by their cell types into capillary, venous, lymphatic, and arterial.

Capillary lesions are present at birth and comprise the familiar "port wine stain" or naevus flammeus. They may be combined with other deeper vascular lesions. Treatment is conservative with frequent utilization of cosmetics and tunable dye lasers.

Venous lesions are most common and often are not noticed until the first year of life. They may be localized or extensive, but all decompress with direct pressure or elevation. Pain is usually secondary to intralesional thrombi or calcification. More extensive lesions are often accompanied by skeletal enlargement and syndromic designations (Fig. 36-4). Management of these low-flow lesions varies with both size and symptoms. Compression garments are the mainstay of therapy. Surgery can safely be performed but should be reserved for large, symptomatic masses.

Lymphatic malformations, often called lymphangiomas and cystic hygromas, are commonly seen on the dorsum of the digit, hand, or forearm. Extensive lesions often extend through the hemithorax and mediastinum (Fig. 36-5). Growth is commensurate with the child. The most common problem relates to skin breakdown over ruptured epidermal vesicles and secondary beta streptococcal infections which are effectively treated with penicillin. Arterial and skeletal architecture is usually normal. Surgical debulking can be

Figure 36-4. Syndromic Associations with Limb Vascular Anomalies

Klippel-Trenaunay: congenital varicose veins with a cutaneous capillary malformation and limb hypertrophy.

Parkes Weber: concurrence of multiple congenital arteriovenous fistulae and an enlarged limb.

Infantile angioectatic hypertrophy: congenital vascular malformations, limb overgrowth and a cutaneous capillary nevus. An unhelpful composite term. Includes Klippel-Trenaunay and Parkes Weber syndromes.

Proteus: partial gigantism of hands or feet, exostoses, macrocephaly, hemihypertrophy, and vascular malformations (usually patchy dermal staining).

Maffucci: dyschondroplasia of limb(s), with enchondromas, associated with a vascular malformation (usually venous or combined venous/lymphatic).

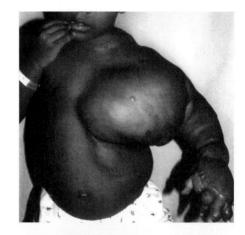

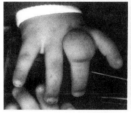 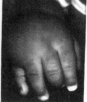 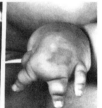

Figure 36-5. Lymphatic Malformations **(Top)** Extensive lesions often extend through the hemithorax and mediastinum. **(Bottom)** Lesions on the dorsum of the hand.

predictably performed. Multiple staged surgical excisions are often required for large lesions. Amputations for gigantic lesions are advised.

Combined venous-lymphatic malformations occur as low-flow lesions. They are often associated with skeletal enlargement or gigantism. Compression therapy is preferred. Surgical approaches are the same as those for pure lymphatic lesions.

Arterial lesions are the most symptomatic and, fortunately, the least common. These malformations are high-flow lesions with arteriovenous shunting, and all present as warm, pulsating, occasionally painful masses (Fig. 36-6). Swelling, ischemic pain, and/or paresthesias are secondary to nerve compression or compartment syndromes. More proximal lesions have often been called "truncal fistulas." The steal caused by the arteriovenous shunting may result in distal gangrene. Bleeding within large lesions may be associated with consumptive coagulopathies, severe pain, nerve compression, ischemic necrosis of skin, and persistent ulceration. Treatment of these difficult lesions is not hopeless but carries risks. Selective embolization runs a high risk of distal gangrene. Radiation is ineffective and may precipitate long-standing skin and other soft-tissue changes. Local scleroinjection therapy is evolving but not useful at this time. Radical surgical resection with appropriate revascularization and/or flap resurfacing utilizing microvascular techniques has definite but limited value. These high-flow arterial lesions are characteristically much larger than expected and involve all tissues within the hand (including bone). Amputation of the most symptomatic, extensive lesions is often necessary.

Epidermal Inclusion Cysts

This common but rarely discussed lesion may present clinically within the first five years of life, but is seen more frequently in adolescents and adults. (Fig. 36-7) Microtrauma,

contusions, and penetrating injuries to the skin drive epithelium into the subcutaneous space where it grows and produces keratin which fills the cyst cavity. The time interval between injury and detection may range from months to years. The result is a mass in the distal digit or palm which is hard, immobile, and may produce destruction of bone by extrinsic pressure. The distal phalanges of the index and long fingers are most commonly involved. Males with this problem outnumber females by a two to one ratio in the adults but there is no sexual preponderance in children. Occasionally these masses are tender and, when large, may cause nerve compression. Motion of the interphalangeal joints is seldom affected.

Treatment consists of surgical removal of the entire epithelial mass with intact capsule. Large osseous defects may require curettage and bone grafts; recurrence is rare.

Enchondroma

This is the most common skeletal tumor in adults and children; there is no sex prevalence. Enchondromas are diagnosed most commonly in the second to fourth decades of life, often as the result of a pathologic fracture. The proximal phalanges and metacarpals of the index and long rays are the most common locations. Radiographs show a radiolucent mass within the diaphysis and/or metaphysis of a bone with a thinned cortex and flecks of calcification. In extreme cases, entire bones may be replaced by these

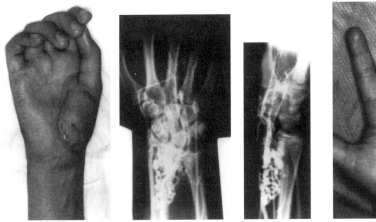

Figure 36-6. **(Left)** Arterial lesion. **(Center and Right)** Involvement of all tissues of the hand, including bone, is characteristic of these lesions.

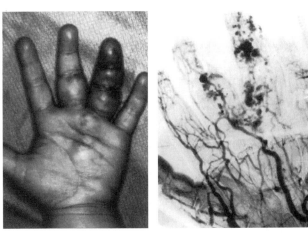

Figure 36-7. Epidermal inclusion cyst.

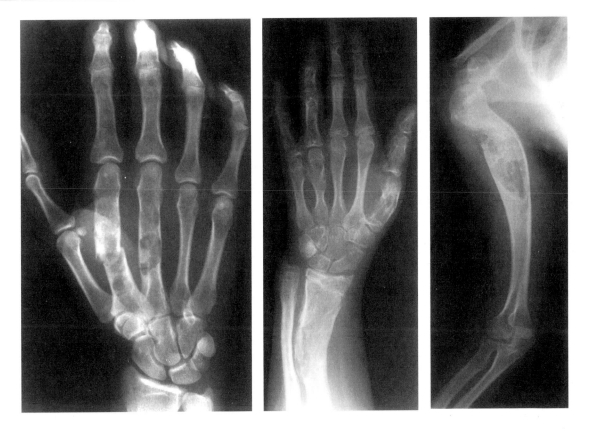

Figure 36-8. **(A)** A pathologic fracture through the index metacarpal is seen in a patient with multiple phalangeal and metacarpal enchondromas. **(B)** Secondary deformities of the distal and radius are seen in another child with the Ollier syndrome. **(C)** Involvement of multiple bones in the upper extremity is common.

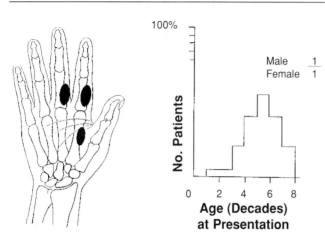

Figure 36-9. Localized nodular tenosynovitis (giant cell tumor of tendon sheath). Adapted with permission from the Regional Review Course, American Society for Surgery of the Hand, 1990.

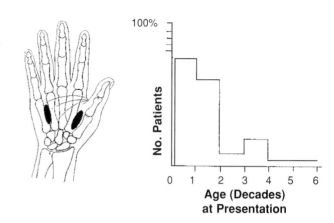

Figure 36-10. Juvenile aponeurotic fibroma.

benign lesions. Pathology shows benign cartilage. Ollier's syndrome consists of multiple enchondromas in a single patient (Fig. 36-8). Those with Maffucci's syndrome have multiple enchondromas as well as venous or combined venous-lymphatic vascular malformations (Fig. 36-4).

Following diagnosis of a pathologic fracture, the most reasonable treatment is conservative immobilization. Several months after the fracture has healed and pain subsides, the preferred treatment consists of curettage and cancellous bone grafting. Curettage alone has many advocates. Grafting of smaller lesions within the metacarpals and phalanges with demineralized bone and larger lesions within the carpals and metacarpals with allograft bone has been reported. The risk of AIDS and hepatitis B always accompanies conventional allografts.

Localized Nodular Tenosynovitis

Nodular tenosynovitis of the tendon sheath, also known as xanthoma or giant cell tumor of the tendon sheath or localized villonodular synovitis, represents the second most common soft-tissue tumor (Figure 36-9) of the pediatric and adult hand. These tumors have an obscure etiology but are believed to be reactive lesions. They are seen rarely in young children, frequently seen in teenagers, and are most frequently seen in adults, without sexual prevalence. There is usually no antecedent history of trauma. These are considered benign tumors in contrast to giant cell tumors of bone.

These tumors are hard, immobile masses found along the fingers, often with intra-articular extensions into interphalangeal joints. They are usually oblique, encapsulated, multilobulated, and variable in size. Calcification and/or bone erosion may be present on radiograph. Although they are painless, the mass of these tumors may result in nerve compression and loss of motion. Pathologically, they present a yellow-tan color. Histologically, they consist of multinucle-

ated giant cells, histiocytes with lipoid globules within their cytoplasm, spindle cells, and reticulin; they are benign.

Treatment consists of surgical removal. Because these lesions are often much larger than expected, the operation must remove of all unexpected extensions, particularly those that extend along vincular vessels into interphalangeal joints.

Juvenile Aponeurotic Fibroma

Although this tumor is often seen in the foot, ankle, back, and shoulder, it presents in the hand and wrist 50% of the time. First described by Keasbey (Keasbey tumor), it typically presents as a painless mass in the palm within the thenar or hypothenar (Fig. 36-10) skin of an older child or teenager. The tumor grows slowly and rarely causes sensory or motor problems. Males outnumber females by a two to one ratio. The stippled calcification seen on radiographs may represent degenerated portions of aponeurotic tissue. Pathologists prefer the term calcifying aponeurotic fibroma. Histology shows a highly cellular proliferative lesion, infiltration of surrounding fat and muscle, dense collagen deposits, and calcification. This is a benign lesion without distant metastases. The diagnosis of juvenile aponeurotic fibroma is frequently confused with a malignancy.

Treatment consists of wide surgical excision but not a damaging radical resection. Incomplete removal is accompanied by a high recurrence rate. (Almost half of the cases in the surgical literature have reported a recurrence.)

Infantile Digital Fibroma (Digital Fibroma of Childhood)

This unusual tumor is seen only in children. Also called the recurrent digital fibroma and the digital fibroma of childhood, these lesions appear early in life along the dorsal surface or side of the ulnar three digits. (Figs. 36-11 and 36-12) Thumb and index fingers are usually not involved.

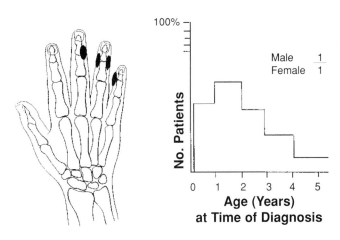

Figure 36-11. Digital fibroma of childhood (infantile digital fibroma) (recurring digital fibroma).

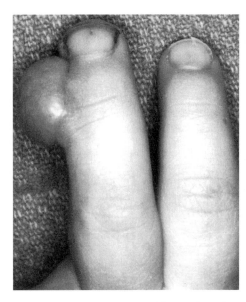

Figure 36-12. A rapidly growing digital fibroma in a six-month-old child that was treated with wide excision and a skin graft.

These lesions may undergo a rapid growth within a short period of time. Histology reveals a deep dermal origin and intracytoplasmic inclusion bodies not seen in other fibrous proliferative disorders. These inclusions may contain a virus, which has never been identified, or the products of cell degradation. This curious tumor has no adult counterpart. The inclusion bodies and characteristic location of the mass distinguish this tumor from the juvenile aponeurotic fibroma.

Preferred treatment consists of wide surgical excision. Resurfacing with skin grafts, and occasionally local flaps, may be needed. A recurrence rate of up to 50% has been reported in several series. Recurrence is often initially confused with hypertrophic scar tissue. No large series have ever been reported.

Rhabdomyosarcoma

Less than 1% of all tumors of the hand and wrist are malignant. Osteogenic sarcoma, the most common skeletal malignancy, occurs more frequently than rhabdomyosarcoma. Pediatric soft-tissue sarcomas are found much more frequently in the head and neck region. Males outnumber females by a three to one ratio. Upper and lower extremity lesions occur with equal frequency, and present as hard, painless, rapidly growing masses. Parents usually link it to some previous trauma. CT and MRI scans show a homogeneous mass that may involve contiguous structures. Biopsy provides the definitive diagnosis. The alveolar histologic group of tumors has a more favorable prognosis than the embryonal subtype.

Present treatment combines chemotherapy, radiation therapy, and surgical ablation. Protocols vary depending upon the histological grade and regional nodal involvement. Wide resection combined with regional node dissection provides an 80%, five-year survival in children with no lymphatic spread and a 46% rate for those with positive nodes. Nodal involvement is a major prognostic sign. Relapse is heralded by distant spread and not local recurrence.

Annotated Bibliography

Adani R, Calo M, Torricelli P, Squarzina PB, Caroli A: The value of computed tomography in the diagnosis of soft-tissue swellings of the hand. *J Hand Surg,* 15(B): 229-232, 1990.

Twenty soft-tissue masses, excluding ganglion cysts, were examined. Lipomas, cystic lesions, and giant cell tumors permitted accurate diagnoses. Vascular lesions were better delineated with angiography. Benign chondromatosis and soft-tissue chondrosarcoma were similar and could not be differentiated by CT alone. CT scans proved to be a valuable tool in assessment.

Azouz EM, Kozlowski K, Masel J: soft-tissue tumors of the hand and wrist of children. *J Canad Assn Radiol,* 40:251-255,1989.

Twenty-three children with soft-tissue tumors were reported. Ganglia were excluded. Tumors of blood and lymphatic vessel origin accounted for nine patients, xanthomas in four patients, and tumoral calcinosis in four. There was one malignancy, a rhabdomyosarcoma. Plain radiographs were the first and often the only test needed. CT, MRI, and angiography were used only if the diagnosis was in doubt.

Binkovitz LA, Berquist TH, McLeod RA: Masses of the hand and wrist: detection and characterization with MR imaging. *Am J Radiol*, 154:323-326, 1990.

High-spatial resolution studies were done in 131 patients using a small local coil or extremity volume coil. Twenty-five patients had either palpable masses or deep suspected masses. Of the 16 benign lesions, the correct diagnosis was suggested in nine (56%). All six malignant tumors were diagnosed correctly. One ganglion cyst was mistaken for a joint effusion. MR imaging is an accurate means of detecting the delineating mass lesions of the hand and wrist.

Hoglund M, Tordai P, Engkvist O: Ultrasonography for the diagnosis of soft-tissue conditions in the hand. *Scand J Plast Reconstr Surg*, 25:225-231, 1991.

Ultrasonographic diagnosis of the hand has proved to be valuable for the diagnosis of ganglion cysts, tendon ruptures, synovitis, tumors, and the presence of foreign bodies. More experience is necessary for the delineation of nerve compressions and epiphyseal plate disorders.

Schmitt R, Marmuth-Metz M, Lanz U, Lucas D, Feyerabend T, Schindler G: Computer tomographie von weichteiltumoren der hand und des unterarmes. *Radiologe*, 30(4):185-192, 1990. (Published in German)

Computed tomography in 32 patients with 24 hand and eight forearm masses was accurate in delineating benign and malignant diagnoses. All were correctly delineated with regard to localization, size, and infiltration of the surrounding tissue. There were two malignancies. One false positive malignancy was later diagnosed as an aggressive fibromatosis. Scar tissue and soft-tissue sarcomas had similar appearance and were difficult to delineate.

Ganglion Cysts

Flugel M, Kessler K: Follow up of 425 patients operated for ganglion cyst. *Handchir Mikrochir Plast Chir*, 18:47-52, 1986.

Of 425 patients operated upon for ganglion cysts, 348 were available for follow up, which ranged from 23 to 95 months. Recurrence was noted in 75 patients (21.6%) with 47 dorsal carpal and 16 palmar ganglia. Three-fourths of the recurrences occurred within the first year. Postoperative symptoms included pain with heavy activity (38.2%), limited motion (11%), and sensitivity to temperature changes (13.5%). The authors recommended that these lesions be primarily removed by experienced hand surgeons.

MacCollum MS: Dorsal wrist ganglions in children. Clinical notes. *J Hand Surg*, 2:325, 1977.

Of 21 children with ganglion cysts (location not specified), seven had surgical excision with two recurrences. Of the remaining 14 patients treated conservatively, nine noted spontaneous disappearance within four months to five years. Seven of the 21 patients complained of pain at the time of diagnosis.

Richman JA, Gelberman RH, Engber WD, Salamon PB, Bean DJ: Ganglions of the wrist and digits - results of treatment by aspiration and cyst wall puncture. *J Hand Surg*, 12(A):1041-1043, 1987.

Eighty-seven wrist and digital ganglion cysts were aspirated; half were immobilized. A successful outcome was found in 37% of all patients. Recurrence was 69% in digital ganglions, 43% in palmar (volar) wrist ganglions, and 27% for dorsal wrist cysts. Recurrence was slightly less in wrist lesions immobilized post-puncture.

Zubowicz VN, Ishii CH: Management of ganglion cysts of the hand by simple aspiration *J Hand Surg*, 12(A):618-620, 1987.

Forty-seven patients were treated successfully with 1 (N=35), 2 (N=3), or 3 (N=2) aspirations with an 85% nonrecurrence rate. The remaining seven patients were offered surgery. Cost savings are emphasized.

Vascular Anomalies: Hemangioma and Malformation

Apfelberg DB, Maser MR, Lash H, White DN: YAG laser resection of complicated hemangiomas of the hand and upper extremity. *J Hand Surg*, 15(A):765-773, 1990.

The YAG laser with saphire scalpel enables partial or complete removal of complicated vascular lesions of the upper extremity that are not amenable to routine surgical excision. A 1-mm rim of tissue must be excised at the conclusion of the procedure to avoid wound-healing complications.

Ezekowitz MB, Mulliken JB, Folkman J: Interferon alfa-2a therapy for life-threatening hemangiomas of infancy. *NEJ Med*, 326(22):1455-1463, 1992.

Eighteen of 20 infants with life-threatening lesions involving multiple organ systems responded to daily subcutaneous injections of interferon alfa-2a (up to three million units per square meter of body surface per day). This substance induces regression. The mechanism is unknown. There was no long-term toxicity at 16 months.

Finn MC, Glowacki J, Mulliken JB: Congenital vascular lesions: clinical application of a new classification. *J Ped Surg*, 18:894, 1983.

A review of 297 patients with 375 hemangiomas was studied over a 24-year period. Seven percent involved the upper limb. Only 40% were evident at birth but all began to proliferate by three to four months of age. Involution started between two and four years of age and was complete by age six in the majority of lesions. Better cosmetic results were obtained in those lesions that involuted early. Malformations were usually present at birth and did not change in size as they grew commensurately with the children.

Mulliken JB, Young AE: *Vascular birthmarks: hemangiomas and malformations*. Philadelphia, WB Saunders Co., 1988.

This text is devoted entirely to vascular lesions. What is known about the folklore, classification, biology, natural history, and treatment of different lesions in all regions of the body is presented in detail. One chapter deals exclusively with the upper limb. Specific treatment recommendations are made for each type of malformation. This book contains the most authoritative and complete discussion of vascular lesions available in the medical literature.

Peeters FLM: Therapeutic embolization in angiomas and tumors. *Diagn Imaging*, 49:193-205, 1980.

Of four patients embolized with gelfoam, three had extremity lesions. One angiogram of an extensive low-flow venous malformation in the hand shows slight decrease in size and obliteration of channels at the distal phalangeal level. Potential ischemic nerve injury and the resorption characteristics of gelfoam are discussed. This method is most useful as an adjunct to planned surgery.

Stober VR: The F. P. Weber syndrome in the hand: clinical presentation, diagnosis, and therapy. *Handchir Mikrochir Plast Chir,* 21:107-110, 1989.

The confusion between the Parkes-Weber syndrome (gigantism and congenital venous malformations) and the Klippel-Trenaunay syndrome (triad of gigantism, nevus flammeus, varices) is discussed. Five of eight patients diagnosed with the Parkes-Weber syndrome were treated successfully with resection of malformation and skeletization of digital vessels to the involved digits. Simple surgical ligation is no longer recommended.

Upton J, Mulliken JB, Murray JE: Classification and rationale for management of vascular anomalies in the upper extremity. *J Hand Surg,* 10(A):970-974, 1985.

Vascular anomalies are classified as hemangioma or malformations (capillary, venous, lymphatic, or combinations) according to their endothelial characteristics and clinical appearance. The rationale for treatment of each group is outlined.

Epidermal Inclusion Cysts

Byers P, Salm R: Epidermal inclusion cysts of phalanges. *J Bone Joint Surg,* 48(B):544-581, 1966.

Four cases of inclusion cysts involving bone are presented, all with some type of antecedent trauma which may have occurred years before the cyst manifested itself clinically. Radiographs showed an expanding lesion with a rim of sclerosis when involving bone. The natural history is reviewed.

Posch JL: In Flynn, JE,(ed), *Hand Surgery,* 2d ed, Baltimore, Williams and Wilkins, 1976.

In a series of 1,499 hand tumors, inclusion cysts are the third most common lesion comprising a 5% total in adults and children.

Enchondroma

Bauer RD, Posner MA: Treatment of enchondromas of the hand with allograft bone. *J Hand Surg,* 1113(A): 908-916, 1988.

Twelve patients received allograft bone in 15 separate operations. In 16 patients cancellous autogenous bone was obtained from the patient's iliac crest. Results were similar in both groups. Excellent or good results were achieved in all allograft patients and in 93% of those receiving autogenous bone.

Hasselgren G, Forssblad P, Tomvall A: Bone grafting unneccessary in the treatment of enchondromas in the hand. *J Hand Surg,* 16(A):1139-1142, 1991.

Twenty-eight consecutive patients with enchondromas were treated with simple curettage over a 20-year period. The majority of tumors were classified as monostatic, monocentric, and nonexpanding. All demonstrated new bone formation, including 15 with excellent bone formation, nine with good bone formation, and four with scanty bone formation. There were no recurrences or pathologic fractures.

Kuur E, Hansen SL, Lindequist S: Treatment of solitary enchondromas in fingers. *J Hand Surg,* 14(B):109-112, 1989.

Of 21 patients with enchondromas, 15 were treated with curettage and cancellous bone grafting, 5 with curettage alone, and one with amputation for an extensive lesion. After a period of 13 months to nine years, all 20 patients with remaining digits were pain free. Eleven of the 15 grafted patients had complete filling of their bone defects, three had persistent defects that did not interfere with function.

Tordai P, Hoglund M, Lugnegard H: Is the treatment of enchondroma in the hand by simple curettage a rewarding method? *J Hand Surg,* 15(B):331-334, 1990.

Forty-six enchondromas were treated by simple curettage on an outpatient basis. Radiographs indicated that 82% had bone defects smaller than 3 mm in diameter, 16% were left with bone defects of 4 mm to 10 mm in diameter, and 2% had recurrence. Follow up ranged from three to 12 years. Simple curettage is useful for obliteration of small lesions at risk for pathologic fractrure.

Upton J, Glowacki J: Hand reconstruction with demineralized bone: a series of 26 implants in 12 patients. *J Hand Surg,* 17(A):704-713, 1992.

A series of 26 demineralized implants was used. Most of the phalangeal and metacarpal defects were large and associated with secondary enchondromas. Time to healing and obliteration of all skeletal defects were similar to cancellous bone grafting.

Localized Nodular Tenosynovitis

Phalen GS, McCormack LJ, Gazale WJ: Giant cell tumor of tendon sheath in the hand. *Clin Orthop,* 15:140-51, 1959.

Of 56 patients evaluated with giant cell tumors of tendon sheaths, nine were children. The recurrence rate in 41 patients followed for eight to 10 years was 25% (nine patients). The natural history, histology, and pathogenesis of these slow-growing lesions are discussed. The authors conclude that these tumors are of synovial cells and that the term benign synovioma is appropriate.

Fyfe IS, MacFarlane A: Pigmented villonodular synovitis of the hand. *Hand,* 12(2):179-188, 1980.

A series of 51 lesions, including two in children, was reviewed. Females outnumbered males by a two to one margin. Out of 51 tumors, 35 were volar and 16 were dorsal. Degenerative joint changes were present in older patients. All lesions were excised and nine of 51 (19%) recurred one or more times. This is an excellent short review with an adequate bibliography.

Jones FE, Soule EH, Coventry MB: Fibrous xanthoma of synovium—a study of 118 cases. *J Bone Joint Surg,* 51(A):76-86, 1969.

This frequently quoted reference presents 118 lesions seen at the Mayo Clinic over a nine-year period. Ninety-one involved digits and most were located adjacent to the DIP joints. Radiographic changes were seen in 53 (45%). Postoperative recurrence was seen in 17 patients (10%). The etiologic significance of trauma and degenerative joint disease is discussed. Xanthomas and pigmented villonodular synovitis are thought to be different manifestations of the same disease process.

Moore JR, Weiland AJ, Curtis RM: Localized nodular tenosynovitis: experience with 115 cases. *J Hand Surg,* 9(A):412-417, 1984.

A recurrence rate of 9% was reported in a large series of cases involving the hand. Less than 10% were found in children. Bone deformation was common, but infiltration was not seen. Thorough excision with joint exploration was recommended.

Juvenile Aponeurotic Fibroma

Allen PW, Enzinger FM: Juvenile aponeurotic fibroma. *Cancer,* 26:857-867, 1970.

This study presents the histologic characteristics of the tumor. Recurrence rate does not decrease with age as seven of seven children under the age of five had recurrences.

Carroll RE: Juvenile aponeurotic fibroma. *Hand Clin,* 3:219-224, 1987.

A report of 13 cases emphasizes the early presentation in infants and young children, slow growth, and lack of symptoms. Surgery included wide excision in six patients, excision and skin graft in six patients, and amputation in one child.

Mehregan AH: Superficial fibrous tumors in childhood. *J Cutan Path,* 8:321-334, 1981.

A review is made of superficial fibrous tumors of childhood and differences between the pattern of fibrous tumor proliferation in children and adults are discussed. The tumors of childhood and infancy include the recurring digital fibrous tumor, juvenile aponeurotic fibroma, juvenile hyalin fibromatosis, fibrous hamartoma of infancy among others. Palmoplantar fibromatosis and fibrosarcoma may appear in all ages. Dupuytren's contracture is not observed early in life. Histiocytomas and dermatofibromas are common in adults and rare in children.

Sprecht EE, Stahele LT: Juvenile aponeurotic fibroma. *J Hand Surg,* 2:256-257, 1977.

A review of 66 reported cases showed that 45 were located in the hand or forearm and that 57 presented before the age of 20 years. A highly cellular pleomorphic histology does not show mitosis but is often mistaken for a malignancy. No instances of metastasis have been recorded. Excision without sacrifice of vital structures is recommended.

Digital Fibroma of Childhood (Infantile Digital Fibroma)

Falco N, Upton J: Infantile digital fibromas. *J Hand Surg.*

Fifteen digital lesions in seven pediatric patients were excised with a recurrence in one (7%). This unique tumor has a multicentric origin as five separate masses were seen in one patient. Diagnosis was confirmed by intracytoplasmic inclusion bodies. Local flaps and full-thickness hypothenar skin grafts were used to cover large excision sites.

Kankatus Y: Infantile digital fibromatosis. Immuno-histochemical and ultrastructural observations of cytoplasmic inclusions. *Cancer,* 61:500-507, 1988.

Ultrastructural studies have shown that the inclusions seen in these cells may not be viral in origin but represent altered fibroblast metabolism and consist of degradation products of actin, actin myosin complexes, or other cytoskeletal proteins.

Rayner CR: Soft-tissue tumours of the hand. Review article. *J Hand Surg,* 16(B):125-126, 1991.

In a short review, an experienced surgeon emphasizes the confusion with hypertrophic scarring, the rapid growth, location along the sides of digits, and the pressure from parents for excision. Radical excision with a diagnosis of "juvenile sarcoma" should be avoided with self-limiting lesions. Diagnosis of fibrous lesions in the hand is difficult.

Tizian C, Berger A, Schneider W, Vykoupil KF: The differential diagnosis of juvenile digital fibromatosis. *J Hand Surg,* 10(B):418, 1985.

The difficulties of diagnosis of childhood fibromatoses are discussed. The juvenile digital fibroma has a characteristic natural history and histology.

Rhabdomyosarcoma

Kuschner SH, Menendez LR, Stephens S, Gellman H: Malignant tumors of the upper extremity in children. *Orthop Rev,* 19:411-417, 1991.

Of 422 primary malignant tumors of bone and soft-tissue seen in one institution over a 20-year period, 29 involved the upper extremity. There were 13 patients with osteosarcoma, of whom nine were dead. All four patients with Ewing's sarcoma were dead. Of three patients with chondrosarcoma, all treated with surgery, one was lost to follow up and two others were disease free. Two of the nine patients with soft-tissue were dead. Both had spindle cell lesions of the shoulder. Three patients with rhabdosarcoma were disease free at eight, 13, and 16 years after wide resection.

Mandell L, Ghavimi R, LaQuaglia M, Exelby P: Prognostic significance of regional lymph node involvement in childhood extremity rhabdomyosarcoma. *Med Ped Oncol,* 18:466-471, 1990.

Twenty seven patients with 11 upper and 16 lower extremity tumors are presented. Median follow up was 9.2 years. After combined modality treatment, overall survival was 48%(13/27). Excluding those patients with M1 disease, the survival rate was N0, 11/12; N1, 1/10. The first sign of relapse in M0 patients was distant disease in 8/10 cases. Regional node involvement is an important prognostic factor.

Matev I, Stoytscheff K: Congenital sarcoma in the forearm: a long term follow up of a case. *J Hand Surg,* 16(B):346-348, 1991.

A child with congenital fibrosarcoma of the forearm, well differentiated type, is described. Early radical extirpation of the lesion with periosteum led to an apparent cure 15-years postoperatively. Radiation was not employed. Growth was normal.

IX

Pediatric Hand

37

Trauma and Infections of the Hand and Wrist in Children

Terry R. Light, MD

Introduction

The child's hand is vulnerable to injury. The innate curiosity of children, their limited experience, and the peculiar vulnerabilities of the immature hand contribute to these injuries. In nonindustrialized societies, burns of the palmar surface of the pediatric hand are frequent, usually as a result of a fall into an open cooking fire. Industrialized society brings with it other injuries such as those that occur when a child's hand or finger becomes caught in the flywheel of an exercise bicycle or sustains a friction burn from a home treadmill. Pans of boiling water, hot plates, and space heaters often attract the inexperienced hands of young children.

With the encouragement of parents and coaches, children are participating in athletics at an earlier, more vulnerable age. Their hands and wrists are at risk in sports activity, particularly when they are forced to mimic intense adult training regimens. Football, basketball, gymnastics, and downhill skiing are particularly hazardous for the immature hand. Inadequate parental supervision or neglect may be a factor in injuries such as flexor tendon laceration due to knife injuries incurred while carving a pumpkin. Other pediatric hand injuries are the result of parentally inflicted child abuse.

The immature hand is a dynamic, growing composite of many organs. The treatment of children's hand injuries is often different from the treatment of similar injuries in adults. Subsequent growth may correct angulation of fractures that have healed with deformity that would be deemed unacceptable in an adult. In contrast, injury to skeletal growth mechanisms, whether as the result of fracture, infection, or thermal injury may result in deformity that is apparent only with subsequent growth of uninjured elements. The ultimate expression of growth mechanism injuries are more severe when the injury occurs in the younger child. Care of pediatric hand injuries may require monitoring until skeletal maturity or until the viability and normalcy of physeal function can be documented. When longitudinal scar growth lags behind the growth of normal phalangeal elements, contracture results.

The diagnosis of injury is often suggested by the child's reluctance to use the affected hand or finger. Normally there is a cascade of increasing digital flexion, with the middle finger flexed to a greater degree than the index finger, while the ring is flexed more than the middle, and the little finger is flexed more than any of the other three fingers. The altered resting posture of the fingers may suggest a flexor tendon injury (Fig. 37-1). Nerve injury may be more difficult to detect. Because digital arteries accompany digital nerves, pediatric hand wounds that demonstrate pulsatile bleeding usually should be explored under anesthesia, even

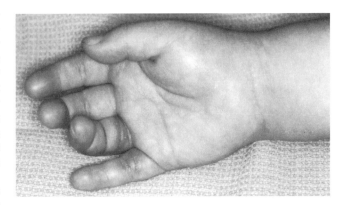

Figure 37-1. This three-year-old girl lacerated the flexor digitorum profundus of the little finger when her hand slipped onto the blade of the knife she was using to carve a pumpkin.

though distal circulation may be entirely satisfactory. If the location of a laceration suggests the possibility of injury to deep structures and the integrity of that structure cannot be proven by clinical examination, the wound should be explored under appropriate anesthesia.

Digital Fractures and Dislocations

The ligaments that support the joints of the immature hand are more resistant to disruption than their adult counterparts. Pure ligamentous injuries are uncommon in children. Conversely, the epiphysis is vulnerable to avulsion disruption. This vulnerability is greatest at the metacarpophalangeal joint where the collateral ligaments insert almost entirely on the epiphysis of the proximal phalanx. In the interphalangeal joints, the collateral ligaments insert on both the epiphysis and metaphysis. This difference in collateral ligament insertion may explain the greater vulnerability of the proximal phalanx to physeal injury. The extensor tendon inserts into epiphyseal bone at the distal phalanx (terminal tendon) and at the middle phalanx level (central slip) while the flexor tendons insert primarily on the metaphysis of the middle and distal phalanges.

Distal Phalanx Fractures

Pediatric distal phalangeal crush injuries are treated in the same manner as adult injuries. In most cases, soft-tissue loss of the distal phalanx may be treated in an open fashion with expectation of excellent healing. Flap coverage is elected when the distal phalangeal skeleton is protruding from the wound. Local V-Y flaps may be useful in mobilizing local sensate skin to provide coverage of protruding bone without shortening the bone. The lateral flaps (described by Kutler) are best in transverse loss, while the palmar flap (described by Atasoy) may be useful in dorsal oblique soft-tissue loss. The thenar flap is particularly useful in the pediatric patient with loss of a major portion of the distal phalanx palmar coverage since residual proximal interphalangeal joint stiffness, a frequent complication in adults, is rare in children.

Displaced Salter I or Salter II fractures occurring in the distal phalanx are regarded as pediatric mallet injuries. The pull of the flexor digitorum profundus inserting on the metaphysis of the distal phalanx tends to flex the distal segment while the insertion of the terminal extensor on the epiphysis tends to hold the proximal fragment in extension, or may result in dorsal and proximal retraction of the articular epiphyseal segment (Fig. 37-2). On rare occasions, the epiphysis may be extruded without attachment to either the extensor or flexor mechanism.

Open distal phalangeal pediatric fractures are often undertreated with adverse consequences. Crush injuries in children younger than age four often have unrecognized longitudinal fractures that may be unappreciated on standard radiographs taken immediately after injury. A rent in the dorsal periosteum may not be apparent unless the proximal nail is retracted distally or the entire nail is removed. These injuries are often overlooked because the proximal nail has flipped out of place to lie in front of the eponychial fold. The displaced nail obscures the underlying nail matrix laceration. Once the nail has been retracted or removed, the fracture site should be debrided and irrigated. The fracture is reduced. The nail bed is repaired and the nail is replaced. If the reduction is judged unstable, a Kirschner wire may be placed across the fracture site, through the epiphysis, and into the middle phalanx, fixing the distal interphalangeal joint in full extension. If an open distal phalangeal fracture is ignored or unrecognized, osteomyelitis is a documented complication (Fig. 37-3).

Salter III fractures of the distal phalanx tend to occur in adolescents with the terminal tendon avulsing a dorsal epiphyseal fragment. Treatment is similar to the adult mallet injury, since growth deformity is unlikely with so little additional growth expected from the adolescent distal phalanx. Nonoperative management, consisting of splinting the joint in extension for four to six weeks, is usually satisfactory.

Proximal and Middle Phalanx Fractures

Fractures of either the proximal or middle phalangeal neck, also referred to as subcondylar fractures, are usually the result of a crush injury. Though these injuries may appear minimally displaced on the AP view, the true lateral radiograph will often demonstrate hyperextension of the condylar fragment (Fig. 37-4). The potential for these fractures to remodel is limited since they are a distance from the physis. Accurate reduction of subcondylar fractures is essential to restoring digital flexion. This usually requires open reduction and internal fixation, most often with small-caliber K-wires (0.028 or 0.035).

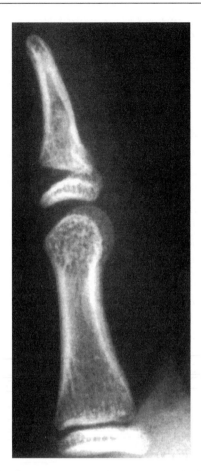

Figure 37-2. Because the flexor digitorum profundus inserts on the metaphysis and the terminal tendon inserts on the epiphysis of the distal phalanx, this Salter I fracture site in a 13-year-old girl tends to gap dorsally as the fragments displace in response to tendon forces.

When phalangeal neck fractures heal in a displaced, hyperextended position, digital flexion is compromised. Rather than attempting to perform an osteotomy on the healed phalanx, flexion can be restored by resection of bone along the palmar edge of the deformed phalanx. By reconstructing and recontouring the subcondylar fossa, the volar edge of the phalanx is free to flex and no longer impinges on the proximal phalanx with digital flexion.

Displaced Salter Type III injuries may occur when the central slip avulses a fragment of the dorsal middle phalangeal epiphysis. Accurate replacement of this fragment is required to prevent articular incongruity as well as boutonnière deformity.

Fractures of the proximal or middle phalangeal shafts are uncommon in children since tubular diaphyseal bone is stronger and more resilient than the adjacent metaphyseal, physeal, and epiphyseal bone. Physeal injuries are most common at the proximal phalangeal level. Abduction of the little finger often results in a displaced Salter II fracture of the proximal phalanx (the so called "extra-octave" fracture). Closed treatment is sufficient to correct resultant

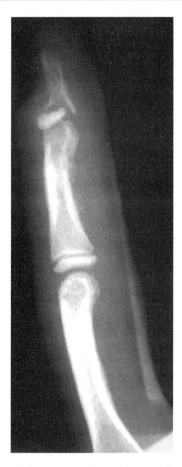

Figure 37-3. Failure to appreciate and appropriately explore, irrigate, and debride this open Salter I fracture resulted in osteomyelitis of the distal phalanx.

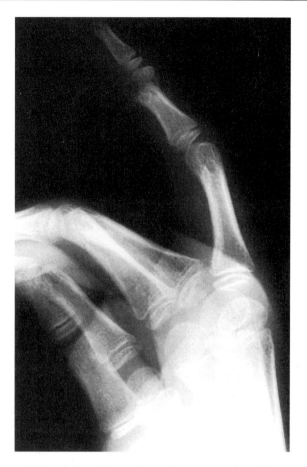

Figure 37-4. Subcondylar phalangeal fractures tend to displace into hyperextension, a position that will block flexion at the adjacent joint.

angulation. Abduction and torsion of other digits may produce Salter II, III, or IV injury patterns (Fig. 37-5). When intra-articular or physeal displacement of Type III or IV fractures results, open reduction is indicated.

Metacarpal Fractures

Metacarpal head fractures usually are the result of an axial crushing force applied to the distal end of the metacarpal. These injuries occur when the metacarpophalangeal joint is flexed, exposing the head to trauma. Decreased longitudinal growth of the metacarpal may result from axial compression physeal injury, but may not become evident until growth abnormality is noted. Salter II fractures of the thumb metacarpal base is a common physeal injury pattern. Closed reduction and cast application usually allows satisfactory healing.

Salter III fractures of the thumb metacarpal base may require open treatment or percutaneous pin fixation.

Interphalangeal Joint Dislocations

Distal and proximal interphalangeal joint dislocations usually can be reduced by closed means. Failure to achieve a closed reduction implies interposition of soft-tissue (eg, volar plate or tendon) in the joint space. Interphalangeal joint dislocations should be splinted in full extension after reduction. Active flexion out of the splint is allowed at seven days. Splint protection is recommended during athletic activity for three weeks after reduction.

Metacarpophalangeal Joint Dislocation

Dislocation of the metacarpophalangeal joint occurs more often in children than in adults. This predisposition has been attributed to the physical characteristics of the soft-tissue support of the joint in children. The collateral ligaments of children are resilient enough to remain intact without avulsion or disruption.

When closed metacarpophalangeal joint dislocations occur in the fingers, the index finger is most often affected, the little finger less frequently, and the middle finger rarely. The volar plate becomes entrapped in the joint space and prevents closed reduction of the joint. Open reduction requires removal of the volar plate from the joint. Associated osteochondral fragments should be sought (Fig. 37-6). Open reduction may be obtained through either a

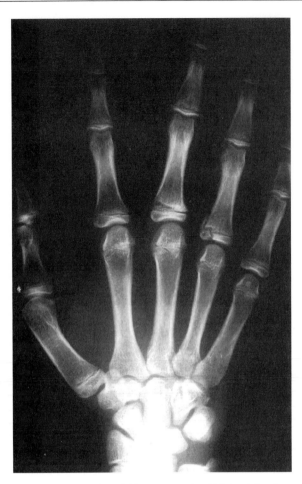

Figure 37-5. Abduction of this youngster's middle and ring fingers by his brother resulted in a Salter I fracture of the middle phalanx and a Salter III fracture of the ring finger. He presented for evaluation one month after the injury.

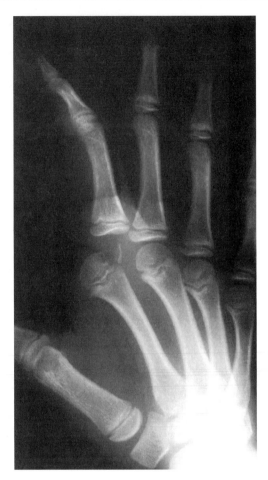

Figure 37-6. Complex dislocation of the index metacarpal in this child was associated with an osteochondral fracture of the metacarpal head.

palmar or dorsal approach. The palmar approach affords direct visualization of vulnerable, displaced neurovascular structures while the dorsal extensor tendon splitting approach exposes dorsal osteochondral fractures. Fractures of the head as well as disruption of metacarpal head vascularity may compromise long-term joint function.

When metacarpophalangeal joint dislocations occur in the thumb, the joint is often reducible by closed techniques. Because of the resiliency of ligaments in children, thumb metacarpophalangeal joint ulnar collateral ligament instability ("gamekeeper's thumb") is usually the result of an avulsion fracture rather than a disrupted ligament. An abduction force on the thumb results in an epiphyseal fracture of the ulnar proximal phalanx. This fracture usually is a Salter-Harris Type III injury. Open reduction and nonthreaded K-wire fixation of the displaced epiphyseal fragment is needed.

Wrist Injuries

Carpal Injuries

The immature carpus is primarily composed of cartilage and is relatively resistant to injury. The cartilaginous carpus is able to absorb compressive force without fracture. When fracture does occur, it is usually the result of considerable violence. Because substantial force is needed to fracture immature carpal bones, many of these injuries involve more than a single carpal bone or involve both the distal radius and the carpus. As the child reaches adolescence and the majority of the carpal is ossified, the patterns of carpal injury begin to resemble those seen in adults.

The most commonly fractured immature carpal bone is the scaphoid. Because the scaphoid is entirely cartilaginous until approximately five years of age, fracture is unlikely in the very young. Between six and 13 years of age, the distal pole ossifies while the proximal pole remains cartilaginous. Scaphoid fractures occur most commonly from age 10 to skeletal maturity. Most adolescent scaphoid fractures involve the distal scaphoid. The most common pattern is an avulsion fracture of the scaphoid tubercle. These tubercle fractures involve a distal radial fragment that unites after cast immobilization. Transverse scaphoid fractures may occur through the junction between the ossified and unossified scaphoid. Nonunion of the pediatric scaphoid is uncommon (Fig. 37-7). It is possible, though unproven, that the so-called bipartite scaphoid represents an unrecognized fracture of the immature scaphoid.

Ligamentous Injuries

Reports of ligamentous injury of the immature wrist are sparse. This probably reflects the fact that these injuries are both rare and difficult to diagnose. Because immature carpal bones are incompletely ossified, it is often impossible to use usual radiographic criteria of instability. The axis of cartilaginous carpal bones is difficult to define when areas of carpal ossification are often circular and eccentrically located within the cartilaginous carpal bone. Further, this eccentric ossification frustrates attempts to detect joint space widening due to instability.

Distal Radius

Fractures of the radius are usually the result of a single traumatic event. When metaphyseal fractures heal with residual angulation, further growth will correct deformity in both the AP and lateral planes.

Two different injuries to the growth mechanism of the distal radius have recently been identified. Each pattern has been described in young gymnasts engaged in repetitive axial loading of the distal radius. These injuries most often occur as a result of gymnastic activity such as floor exercise. The first type of injury occurs in gymnasts between 14 and 16 years of age who are practicing more than 36 hours per week. These adolescents present with pain on dorsiflexion and wrist stiffness. Radiographs demonstrate physeal widening, cystic changes, and metaphyseal beaking of the distal radius, and in some cases of the distal ulna. Cessation of all gymnastic activity leads to resolution of symptoms without long-term sequelae.

The second form of radial injury results in premature closure of the distal radial physis. Physeal closure is usually not evident until a few years after the injury is sustained, again as a result of extensive gymnastic activity. The continued growth of the ulna while the radius length is static results in the ulna's protruding beyond the articular surface of the distal radius. Though the patient usually complains of the painful, unsightly distal ulna, comparative radiographs of both forearms reveal the ulnae to be of similar length and the affected radius to be shorter than the contralateral radius. Impingement of the ulna upon the carpus may result in ulnar-sided wrist pain. Prior to skeletal maturity the unilateral arrest of the distal radial physis may create a Madelung-like appearance if the ulnar aspect of the physis arrests while the more radial physis remains viable.

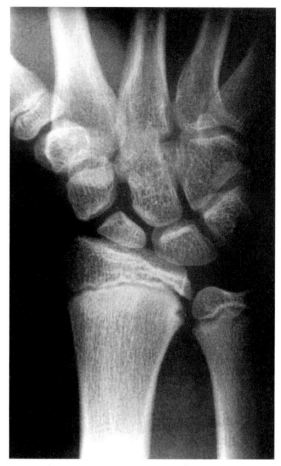

Figure 37-7.   Nonunion of this immature scaphoid was the consequence of injury to the partially ossified scaphoid at age 5+9/12, five years prior to this radiograph.   Reproduced with permission from Larson B, Light T, Ogden J: Fracture and ischemic necrosis of the immature scaphoid. *J. Hand Surg,* 12A:122-127, 1987.

Ulnar shortening osteotomy is usually necessary. As in adults, secure internal fixation of coapted bone surfaces is essential to assure prompt osteotomy healing. If further ulnar growth is anticipated, distal ulnar epiphysiodesis should also be carried out.

Thermal Injury

Burn

Adult burns of the hand tend to be flame burns which are deeper than the scald burns that typically involve the child's hand. Fortunately, many pediatric scald burns are superficial and often heal spontaneously with simple management. Most pediatric scald burns involve the dorsum of the hand and forearm and are the result of spilled hot water. Children may also suffer contact burns, as when the palmar surface of the hand and fingers touches hot objects such as an iron, hot plate, or space heater. These are often deep injuries requiring extensive treatment.

Skin grafts, when needed, may be harvested from many sites; the anterior thigh is most frequently used. The scalp donor site heals quickly and with less pain and residual deformity than other, more visible sites.

Because children form hypertrophic scars more readily than adults, ongoing treatment and follow up are needed until skeletal maturity. Tethering scar may lead to secondary deformities, such as joint contracture, subluxation, or dislocation. Compression garments with molded inserts are often of value to soften scars and prevent contracture. Repeated operations may be necessary over a number of years to address tethering scar.

Though the soft tissues of the digit may be viable, arrest of the phalangeal or metacarpal physes may occur as a result of thermal injury. In other hands, previously unossified epiphyses appear, mature, and fuse at an accelerated rate after a burn. This accelerated development is presumably the result of increased local vascularity, much as one sees in juvenile rheumatoid arthritis.

During the first year after the burn, periosteal new bone formation may be seen in bones beneath areas of soft-tissue burn, presumably reflecting chronic inflammation.

Frostbite

When frostbite involves the immature hand, the distal, and less commonly, the middle and proximal phalanges of the fingers are most vulnerable to injury. The thumb, a shorter digit often clutched in the palm, is usually spared. Though rewarming at 110° may result in normal-appearing viable fingers of full length, the physes may sustain irreparable damage. These physeal injuries result in epiphyseal arrest and often destruction of the epiphysis itself (Fig. 37-8). This leads to proximal joint incongruity and ultimately, destruction of the distal articular surface. The affected interphalangeal joints may become swollen. Angular deformity is common. Nail abnormalities are often associated with distal phalangeal physeal arrest.

Viral Infection

Herpes simplex (not herpes progenitalis) infections of the hand are most common in children between six months and six years of age. While adult herpes simplex infections are most frequently seen in medical or dental workers or in individuals with cancer or acquired immunodeficiency, children with herpetic lesions may, in contrast, have no intercurrent illness. Concomitant oral lesions (herpetic stomatitis) are frequently encountered in children. The clinical picture in children is characterized by painful fluid-filled vesicles, usually on the distal phalanx of a digit (Fig. 37-9). A Tzanik smear of fluid aspirated from a vesicle establishes the diagnosis by demonstrating intracellular viral particles; cultures of fluid aspirate confirms the diagnosis. After a number of days the vesicles spontaneously rupture. A painless crust forms as the viral infection resolves. Broad spectrum oral antibiotic prophylaxis may

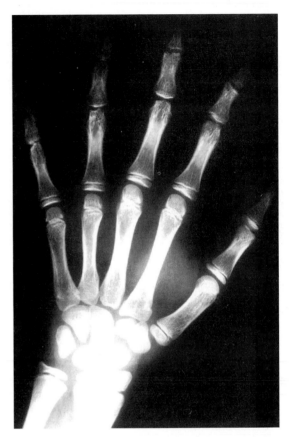

Figure 37-8. Frostbite injury a few years previous has resulted in premature closure of the index, middle, ring, and little finger middle and distal phalangeal physes. The thumb was spared physeal injury.

help prevent secondary bacterial infection after vesicle rupture. Recurrence is noted in approximately one-fifth of cases, and occurs in the same distribution as the original infection, reflecting the persistence of the herpes simplex virus in the corresponding anterior horn cells.

Child Abuse

The hand may be the primary or incidental target of child abuse. The hand can be burned either by immersion in hot liquids or by contact with a hot object (such as an iron or a cigarette). Immersion injuries typically involve a demarcated glove-like pattern and are most common in younger children (Fig. 37-10). With accidental immersion, splash marks are typical; when the hand has been forcibly held in the liquid, splash marks are uncommon. Intentional cigarette burns to the hand result in one centimeter diameter, nearly perfectly round lesions; these may be misdiagnosed as impetigo.

The older child's hand may be incidentally injured when the hand is raised to protect to face or body from being struck or stabbed. The treating physician has a responsibil-

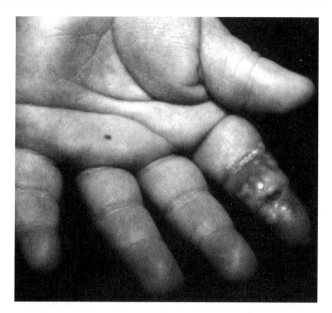

Figure 37-9. Multiple clear fluid-filled vesicles were evident on the palmar aspect of this 11-month-old infant's index finger, herpetic infection. Reproduced with permission from Behr J, et al: Herpetic infections in the fingers of infants. *J Bone Joint Surg,* 1987:137-139.

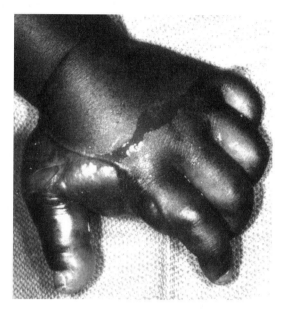

Figure 37-10. This retarded institutionalized child sustained an immersion injury of the radial border of the hand when he was "punished" by a caretaker.

ity to report suspicious injuries. Most physical abuse injuries are bruises, hematomas and abrasions, whose effects fade with time. The physician must recognize the need for intervention, to both deal with the more permanent psychological effects of abuse and to prevent future, potentially fatal abuse.

Annotated Bibliography

Overview

Beatty E, Light TR, Belsole RJ, Ogden JA: Wrist and skeletal injuries in children. *Hand Clin,* 6(4):723-738, 1990.

Considers physeal and periosteal response to fracture and thermal injuries.

Campbell RM: Operative treatment of fractures and dislocations of the hand and wrist region in children. *Orthop Clin North Am,* 21(2):217-243, 1990.

Defines indications for open reduction and internal fixation of pediatric hand and wrist fractures and dislocations. Detailed discussion of technique at ORIF of displaced supracondylar fractures of the phalangeal neck.

Markiewitz AD, Andrish JT: Hand and wrist injuries in the preadolescent athlete 1992; *Clin Sports Med,* 11:203-224.

Injuries to immature athletes more common in football, wrestling, gymnastics, and basketball.

Simmons BP, Lovallo JL: Hand and wrist injuries in children. *Clin Sports Med,* 7:495-512, 1988.

As childhood athletic participation has increased in recent years, the frequency of pediatric hand and wrist injuries has also increased.

Digital Injuries

Hankin FM, Janda DH: Tendon and ligament attachments in relationship to growth plates in a child's hand. *J Hand Surg,* 14B:315-318, 1989.

Dissection of an eight-year-old child's hand defines point of insertion of tendons and ligaments.

Light TR, Ogden JA: Complex dislocation of the index metacarpophalangeal joint in children. *J Pediatr Orthop,* 8:300-305, 1988.

Four cases in children.

Light TR, Ogden JA: Metacarpal epiphyseal fractures. *J Hand Surg,* 12A:460-464, 1987.

Injury due to axial loading of flexed head. Of five cases described, three resulted in longitudinal growth arrest.

Savage R: Complete detachment of the epiphysis of the distal phalanx. *J Hand Surg,* 15B:126-128, 1990.

Case report of distal phalanx epiphysis fracture separation.

Simmons BP, Peters TT: Subcondylar fossa reconstruction for malunions of the proximal phalanx in children. *J Hand Surg,* 12A:1079-1082, 1987.

Three patients increased average flexion from 43° (30°- 65°) preoperatively to 85° (75°- 90°) postoperatively.

Torre BA: Epiphyseal injuries of the small joints of the hand. *Hand Clin,* 4:113-121.

Anatomic and treatment considerations in phalangeal and metacarpal physeal injuries.

Carpal Injuries

Albanese SA, Palmer AK, Kerr DR, Carpenter CW, Lisi D, Levinsohn EM: Wrist pain and distal growth plate closure of the radius in gymnasts. *Ped Orthop,* 9:23-28, 1989.

Three cases of competitive gymnasts detailed.

Carter SR, Aldridge MJ, Fitzgerald R, Davies AM: Stress changes of the wrist in adolescent gymnasts. *Br J Radiology,* 61: 109-112, 1988.

Eight gymnasts and one roller skater developed bilateral radial physeal changes due to chronic repetitive shear on the hyperextended wrist.

Light TR: Injury to the immature carpus. *Hand Clin,* 4:415-424, 1988.

Pediatric carpal fractures, ligamentous injury, and ischemic necrosis are uncommon occurrences. Eccentric carpal ossification patterns influence injury patterns and complicate radiographic evaluation.

Tolat, AR, Sanderson PL, DeSmet L, Stanley JK: The gymnast's wrist: acquired positive ulnar variance following chronic epiphyseal injury. *J Hand Surg,* 17B:678-681, 1992.

Arthroscopy of the wrist was used to evaluate three of five cases of distal radial physeal arrest in teenage female gymnasts.

Zimmerman NB, Weiland AJ: Scapholunate dissociation in the skeletally immature carpus. *J Hand Surg,* 15A:701-705, 1990.

Case report of a 13-year-old boy whose scapholunate dissociation was treated with soft-tissue reconstruction.

Thermal Injury

Clarke HM, Wittpenn GP, McLeod AME, Candlish SE, Guernsey CJ, Weleff DK, Zuker RM: Acute management of pediatric hand burns. *Hand Clin,* 6:221-232, 1990.

Fifty-six patients with 64 burns distal to the elbow. Advocates open treatment of most pediatric hand burns with twice-daily dressing changes, splinting, therapy, psychosocial support, and pain management.

Dado DV, Angelats J: Management of burns of the hands in children. *Hand Clin,* 6(4):711-721, 1990.

Emphasizes need for ongoing evaluation of growing healed burned hand. Notes the characteristics of burns due to child abuse.

Mooney MR, Reed MH: Growth disturbances in the hands following thermal injuries in children. 1. Flame Burns. *J Canadian Assn Radiol,* 39:91-94, 1988.

Five cases each had premature phalangeal or metacarpal physeal closure. Periosteal reaction was a frequent finding.

Mooney MR, Reed MH: Growth disturbance in the hands following thermal injuries in children. 2. Frostbite. *J Canadian Assn Radiol,* 39:95-99, 1988.

All nine patients demonstrated distal phalangeal physeal arrest and phalangeal shortening while seven had evidence of middle phalangeal growth disturbances.

Infection

Walker LG, Simmons BP: Pediatric herpetic hand infections. *J Hand Surgery,* 15A:176-180, 1990.

Among 14 cases seen between five months and six years of age, 80% had associated oral lesions.

Child Abuse

Johnson CF, Kaufman KL: The hand as a target organ: in child abuse. *Clin Ped,* 29(2):66-72, 1990.

Ninety-four of 944 cases of child abuse involved the hand. Of 19 isolated hand injuries, eight were burns, two bruises, two human bites, two fractures, two erythema, and one laceration. Sixty-five percent of all pediatric hand abuse lesions are the result of contusion or hematoma. The hand is often injured in older children trying to protect face or other body parts from being struck.

Compson JP: Trans-carpal injuries associated with distal radial fractures in children: a series of three cases. *J Hand Surg,* 17B: 311-314.

Three cases of transcarpal injury associated with ipsilateral distal radial fracture are described. Two cases involved both the scaphoid and the capitate while the remaining case involved the scaphoid and the triquetrum. Multiple radiographic views may be necessary to detect all fracture lines.

38

Congenital

Graham D. Lister, MD

Failure of Formation of Parts (incidence 12.2% after Cheng)

Failure of formation has been divided into transverse and longitudinal. Transverse deficiencies have been restricted to include all congenital amputations, from absence of the fingers (aphalangia) to absence of the entire upper extremity (amelia). All other failures of formation are considered to be longitudinal deficiencies. Hence intercalated defects—phocomelia—are classified as longitudinal, since the peripheral limb that is present invariably shows anomalies.

Transverse Absence: Carpus, Metacarpus, and Phalanges

The absence of digits may present as a result of several congenital anomalies, the most common being true transverse absence; cleft hand; amputations from constriction ring syndrome; and symbrachydactyly. Symbrachydactyly is unilateral, non-genetic, and has no foot involvement. The "nubbins" of fingers demonstrate nails and a rudimentary skeleton. When oligodactylous, the digits present are on the radial side of the hand. These features contrast with true cleft hand (see below).

Surgical management of transverse absence may include any, all, or none of the following: free phalangeal transfer; ulnar post construction; ormicrovascular toe-to-hand transfer.

Phalangeal transfer can be undertaken if a) there is a suitable soft-tissue envelope, usually present only in symbrachydactyly; b) there is adequate bony support; and c) the child is under 15 months of age, since beyond this age growth of the free graft becomes progressively less likely. Survival of such transfers has been reported in 100% of 69 transfers and appears to be due to preservation of the periosteum and stabilization of the transfer, either by bony union or attachment of the collateral ligaments.

In the absence of adequate skin envelopes for phalangeal transfer, metacarpal remnants can be put to good use, especially the first and fifth (or fourth). The ulnar remnant can be lengthened by interposition or "on top" corticocancellous bone grafting. Transverse absence of the thumb, and less commonly of other digits, at the metacarpal level may be managed by the microsurgical transfer of the second toe. While it is technically possible to achieve survival, the acquisition of function is even more difficult in congenital absence than following traumatic loss of fingers (except in constriction ring amputation which mimics trauma) because of the vestigial nature of all structures in the hand.

For these reasons, complex reconstruction is more strongly indicated in bilateral transverse absence. If undertaken in unilateral, surgery should be performed early in life (during the first year if possible) since the infant becomes less and less likely as it grows older to incorporate the still impaired hand limb into manual handling.

Longitudinal Absence: Distal-Radial Club Hand

This condition may be associated with other anomalies, most commonly cardiac (in 10% to 13% of patients), as in the Holt-Oram syndrome, and varying blood dyscrasias. In the TAR syndrome (thrombocytopenia-absent radii), survival, formerly only 60%, has been improved by platelet transfusion. Fanconi's anemia is the next most serious dyscrasia, associated with progressive pancytopenia and an increased predisposition to malignancy. It is often not apparent in infancy and less pronounced cases may never be diagnosed. Identification in the pre-anaemic stage can be achieved by tests on the peripheral blood and by amniocentesis. All radially dysplastic infants should be so assessed, for early diagnosis allows for appropriate genetic counselling since there is a one in four chance of Fanconi syndrome developing later in children, and also for intrauterine testing during later pregnancies. Such testing both warns of further affected children and offers the possibility of umbilical cord transfusion from those not affected to their older Fanconi sibling. In radial club hand, both extremities are affected in 50% to 72% of cases, depending on the series. The thumb may be normal, hypoplastic, rudimentary, or absent, the incidence varying widely in different series. The elbow of the child with radial club hand may show fixed extension. Passive motion usually improves with manipulation, as does that of the deviated wrist. Such therapy by a parent is superior to application of a splint. The wrist should not be centralized where residual lack of elbow flexion would prevent the corrected hand from reaching the head. The proximal interphalangeal joints show a reduced range of motion, in one series averaging index (24°), middle (35°), ring (57°), small (78°). Despite this reduced motion, true symphalangism rarely occurs. Muscles throughout the upper limb are often deficient. On the extensor aspect, the extensor digitorum may be fused to the wrist extensors. The long flexors, especially the superficial, may be incomplete, atrophic, or fused. Others commonly affected are pectoralis major, biceps, brachioradialis, supinator, extensor carpi radialis, flexor carpi radialis and the muscles of the thumb. Radiologic examination shows the following:

A. Radius stage
  I. Deficient distal radial epiphysis
  II. Complete but short = hypoplasia
  III. Present proximally = partial aplasia
  IV. Completely absent = total aplasia
B. Ulna curved, thickened and only 60% of normal length
C. Humerus also shorter than normal
D. Carpal bone fusions and absence

If elbow flexion has been achieved, centralization or radialization of the carpus on the ulna should be undertaken at six to 12 months of age. The former, more common procedure is achieved by varying amounts of carpal excision, shortening of extensor carpi ulnaris and, where necessary, by angulation closing wedge osteotomy of the curved ulna. Centralization should aim to preserve the distal ulnar epiphysis, although premature fusion is a recognized complication.

Longitudinal Absence: Distal Ulnar = Ulnar Club Hand

Ulnar club hand occurs less frequently than does radial club hand, by a factor varying from 1/3.6 to 1/10. It is characterized by deficiencies on the ulnar side of the hand and forearm and by a varying degree of dysfunction in the elbow. It differs from radial club hand in that in ulnar club hand the wrist is stable, the elbow is not. The anomalies associated with ulnar club hand tend to be of the musculoskeletal system as opposed to the visceral and hematopoietic problems that may accompany the radial deficiency. Several classifications of ulnar club hand have been proposed and Bayne has rationalized these:

I. Hypoplasia of the ulna (both ulnar epiphyses present)
II. Partial aplasia of the ulna (absence of the distal or middle third)
III. Total aplasia of the ulna
IV. Radiohumeral synostosis

Digits are absent from the ulnar side of the hand and in those present, are syndactylized. If digits are absent, carpal bones are also, in the order of frequency of pisiform, hamate, triquetrum, capitate. The forearm and wrist are ulnar deviated. In all except type IV, the elbow is potentially unstable; there may also be radial head dislocation. An ulnar anlage, a fibrocartilaginous band which attaches the carpus distally to the ulna or, if the ulna is absent, to the humerus proximally, is present in types II and IV, not in I and III. In types II and IV, some authors maintain that the ulnar anlage should be excised before six months of age; others of equal authority, believe it should not. In cases of type IV, an osteotomy of the radius may be required to obtain extension of the arm, and to correct the internal rotation which may accompany the radiohumeral synostosis. Syndactyly release and rotation osteotomy of the fingers should be performed during the first year of life. In later cases of type II, the subluxation of the radial head may require radial head resection, with creation of a one-bone forearm if there is insufficient proximal ulna to stabilize the forearm.

Longitudinal Absence: Distal Central = Cleft Hand

Until recently classified as typical or atypical, it is now agreed that atypical is related to symbrachydactyly. The true cleft hand is often bilateral, familial, and involves the feet.

The typical cleft hand can vary in severity from a simple cleft between middle and ring fingers, to absence of the middle finger, to progressive hypoplasia of radial digits, to an oligodactylous syndactyly of ulnar digits. These features contrast with symbrachydactyly (see above). Mild forms of cleft show a degree of adduction contracture of the thumb. Transverse bones may be present in the metacarpus, their presence and growth serving to make the cleft wider. Since the syndactyly, when it exists, is between digits of unequal length in the first and the fourth web space, early correction is required to prevent further deformity of the longer digit. Reconstruction of the thumb may require simple deepening of the first web space, tendon transfers, rotational osteotomy, or even full pollicization. The skin from the cleft can be transferred, with some difficulty, as a palmar based flap into the first web thus combining the two procedures of cleft closure and first space widening. This aim can be achieved more simply by sliding the index towards the ring in a slot of palmar and dorsal V-shaped flaps, as described by Miura. Transverse bones should be excised, taking care not to be so radical as to disturb the metacarpophalangeal joint of a digit to be preserved, a joint in which the transverse bone may be intimately involved.

Failure of Differention of Parts (incidence 31.3%)

Radioulnar Synostosis

This condition occurs at the proximal forearm in the large majority and is bilateral in 60% of cases. Examination reveals a fixed pronation deformity which exceeds 50° in 50% of cases. Some compensation for this limitation is provided by hypermobility of the wrist, which permits up to 50° of rotation. The radius is heavy and bowed, the ulna straight and narrow. Where a case is unilateral and minor, no treatment is indicated. In severe cases, a rotational osteotomy through the synostosis should be performed at age five. In unilateral cases the limb is placed at 10° to 20° of pronation, in bilateral the dominant is fixed at 30° to 45° of pronation, the nondominant at 20° to 35° of supination.

Symphalangism

Symphalangism (congenital stiffness of a finger at any joint) affects mainly the proximal interphalangeal joint and is commonly associated with varying degrees of shortness of the middle phalanx. Hereditary symphalangism is transmitted as an autosomal dominant trait, is often associated with correctable hearing loss, and is more common in ulnar than in radial digits. Nonhereditary symphalangism occurs in association with syndactyly, Apert's syndrome, Poland's syndrome, and anomalies of the feet, in that order of incidence. Radiologic evaluation may be confusing, for the middle phalangeal epiphysis may appear to be a joint space. Indications for surgery in infancy do not exist. Both function and appearance may be improved by an angulation osteotomy in late adolescence, once the epiphysis has fused.

Camptodactyly

A congenital flexion deformity of the digit, usually at the proximal interphalangeal joint, camptodactyly is most commonly encountered in the small finger. There are two types, one which appears in infancy and affects the sexes equally and one which usually first presents in girls in their early adolescence. Both types of deformity may become much more marked during the teenage growth spurt. Function is rarely, if ever, affected. Most cases are due to either an abnormal insertion of the lumbrical or an abnormal origin and/or insertion of the superficialis. Radiologic examination may show characteristic changes:

I. The neck of the proximal phalanx shows an indentation corresponding to the anterior lip of the base of the middle phalanx when in full flexion

II. The base of the middle phalanx is wider than normal in an antero-posterior direction

III. The head of the proximal phalanx, rather than being a full, smooth arc of a circle matching other heads and congruous with the base of the middle phalanx, has a blunt-pointed configuration such as would be produced by grinding off the palmar surface of the head.

When the radiologic findings are well established, soft-tissue procedures are unlikely to restore extension and are contraindicated. When the radiograph shows a normal bony outline, the palmar aspect of the digit should be explored, seeking in particular anomalies of the lumbrical and/or superficialis. Where flexion of the metacarpophalangeal joint produces full active proximal interphalangeal joint extension, release of the abnormal tendon with transfer to the radial lateral band is indicated. Camptodactyly of several digits is seen in arthrogryposis, has a much more complex anatomy, and is relatively intractable; full thickness skin grafts, tendon lengthening, and capsulectomy may give limited improvement.

Clinodactyly

This is curvature of a digit in a radioulnar plane. It is most commonly seen in the small finger and next frequently in the triphalangeal thumb. In most instances finger curvature turns the tip of the digit towards the midline of the hand and is due to a deformity of the middle phalanx. The two articular surfaces of any phalanx should be parallel in an antero-posterior projection. In clinodactyly, they are not. There are three different forms of clinodactyly:

I. Minor angulation normal length—very common

II. Minor angulation short phalanx—present in 25% of children with Down's syndrome, only 3% in others

III. Marked angulation—delta phalanx

The delta phalanx comes about as a result of an abnormal epiphysis, which extends from one end of the normal proximal epiphysis around and along the short side a "J-shaped epiphysis," usually continuing to form an abnormal distal epiphysis to the bone, thus creating a "C-shaped epiphysis" and a "longitudinally bracketed diaphysis." When the epiphysis is not ossified, the presence of a delta phalanx is suggested by displacement of the diaphysis towards the convex side of the clinodactylous digit. The delta phalanx is usually seen in infancy. When the digit is too long, especially where the phalanx is an additional one, as in triphalangeal thumb, then early excision should be performed. The ligaments should be preserved and repaired. When the delta phalanx replaces a normal constituent of a consequently short finger, opening wedge osteotomy should be performed. This not only straightens and lengthens the digit it also breaks the continuity of the abnormal epiphysis.

Flexed Thumb

The two main causes are trigger thumb and clasped thumb, distinguished by the fact that the fixed flexion in the first is of the interphalangeal joint alone, while in the latter the metacarpophalangeal joint is affected also.

Trigger digits may involve the fingers as well as the thumb, may not be due solely to problems at the A1 pulley, and may prove relatively intractable. However, by far the majority of congenital cases involve the thumb alone and, if they do not resolve spontaneously, will respond immediately to release of the A1 pulley.

Clasped thumb falls into two groups: supple, due solely to weak or absent extensors pollicis; and complex, which has hypoplastic extensor tendons, flexion contracture of the metacarpophalangeal joint, ulnar collateral ligament laxity, thenar muscle absence or hypoplasia, adduction contracture of the carpometacarpal joint, and inadequate skin in the first web space. The complex clasped thumb is often associated with the ulnar deviation and flexion contracture at the metacarpophalangeal joints and wrist dorsiflexion characteristic of a "wind-blown hand," or congenital ulnar drift of the fingers. If this complex exists in conjunction with typical facial deformities, the condition is known as "whistling face syndrome" or Freeman-Sheldon syndrome. Complex clasped thumb has been reported to have a high association with arthrogryposis.

Supple clasped thumb diagnosed in infancy should be splinted for three months in extension and then reassessed. If extension is present, but weak, splinting should continue. If it is not, then a tendon transfer is required. The common choice for transfer, the extensor indicis, may be absent and an alternative must be sought during examination. Complex clasped thumb requires extensive release on the palmar aspect. Full and free extension may only be achieved when the first dorsal interosseous, the adductor pollicis and both heads of the flexor pollicis brevis have been released. The flexor pollicis longus may be short and require step-cut lengthening. A transposition flap is often required to maintain the release achieved with a full thickness graft on the secondary defect. The ulnar collateral ligament of the metacarpophalangeal joint of the thumb may need added strength. Finally, transfers may be required both for extension and, in cases with thenar atrophy, opposition.

Arthrogryposis

Arthrogryposis (curved joints) is due to a defect in the motor unit as a whole, at some point between the anterior horn cells and the muscle itself. It has thus been divided into neurogenic and myopathic, the former constituting over 90% of cases. The resultant severe muscle weakness occurs early in fetal life, producing immobility of joints which proceed to contractures. The contractures are present at birth and do not progress thereafter. Involvement may be minimal, moderate, or severe; it is symmetrical; upper and lower extremities are equally impaired. These patients may be categorized by a classification useful in planning treatment:

I. Single localized deformities, forearm pronation contracture, complex clasped thumb, loss of wrist and/or finger extensors, intrinsic contracture

II. Full expression of arthrogryposis with absence of shoulder musculature, thin tubular limbs, elbows fixed, usually in extension, sometimes flexion, wrist fixed in flexion and ulnar deviation, fingers fixed usually in intrinsic plus posture, thumb adducted, skin thick and shiny with no creases

III. Same as II with added anomalies including polydactyly and involvement of systems others than the neuromusculoskeletal

In group I cases, correction of the isolated deformity is usually achieved surgically. In the more complex groups II and III, efforts are directed at overcoming contractures and replacing essential motors that are not functioning. The minimal goals are to achieve function in elbow extension on at least one side to assist in pushing off and using crutches, and in elbow flexion on at least one side for eating and hygiene. Initially contractures are addressed by progressive casting, splints, and stretching exercises. If these are unsuccessful, then surgical correction may be achieved by capsulectomy or, in more severe cases, skeletal adjustment. For internal rotation of the shoulder this would require a rotational osteotomy; for flexion contracture of the wrist, proximal row carpectomy. The most significant active transfer is that to retrieve elbow flexion, if a satisfactory muscle can be found. Wrist extension, once achieved, is also maintained by transfer if one is available. Finger posture will be improved by successful management of the wrist and further splinting, but occasionally arthrodesis of the proximal interphalangeal joints will be required. It is most important that essential functions not be impaired by operative procedures such as tendon transfers, particularly in the more complex groups II and III, in which function is often marginal.

Syndactyly

This most common condition is classified as complete, in which the involved digits are united as far as the distal phalanx, or incomplete, in which they are united farther than the midpoint of the proximal phalanx but short of the distal phalanx; complex, in which bony union exists between the involved digits; or simple, in which no such bony union exists. Acrosyndactyly, in which fusion is present between the more distal portions of the digits, and in which there frequently is some proximal fenestration from dorsal to palmar surfaces, occurs as a manifestation of constriction ring syndrome. When syndactyly presents alone (endogenous) it is transmitted by a dominant gene, but with reduced penetrance and variable expression, so that a family history is present in from 10% to 40% of patients, depending on the series. Fifty percent of such cases are bilaterally symmetrical. The incidence of ray involvement can best be recalled by the mnemonic "5.15.50.30":

- Thumb-index (5%)
- Index-middle (15%)
- Middle-ring (50%)
- Ring-small (30%)

Anomalies of tendons, nerves, and vessels occur with increasing frequency the more complete a syndactyly. Even in the most simple complete syndactyly, the bifurcations of both nerve and artery lie distal to the normal location.

Poland's syndrome is a rare, nongenetic disorder characterized by four features:

I. Unilateral shortening of the digits, mainly the index, long and ring, due largely to shortness or absence of the middle phalanx

II. Syndactyly of the shortened digits, usually of a simple, complete type

III. Hypoplasia of the hand, and, to a lesser degree, of the forearm

IV. Absence of the sternocostal head of the pectoralis major muscle on the same side, associated in a decreasing proportion with

   a. Absence of the pectoralis minor

   b. Hypoplasia of the breast and nipple (33% of affected females)

   c. Contraction of the anterior axillary fold

   d. Absence of serratus anterior, latissimus dorsi, and deltoid

   e. Rib deficiencies, thoracic scoliosis, and dextrocardia

Apert's syndrome is characterized by acrocephaly with hypertelorism and bilateral complex syndactyly with symphalangism. The index, middle, and ring fingers frequently share a common nail. The thumb is involved in the syndactyly in one-third of cases; it often demonstrates a delta proximal phalanx with resultant radial deviation.

Certain general rules apply to syndactyly release; there may be exceptions in specific cases. Early separation is indicated in acrosyndactyly, in which the distal bond alone should be released as soon as possible after birth, and in syndactyly between rays of unequal length, which should be formally separated by six months of age. Where two digits have a common nail, syndactyly separation should be preceded by nail division with introduction of additional skin using a thenar flap. The sinus fenestration present in acrosyndactyly is always too far distal to form the new web space but must always be excised during division. Syndactyly release should not be performed simultaneously on adjacent webs, that is, on both sides of one digit. The new web must always be constructed of local skin. Full thickness skin grafts are always required, except in the most minor of incomplete cases.

Duplication (incidence 35.9%)

Polydactyly

Duplication of the small finger, in strong contrast to that of the thumb, is usually the result of an autosomal recessive trait and is often part of a syndrome. Its presence therefore dictates the need for a full physical examination. The radial aspect of the hand is involved a little more than the ulnar and both are much more common than central polydactyly. The latter is almost always associated with syndactyly and often shows disorganization of the skeleton.

Duplication of the thumb can occur at any level and is classified by type in the following way:

I.	BIFID distal phalanx	2%
II.	Distal phalanx DUPLICATED	15%

III. BIFID proximal phalanx   6%
IV. Proximal phalanx DUPLICATED   43%
  V. BIFID metacarpal   10%
VI. Metacarpal DUPLICATED   4%
VII. TRIPHALANGIA, in either or both thumbs   20%

By contrast with ulnar polydactyly, thumb duplication is usually unilateral and sporadic, except for type VII, triphalangia, which results from a dominant gene.

In types I and II in which the thumbs are usually of equal size, the Bilhaut-Cloquet sharing procedure can be performed. Since the thumbs are usually small, a little more than half should be taken from each. The difficulties associated with this procedure are residual nail deformity and unintentional epiphysiodesis. If the thumbs are of almost normal size, the first problem can be avoided by taking the entire nail from only one of them, discarding that from the other. The second problem is avoided by accurate matching of the epiphyseal plate, disregarding any incongruity in the joint surface that can be shaved down later in the procedure; the two epiphyses are rarely of equal thickness.

In the more proximal types, size, deviation, function, or passive mobility may make the choice easy. Where the thumbs are equal in all respects, however, then the choice may await exploration before a final decision is made on the basis of tendon and nerve anatomy. In the duplicated types IV and VI (especially the former which is also the most common) the surgeon should favor retention of the ulnar thumb, thereby avoiding reconstruction of the ulnar collateral ligament so important for thumb stability. Certain steps are indicated in type IV to ensure the best result:

1. Exploration and appropriate realignment of the insertions of both flexor and extensor tendons
2. Division of anomalous connections between flexor and extensor tendons
3. Shaving of the metacarpal head on the side of excision of the duplicate in order to eliminate an unsightly prominence
4. Preservation of both ligaments–that between the two duplicated proximal phalanges and that between the metacarpal and the discarded phalanx–for reconstruction of the one collateral
5. Reattachment of the intrinsic muscles

Triphalangeal thumb may present as part of a type VII duplication or as an isolated entity. It may be inherited as a dominant trait. The additional phalanx lies between the proximal and distal phalanges and may be a delta phalanx, producing increasing deviation (see above) or a rectangular phalanx, which may be short or of normal length. In the latter two types, the metacarpal is longer than normal, adding even more length to the already lengthened thumb. A delta phalanx should be totally excised as early as possible and the soft tissues reconstructed. If the patient is seen late, arthrodesis of one joint with wedge osteotomy is required. A rectangular phalanx is treated by resection and arthrodesis of the distal joint, where necessary accompanied by an opponensplasty, widening of the first web space and shortening of the metacarpal. The closer the triphalangeal thumb comes to being a five-fingered hand, the more should formal pollicization be considered (see below).

Central Polydactyly

This, the least common of the duplications, affects the ring finger in more than half of the cases and the middle and index fingers in about an equal number of cases. It is frequently associated with syndactyly, thereby producing a "hidden central polydactyly," and is the most difficult polydactyly to treat. This is because it is intimately involved anatomically with both of the digits between which it lies, and also because they are impaired to a differing degree. Early surgery is indicated since deviation of the digits to be retained only worsens and correction becomes more difficult with time. It is important to emphasize to the parents a number of points:

- Impairment of motion may be due to the interposed extra digit or to an indeterminable degree of limitation in the apparently normal digits alongside, even to the point of symphalangism, the implications of which must be explained.
- Tendons and nerves may be shared between two or even three digits in central polydactyly.
- Deviation of the "normal" digits which may be evident or concealed may require ligament reconstruction with simultaneous or subsequent angulation osteotomy.
- The anomalies existing within an apparently simple complete syndactyly may be so great that only one functional finger can be obtained from the three digital skeletons available.

Overgrowth (incidence 0.5%)

Macrodactyly

Macrodactyly is a nonhereditary congenital enlargement of a digit. It is unilateral in 90% of cases. In 70% of those afflicted the condition affects more than one digit, those always being adjacent and corresponding to the territory of one or more peripheral nerves, most commonly the median. The enlargement is more pronounced distally than proximally, thus phalanges are affected more frequently than metacarpals. All tissues that respond late in development to neurogenic influence are enlarged: nerves, fat, skin appendages, and bone. Two types of macrodactyly have been described:

- Static—present at birth, the enlargement keeps pace with growth of the normal digits.
- Progressive—sometimes not apparent until as late as two years of age, this form is more aggressive, growing more quickly than adjacent digits and involving the adjacent palm.

Joint stiffness becomes more severe with age and excessive growth. Deviation is a common accompaniment, due to uneven overgrowth of the two borders of the digit. In adult patients, compression of the enlarged median nerve may lead to carpal tunnel syndrome. Ulceration of the fingertips may be evidence of impaired neuro-vascular status.

The severely affected single digit that has little motion, gross curvature, and poor circulation should be amputated. When the thumb or multiple digits are affected, epiphyseal ablation and osteotomies (both shortening, to reduce length, and angulatory, to correct deviation) will give modest reduction. Further shortening with nail preservation and longitudinal narrowing osteotomies are often required. Nerve stripping and extensive defatting to the extent of creating "flap grafts" achieve some meager soft-tissue reduction. Many operations are required and each reduces blood and nerve supply and contributes to scarring and stiffness.

Undergrowth (incidence 4.3%)

Hypoplasia and Aplasia of the Thumb

Hypoplasia of the thumb has been classified by Blauth:

Grade I   Minor hypoplasia, in which all elements are present, the thumb being overall somewhat smaller than normal

Grade II   Adduction contracture of the first web space
           Laxity of the ulnar collateral ligament of the metacarpophalangeal joint
           Hypoplasia of the thenar muscles
           Normal skeleton, with respect to articulations

Grade III Significant hypoplasia, with aplasia of intrinsics
           Rudimentary extrinsic tendons, if any
           Skeletal hypoplasia, especially of the vestigial carpometacarpal joint

Grade IV   Floating thumb (pouce flottant), a vestigial, totally uncontrolled digit attached just proximal to the metacarpophalangeal joint of the index finger

Grade V   Total absence

Hypoplasia, especially of grade II, may be associated with the following:

I.   Duplication of the thumb
II. Triphalangia, with or without delta phalanx
III. Anomalies of tendons and muscles, including:
    a. Flexor pollicis longus, which may be absent, rudimentary or attached to the extensor tendon—the pollex abductus
    b. Eccentric insertion of extrinsic motors on the distal phalanx with resultant deviation of the distal phalanx, early or late
    c. Anomalous extensors
    d. Aplasia of the thenar muscles.

Where flexion creases are absent or rudimentary, abduction at the metacarpophalangeal joint may be seen and the tendon of the anomalous flexor pollicis longus of a pollex abductus palpated where it crosses the hypoplastic thenar area.

In Blauth grade I, no treatment is required. In grades III, IV, and V, pollicization of the index finger gives the best functional thumb. Parents may express reluctance to sacrifice a hypoplastic thumb, especially of grade III; however, the deficiencies of skeleton, joints, motors, and size can never be restored. Grade II hypoplasia requires exploration of flexor and extensor tendons and correction of any anomalies; release of the first web space; opponensplasty; and stabilization of the metacarpophalangeal joint. Tendon anomalies are most significant on the flexor surface. In 27% of one series, pollex abductus, an anomalous attachment from flexor to extensor, was located. Such a tendon

slip should be removed. Of the 27%, 30% showed an abnormal origin of the first lumbrical from the anomalous flexor of the thumb. This also should be sought and removed, as its action narrows the first web space further. Flexor pollicis longus, if absent or grossly anomalous, may require replacement using immediate or two-stage tendon graft. In such circumstances, and even in some cases where the flexor is adequate, pulley reconstruction will be required at the level of the proximal phalanx. Release of the web space may be achieved with a two-flap or four-flap Z-plasty, but frequently additional skin is required.

Opponensplasty is most frequently achieved by use of the flexor digitorum superficialis. Stabilization of the metacarpophalangeal joint is undertaken by fusion, leaving the epiphyseal plate undisturbed; reconstruction, using the distal end of the opponensplasty tendon; or tendon graft attachment to the vestigial ligament or through bone.

Constriction Ring Syndrome (incidence 6.5%)

This condition occurs sporadically, there being no evidence of heredity. It may manifest itself in four ways:
1. Simple constriction rings
2. Rings accompanied by distal deformity, with or without lymphoedema
3. Rings accompanied by distal fusion—acrosyndactyly
4. Amputations

In the severe cases even where no emergency exists, both circulation and neurological function are impaired. Early release of constriction rings is required in the immediate neonatal period where edema is gross. Contrary to traditional teaching, there is no hazard in multiple, circumferential Z-plasties, incorporating both skin, subcutaneous tissue, and fascia. Amputation fortunately usually occurs in only one or two fingers and good function can be achieved with the remaining digits, which may be enhanced by ray resection of the residual stumps. Partial aplasia of the thumb is treated by one of the following procedures: phalangization; metacarpal lengthening; toe-to-hand transfer; or pollicization of another shortened digit. The considerations involved in choosing the correct procedure are existing length, intrinsic function, presence of a basal joint, and the condition of the other digits.

Recent Advances

In classification, the decision to eliminate the distinction between typical and atypical cleft hand, recognizing all of the latter as symbrachydactyly, is to be applauded. Ogino's demonstration of the apparent embryologic association between cleft hand, central polydactyly, and syndactyly awaits further confirmation and raises doubts, if proven, about the current classification used herein.

In investigation, the use of improved imaging techniques, including enhanced fetal sonography, digital subtraction angiography, and magnetic resonance imaging, promise earlier, more detailed information for the surgeon.

In surgical treatment, the merits of earlier surgery and microsurgical toe transfer in carefully selected cases are relatively well established. Corticotomy and distraction of short bones (such as the ulnar in radial club hand, which has given an increase of 10 cm in one case and 47.8% lengthening in one series, both with no loss of function) is promising but requires more study before clear indications can be established.

Annotated Bibliography

Alter BP: Arm anomalies and bone marrow failure may go hand in hand. *J Hand Surg,* 17:566-571, 1992.

Children with congenital hand differences may have inherited bone marrow failure syndromes, most notably Fanconi's anemia, Diamond Blackfan syndrome and thrombocytopenia-absent radii (TAR) syndrome. These are often not apparent at birth or even at surgery, but evidenced by increased mean corpuscular volume and steady decline in hemoglobin levels and platelet counts.

Auerbach AD, Liu Q, Ghosh MS, Pollack GW, Douglas GW, Broxmeyer HE: Prenatal identification of potential donors for umbilical cord blood transplantation for Fanconi's anemia. *Transfusion,* 30:682-687, 1990.

Umbilical cord blood is successfully used for transplantation instead of bone marrow in the treatment of Fanconi's anemia. This, and the possibility of using umbilical cord blood in place of bone marrow as a source of transplantable cells for treating certain hematopoietic diseases, is discussed.

Brons JT, van der Harten, van Giejn HP, Wladimiroff JW, et al: Prenatal ultrasonographic diagnosis of radial-ray reduction malformations. *Prenat Diagn,* 10:279-288, 1990.

Radial-ray reduction malformations (RRRM) may be isolated or occur in association with other congenital anomalies. Data is reviewed from seven fetuses born with RRRM, six of which had associated lethal abnormalities. Guidelines are given and discussed for a diagnostic approach before and after birth for the infant with RRRM.

Buck-Gramcko D: Radialization as a new treatment for radial club hand. *J Hand Surg,* 10:964-968, 1985.

In "radialization," as opposed to centralization, the radial carpal bones are brought over the head of the ulna, without carpal bone resection, and pinned in some overcorrection, which is maintained by transfer of the flexor and extensor carpi radialis to the ulnar side of the hand.

Buck-Gramcko D: Congenital malformations (editorial). *J Hand Surg,* 15:150-152, 1990.

Comments are made on the papers of Ogino, Siegert, and others, and of Hadidi and others (see below). With respect to arteriography, the author, on the basis of his experience of over 2,500 operations on congenital differences of the hand, states that the risks outweigh the possible advantages. On the subject of the outcome of syndactyly correction, he states that unsatisfactory results are caused by incorrect incisions or by disturbances in wound healing.

Cheng JC, Chow SK, Leung PC: Classification of 578 cases of congenital upper limb anomalies with the IFSSH system – 10 years' experience. *J Hand Surg,* 12:1055-1060, 1987.

In a review of 728 congenital differences of the upper extremity seen over a 10-year period, the incidence of the seven IFSSH groups was that given in the above text. Many common differences had not been included in the IFSSH classification, and difficulties were encountered in classifying multiple disorders.

Delaney TJ, Eswar S: Carpal coalitions. *J Hand Surg,* 17:28-31, 1992.

This series of 36 cases, the largest in the literature, showed 32 lunatotriquetral, two capitohamate, one scapholunate, and one capitotrapezoid. It also confirmed that they are asymptomatic, often bilateral, and are much more common in blacks than in whites.

Eaton CJ, Lister GD: Toe transfer for congenital hand defects. *Microsurg,* 12:186-95, 1991.

This review, with 134 references, emphasizes that toe transfer offers most favorable results in constriction ring amputation, when the child is under two years of age and the digit being replaced is the thumb. Details of operative technique as described by different authors are given. Management of postoperative spasm is analyzed. Return of sensibility is more predictable than is the achievement of motion.

Gilbert A: Congenital absence of the thumb and digits. *J Hand Surg Br,* 14:6-17, 1989.

The author reviews his wide experience in absence of digits with a normal thumb; cleft hand; thumb aplasia; absence of thumb and digits treated variously by bone graft, toe phalanx transfer, pollicization, and microvascular toe transfer. With respect to the latter, he reports three failures from 97 cases, 83° of total mobility and 85% of expected growth.

Hadidi AT, Kaddah NT, Zaki MS, Sami A, Aal NA: Congenital malformations of the hand. A study of the vascular pattern. *J Hand Surg Br,* 15:171-180, 1990.

Comparison of three techniques in 65 children, whose ages ranged from 13 days to nine years, showed that direct exposure of the brachial artery through a 1-cm incision gave the best, safest, and quickest results. In transverse deficiencies, the median artery was always present, an atypical superficial arch always accompanied radial deficiencies, the ulnar artery was dominant in all cases of ulnar ray deficiency, and the sole artery to the dominant thumb in duplication may pass very close to the one to be excised.

Jennings JF, Peimer CA, Sherwin FS: Reduction osteotomy for triphalangeal thumb: an 11-year review. *J Hand Surg,* 17:8-14, 1992.

Reduction osteotomy of 13 triphalangeal thumbs followed for an average of 65 months showed active motion of 63° at the interphalangeal joint and 79° at the metacarpophalangeal joint.

Reduction osteotomy of 13 triphalangeal thumbs followed for an average of 65 months showed active motion of 63° at the interphalangeal joint and 79° at the metacarpophalangeal joint.

Ledesma-Medina J, Bender TM, Oh KS: Radiographic manifestations of anomalies of the limbs. *Radiol Clin North Am,* 29:383-405, 1991.

A review of embyology, etiology, and classification of limb anomalies with a focus on the role of plain radiographs in the diagnosis and treatment of various upper and lower limb anomalies.

Light TR (ed): The pediatric upper extremity. *Hand Clin,* 6(4):551-738, 1990.

This overview has chapters on syndactyly, polydactyly, radial dysplasia, digital augmentation in transverse absence, thumb hypoplasia, phalangeal transfer, cleft hand, and the "super digit."

Light TR, Manske PR: Congenital malformations and deformities of the hand. *AAOS Instr Course Lect,* 38:31-71, 1989.

This instructional course lecture reviews congenital deformities or malformations of the hand and the surgical reconstruction recommended. A strong emphasis is placed on the need to individualize goals and techniques to balance both function and appearance.

Lister G: Pollex abductus in hypoplasia and duplication of the thumb. *J Hand Surg,* 16:626-633, 1991.

The anomalous connection between flexor and extensor tendons of the thumb known as pollex abductus was found in 20 cases, 35.5% of all cases of thumb hypoplasia Blauth Type II and 21.4% of Wassel types III, IV and V duplication. In six of 11 thumb hypoplasia cases, an anomalous M. lumbricalis pollicis was found passing from the flexor pollicis longus to the extensor hood of the index finger.

Manske PR: Treatment of duplicated thumb using a ligamentous/periosteal flap. *J Hand Surg,* 14:728-733, 1989.

The importance of elevation of a ligament-periosteal flap from, and reduction osteotomy of, the proximal bone with ligament reconstruction in achieving a stable thumb is emphasized. Three of 22 thumbs required later arthrodesis due to the instability of the opposite ligament.

Manske PR (ed): Thumb reconstruction. *Hand Clin,* 8(1):1-196, 1992.

This review volume contains chapters on the windblown hand, pre-axial polydactyly, and the congenitally deficient thumb.

Mantero R, Rossello MI, Grandis C: Digital subtraction angiography in preoperative examination of congenital hand malformations. *J Hand Surg,* 14:351-352, 1989.

Using the approach favored by Hadidi and others (see above), digital subtraction angiograms were performed on 34 patients in five years. The most common variations seen were distalization of the digital arterial bifurcation, agenesis of one or both palmar arches, digital monoarterialization, hypoplasia of proper digital arteries, and single vessel forearms.

Miura T, Nakamura R, Horii E: Congenital hand anomalies in Japan: a family study. *J Hand Surg,* 15:439-444, 1990.

In a study of 1,024 patients, postaxial polydactyly showed familial recurrence 33%, symphalangism and Kirner's deformity 23%, syndactyly 18%, radioulnar synostosis 9%, radial ray deficiency 8%, cleft hand 7%, and duplicated thumb 5%. None of the relatives had ulnar deficiency or symbrachydactyly.

Netscher DT, Scheker LR: Timing and decision-making in the treatment of congenital upper extremity deformities. *Clin Plast Surg,* 17:113-131, 1990.

Urgent surgery, which is required in severe constriction ring syndrome causing lymphedema and aplasia cutis, should be done in the first five weeks. Less pressing conditions, complex syndactyly, syndactyly between digits of unequal length, radial club hand, and delta phalanx should be corrected once the child develops active immunity at six months. All surgery should be completed by the end of the second year at the latest.

Ogino T: Teratogenic relationship between polydactyly, syndactyly, and cleft hand. *J Hand Surg Br,* 15:201-209, 1990.

These three conditions, which lie in different groups of the IFSSH classification, are shown experimentally in rats and in a review of 75 patients to arise probably from the same teratogenic factor acting at the same developmental period.

Siegert JJ, Cooney WP, Dobyns JH: Management of simple camptodactyly. *J Hand Surg Br,* 5:15:181-189, 1990.

A review of 57 patients showed 18% good or excellent results following surgery compared with 66% following conservative management. Sixteen of 21 patients treated operatively lost flexion. The authors recommend conservative treatment where the extension deficit is less than 60%.

Smith RJ: Congenital deformities of the hand. *Hand Clin,* 1(3):371-594, 1985.

This overview, edited by Richard Smith, considers future development of preventive surgery, upper limb development, etiology and associated malformations, distraction lengthening, microsurgery, congenital ulnar drift, pseudarthrosis, cleft hand, ulnar deficiency, macrodactyly, polydactyly, clasped thumb, and a different classification of thumb hypoplasia.

Tsuge K: Treatment of macrodactyly. *J Hand Surg,* 10:968-969, 1985.

This author reports his experience in treating 30 cases of macrodactyly over 30 years. In minimal cases, he recommends total removal of the hypertrophic nerve and excision of the epiphyseal plate, with wedge osteotomy where necessary. In advanced cases, Tsuge excises the tip, reduces the nail, and excises the metacarpophalangeal joint.

Upton J, Zuker RM: Apert syndrome. *Clin Plast Surg,* 18:217-435, 1991.

This overview of Apert syndrome includes chapters on classification and pathological anatomy of limb anomalies, syndactyly correction, and management of the shoulder, elbow, forearm and thumb.

Upton J, Tan C: Correction of constriction rings. *J Hand Surg,* 16:947-953, 1991.

In a review of 116 constriction rings, the authors recommend mobilizing subcutaneous fat and fascial flaps as well as employing the customary Z-plasty flaps. Comparing 55 rings treated by this method with 61 treated traditionally, the authors found complications to be less and the results superior.

Wilson MR, Louis DS, Stevenson TR: Poland's syndrome: variable expression and associated anomalies. *J Hand Surg,* 13:880-882, 1988.

A series of 20 patients showed, apart from generalized hypoplasia and syndactyly, missing digits in two, hypoplastic metacarpals or phalanges in 11 and flexor tendon absence in one. Thirty-one other anomalies were seen in this group apart from those generally associated with Poland's syndrome.

Wood VE, Biondi J: Treatment of the windblown hand. *J Hand Surg,* 15:431-438, 1990.

Congenital ulnar drift or windblown hand is a rare occurrence

39

Cerebral Palsy in the Upper Extremity

James H. House, MD

Introduction

Cerebral palsy may be described as a nonprogressive central nervous system lesion, usually resulting from anoxic injury in the perinatal period. The prevalence of cerebral palsy in children has been estimated at five per 1,000. Cerebral palsy has been classified by the type of motor deficiency, including athetotic/dystonic, spastic, atonic, and mixed disorder. Spastic cerebral palsy accounts for roughly one-third, and it is that subgroup which is most predictably improved by surgical intervention. Upper extremity function in an individual with cerebral palsy is compromised in several ways: lack of voluntary control, sensibility deficiencies, muscular imbalances including both spasticity and weakness, joint contractures, and articular instabilities. The typical upper extremity posture is one of shoulder internal rotation and adduction, elbow flexion, forearm pronation, wrist flexion and ulnar deviation, and thumb adduction and flexion (thumb-in-palm deformity). Occasionally, a dynamic finger swan neck deformity is observed secondary to intrinsic muscle spasticity. Shoulder and elbow deformities make it difficult to position the hand in space. Wrist and digital deformities may impair grasp and release.

In selected individuals, surgery can improve hand function. The ideal surgical candidate is a motivated, intelligent individual who has good sensibility, and most importantly, demonstrates voluntary use of the extremity. Some degree of sensory impairment is usually present. Sensibility is assessed with stereognosis testing, graphesthesia, two-point discrimination, and proprioception. Stereognosis and graphesthesia require the synsthesis of multiple sensory inputs at the cortical level and are excellent techniques for sensibility evaluation. The better the sensibility, the more useful the extremity, and the more predictable the results of surgical intervention. However, hand/eye coordination can compensate to some degree for poor sensibility.

An individual's IQ is an important consideration. For the most part, this relates to postoperative care. Goldner has suggested that an IQ of 70 or more is necessary for such compliance, although he does not use this as an absolute cut-off. Green has observed a direct correlation between a higher IQ and good surgical results. However, the validity of IQ testing by standard means in patients with cerebral palsy has been questioned. Most surgeons feel that IQ should play a role in surgical decision making, but should not be the sole criterion. It should be emphasized that serial examinations should be performed to accurately evaluate the individual and make plans for surgery.

Physical examination should consist of observation, assessment of joint mobility and muscular contracture, muscle strength, and sensibility of the extremity. The individual is observed for speed and precision of movement, grasp and release with the hand, and the degree to which the hand is utilized. Isolation and specific muscle group strength testing are ideal; however, this is often difficult. Because muscle strength may be masked by overactivity of antagonistic muscle groups, selective muscle or peripheral nerve blocks may facilitate the motor examination. An example would be that of spastic wrist and digital flexors, which may mask the presence of active wrist and digital extensor power. Median nerve block at the elbow temporarily eliminates the activity of these spastic muscles, and previously unidentifiable active wrist extension strength may be recognized. This bears significantly on reconstructive technique selection.

Dynamic electromyography has been employed to help identify muscle activity patterns and the appropriateness of muscle group transfers. In general, transfers are more effective if the transferred muscle group fires in phase with the recipient muscle group. Continuous electromyographic activity is not a contraindication to muscle transfer, and there is some evidence to suggest that these groups may adopt a phasic pattern after transfer.

Nonsurgical Treatment

Physical therapy and occupational therapy are valuable modalities in the postoperative treatment of patients. The role of occupational therapy preoperatively is less defined. A recent study investigating the effectiveness of intensive neurodevelopmental therapy and inhibitive casting (casting over a specific joint, maintaining the joint in a functional tone-inhibiting posture) found that the combination of these two modalities improved the quality of upper extremity movement and range of motion. No immediate benefits from intensive therapy alone were found. Another study has demonstrated improved function and arm/hand position with inhibitory upper extremity casting in young children with hemiplegic cerebral palsy. It is generally felt that inhibitory casting and splint support is valuable in the child younger than four years of age. There is no universal agreement on the beneficial effects of bracing in this population, but nighttime use of wrist and digital extension splints may promote lengthening of muscle-tendon units during growth. No study has demonstrated a decrease in spasticity with bracing, and resistance applied against spastic muscles may serve to strengthen them. A dorsal-based wrist extension splint may be useful as a functional splint. Unless accurately designed, braces and splints can impede rather than facilitate extremity function.

Pharmacologic manipulation of spasticity has had limited success. Oral agents have included the benzodiazapenes, Dantrolene® and L-Dopamine®. No controlled studies have demonstrated their usefulness. The role, if any, of these agents for upper extremity spasticity is unproven. A recent study investigated the intrathecal use of Baclofen® in a randomized double-blind fashion. Muscle tone in the lower extremities was significantly diminished, but upper extremity tone and function were not significantly affected. Neuromuscular blocking agents have been used in a therapeutic as well as a diagnostic fashion. Reversible neuromuscular blocking agents such as 45% ethanol and Botulinum-A toxin have been employed to provide long-term inactivation of spastic muscles groups. These agents are introduced directly into the desired muscle belly and may have a duration of action lasting from six to 20 weeks. The use of Botulinum-A toxin is presently limited to experimental protocols.

Surgical Treatment

Elbow

Elbow flexion contractures of less than 45° to 60° that are minimally increased with activity or anxiety are usually not functionally disabling and do not require intervention. Deformities greater than 60° flexion that worsen with activity may benefit from surgery. Surgical alternatives include lengthening of the biceps tendon distally, usually in the form of Z-plasty, and fractional lengthening of the brachialis at the musculotendinous junction. These two combined procedures can achieve 40° or more of correction. Release of the flexor-pronator origin diminishes elbow flexion contracture, but this procedure has the additional effect of weakening wrist and digital flexors. These additional effects may or may not be desirable. Many surgeons choose to address wrist and digital flexor spasticity distally, where individual muscle groups can be selectively lengthened. Also, lengthening of the biceps tendon may lead to worsening of a forearm pronation deformity if present and not concomitantly addressed.

Forearm

Forearm pronation deformity is due to spasticity in the pronator teres and pronator quadratus muscle groups. When severe, this deformity makes useful positioning of the hand for many activities difficult. Grasping a walker or a cane, balancing objects in the palm, and accepting change are activities that require some forearm supination. Surgical procedures that have been designed to reduce forearm pronation deformity or improve active supination include release of the lacertus fibrosis, release of the pronator teres insertion, pronator teres rerouting, flexor-pronator slide, and pronator quadratus recession. Addressing the pronator quadratus contracture is seldom necessary after release or transfer of the pronator teres. Long-standing pronation contracture of the forearm leads to relative shortening of the lacertus fibrosis (biceps aponeurosis). If this structure is taut with attempted forearm supination it should be released, thereby allowing the biceps to be a more effective supinator. A recent study has compared release of the pronator teres from its radial insertion with rerouting through the interosseous membrane and reinsertion on the anterolateral of the radius. This study demonstrated improved active supination in the pronator transfer group, with an average gain in supination of 54° for the pronator teres release, and 78° for pronator teres rerouting. Flexor-pronator origin release diminishes forearm pronation deformity. If wrist flexion deformity exists, and flexor carpi ulnaris (FCU) transfer is planned to supplement wrist extension, transfer to the extensor carpi radialis longus (ECRL) or brachioradialis (ECRB) (as described by Manske) provides some active forearm supination.

Wrist

The wrist usually is held in a position of flexion and ulnar deviation. Principal deforming forces are the flexor carpi radialis and flexor carpi ulnaris muscles. When the forearm is positioned in pronation, the extensor carpi ulnaris is a strong ulnar deviator of the wrist. Wrist flexion deformity places the digital flexors at a mechanical disadvantage and significantly weakens grasp. The digital flexors themselves may contribute to the wrist flexion deformity. This is likely if the interphalangeal joints of the fingers are tightly flexed when the wrist and metacarpophalangeal joints are maintained in neutral position.

Surgical alternatives include wrist flexor lengthening, flexor origin slide, tendon transfer to improve wrist extension, proximal row carpectomy, and wrist fusion with or without carpal shortening. In general, wrist arthrodesis is avoided if possible. The tenodesis effect of wrist extention-flexion facilitates and grasp and release, and this is lost with wrist fusion. If active digital and wrist extension is present, the flexor carpi ulnaris may be detached or fractionally lengthened. This determination may require myoneural or peripheral nerve block, as spasticity in the wrist and digital flexors may mask any wrist or digital extensor power. In severe spasticity the flexor carpi radialis may require fractional lengthening. It is important not to release or transfer both FCU and FCR, as this eliminates active wrist flexion.

When weak or absent wrist extension is present with wrist flexion deformity, tendon transfers to augment wrist extension may be performed. Available motors include the flexor carpi ulnaris, flexor carpi radialis, flexor digitorum superficialis, extensor carpi ulnaris, brachioradialis, and pronator teres. Green described transfer of the flexor carpi ulnaris to the radial wrist extensors in 1942 and 1962. This is one of the most frequently used transfers for augmentation of wrist extension in cerebral palsy. However, the danger of over-correction with wrist extension deformity exists. If digital extension is weak with the wrist maintained in neutral, and wrist flexion with the tenodesis effect is required for digital opening, release is impaired. A recent long-term follow-up study on tendon transfers to the wrist and digital extensors demonstrated extension contractures with impaired release in five of 12 patients with FCU-to-ECRB transfers. The authors concluded that transfer to the central wrist extensor was not indicated unless the individual's preoperative difficulty was isolated to grasp and active digital extension is present with the wrist stabilized.

Another recent study examined 14 patients who had undergone FCU to radial wrist extensor transfer. All patients in this study group who demonstrated active digital extension with the wrist positioned in neutral preoperatively had excellent results with this tendon transfer. Two patients who had no active finger extension preoperatively had unsatisfactory results following transfer. The authors conclude that transfer is indicated when active digital extension is possible with the wrist maintained in neutral, but active wrist extension to neutral is not present. A recent report has compared the flexor carpi ulnaris and brachioradialis in wrist extension transfer. The authors conclude that both transfers can provide good active wrist extension. Retention of the flexor carpi ulnaris preserves good strong wrist flexion, and leaves the flexor carpi radialis available for later transfer or possible transfer to augment thumb abduction extension. Wrist extension deformity occurred in four patients treated with FCU-to-ECRB transfer. This was not observed with transfer of the brachioradialis. An additional advantage of brachioradialis transfer is that this muscle crosses both the elbow and the wrist, and exhibits a multiplier effect with elbow motion.

If a large ulnar deviation component exists, extensor carpi ulnaris may be transferred to extensor carpi radialis brevis in association with fractional lengthening of the flexor carpi ulnaris. Transfer of flexor carpi ulnaris to extensor digitorum communis is indicated when weak digital extension coexists with weak wrist extension. This transfer improves wrist extension and does not impair digital extension and release.

Wrist arthrodesis has limited indications in spastic cerebral palsy, and should be considered a salvage procedure. Indications include: (1) the presence of strong finger flexion and extension that is independent of wrist position, with poor wrist control; (2) severe flexion deformity of the wrist with very weak hand and wrist muscles; and (3) athetotic/dystonic patient who demonstrates improved digital function when the wrist is immobilized with a cast or brace. The severely contracted wrist in an older individual may require carpectomy and/or flexor tendon lengthening in association with wrist arthrodesis.

Fingers

Fingers are often held in a flexed posture as a result of spasticity and contracture of the flexor digitorum superficialis and flexor digitorum profundus muscles. The degree of this spasticity becomes clinically apparent when the wrist and metacarpal phalangeal joints are passively maintained in neutral position. Flexor spasticity interferes with hand function by impeding release. When flexion deformity is severe enough to impair release, surgical intervention may be considered. Treatment alternatives include flexor-pronator origin release, specific lengthening of musculotendinous units by either fractional lengthening or Z-lengthening, sublimis to profundus tendon transfer, or finger flexor transfer for augmentation of wrist, finger, or thumb extension. The flexor-pronator origin slide effectively lengthens the flexor digitorum superficialis muscle, at least in part, but also lengthens pronator teres and flexor carpi radialis. Anterior transfer of the ulnar nerve is required to permit distal slide of the flexor carpi ulnaris and flexor digitorum profundus tendons from the proximal forearm. Finger flex-

ion deformity can be corrected by distal fractional lengthening, but more precise lengthening can be accomplished by direct Z-lengthening of involved tendons. A rough guideline for lengthening at this level is 0.5 millimeters for every degree of flexion contracture present. Once the flexor digitorum superficialis has been lengthened, it is usually found that the flexor digitorum profundus does not require surgical attention. If mild to moderate flexor tightness remains, stretching and night splinting are sufficient management. Excessive lengthening weakens flexor power, impairs grasp, and can produce swan neck deformities. Superficialis-to-profundus transfer has the disadvantage of weakening grasp, and is probably most applicable in patients with limited functional potential who have tightly clenched fists and difficulty with upper extremity hygiene.

An alternative to lengthening of the flexor digitorum superficialis tendons is their transfer to augment wrist, finger, or thumb extension. Ideally, the tendons should have grade four or better strength (Medical Research Council Grade 0 to 5, where Grade 5 is normal, Grade 3 is antigravity). The remaining flexor digitorum profundus tendons should have 50% or greater strength. The tendons are transferred through the interosseous membrane. It is preferable for the tendons to be active in one phase only, although continuous activity does not preclude successful transfer, as described above.

Hyperextension deformity of the proximal interphalangeal joints (swan neck deformity) is due to over-activity of the intrinsic muscles, augmented by pull of the extensor digitorum communis via a tenodesis effect when the wrist is postured in flexion. Surgical intervention is indicated with severe hyperextension, or when the proximal interphalangeal joints lock in extension. Milder degrees of deformity may respond to balancing of the wrist and metacarpophalangeal joints. When surgery is required, several alternatives exist. These include tongue-in-groove lengthening of the EDC and lateral bands at the level of the proximal phalanx (Goldner technique), palmar capsulodesis with volar plate advancement, or flexor digitorum superficialis tenodesis as described by Swanson.

Thumb-in-palm Deformity

The thumb-in-palm deformity is characterized by metacarpal flexion and adduction, metacarpophalangeal joint flexion or hyperextension, and usually, interphalangeal joint flexion. (Interphalangeal joint hyperextension may be observed in individuals with active extensor pollicialongus and adductor spasticity.) Thumb deformity results from spasticity and contracture of the adductor pollicis, first dorsal interosseous, flexor pollicis brevis, and flexor pollicis longus. The extensor pollicis longus, extensor pollicis brevis, and/or abductor pollicis longus are often weak or functionally ineffective.

The thumb-in-palm deformity has been divided into four types: (1) simple metacarpal adduction; (2) metacarpal adduction and metacarpophalangeal joint flexion; (3) metacarpal adduction with hyperextension instability of the metacarpophalangeal joint; and (4) metacarpal adduction, metacarpophalangeal and interphalangeal joint flexion. The thumb-in-palm deformity is perhaps the most functionally disabling deformity associated with cerebral palsy of the upper extremity, because it impairs the ability of the hand to accept, grasp, and release objects.

Appropriate surgical reconstruction requires selective release or lengthening of the contracted adductor pollicis, first dorsal interosseous, flexor pollicis brevis, and flexor pollicis longus muscles, as well as augmentation of active thumb abduction and extension. The goals of surgery should be to release contracted muscles and to allow functional positioning of the thumb, to improve muscular balance about the thumb, and to provide articular stability for grasp and pinch.

Release of contracted muscles can be done in one of three ways: (1) release of the tendinous insertion, (2) fractional intramuscular tendon release, or (3) release of muscular origin. The latter technique has the advantage of providing muscle lengthening with preservation of strength. Occasionally, thumb index web space skin contracture is present in addition to muscle fascial contracture. This may be corrected with a four-flap Z-plasty deepening. Muscular release may not be necessary if the thumb is easily abducted and extended passively, but tendon transfer may be indicated to improve active extension.

Instability of the thumb metacarpophalangeal joint with hyperextension is an indication for stabilization, accomplished either by arthrodesis or capsulodesis. This instability can be aggravated by poorly designed thumb extension splints. Significant instability is probably best addressed by arthrodesis. A recent review of thumb metacarpophalangeal joint fusion for instability of this joint, performed in skeletally immature individuals, showed no significant disturbance of thumb growth.

If flexor pollicis longus contributes to persistent adduction deformity and interphalangeal joint flexion deformity, tendon lengthening is indicated, usually in a Z-fashion in the forearm. In patients with severe deformity, flexor pollicis longus lengthening is also accompanied by interphalangeal joint arthrodesis to avoid weakness of pinch.

Restoration of dynamic balance of the thumb may also be achieved by shortening of the abductor pollicis longus and extensor pollicis brevis tendons. However, tendon transfers are used more commonly. Rerouting the extensor pollicis longus to provide a more radially oriented pull augments thumb abduction as well as extension. If hyperextension of the metacarpophalangeal joint is aggravated by transfers inserted into the extensor pollicis longus or brevis, concomitant metacarpophalangeal stabilization is indicated. Motors available for transfer to abductor pollicis longus or extensor pollicis longus include brachioradialis, palmaris longus, or the flexor digitorum superficialis. The brachioradialis is prone to develop adhesions along the course of its tendon and gives only a limited range of active excursion.

Summary

Individuals with cerebral palsy have a characteristic upper extremity posture that consists of elbow flexion, forearm pronation, wrist flexion and ulnar deviation, thumb-in-palm deformity, and occasionally swan neck deformities of the fingers. Individuals with the spastic type of cerebral palsy respond most predictably to surgical intervention. Athetosis and dystonia respond much less predictably to tendon transfer and muscle-balancing procedures, but joint-stabilizing procedures may be useful. The ideal candidate for surgery is a motivated, intelligent individual who retains voluntary control of grasp and release, has good sensibility of the extremity, and tries to use the limb in spite of deformity. Serial examinations are necessary to accurately define muscle strength, coordination, and sensibility.

The child should be observed and splinted at night (if needed) to prevent progression of deformity but not be considered for surgery, until at least age four. The goal of the surgical intervention is to maximize upper extremity function by facilitating the individual's ability to position the hand in space, and to perform grasp and release activities. Carefully planned and performed surgery should accomplish this goal.

Annotated Bibliography

Albright AL, Cervi A, Singletary J: Intrathecal Baclofen for spasticity in cerebral palsy. *JAMA,* 265:1418-1422, 1991.

Seventeen patients with congenital spastic cerebral palsy received intrathecal injection of varying does of Baclofen® in a randomized double-blind fashion. Muscle tone in the lower extremities was significantly decreased within two hours after injection and remained lower than baseline eight hours after injection. Upper extremity tone and function were not significantly affected.

Currie DM, Mendiola A: Cortical thumb orthosis for children with spastic hemiplegic cerebral palsy. *Archives of Phys Med Rehab,* 68:214-216, 1987.

Five children between the ages of 20 and 26 months with mild to moderate spastic hemiplegic cerebral palsy were provided with a thumb orthosis to place the thumb in a more functional position. The orthosis was successful in all five children, effectively changing the position of the thumb and improving prehension pattern to that of a radial grasp.

Goldner JL, Koman AL, Gelberman RH, Levin S, Goldner RD: Arthrodesis of the metacarpophalangeal joint of the thumb in children and adults. *Clin Orthop Rel Res,* 253:75-89, 1990.

Instability of the metacarpophalangeal joint of the thumb in patients with thumb-in-palm deformity was treated by arthrodesis with or without soft-tissue procedures. Sixty-eight of these individuals were skeletally immature. Fifty of these patients were followed to maturity, and 44 demonstrated measurable improvement in function. There were no significant disturbances in growth in those thumbs that had joint fusion with open physes.

Goldner JL: Surgical reconstruction of the upper extremity in cerebral palsy. *Hand Clin,* 4:223-265, 1988

The author provides a comprehensive review of reconstructive procedures for cerebral palsy of the upper extremity.

Green WT, Banks HH: Flexor carpi ulnaris transplant and its use in cerebral palsy. *J Bone Joint Surg,* 44A:1343-1352, 1962.

Thirty-nine patients with spastic paralysis underwent FCU-to-ECRL or ECRB transfer to improve wrist extension and forearm supination. Twenty-four were rated as good or excellent, 13 fair, and two as poor. Factors associated with better results included reasonable finger control; passive flexibility of the hand, wrist, and forearm; good stereognosis; reasonable intelligence; high motivation; and a thorough postoperative regimen.

Hoffer MN, Lehman M, Mitani M: Long-term follow up on tendon transfers to the extensors of the wrist and fingers in patients with cerebral palsy. *J Hand Surg,* 11A:836-840, 1986.

Thirty-eight patients with cerebral palsy who had undergone tendon transfers to improve wrist and finger extension were reviewed. Ten patients who had poor hand placement sensibility and motor control preoperatively demonstrated no functional improvement; the remaining 28 improved function. Five of 12 patients undergoing transfer to the wrist extensors demonstrated wrist-extension contractures with impaired release. This was not seen in transfers to the finger extensors.

House JH, Gwathmey FG: Flexor carpi ulnaris and brachioradialis as a wrist-extension transfer in cerebral palsy. *Minnesota Medicine,* 61:481-484, 1978.

This article reviews 54 cerebral palsy patients who had undergone wrist-extension augmentation using either flexor carpi ulnaris or brachioradialis. Six of 32 patients who underwent flexor carpi ulnaris to wrist-extensor transfer achieved a poor result, defined as less than 15° of active wrist extension, or an extension posture with loss of active flexion. This was seen in only three of the 22 patients in whom the brachioradialis was transferred to wrist extensors. The authors conclude that brachioradialis is probably the best muscle to select for transfer when augmentation of wrist extension is all that is necessary to provide wrist balance.

House JH, Gwathmey FW, Fidler MO: A dynamic approach to the thumb-in-palm deformity in cerebral palsy. *J Bone Surg,* 63A:216-225, 1981.

Fifty-six patients with spastic cerebral palsy underwent 165 surgical procedures for correction of thumb deformities that were classified into four types. Voluntary muscle control and sensibility were the most important factors in predicting successful surgery. Various combinations of releases, tendon transfers, and joint stabilizations resulted in measurable and predictable improvement in function.

Koman LA, Gelberman RH, Toby EB, Poehling GG: Cerebral palsy. Management of the upper extremity. *Clin Orthop Rel Res,* 253:62-74, 1990.

The authors review the evaluation, nonsurgical, and operative treatment for upper extremity cerebral palsy.

Law M, Cadman D, Rosenbaum P, Walter S, Russell D, DeMatteo C: Neuro-developmental therapy and upper extremity inhibitive casting for children with cerebral palsy. *Dev Med Child Neurol,* 33:379-387, 1991.

The authors review the treatment of 73 children with spastic cerebral plasy between the ages of 18 months and eight years. Casting with neurodevelopmental therapy improved the quality of upper extremity movement and range of motion. There appear to be no immediate benefits from intensive physical therapy alone.

Manske PR: Cerebral palsy of the upper extremity. *Hand Clin,* 6:697-709, 1990.

The most important aspect of surgical planning is to determine whether or not the individual demonstrates voluntary use of the upper extremity. Surgical concepts should be kept simple, and principally include release of spastic muscles and augmentation tendon transfers to maintain an improved functional position. Transfer of muscles that contribute to the deformity will allow them to correct the deformity and fire in phase without extensive postoperative training.

Manske, PR: A redirection of extensor pollicis longus in the treatment of spastic thumb-in-palm deformity. *J Hand Surg,* 10A:553-560, 1985.

Twenty patients with thumb-in-palm deformity were treated by surgical redirection of the EPL through the first dorsal wrist compartment in combination with spastic intrinsic muscle release. Eighteen patients were able to grasp with the thumb outside of the clenched fist and noted improvement in functional activities.

Strecker WB, Emmanuel JP, Dailey L, Manske PR: Comparison of pronator tenotomy and pronator rerouting in children with spastic cerebral palsy. *J Hand Surg,* 13A:540-543, 1988.

Forty-one patients with cerebral palsy and pronation contracture of the forearm were treated with pronator teres rerouting compared with 16 patients who were treated with pronator teres tenotomy. The average gain in supination was 78° for rerouting and 54° for tenotomy.

Szabo RM, Gelberman RH: Operative treatment of cerebral palsy. *Hand Clin,* 1:525-543, 1985.

The authors describe surgical approaches to upper extremity deformity in cerebral palsy, and emphasize the importance of careful serial examinations of the patient and an individualized plan of approach. Contractures and spasticity can be diminished so as to provide the ability to perform certain coordinated actions that will help improve the patient's activities of daily living.

Thometz JD, Tachdjian M: Long-term follow-up of the flexor carpi ulnaris transfer in spastic hemiplegic children. *J Ped Orthop,* 8:407-412, 1988.

Twenty-five patients who had undergone flexor carpi ulnaris to radial wrist extensor transfer were studied retrospectively. Of the five poor results, two patients required surgery to correct a supination dorsiflexion contracture. This transfer is quite effective in improving wrist dorsiflexion, although significant loss of active palmar flexion was often noted. The authors recommend that to be considered for this transfer, patients should have good digital extension with the wrist held in passive extension.

Johnson KA, Wenner SM: Transfer of the flexor carpi ulnaris to the radial wrist extensors in cerebral palsy. *J Hand Surg,* 13A:231-233, 1988.

Patients with cerebral palsy who have active finger extension with the wrist passively extended but poor active wrist extension are likely to benefit from transfer of the flexor carpi ulnaris to the wrist extensors. Patients who are unable to actively extend their fingers to neutral regardless of wrist position are unlikely to benefit from this transfer.

Yasukawa A: Upper extremity casting: Adjunct treatment for a child with cerebral palsy hemiplegia. *Am J Occup Ther,* 44:840-846, 1990.

Early management of children with hemiplegic cerebral palsy is important in optimizing overall function. Inhibitory upper extremity casting can enhance function and improve arm-hand position.

X
Other Conditions

40

Infections

Allen T. Bishop, MD

Introduction

Infections of the hand may involve any tissue including skin and subcutaneous tissue, tendon sheaths, joints, and bone. A wide variety of pathogens cause hand infections, including viruses, mycoplasma, bacteria, yeast, and fungi. Infections that are inadequately treated may result in permanent disability and prolonged morbidity, and some are life-threatening. Occasionally an infection may be the initial manifestation of serious systemic disease. An appreciation of the variety and extent of pathology is important to avoid delay or missed diagnosis and inappropriate treatment. In many instances both surgical treatment and antibiotic therapy are necessary to eradicate an established infection. Selection of antibiotics must take into account the polymicrobial nature of traumatic wounds, and the possible agents causing chronic indolent or opportunistic infections in immunocompromised hosts.

Infection

Principles

Management of potential or established hand infections requires consideration of a variety of host and organism-specific factors. Systemic disease may alter the ability of the host to fight infection, allowing development of infection by normally nonvirulent organisms and more extensive or severe infection of normal pathogens. Examples of conditions with altered immune status include diabetes mellitus, particularly with impaired renal status, malignant hematologic or lymphoreticular disorders, and HIV infection. Steroid, immunosuppressive, or cytotoxic agents used in patients with organ transplants, rheumatologic disease, and malignancy increase the risk of infection and increase the virulence of potential infectious agents. Local conditions also affect potential for infection, including contaminated open wounds or fractures, prior mastectomy, or chronic edema and impaired circulation. Routine use of antibiotics in managing open fractures of the fingers is less common than in open fractures of the long bones, although the effectiveness of antibiotics in grossly contaminated or marginally viable wounds has been established. Isolated soft-tissue wounds in the upper extremity may be treated with local care alone without the increased risk of infection.

Vigorous irrigation and debridement is adequate primary treatment for open phalangeal fractures in fingers with intact digital arteries. Early treatment with antibiotics may play a role in helping prevent infections of the fingers in patients who have significant amounts of devitalized tissue or who are noncompliant in follow-up care. The infection rate of open hand fractures increases with delay in treatment greater than 24 hours, wound contamination, or systemic illness. It is not necessarily increased by internal fixation, immediate wound closure, large wound size, tendon/nerve/vascular injury, or high-energy mechanism. Open contaminated wounds may be effectively managed by debridement, culture, and expectant treatment with intravenous cefazolin (1g IV q8h) and penicillin G (2 MU IV q4h). If the wound is caused by intravenous drug abuse, is a severe crush injury, or is contaminated, gentamycin is added.

Infectious Agents

Because hand infections may be caused by a variety of agents, it is important that the infected material be obtained for special stains and culture before instituting a definitive antibiotic regimen. Only culture of infected material can provide precise species identification and antibiotic sensitivities. When specific organisms are suspected, the laboratory should be alerted, since special techniques are required for many mycoplasma, mycobacteria, and fungi, as well as for the common bite wound pathogens Eikenella corrodens (humans) and Pasteurella multocida (animals). While awaiting culture results, empiric antibiotic therapy is a practical initial approach. Selection of chemotherapeutic drugs may be aided by examination of infected material by special stains. The Gram stain is best for identifying bacteria. When fungi are present, they are gram-positive (dark blue); gram-negative bacteria stain red. The Ziehl-Neelsen stain is used for Mycobacteria and Nocardia species. Fungal examination is done with potassium hydroxide, Giemsa, or a silver stain. Hyphae, spores, and mycelia are more easily identified than mycobacteria. Herpes simplex may be seen with a Tzank smear of fluid from ruptured vesicles. Selection of appropriate antibiotics for specific clinical situations is shown in Table 40-1.

Bite Infections

Animal Bites

Animal bites account for 1% of all ER visits and $30 million in healthcare costs annually. According to the Public Health Service, more than one million animal bites requiring medical attention occur in the U.S. each year. Most of these wounds (80% to 90%) are dog bites. One to two percent of these require hospitalization. Children are especially prone to animal bites on their fingers. The dominant hand is most commonly injured.

Most studies of animal-bite wounds have focused on the isolation of Pasteurella multocida, disregarding the role of anaerobes. Recent studies of the gingival canine flora and

Table 40-1   Antibotics Used in Treating Infections

Situation	Organism	Empiric Therapy
Animal bite	α-hemolytic streptococcus Pasteurella multocida, S. aureus	Ampicillin-sulbactam 39g q 6 hr IV or Amoxicillin-clavulanic acid 500 mg q 8 hr po(l9);(11)
Human bite	α-hemolytic streptococcus, Eikenella corrodens, anaerobes, S. aureus	Same(l9);(11)
Drug addicts	Methicillin-resistant S. aureus, group A ß-hemolytic streptococcus	Vancomycin 500 mg IV q6h
Necrotizing fasciitis	group A ß-hemolytic streptococcus, staphylococcus, gram-negative aerobes, anaerobes	Penicillin 2 million U q2 hr IV (erythromycin if allergy), clindamycin, gentamycin(23)
Simple laceration, open fracture of phalanges without crush, contamination, soft-tissue loss, delay in treatment		None necessary with adequate surgical care
Herpetic whitlow	Herpes simplex	Observation, oral, or intravenous acyclovir
Mycobacteria	M. tuberculosis	Isoniazid 10-15 mg/kg/day, up to 300 mg/day rifampin 10-15 mg/kg/day up to 600 mg/day + pyrazinamide and ethambutol(26,64)
	Runyon group I (Photochromogens) M. marinum M. kansasii	above, or ciprofloxacin, minocycline, doxycycline with ethambutol and rifabutine
	Runyan group III (nonchromogens) M. avium-intra-cellulare, M. terrae	Multiple drug therapy, including ethambutol, cycloserine, imipenem, clofazamine, amikacin, ciprofloxacin or ethionamide(65)
	Runyon group IV (rapid growers: M. fortuitum, chelonei, ulcerans)	amikacin or kanamycin doxycycline or minocycline(40)
Fungal infections	Sporothrix, Actinomyces, Aspergillus, Blastomyces, Cryptococcus, Histoplasma, Candida, Nocardia, Coccidioides	Consult infectious disease specialist
Open contaminated wound	alpha-hemolytic streptococci, staphylococcus, anaerobes, gram-negative bacilli	Cefazolin 1 g q 8 hr, penicillin G 2 million units q 4 h (bite wounds, animal exposure), and gentamycin (severe crush, contamination)(7)

of dog-bite wounds, however, point toward an oral flora of multiple organisms, most of which are potential pathogens. Goldstein and associates isolated P. multocida from only 26% of dog-bite wounds in adults. The most common aerobic isolates were alpha-hemolytic streptococci (46%) and S. aureus (13%). Anaerobic pathogens were present in 41% of wounds, including Bacteroides and Fusobacterium species. Cat-scratch disease may follow a bite or scratch from a cat, dog, or monkey and is due to a newly named motile, gram-negative bacteria, Afipia felis. One case each of mycoplasma tenosynovitis and Sporothrix infection have been reported following cat bites. Most animal bites cause mixed infections with both aerobic and anaerobic bacteria.

Animal bites have a high infection potential for a variety of reasons including the puncture nature of the wound, devitalizing crush injury of adjacent tissue, and introduction of large numbers of oral flora into the wound. Risk of infection is heightened by advanced patient age, delay in treatment of more than 12 hours, and in deeper or more severe wounds. Cat bites and scratches are more likely to become infected than dog bites. Bites of nondomestic animals are less common but have similar risks. Insect, arthropod, and snake bites less commonly become infected. Snake venom is sterile, although the oral flora of the snake reflects the fecal flora of its prey. Venom is inhibitory to aerobic but not anaerobic bacteria.

Human Bites

The most striking difference in the microbial flora of human- and animal-bite wounds is the higher number of mean isolates per wound in human bites, the difference made up mostly of higher numbers of anaerobic bacteria. Occasionally, human bites can transmit an infectious disease, such as hepatitis B, scarlet fever, tuberculosis, syphilis, or actinomycosis. Theoretically, HIV may also be transmitted. The incidence of Eikenella corrodens in human-bite hand infections has been reported to vary from 7% to 29%. As in animal bites, alpha hemolytic streptococcus and S. aureus are the most common organisms isolated from infected bite wounds. ß-lactamase producing strains are found in many of these wounds, including S. aureus and Bacteroides species. The presence of anaerobic spirochetes and fusiform bacilli isolated from bites correlates with a less favorable prognosis. Penicillin-resistant, gram-negative rods, alone or in mixed culture, were reported in about one-third of bite-wound cultures. Anaerobic bacteria are also far more prevalent in human-bite infections than previously recognized. Two types of human-bite injury occur: actual direct bites to the hand and the clenched fist or knuckle-tooth wound (Figs. 40-1 and 40-2). The direct bite wound occurs as one would bite a carrot, and the knuckle-tooth wound by hitting one's opponent in the mouth.

Treatment of Bite Wounds

Appropriate treatment depends upon wound location, elapsed time since injury (< or > eight hours), and presence or absence of obvious infection. Bite injuries are emergency injuries. Mismanagement may lead to disastrous results; therefore, treatment must be early, correct, and comprehensive.

clenched-fist injuries occur with the joint flexed, these wounds must be explored with the metacarpophalangeal joint flexed to determine the extent of injury. All early wounds should be cleansed, irrigated with a large volume of fluid using a blunt needle or plastic IV catheter, debrided of devitalized tissue, and wound edges excised. Wounds on the hand should never be closed primarily. Oral antibiotics and appropriate tetanus prophylaxis are given, and a compressive dressing with a splint applied in the "safe" position. The wound should be reevaluated in 12 to 24 hours, and soaks or whirlpool treatments and range of motion begun. Failure to provide appropriate prophylactic antibiotic results in an infection rate of nearly 50%. Involvement of bone, joint, tendon, or nerve requires admission as does the presence of sepsis, extensive cellulitis, and unreliable or incompetent patients. Wild animal bites usually require rabies prophylaxis.

An infected bite wound may present with a history of rapid progression (over six to 24 hours), redness and swelling, clear or purulent discharge, enlargement of adjacent lymph nodes, and a reduced range of motion of the affected extremity. Septic arthritis reveals fusiform swelling, diffuse joint tenderness, and pain with minimal joint motion. Treatment is administered as above, with operative irrigation and debridement and admission for intravenous antibiotics.

Selection of antibiotics ultimately is dictated by culture and sensitivity data. Empiric treatment must be started immediately. Because of the large number of ß-lactamase-producing isolates, penicillin is not adequate treatment, and first-generation cephalosporins do not reliably cover Pasteurella multocida, Eikenella corrodens, or anaerobes. The combination of a penicillin and a ß-lactamase inhibitor provides adequate coverage of bite wound isolates, and is the treatment of choice. Tetracycline has good *in vitro* activity against most isolates and, along with doxycycline and minocycline, may be the best therapeutic alternative in penicillin-allergic patients.

Necrotizing Fasciitis

Necrotizing fasciitis is a limb- and life-threatening infection caused by a variety of aerobic and anaerobic bacteria. Necrotizing fasciitis was recognized as early as the American Civil War and referred to by Jones as hospital gangrene. Meleney accurately described this infection in 1924 based on 20 patients with streptococcal infection. In 1952, Wilson introduced the currently preferred term of necrotizing fasciitis to emphasize the constant feature of necrotic fascia with spread of infection along fascial planes and the nonspecificity of the bacterial etiology. Although most cases can be attributed to streptococcal and staphylococcal organisms, a mixture of facultative and anaerobic organisms can also lead to this type of infection.

Giuliano described two groups of necrotizing fasciitis based upon culture results. Type I consisted of a combination of anaerobic bacteria and facultative anaerobic bacteria such as Enterobacteriaceae, and streptococci other than group A. Type II consisted of cases in which group A streptococci were isolated or in combination with Staphylococcus aureus or Staphylococcus epidermidis. In his series, most

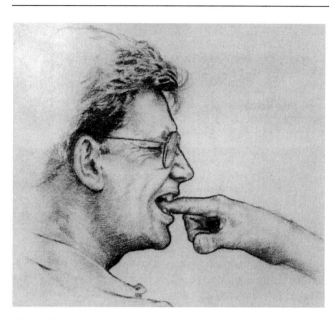

Figure 40-1.   A direct human bite.

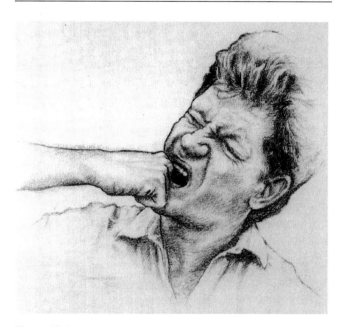

Figure 40-2.   A clenched-fist or knuckle tooth injury occurs in a fight, resulting in a penetrating wound overlying the metacarpophalangeal joint.

Patients with early bite wounds without signs of infection may be treated as outpatients provided the bite has not penetrated a joint capsule or injured a tendon. A thorough history and physical exam are performed and a radiograph obtained to rule out fracture, gas, or foreign body. As

were Type I, and only 19% were Type II. In another study, 52% of patients had a single organism. Most commonly, particularly in the past decade, Group A ß-hemolytic Streptococci have been isolated from fasciitis wounds. The polymicrobial infections tend to have a longer incubation period than monomicrobial infections, making them more difficult to diagnose. No differences in survival have been observed attributable to bacteriology.

Predisposing factors may include diabetes mellitus, arteriosclerosis and peripheral vascular disease, alcoholism, malignancy, polymyositis, IV drug abuse, and postpartum state. Minor trauma such as abrasions, lacerations, insect bites, hypodermic needle injections, or surgical incisions may result in infection.

The infection may appear at first to be a benign, low-grade cellulitis, but as bacterial enzymes elevate soft-tissue planes, rapid advance of the infection occurs with concomitant soft-tissue necrosis. Patients initially present with cellulitis, soft-tissue swelling, fever, and pain. Hemodynamic instability and multisystem organ failure similar to toxic shock syndrome are often present. Skin bullae, crepitus, skin necrosis, and high fever are frequently absent at presentation.

The infectious process involves the fascia, which liquefies. At surgery, necrotic fat weeps muddy brown serous fluid, and thrombosis of subcutaneous vessels is usually present (Fig. 40-3). Inspection of the underlying muscle is imperative because of the occasional presence of myositis and myonecrosis. Only radical surgical debridement can control the infection. Delayed or incomplete excision may lead to disseminated infection. All necrotic skin, fat, fascia, and muscle must be debrided and fasciotomy extended well beyond the area of cellulitis to contain the infection. Early redebridement in 12 to 24 hours should be performed and repeated as necessary. Multiple debridements and ultimately skin grafts are required in most cases. Broad-spectrum antibiotic coverage is begun empirically, including penicillin, clindamycin or metronidazole, and an aminoglycoside. Hemodynamic monitoring with a Swan-Ganz catheter with fluid resuscitation and dopamine support is indicated, as well as nutritional supplements. Amputation may be necessary in medically unstable patients or for those limbs demonstrating progression of infection at re-exploration. Enhanced fibrin deposition and vascular occlusions in the skin are the basis for most complications present in necrotizing fasciitis. Increased morbidity and mortality occur with delayed surgery. When the diagnosis is in doubt, a bedside diagnostic incision with local anesthesia may be needed to further reduce morbidity. Mortality rates reported from 1924 to the present range from 8.7% to 73.0%, with a mean rate of 32.2%. Increased rates occur with old age, peripheral vascular disease, and diabetes.

Mycobacterial Infections

Mycobacterium Tuberculosis Infection

Tenosynovitis attributed to tuberculosis has been reported since 1777, and subsequent descriptions have been provided

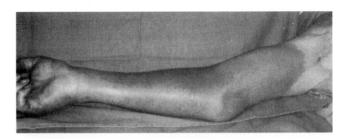
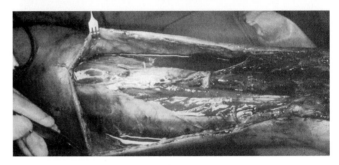

Figure 40-3.   Necrotizing fasciitis arising from a peripheral IV catheter. **(Top)** Rapidly advancing cellulitis clinically; **(Bottom)** typical fascial necrosis with serous exudate in the subcutaneous tissues.

by historical figures including Dupuytren and Virchow. Now, tenosynovial tuberculosis is rare and seldom mentioned in standard medical or surgical texts. Like other mycobacterial infections, tuberculosis in the hand is an indolent process resulting in gradually progressive diffuse digital swelling (dactylitis) and chronic tenosynovitis reminiscent of rheumatoid arthritis. Signs of acute inflammation such as warmth and pain are not prominent. Radiographs demonstrate soft-tissue swelling. The Mantoux skin test is positive, and the sedimentation rate elevated. Malnutrition, advanced age, immunosuppression, ethanol abuse, and history of pulmonary tuberculosis are risk factors for musculoskeletal infection. Treatment includes surgical tenosynovectomy for both diagnosis and treatment, with postoperative chemotherapy with isoniazid, rifampin, and pyrazinamide for several months.

Atypical Mycobacterial Infection

Atypical mycobacteria are widely distributed in nature, and are infrequently human pathogens. The mycobacteria are grouped by the Runyon classification according to pigmentation and growth characteristics (Table 40-2). Most have been implicated in infections, although M. marinum, M. kansasii, M. terrae and M. avium-intracellulare are most common. Musculoskeletal manifestation of infection involves the wrist and hand in almost 50% of cases.

Mycobacterium marinum is endogenous to both freshwater and saltwater fish, and proliferates in freshwater or saltwater enclosures, especially when the water is not frequently replenished. All types of bathing places, aquaria,

Table 40-2   Runyon Classification of Mycobacteria

Type	Characteristic
Group I M. marinum M. kansasii	Photochromogens (cream colored colonies turning yellow on exposure to light)
Group II M. gordonae M. szulgai	Scotochromogens (produce orange pigment independent of light)
Group III M. avium-intracellulare M. terrae	Nonchromogens (white colonies that do not develop pigment)
Group IV M. fortuitum M. chelonei M. ulcerans	Rapid growers (form cream-colored colonies in 1 week or less, compared with the 10 to 28 days required by the other groups) Resistant to most antituberculosis drugs, but often susceptible to amikacin, doxycycline, erythromycin, kanamycin

fish farms, and fish tanks qualify as potential sources of infection. Fish, shrimp, snails, and crabs may become infected and transfer the organism to man. M. marinum may cause infection varying from subcutaneous granulomas with sinus tracts to sporotrichoid-like nodules, tenosynovitis, bursitis, arthritis, and osteomyelitis. There is usually a history of a puncture wound or trauma within six months of the onset of symptoms that could have allowed the organism to violate the skin barrier. Patients are usually healthy and have no underlying diseases. The typical swimming pool granuloma is a localized superficial granuloma involving little more than deep dermis and presenting as an ulcerated nodule. Flexor tenosynovitis involving a digit, the wrist, or both is common. Symptoms of carpal tunnel syndrome may be present.

M. avium-intracellulare is an organism found in soil, water, and domestic poultry. In humans it may cause pulmonary disease, localized skin and subcutaneous infections, arthritis, osteomyelitis, and disseminated sepsis. Before 1982, disseminated sepsis was extremely rare. However, M. avium-intracellulare has become the most frequently isolated organism in patients terminally ill with AIDS. Primary musculoskeletal disease remains rare, although multifocal osteomyelitis may occur in immunocompromised hosts and young children. Focal septic arthritis or osteomyelitis is even more uncommon. History of puncture wounds, closed trauma, treatment with oral corticosteroids, or local steroid injections and immunodeficiency are risk factors. The organism is difficult to eradicate because of multiple drug resistance and the immunocompromised nature of most of its hosts. No combination of chemotherapy appears particularly effective in M. avium-intracellulare infection, including the use of five or more agents.

Other mycobacteria have been reported to cause hand infections, including M. kansasii and M. terrae. Most cases have been pulmonary, but hand infections from penetrating wounds from pins, fish fins, wooden splinters or while gardening have occurred. M. fortuitum has been isolated from soil, house dust, milk, and saliva, as well as fish, frogs, and cattle. M. fortuitum infections have been associated with trauma and prosthetic devices and can infect operative incisions. Clinically, M. fortuitum infections may present in the hand as indolent subcutaneous masses, cold abscesses, tenosynovitis, or joint synovitis. Other species causing hand infections include M. malmoense, M. chelonei, and M. szulgai.

Diagnosis

Because of the indolent nature of mycobacterial infection, lack of clinical suspicion, and special growth requirements, diagnosis is usually delayed. Indolent inflammation following a puncture wound or arising in an immunocompromised host should suggest the possibility of an atypical mycobacterial infection. Tuberculin skin testing is not a reliable indicator of these infections. Diagnosis in all instances requires biopsy for histopathology of the involved tissue as well as culture submission for tuberculosis, atypical mycobacteria and fungi, and aerobic and anaerobic bacteria. Requests for sensitivities to antibiotics must be stressed because of widely varying resistance to chemotherapeutic agents. At the time of biopsy, histologic examination should be performed, although synovial lesions may not be diagnostic. Forms and components of the inflammatory reaction from M. marinum-infected tissue include diffuse granulomatous inflammation, focal granulomatous inflammation, fibrous exudates and caseation, and acid-fast bacilli seen on Ziehl-Neelsen stained sections. Synovial lesions may resemble rheumatoid disease, although careful examination reveals the presence of small, well-formed granulomas consisting of nodular collections of epithelioid cells, and multinucleated giant cells. In addition, poorly formed granulomas and several dense collections of plasma cells may be observed.

Growth in culture requires special media and temperatures. For example, M. marinum is a rapidly growing photochromogen, requiring two to eight weeks in culture with best growth at 30° to 32° C. Little or no growth occurs at 37°. M. fortuitum is distinguished in the laboratory by growth of nonpigmented colonies within 48 hours at 20° C on Lowenstein-Jensen medium. Isolation of mycobacteria from a hand should prompt a search for pulmonary foci by chest roentgenogram, as infection may occur by either hematogenous spread or direct inoculation.

Treatment

Although spontaneous healing of cutaneous lesions has been mentioned in the literature, tenosynovitis will not heal spontaneously. At the present time, treatment recommendations for most of these infections include both surgical debridement and postoperative pharmacologic therapy. Abscesses require drainage, and synovectomy of involved joints and tendon sheaths is probably necessary (Fig. 40-4).

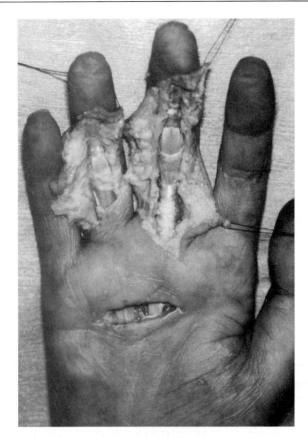

Figure 40-4. Mycobacterium marinum tenosynovitis. The proliferative tenosynovium bears a clinical resemblance to rheumatoid tenosynovitis.

Superficial (cutaneous) infections may be satisfactorily managed by debridement alone. The length of postoperative chemotherapy depends in part on the antibiotic resistance of the organism, but commonly is continued for several months. Institution of drug therapy in most instances should begin immediately following surgery, although empiric treatment may need to be modified once sensitivities are obtained. The rapid growers M. fortuitum and M. chelonei are resistant to conventional mycobacterial agents, but may be susceptible to amikacin, doxycycline and others (see Table 40-1). M. terrae is resistant to drug therapy, and M. avium-intracellulare responds poorly to regimens of five or more agents in immunocompromised patients. Consultation with an infectious disease specialist is indicated in the postoperative management of mycobacterial infections.

Fungal Infections

Fungal involvement of the hand may be broadly divided into cutaneous, subcutaneous, and deep infections. The organisms involved may be true pathogens, capable of infecting normal hosts, or opportunists. These fungi cause infection in patients with immune compromise, such as diabetics, patients using steroids or immunosuppressives, or those having a myeloproliferative disorder, or HIV infection.

Cutaneous Infections

Examples of cutaneous infection include chronic paronychia, onychomycosis, and tinea manuum. Chronic infection of the nail fold is most frequently caused by Candida albicans, resulting in thickening and chronic inflammation in the eponychial area. A history of occupational activity requiring frequent exposure of the hands to moisture is common. Acute flare-ups are often due to bacterial superinfection. Topical antifungal agents such as tolnaftate clotrimazole may effect a cure, along with avoidance of moisture. Nail plate removal or marsupialization may be necessary if this does not work.

Onychomycosis is a destructive or deforming infection of the nail plate caused by fungal invasion. Dermatophytes including Trichophyton rubrum are the most common cause. Nondermatophytes and Candida make up a minority of nail plate infections. Onychomycosis may be treated with topical agents such as Tinactin, Lotrimin, or Halotex. Systemic therapy with griseofulvin, ketoconazole, or terbinafine over several months may be effective, but with potential for liver, renal, and bone marrow toxicity.

Tinea manuum is a fungal infection of the glabrous skin of the hand. All species of dermatophytes are capable of producing skin lesions, but T. rubrum is the most common agent. Lesions are interdigital in location, and vary from hyperkeratotic scaling lesions to areas of acute inflammation with vesicles. The "id" reaction, an allergic response to circulating fungal antigens due to dermatophyte infection in the feet, may appear similar to tinea manuum. Cladosporium werneckii produces brown to black discoloration of the stratum corneum, referred to as tinea nigra. The typical lesions are macules one to five centimeters in size. These lesions may resemble malignant melanoma, and occur primarily in the tropics or southern coastal regions of the United States. A history of travel or residence in the endemic area assist in diagnosis. Keratolytic agents such as Whitfield's ointment and topical imidazoles are helpful along with topical antifungal agents.

Subcutaneous

Subcutaneous infection is commonly caused by Sporothrix schenckii. The most common form of sporotrichosis is the lymphocutaneous variety, although deep infections also occur. Most result from handling plants or soil, with the recollection of a penetrating injury from a thorn, scratch, animal bite, or wood sliver. Sporotrichosis skin lesions begin with a papule at the site of inoculation, with subsequent development of metastatic lesions along lymphatic channels. These channels become indurated and cordlike, with the development of violaceous abscesses which drain seropurulent material.

Deep Infection

Deep fungal infections of the upper extremity have three common presentations: tenosynovial infections of the flexor or extensor compartments, septic arthritis, or osteomyelitis. Definitive diagnosis requires identification of the organism on specific fungal cultures. True pathogens include histoplasmosis, blastomycosis, coccidioidomycosis, and paracoccidioidomycosis. Opportunistic infections include aspergillosis, candidiasis, mucormycosis, and cryptococcosis. Histoplasmosis is caused by histoplasma capsulatum and is endemic as a subclinical primary pulmonary infection in the Mississippi-Ohio River valley region. Cases of tenosynovial infection have been reported. Blastomycosis occurs in the same region of North America, but at a lower incidence. Cutaneous lesions may occur with systemic infection, including subcutaneous nodules that may develop draining peripheral ulcerations. Septic arthritis and lytic epiphyseal lesions may also be commonly seen. Coccidioidomycosis is a rare fungal infection found in arid regions of the southwestern United States and northern Mexico. A self-limiting pulmonary infection, hematogenous spread to the upper extremity occurs in a minority of patients, causing metaphyseal osteomyelitis or septic arthritis. Treatment of deep infection, including opportunistic infections, should combine surgical debridement and intravenous antifungal agents such as amphotericin B.

HIV Infection

General Information

The human immunodeficiency virus, or HIV, is an RNA retrovirus with a mode of transmission similar to hepatitis B, via percutaneous inoculation, open wound contact, nonintact skin or mucous membranes. Other methods of transmission such as by contact with intact skin cannot be entirely ruled out, but are presently unproven. As of 1990, the World Health Organization estimated that a total of five million people had HIV infection, of whom 600,000 had AIDS with 300,000 fatalities. The infection is rapidly spreading. By 2000, 15 million infections are projected.

Infection with HIV follows a natural progression reflecting the severity of the disease process. A currently advocated classification system for HIV infection includes four principal groups (Table 40-3). Group I includes patients with transient signs that appear at the time of initial infection with HIV. Group II includes patients who have no

Table 40-3 Summary of Classification System for HIV Infection

Group	
I	Acute infection
II	Asymptomatic infection
III	Persistent generalized lymphadenopathy
IV	Other disease
Subgroup	
A	Constitutional disease
B	Neurologic disease
C	Secondary infectious disease
D	Secondary cancers
E	Other conditions

signs or symptoms of HIV. Group III includes those with persistent generalized lymphadenopathy, and group IV with associated diseases.

In a recent survey, 93% of orthopaedic surgeons interviewed had treated an HIV-infected patient in the past year. Current concerns regarding HIV infection include risk to healthcare workers, risk to patients from surgical procedures, and associated complications of HIV including opportunistic infection and Kaposi's sarcoma.

Risk to Healthcare Workers

As of 1988, 169 healthcare workers were known to have acquired HIV without having a risk factor other than occupation. The risk to healthcare workers of acquiring HIV infection has been estimated by several authors. For surgeons, contact of broken skin or mucus membranes with contaminated body fluids is the most likely mode of transmission. Because the virus targets Langerhans cells in epithelium, Day has postulated the ability of the virus to infect through intact skin as well. Lacerations or puncture wounds from sharp injuries are known to occasionally result in HIV infection. Best estimates of risk from a single contaminated needle stick is 0.4% to 0.5%, or about one in 200. The possible risk from aerosols related to cautery and power equipment is unknown. The prevalence of sharp injury in the operating room has been estimated to be approximately 5% by Hussain, or about 4.2 punctures per 1000 operating hours (a typical amount of operating time/year for a busy surgeon) by Lowenfels. Acquiring an HIV infection in the operating room also depends upon prevalence of HIV infection in a surgeon's patient population. The product of prevalence, incidence of sharp injury, and risk of transmission from a single injury provides an estimate of likelihood of infection. Risk has been estimated to be 1% to 2% over a 30-year career in New York, but 4% in the practice of one San Francisco orthopaedic surgeon. At the present time, the Centers for Disease Control and Prevention are recommending a program of universal precautions, treating every operative case as HIV-positive. While some authors have embraced this policy, others feel that the presence of identifiable risk factors should dictate additional special precautions, particularly in emergency surgery. There does not seem to be any substantial benefit to routinely determining the HIV status of all patients admitted for elective surgical procedures. Precautions should include double gloves, masks, face shields, hourly checks of gloves, mask, and gown for penetration, and minimizing the number of personnel involved in high-risk patients, especially inexperienced individuals. A minimum number of instruments should be used, passing scalpels between surgeon and nurse in a basin.

Risk to Patients

The major risk to patients has been transmission of the virus though blood products, but transmission via bone allografts, fibrin glue, and infected healthcare workers might also occur. Current estimates of the risk of HIV infection from the transfusion of blood or components vary from 1/140,000 to 1/250,000. The major route of transmission in these instances is via blood collected during the interval between HIV infection and the development of detectable circulating antibody to the AIDS virus. With appropriate screening including history of risk behavior, screen of police records, ELISA, and Western blot studies of donors (including post-donation screens of living donors) and omission of patients with infection or penetrating trauma, the risk of HIV transmission with bone allograft donation is about 1/10,000. Fibrin glue preparations made with effort to select plasma donors and with pasteurization allow the production of a product with virtually no risk of transmission of viral infections. The risk of transmission from infected healthcare workers is thought to be low, but no data are currently available to estimate risk. The only known case, a Florida dentist, transmitted the virus to five patients.

Hand Infection and HIV

Infections of the upper extremity in HIV infected patients in most cases are neither severe nor unusual, although the virulence of the infecting agent is enhanced by the immunocompromised state of the patient. Infection may be viral (herpes simplex and CMV), fungal (candidiasis, cryptococcus, histoplasmosis, aspergillosis), protozoal, or mycobacterial. Most opportunistic infections reported are pulmonary, gastrointestinal, or disseminated. Infections of the hand may occur early in the disease process, and may suggest the development of AIDS in a patient at risk. In Glickel's series, herpes infections were most common, and required antiviral medication for resolution. Cellulitis responded to intravenous antibiotics, and osteomyelitis to debridement and antibacterial chemotherapy. Disseminated fungal and mycobacterial disease may also involve the musculoskeletal system.

Following elective orthopaedic procedures, including open reduction and internal fixation of fractures, HIV-infected patients have a significantly higher risk of postoperative infection with usual pathogens. Patients respond to conventional antibiotic treatment in such instances. A reduced CD4 lymphocyte count, which correlates with disease progression, may be predictive of increased risk of infection.

Annotated Bibliography

Brook I: Human and animal bite infections. *J Fam Pract,* 28(6):713-718, 1989.

A review of human and animal bite wounds, including incidence, bacteriology, diagnosis, and treatment.

Buck BE, Malinin TI: Bone transplantation and human immunodeficiency virus. An estimate of risk of acquired immunodeficiency syndrome (AIDS). *Clin Orthop,* 240:129-136, 1989.

The possibility of transplanting a bone allograft from a donor infected with human immunodeficiency virus is remote, provided there is a combination of rigorous donor selection and exclusion, screening for the HIV antigen and antibody, and histopathologic studies of donor tissues. The chance of obtaining a bone allograft from an HIV-infected donor who failed to be excluded by the above techniques is calculated to be one in well over a million, using average estimates. On the other hand, if adequate precautions are not taken (for example, by testing only for antibodies to HIV), the risk might be as high as one in 161.

Bush DC, Schneider LH: Tuberculosis of the hand and wrist. *J Hand Surg,* 9A:391-398, 1984.

Eleven cases of M. tuberculosis of the hand and wrist were reviewed. Most patients had a significant delay in the diagnosis of infection and had no history of pulmonary involvement. Flexor or extensor tenosynovitis was most common, and responded to combined surgical debridement and antituberculosis therapy.

Centers for Disease Control. Guidelines for prevention of human immunodificiency virus and hepatitis B virus to health-care and public safety workers. *MMWR,* 38(suppl S6):4-5, 31-33, 1989.

This report contains the CDC's recommendations for protection of healthcare workers, including surgeons and operating room personnel.

Collins RJ, Chow SP, Ip FK, Leung YK: Synovial involvement by Mycobacterium marinum. A histopathological study of 25 culture-proven cases. *Pathology,* 20(4):340-345, 1988.

This series of culture-proven cases demonstrates that a wide spectrum of pathological lesions may be seen in the synovium and adjacent tissues in patients infected by M. marinum. Variations in the morphology of the inflammatory reaction occur, ranging from the common nonspecific diffuse form, to lesser areas of focal noncaseating lesions, to rarer focal caseating types of granulomatous reaction, and can include an acute inflammatory cell component. Fibrinous exudate on the synovial surface is a recurrent feature and is often the site harboring most acid-fast bacilli.

Francel TJ, Marshall KA, Savage RC: Hand infections in the diabetic and the diabetic renal transplant recipient. *Ann Plast Surg,* 24(4):304-309, 1990.

Diabetics with hand infections tend to suffer more morbidity from hand infections, with higher incidence of deep-space infections, osteomyelitis, tenosynovitis, and need for amputation. Mixed flora were most commonly isolated. Renal transplantation patients were most at risk because of additional immune compromise.

Glickel SZ: Hand infections in patients with acquired immunodeficiency syndrome. *J Hand Surg,* 13A(5):770-775, 1988.

Hand infections occurring in eight HIV-infected patients were not truly opportunistic, but rather unusual in presentation and course of the infection. Virulence of the infectious agent was enhanced in the immunocompromised host. Herpetic whitlow required intravenous antiviral therapy for cure.

Giuliano A, Lewis F Jr., Hadley K, et al: Bacteriology of necrotizing fasciitis. *Am J Surg,* 143:52-56, 1977.

Sixteen patients with necrotizing fasciitis were studied. The clinical observations of necrosis of fascia, subcutaneous fat, and skin with thrombosis of the microvasculature, and absence of myonecrosis were clearly apparent in these patients. Two clear-cut groups of culture and Gram-stain results were found, suggesting that the clinical entity of necrotizing fasciitis can occur after infection by different infecting organisms. The cultivation of Streptococcus pyogenes (Group A), either alone or in combination with staphylococcus, in three patients conforms to the culture results found by Meleney in his original description.

Greene WB, De Gnore LT, White GC: Orthopaedic procedures and prognosis in hemophilic patients who are seropositive for human immunodeficiency virus. *J Bone Joint Surg,* 72(1):2-11, 1990.

Thirty patients who had hemophilia and were seropositive for the human immunodeficiency virus were evaluated. The preoperative CD4 lymphocyte count was decreased to an average of 336 x 10(9) per liter (range, 27 to 708 x 10(9) per liter). After 26 orthopaedic operations in patients who had no previous bacterial infection, a nosocomial infection (cellulitis in the forearm, at the site of an intravenous catheter) developed in only one patient, but five patients had an abnormal postoperative fever that was not accompanied by the expected increase in the white blood cell count. The preoperative CD4 lymphocyte count was significantly reduced in the patients who had an abnormal elevation in body temperature (p < 0.004). Preoperative evaluation of the CD4 lymphocyte count and the response to intradermal skin-test antigens in patients who are at risk for infection postoperatively provides additional information concerning immunological competence. With these data, the possible risk of infection in patients who are seropositive for the human immunodeficiency virus can be estimated more accurately.

Goldstein EJ, Citron DM: Comparative activities of cefuoxime, amoxicillin-clavulanic acid, ciprofloxacin, enoxacin, and ofloxacin against aerobic and anaerobic bacteria isolated from bite wounds. *Antimicrob Agents Chemother,* 32(8):1143-1148, 1988.

The *in vitro* activities of 10 oral antimicrobial agents were studied against 147 aerobic and 61 anaerobic bacteria isolated from bite wounds. Cefuroxime was generally greater than fourfold more active than cephalexin and cefadroxil against all aerobic isolates, including Pasteurella multocida. The fluoroquinolones were highly active against most aerobic isolates but were less active against anaerobic isolates. Ciprofloxacin was generally more active than either enoxacin or ofloxacin.

Goldstein EJ: Bite wounds and infection. *Clin Infect Dis,* 14(3):633-638, 1992.

One in every two Americans will be bitten by an animal or by another person. Bites account for approximately 1% of all visits to emergency rooms; injuries inflicted by dogs are most common. The bacteria involved in infection of animal-bite wounds include Pasteurella multocida, Staphylococcus aureus, Staphylococcus intermedius, alpha-hemolytic streptococci, Capnocytophaga canimorsus, and other members of the oral flora. Infections of human bites are associated with alpha-hemolytic streptococci, S. aureus, Eikenella corrodens, Haemophilus species, and (in more than 50% of cases) anaerobic bacteria. The principles of management of bite wounds are discussed.

Hilfenhaus J, Weidmann E. Fibrin glue safety: inactivation of potential viral contaminants by pasteurization of the human plasma components. *Arzneimit-telforschung* 35(11):1617-1619, 1985.

Fibrin glue has become an indispensable tool in neurorrhaphy and nerve grafting, particularly of the brachial plexus. Currently available glues contain clotting factors from human plasma and thus carry the potential risk of transmitting viral infections like hepatitis or acquired immunodeficiency syndrome. Combined efforts in selection of plasma donations as well as pasteurization of the human plasma products allow the manufacturing of a product with virtually no risk of transmission of viral infections. No changes in activity or antigenicity of the clotting factors by the pasteurization procedure have been encountered.

Hitchcock TF, Amadio PC: Fungal infections. *Hand Clin,* 5(4):599-611, 1989.

An excellent review of fungal hand infections.

Hoekman P, Van de Perre P, Nelissen J, Kwisanga B, Bogaerts J, Kanyangabo F: Increased frequency of infection after open reduction of fractures in patients who are seropositive for human immunodeficiency virus. *J Bone Joint Surg,* 73A(5):675-679, 1991.

In this prospective study, 214 patients who had elective operations for fractures were compared. The relative frequency of postoperative infection was significantly higher in patients who were seropositive for HIV and had associated clinical symptoms (four of 17) than in patients who were seronegative (eight of 171) (Fisher exact test, p = 0.01). In all patients who were seropositive and had a postoperative bacterial infection, treatment with antibiotics was effective. The results of this study suggest that people who are seropositive for human immunodeficiency virus and have associated symptoms are at increased risk for postoperative infection.

Hussain SA, Latif AB, Choudhary AA: Risk to surgeons: A survey of accidental injuries during operations. *Br J Surg,* 75:314-316, 1988.

A survey was conducted with the participation of eight consultant general surgeons, two consultant urologists, four consultant orthopaedic surgeons, and four surgical residents to find the incidence of accidental injuries to surgeons and their assistants during operations. Of the total of 2,016 operations over a one-year period there were 112 reported accidental injuries. These included 107 needle stick injuries, four knife cuts and one diathermy burn (5.6%). The authors found that accidental injuries to surgeons during operations were inevitable.

Keyser JJ, Littler JW, Eaton RG: Surgical treatment of infections and lesions of the perionychium. *Hand Clin,* 6(1):137-153, 1990.

This review article discusses the acute and chronic bacterial, viral, and fungal infections involving the perionychium.

Lacy JN, Viegas SF, Calhoun J, Mader JT: Mycobacterium marinum flexor tenosynovitis. *Clin Orthop,* 238:288-293, 1989.

Four culture-positive cases of flexor tenosynovitis of the hand caused by Mycobacterium marinum are reported. The organisms were cultured at 32°. All patients were treated with a combination of flexor tenosynovectomy and antimycobacterial treatment with ethambutol and rifampin. The length of antimycobacterial treatment ranged from nine to 22 months. All four patients responded to treatment with cessation of signs of infection, increased range of motion, and complete wound healing.

Love GL, Melchior E: Synovial hand infection from Mycobacterium terrae. *J Hand Surg Br,* 13(3):335-336, 1988.

A case of extensive synovial infection in the hand due to Mycobacterium terrae is described. The infection is resistant to drug therapy but appears to remain localized.

Lowenfels AB, Wormser GP, Jain R: Frequency of puncture injuries in surgeons and estimated risk of HIV infection. *Arch Surg,* 124(11):1284-1286, 1989.

Two hundred-two surgeons working in New York City were surveyed. Eighty-six percent reported at least one puncture injury in the preceding year, with a median injury rate of 4.2 per 1,000 operating room hours. If the prevalence of HIV infection in surgical patients is 5%, then the estimated 30-year risk of HIV seroconversion is less than 1% for 50% of the group, 1% to 2% for 25% of the group, 2% to 6% for 15% of the surgeons, and greater than 6% for 10% of the surgeons, depending upon their injury rate.

Mennen U, Howells CJ: Human fight-bite injuries of the hand. A study of 100 cases within 18 months. *J Hand Surg Br,* 16(4):431-435, 1991.

One hundred consecutive patients whose fingers had been bitten by another person, or who had cut fingers on a tooth in a fight, were studied. Eighty-two healed completely but 18 eventually needed amputation. Early and thorough debridement is required, plus a suitable mixture of antibiotics. Once infection is established in bone or tendon sheath, amputation is often needed; most infected joints can be saved.

Schecter W, Meyer A, Schecter G, Giuliano A, Newmeyer W, Kilgore E: Necrotizing fasciitis of the upper extremity. *J Hand Surg,* 7(1):15-20, 1982.

Thirty-three cases of necrotizing fasciitis were reported, primarily in an indigent population associated with the abuse of drugs and/or alcohol. Findings resemble a benign, low-grade cellulitis on admission. Group A α-hemolytic Streptococcus was the most common cause (33%). Another third grew mixed flora. Radical debridement of all involved skin, fat, fascia, and muscle is associated with a significant reduction in length of hospital stay and number of operations.

Sudarsky LA, Laschinger MD, Coppa GF, Spencer FC: Improved results from a standardized approach in treating patients with necrotizing fasciitis. *Ann Surg,* 206(5):661-665, 1987.

Thirty-three patients were studied over a three-year period. Predisposing factors included intravenous drug abuse (30%), diabetes (21%), and obesity (18%). Severe pain (94%) and abnormal temperature (88%) were present, whereas laboratory data and X-ray were nonspecific. Gram-positive organisms were most frequently recovered (ß-hemolytic streptococcus 45%). Treatment consisted of antibiotics, surgical debridement, reexploration 24 hours after surgery, nutritional support, and early soft-tissue coverage as needed. Mean duration from admission to operation was 43 hours. Despite antibiotics and aggressive debridement, significant morbidity exists if operation is delayed more than 12 hours.

Swanson TV, Szabo RM, Anderson DD: Open hand fractures: prognosis and classification. *J Hand Surg,* 16(1):101-107, 1991.

Review of 200 open fractures distal to the carpus demonstrated increased infection rate in the presence of wound contamination, delay in treatment greater than 24 hours, or systemic illness. Infection was not increased by presence of internal fixation, immediate wound closure, wound size, tendon/nerve/vascular injury, or high-energy mechanism. The authors recommend use of stable internal fixation regardless of the wound, and immediate wound closure in the absence of any of the above risk factors.

Zubowicz VN, Gravier M: Management of early human bites of the hand: a prospective randomized study. *Plast Reconstr Surg,* 88(1):111-114, 1991.

This prospective, randomized study of 48 early, noninfected human-bite wounds compared the outcome of patients in one of three study groups after standardized ER wound care. The results substantiate that mechanical wound care alone is insufficient therapy, with a 46.7% incidence of infection. Use of antibiotics prevented infection. No difference was seen between use or oral or parenteral administration.

41

Injection and Extravasation Injuries

Alan E. Seyfer, MD

Introduction

Upper extremity injuries are common and those due to infiltrations caused by injections or extravasation from intravenous lines are less frequent and have less standardized treatment protocols. Fortunately, most of these injuries are relatively mild and self-limiting. However, others may be extremely toxic to the tissues, cause large-scale local tissue necrosis, and require radical debridement and coverage with soft-tissue flaps. Frequently, the extravasation is unseen or unpreventable. A catheter may slip from the lumen of a venous access site and the toxic medication may cause local tissue necrosis that is delayed and initially undetected. In some cases, the necrosis is not demarcated until a few weeks following the infiltration across the tissues.

At the cellular level, the acute injury can be due to direct interruption of intracellular metabolism, pH changes, or osmolar changes that destroy the cell. Toxic agents can cause long-term problems related to joint stiffness and permanent scarring secondary to tissue necrosis. This chapter outlines common agents that can cause these injuries and reviews the treatment of such problems.

Types of Injury

It is important to realize that so-called "non-toxic" solutions can also result in infiltration injuries. Electrolyte solutions, especially those containing high concentrations of potassium or calcium salts, may cause an immediate reaction if infiltrated into the tissues. There is usually an early onset of local pain, swelling, and erythema. Unfortunately, this often occurs in infants, who cannot communicate their distress (Fig. 41-1).

Many individuals consider hyperosmolar infiltration to be of no serious consequence. However, if the agent is locally toxic, the swelling and pain increase in area and intensity, and it is evident that the problem is serious. Hyperosmolar fluids cause water to shift across the cell membranes until a new equilibrium is reached; however, the resultant crenation of cells, along with other toxic manifestations of excessive anions and cations, causes a mass destruction of cellular components (Fig. 41-2).

It should also be noted that common electrolyte solutions can cause problems by producing unphysiologic pH changes. The subsequent necrosis of the soft tissues usually demarcates within 72 hours. Total parenteral nutrition is lifesaving therapy but can also cause significant local problems if it infiltrates into the superficial soft tissues due to the high osmolality of the fluid. Vasopressors required to maintain blood pressure can also be toxic to tissues in their undiluted form (Fig. 41-3).

Both old and new chemotherapeutic agents can produce

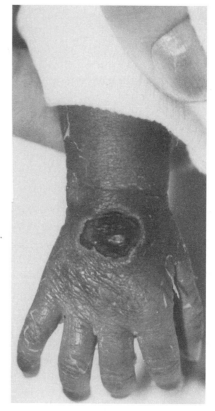

Figure 41-1. This infant sustained local soft tissue necrosis secondary to an infiltration of electrolyte solution.

local tissue necrosis. Powerful agents continue to be tested and often lead to new manifestations of toxicity. Likewise, methods of administration and dosages continue to change, with differing combinations of both old and new agents being given intravenously and by other routes. Most of these toxic agents cause death of neoplastic tissue by direct interdiction of cellular metabolism. Unfortunately, cellular death can also be seen if the agent comes into direct contact with normal tissue cells.

It is believed that most of the antineoplastic agents directly interfere with intracellular metabolism, causing death of individual cells. For example, methotrexate inhibits DNA synthesis through tight binding to the enzyme dihydrofolatereductase, resulting in a depletion of reduced folates and interruption of thymidylate and purine biosynthesis. Its toxicity can be modulated by calcium leucovorin, which may serve as a source of reduced folates. Cisplatin is a platinum

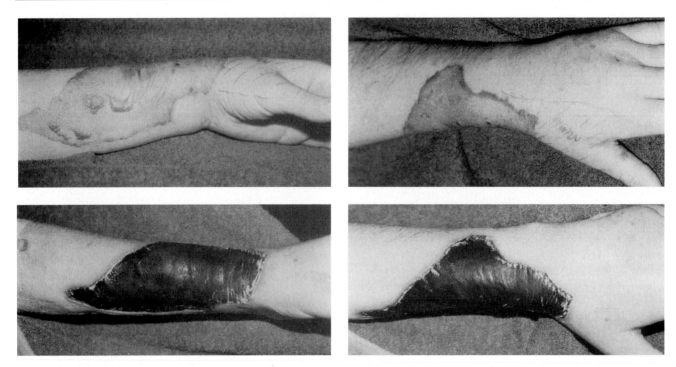

Figure 41-2. **(Top)** This patient was seen in the cardiac intensive care unit within 48 hours of having sustained local infiltration of calcium chloride. There was numbness, indicating a deep injury. **(Bottom)** Several days later, there is obvious demarcation of necrotic margins.

complex that inhibits DNA synthesis by complexing and abnormally cross-linking strands of DNA. Bleomycin is thought to cause breakage of single and double DNA strands. Doxorubicin (Adriamycin) causes tissue necrosis by mechanisms that are, as yet, poorly understood. However, it is toxic to a wide variety of normal and abnormal tissues. Doxorubicin and bleomycin are antibiotics that are isolated from strains of Streptomyces. Bleomycin causes somewhat unusual effects on the hand and soft tissues, even in the absence of direct injury. For example, it can cause dark bands over the nail beds and skin creases (Fig. 41-4).

Newer agents are being developed and can be used alone or in combination to provide optimum antineoplastic activities. For example, there has been promising activity among second-generation platinum coordination complexes. Carboplatin, Ibroplatin, Trimetrexate, and others are being studied. These medications and combinations will have their own set of local and systemic toxicities. The reader is referred to product information manuals for specific details.

As far as the hand/upper extremity surgeon is concerned, all of these medications should be viewed as potentially toxic to local tissues and differing from osmolar/electrolyte solutions in degree only. Nonchemotherapeutic agents tend to cause an immediate reaction that demarcates quickly; chemotherapeutic agents usually cause deeper necrosis that often takes up to three weeks before final demarcation of necrotic margins occurs. With either of these particular problems, it is difficult to predict the margin of necrosis that would require surgical debridement and coverage.

One should also be prepared to see the occasional idiosyncratic reaction associated with chemotherapy. Hypercoagulable states can cause necrosis of the digits following systemic antineoplastic medications (Fig. 41-5). Such problems, although not due to infiltration, can be just as devastating.

Clinical Assessment of Injury

The degree of injury often cannot be accurately defined on the initial examination. When assessing a patient with possible infiltration injury, the first priority is to discontinue the medication immediately and remove the catheter from the injured tissue. The initial examination may be weeks later, however. In either case, the area is gently palpated and the area of induration is measured and marked. A photograph is helpful to assess the time course of injury, and this can be taken immediately following the marking of the skin with a soft felt pen (Fig. 41-6). Any area of erythema and tenderness is noted, and an effort is made to identify the type of solution that was infiltrated into the tissues. If the patient is seen during the acute phase, direct examination of the plastic intravenous medication bag, glass bottle, or other administration set that is labeled with the agent is helpful. Antidotes that have been used in the past (such as isoproterenol or corticosteroid derivatives) have not been effective and have, on occasion, seemed to inflict more damage to the tissues. Injecting anything into swollen, painful tissues will intensify an already critical problem, and

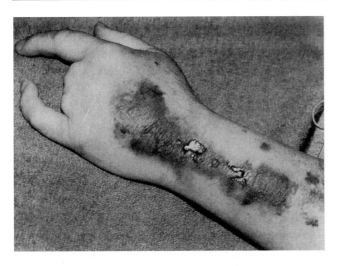

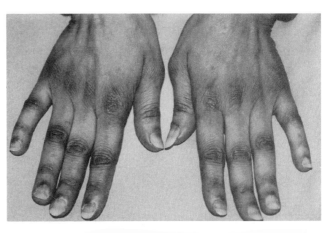

Figure 41-4. Dark coloration of the skin creases and nail-beds also occurs with bleomycin therapy, as well as transient and severe tenderness over the palms and digital pulps.

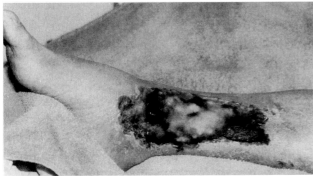

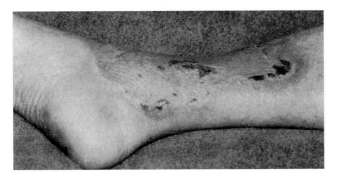

Figure 41-3. **(Top)** This patient sustained local infiltration of dopamine, with resultant superficial necrosis within 72 hours. **(Center and Bottom)** Another dopamine injury is shown that, after debridement, was successfully treated with a meshed, split-thickness skin graft.

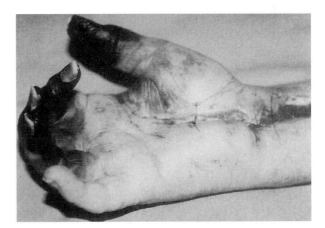

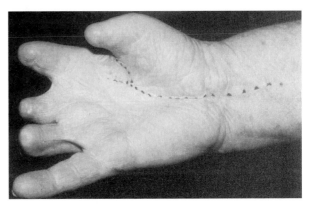

there is no way to ensure that an antidote will hit its target.

Warm packs and other externally applied measures are usually ineffective and can actually exacerbate the problem. Heat application is counterproductive since it causes vasodilatation, increased interstitial edema, increased swelling, and periarticular stiffness. Early application of cool (not cold) compresses during the first few hours seems to alleviate pain and to blunt the edema reaction. There seems to be no advantage after the initial hours.

Figure 41-5. **(Top)** This patient received her usual dosage of adjuvant chemotherapy (Cytoxan, methotrexate, and 5-fluorouracil). Within 24 hours, there was thrombosis of the ulnar and radial arteries, despite no previous history of difficulties. **(Bottom)** The patient sustained digital necrosis and is seen following recovery and healing. The dotted lines indicate areas that were decompressed surgically. She also underwent thrombectomies of the radial and ulnar arteries with balloon catheters.

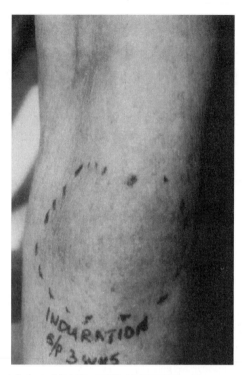

Figure 41-6. This patient is seen three weeks after local infiltration with Adriamycin into the dorsal forearm. There is erythema and induration, marked with a dotted line. This injury was superficial and had reached its peak without full-thickness necrosis. The patient recovered without further problems.

The importance of elevating of the extremity cannot be overemphasized and this should be accomplished as soon as the infiltration is noted.

Nonsurgical Management

As with any injury, emphasis is on full rehabilitation as soon as possible. This means that the injured extremity should be elevated and aggressive physical and occupational therapy should be instituted as soon as possible. The emphasis is on full active and passive range of motion of joints within the affected extremity so that the edema can be minimized and, therefore, periarticular fibrosis can be eliminated. This is a gradual process, but dynamic splinting, soft elastic garments, and exercises within a protected arc of motion are certainly possible early in the course of treatment. These exercises are gradually increased to prevent long-term disability.

Surgical Management

If the area of infiltration is anesthetic, discolored, and without evidence of dermal circulation, early excision may be warranted. These signs correlate with necrosis of the soft tissues and a deep injury. However, it is difficult to gauge the extent of necrosis and to predict the natural course of any specific infiltration injury. With this in mind, it is accept-

able to await demarcation and then proceed with excision of the necrotic area. Coverage of the defect usually involves the application of skin grafts or flaps.

Although immediate excision has been advocated by others, such patients are not often seen by the surgeon until it is apparent to their primary physician that the problem is serious enough to merit a surgical consultation. This can occur anywhere between one and 14 days following the initial injury. Many of these injuries are successfully treated with elevation alone. Since it may be difficult to clinically assess the initial extent of injury, both to the primary physician as well as to the surgical consultant, immediate (within the first week) and empirical excision of the estimated region of necrosis may result in removal of uninjured areas as well. Patients who require debridement can be successfully treated after demarcation occurs and with the expectation that good function will return if this is performed before any chronic and fibrotic changes have occurred. These changes happen several weeks after the initial injury so the surgeon has some leeway with regard to timing of intervention, if any. This author's experience indicates that the area is injured early (possibly within the first few hours of the infiltration).

Infiltrations that are associated with induration and erythema less than 10 cm in diameter tend to have a favorable prognosis. If the area of induration and tenderness does not seem to be fixed to underlying bone and fascia, the depth tends to be superficial and, less serious in nature.

Following the initial assessment of the injury, the patient should be followed closely and the progression or resolution of the induration monitored. With local injury caused by so-called nontoxic electrolyte and hyperosmolar solutions, the area of necrosis often demarcates within 48 to 72 hours, and excision and grafting may be required. It may be necessary to perform serial debridements until the area is cleared of necrotic debris and the underlying tissues can support a split-thickness skin graft or soft-tissue flap. It is best to cover these areas as early as possible to prevent the development of chronic local changes and edema within the soft tissues that could compromise early return to function and rehabilitative efforts. If a skin graft is selected for coverage of the wound, remember that skin grafts do not heal over structures that are devoid of healthy, well vascularized tissue. Grafts that are meshed 1.5:1 and applied unexpanded will heal as a sheet, yet allow sufficient drainage such that the graft will not fail to adhere due to local seromas or hematomas. Meshed grafts also follow irregular contours more effectively and can survive on a contaminated recipient bed (Fig. 41-7).

If significant loss of tissue has occurred that cannot be treated effectively with skin grafting, soft-tissue flaps (regional or distant) may be required to restore functional continuity (Fig. 41-8). It may be possible to use a skin graft for temporary coverage and allow the skin graft to contract. In this way, a later (and smaller area) reconstruction can be performed with soft-tissue flaps, if necessary. There has been a decline in the incidence of these deep, extensive injuries. This is primarily related to increased awareness and the use of more sensitive pressure alarms and venous access sites that use large, freely flowing veins.

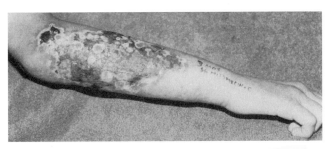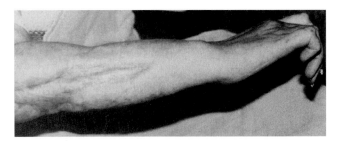

Figure 41-7. **(Left)** This individual was treated with mitomycin-C and is initially seen three months following infiltration of the agent. **(Right)** The necrotic area was excised with two debridements and coverage provided with meshed, unexpanded skin grafts. Due to unavoidable late treatment, there is residual contracture of the metacarpophalangeal joints, although the patient uses the hand in many activities.

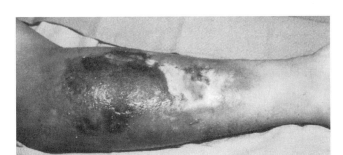

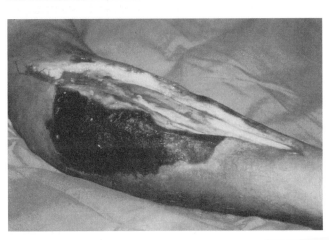

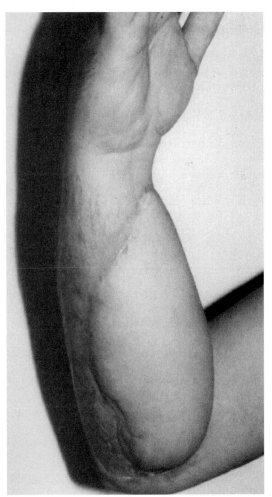

Figure 41-8. **(Top)** Extensive and deep infiltration of doxorubicin (Adriamycin). There was also evidence of increased pressure within the muscular compartments. The patient is initially evaluated two weeks following the injury. **(Bottom)** The compartments were released earlier and the necrosis is demarcated. The muscles were retained and eventually functioned well. **(Right)** An abdominal flap provided coverage, and there was excellent function of the hand.

Special Problems

Another devastating problem is that of a compartment syndrome following infiltration of an intravenous or arterial catheter into the deeper tissues. It can be seen following radial artery access for blood pressure monitoring. IV lines are especially dangerous in children, since pediatric wards may use pressure devices to keep intravenous solutions flowing at optimal levels. If these devices force the infiltrated fluid into the deep compartments, a full-blown compartment syndrome may develop that is initially overlooked.

The compartment syndrome may be diagnosed by insertion of pressure catheters within the affected compartment. However, it is usually apparent that the extremity is "tight" and there is pain on passive stretch of the digits in the affected extremity. If this occurs, it may be necessary to perform a compartment release at the bedside in the intensive care unit. After preparing the area, the skin is gently infiltrated with local anesthetic and, following incision of the skin, incision of the compartments is performed and expanded by gentle digital exploration. It is best to perform this under a short general anesthetic in the operating room, especially when the patient is a child. The usual principles of diagnosis and treatment of compartment syndromes are applicable.

Hydrofluoric acid burns can be disabling. This powerful inorganic acid is widely used in the production of semiconductors, plastics, and solvents. The fluoride ion quickly penetrates the skin, causing liquefaction necrosis to the deep tissue and corrosion of the bone. The destructive process is painful and can last for days as the acid is gradually neutralized into calcium and magnesium salts. Symptoms may not appear for more than an hour following exposure.

The affected area may exhibit swelling, erythema, tenderness, and induration, depending on the duration of contact and concentration of the acid. Immediate and specialized treatment is mandatory if necrosis is to be averted. Anything short of rapid dilution and neutralization of the acid usually fails.

The treatment of choice, according to Dibbell and associates is copious irrigation with cold tap water and an alkaline soap (as first aid); immediate dressing with acid zephiran or hyamine chloride-soaked sponges; and emergent referral for treatment. On arrival for treatment, if the concentration was less than 20%, the zephiran or hyamine chloride soaks are continued for several hours and close follow-up maintained. If the concentration was greater, or if the burns appear to be deep, calcium gluconate injections are administered into the tissues with a 30-gauge needle, in milliliter quantities.

The injection treatment may require regional block anesthetic, but the surgeon must determine whether pain from the acid burn is necessary to guide the location of the injections and the response to them. Approximately 0.5 milliliter of calcium gluconate per square centimeter of burned surface area is a general guide. A rim of uninjured tissue is also injected.

After injection, the area may require debridement. Removal of the fingernail should be done if any doubt exists as to subungual injury, since this is relatively common. The hand is dressed in a bulky, elevated dressing and observed carefully for 48 hours. If the pain recurs, additional calcium gluconate injections are administered. Later reconstructive procedures may be required, despite optimum care.

Bibliography

Adendorff DJ, Lamont A, Davies D: Skin loss in meningococcal septicemia. *Br J Plast Surg,* 3:251-255, 1980.

Bowers DG, Lynch JB: Adriamycin extravasation. *Plast Reconstr Surg,* 61:86-90, 1978.

Chabner B, Myers C, Coleman N, Johns D: The clinical pharmacology of antineoplastic agents. *N Engl J Med,* 292:1159-1168, 1975.

Dibbell DG, Iverson RE, Jones W, et al: Hydrofluoric acid burns of the hand. *J Bone and Joint Surg* 170:52-A:931-936.

Dorr RT, Alberts DS: Modulation of experimental doxorubicin skin toxicity by beta adrenergic compounds. *Cancer Res,* 41:2428-2432, 1981.

Gardland B: Prognostic evaluation in meningococcal disease. A retrospective study of 115 cases. *Int Care Med,* 12:302-307, 1986.

Greenwood BM, Onyewotu II, Whittle HC: Complement and meningococcal infection. *Br Med J,* 1:797-799, 1976.

Harwood KVS, Aisner J: Treatment of chemotherapy extravasation: Current status. *Cancer Treat Rep,* 68:(78):939, 1984.

Larson D: What is the appropriate management of tissue extravasation by antitumor agents. *Plast Reconstr Surg* 75:397-402, 1985.

Lebredo L, Barrie R, Woltering EA: DMSO protects against adriamycin-induced tissue necrosis. *J Surg Res,* 53:62-65, 1992.

Linder RM, et al. Hydrofluoric acid burns of the hand. *J Hand Surg,* 8:32-38, 1983.

Loth TS, Eversmann WW: Treatment methods for extravasations of chemotherapeutic agents: A comparative study. *J Hand Surg,* 11A:388-396, 1986.

Rudolph R, Stein RS, Patillo, RA: Skin ulcers due to adriamycin. *Cancer,* 38(3):1087, 1976.

Seyfer AE, Kiefer R: The management of dermal necrosis after acute Neisseria infections. *Military Medicine,* 154:598-600, 1989.

Seyfer AE, Seaber AV, Combrose F, Urbaniak JR: Coagulation changes in elective surgery and trauma. *Ann Surg,* 193:210, 1981.

Seyfer A, Solimando D: Toxic lesions of the hand associated with chemotherapy. *J Hand Surg,* 8:39-42, 1983.

Seyfer AE: Upper extremity injuries due to medications. *J Hand Surg,* 5:(1):744-750, 1987.

Soho MN, Langer B, Hoshino-Schimizu, et al: Pathogenesis of cutaneous lesions in acute meningococcemia in humans: sight, immunofluorescent, and electron microscopic studies of skin biopsy specimens. *J Infect Dis,* 33:506-514, 1976.

Yagoda A, Mukherji B, Young C, et al: Bleomycin, an antitumor antibiotic. *Ann Intern Med,* 77:861-870, 1972.

Yosowitz P, Ekland DA, Shaw RC, Parsons RW: Peripheral intravenous infiltration necrosis. *Ann Surg,* 182:553-556, 1975.

42

Burn Injuries

John O. Kucan, MD

Introduction

The hands are the most commonly burned area of the body. Although the hands comprise only about 5% of the total body surface area, they are unique by virtue of their functional importance. For this reason, the American Burn Association has categorized hand burns as "major thermal injuries." At first, such a classification may be viewed as an exaggeration, but closer scrutiny permits an appreciation of the singular importance of the hand and the functional consequences of burns. Burns of the hand require specialized care to maximize the potential for optimal functional outcome.

The spectrum of burn injuries to the hands is broad when viewed from the perspectives of etiology and severity. Bilateral injuries are common. In 1958, Moncrief reported that 75% of patients treated at the Brooke Army Medical Center had sustained hand burns, and 80% were bilateral. In the civilian population the incidence of hand burns in conjunction with other burn injuries exceeds 50%. The frequency of such injuries, coupled with a variety of etiologies and severity, produces a spectrum of functional impairments. Treatment assumes a major role in either minimizing or aggravating functional impairments. A basic philosophy that guides treatment from the outset is "circumvent the need for future reconstruction and rehabilitation." Incorporation of this tenet as the foundation of all treatment for burned hands optimizes functional outcomes. The primary goals of treatment are the attainment of stable, pliable soft-tissue coverage, through which preservation and/or restoration of optimal function can be realized.

Analysis of the Problem

Care of the burned hand requires a correct analysis of the problem and the development of an organized and systematic treatment plan. A complete history is the first component of this process. It should include a thorough recounting of the history of the injury, with emphasis on mechanism of injury, and the patient's medical history. Hand dominance, occupation, special activities or hobbies, and the age of the patient should be recorded. A complete physical examination and necessary stabilization of the patient should be achieved.

The burned hand is examined to determine the severity of the injury. An appreciation of the mechanism of injury is a major aid in ascertaining the severity of the injury. The essential elements of this evaluation are determining the depth of the burn wound; the extent or distribution of the burn wound; the presence and degree of edema; circulation; sensibility; the range of motion; and the involvement of underlying structures.

The first priority is restoration or preservation of circulation to the hand. Circumferential burn wounds of the upper extremity, partial thickness and full thickness alike, may result in compartment syndrome and subsequent cessation of nutrient blood flow to the hand.

In general, any circumferential deep partial-thickness or full-thickness burn can result in compartment syndrome. The obligatory edema of burn injury occurring beneath a nonyielding circumferential eschar results in rapidly increasing interstitial pressure and ultimate cessation of nutrient blood flow. Whereas most circumferential upper extremity burns can be treated by escharotomy alone, charred full-thickness (fourth-degree) burns, or those resulting from high-voltage electrical injury, will likely require fasciotomy. The only accurate determinant of both the need for and efficacy of either escharotomy or fasciotomy is direct compartment pressure measurement. Physical examination and Doppler examination can be misleading. Pressures in excess of 30 mm Hg necessitate decompression to restore nutrient blood flow to nerves and muscles. (Fig. 42-1)

Pathophysiology

Thermal injury causes cellular death directly and indirectly because injured cells liberate vasoactive products, which produce edema, vasoconstriction, and tissue necrosis. (Fig. 42-2) Bacterial colonization with subsequent multiplication may further contribute to tissue destruction. (Fig. 42-3)

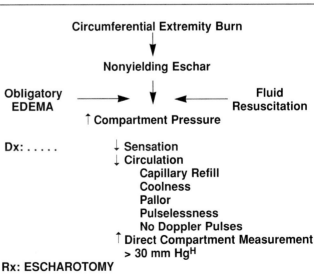

Figure 42-1.

- Histamine
- Serotonin
- Kinins
- Thromboxane
- Prostaglandins
- Free Oxygen Radicals
- Lipid Peroxides

Figure 42-2. Vasoactive Substances Liberated From Damaged Cells

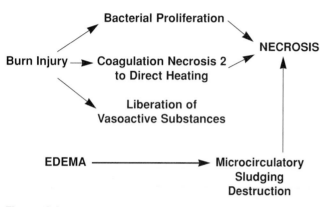

Figure 42-3.

Treatment of the Acutely Burned Hand

Treatment of the burned hand depends upon the injury. First-degree burns require only symptomatic treatment on an outpatient basis. Patients with small circumscribed partial-thickness and full-thickness burns of the hand are admitted at the physician's discretion. All burns of the hand except for minor injuries are best treated in the hospital setting. Hospitalization in cases of bilateral hand burns is generally mandatory.

Treatment of the burned hand is founded upon basic principles which include: protection from further injury; maintenance of circulation; prevention of infection; attainment of expeditious wound closure; preservation of motion; and the achievement of functional rehabilitation.

Prevention of Further Damage

Burn wounds consist of three zones: 1) the "zone of coagulation," an area of irreversible injury, 2) the "zone of stasis," the intermediate region of damaged but potentially salvageable cells, and 3) the "zone of hyperemia," the peripheral, transiently affected area which is destined to heal. Cooling of the burn wound within 30 minutes of injury may help limit injury to "the zone of stasis" and prevent further damage. The prevention of wound maceration or desiccation is essential. Blisters should be aspirated or debrided to remove fluid which contains high levels of thromboxane and other mediators known to be deleterious to the microcirculation within the "zone of stasis."

Maintenance of Circulation

Edema control can be achieved by elevating the injured hand above the level of the heart. The circumferentially burned hand and upper extremity must be observed for the development of compartment syndrome. Prompt decompression by surgical or chemical escharotomy is indicated when compartmental pressures exceed 30 mm Hg.

Surgical escharotomy is performed by incision of the offending circumferential eschar, thus achieving decompression of the hand or arm. This technique requires meticulous hemostasis to prevent potentially exsanguinating hemorrhage. Chemical or enzymatic escharotomy avoids surgical incisions and is an effective alternative to surgical decompression. Advantages of this method over surgical escharotomy include the avoidance of surgical incisions, decreased morbidity, accurate estimation of burn depth, and earlier preparation of the wound for split-thickness skin grafting. The author employs enzymatic escharotomy in lieu of surgical incisions except in the presence of charred full-thickness burns, high-voltage electrical injuries, or in the presence of elevated compartment when more than six hours have elapsed from the time of injury.

Enzymatic debridement employing Travase ointment is an effective alternative to surgical decompression. The enzyme lyses denatured proteins without injury to viable tissues. Prompt decompression, usually within one hour, can be achieved by this method in lieu of surgical incisions. This technique is contraindicated in the presence of dry-leathery, charred, full-thickness burns, high-voltage electrical injuries, or where more than six hours have elapsed from the time of injury in the presence of elevated compartment pressures.

Prevention of Infection

Infection of the burned hand, though uncommon, is nonetheless possible. During the initial edema phase, inactivation of antistreptococcal fatty acids of the skin may increase the likelihood for development of streptococcal cellulitis. Administration of a specific antistreptococcal drug such as penicillin or erythromycin during the edema phase may be indicated. Topical antimicrobial therapy is indicated in deep partial-thickness and full-thickness burns to control bacterial proliferation and prevent wound sepsis. Silver sulfadiazine cream is most commonly employed for this indication. It can be incorporated in a hand dressing, or can be used in conjunction with gortex bags, which permit motion but prevent maceration.

Attainment of Closed Wound

Autologous skin is the only permanent wound cover. Adequate, durable, stable, supple skin cover is essential to normal function. Wound closure options are primarily determined in the hand by the depth of the wound and consist of the following: spontaneous healing < 14 days; early wound excision and split-thickness skin grafting (STSG); delayed spontaneous healing > 14 days; delayed STSG >14 days; e) delayed excision and STSG.

Superficial burn wounds that are expected to heal within 14 days should be protected from desiccation. In general, they require no topical antimicrobials and may be effectively treated by applying semisynthetic skin-substitute (Biobrane) gloves. Alternatives include nonadherent gauze dressings and ointments to maximize dressing adherence to the wounds. Uncomplicated healing and normal function can be expected.

Full-thickness burn injuries of the dorsum of the hand are often managed by early excision to fascia and split-thickness skin grafting. The dorsal veins and paratenon should be preserved and sheet grafts should be employed whenever possible.

Full-thickness burn injuries to the palmar surface are far less common than injuries to the dorsum. These wounds are difficult to excise and close, and the functional outcomes are frequently poor. Circumferential full-thickness burns of the hands are challenging problems in which poor functional outcomes are the rule. The literature fails to define the best treatment for full-thickness burns of the hand. Early aggressive surgical management produces results that are not functionally different from wounds managed by delayed grafting onto a granulating wound.

The majority of burn injuries to the hands are deep dermal burns, and their optimal treatment remains controversial. Proponents of early excision (i.e. intradermal debridement) and split-thickness grafting, claim shorter hospitalization, improved function, fewer complications, and cost reduction. However, two prospective randomized studies and an additional nonrandomized study failed to demonstrate any difference in outcomes between the excised-grafted groups and those patients whose hands were allowed to heal spontaneously. Therefore, the controversy will persist, although the trend toward early excision and grafting is established and is generally accepted for treatment of deep-dermal burn injuries. Enzymatic debridement using the proteolytic enzyme Travase is an effective method for achieving intradermal debridement. The enzyme dissolves devitalized dermis but spares viable tissue. Preparation of the wound bed is accomplished with minimal surgical trauma, and skin-grafting can be applied to a viable dermal recipient bed. (Fig. 42-4)

Partial-thickness burn wounds to the palmar surface of the hand are excised infrequently since most heal spontaneously. If excision is undertaken, the task is made difficult by the absence of a defined surgical plane and may produce significant blood loss, which can be minimized by use of a tourniquet. The arm and hand should not be exsanguinated prior to inflation because the pooled blood aids in the recognition of the viable tissue plane in the course of debridement of both dorsal and palmar burns. Correct splinting of the palm in the antideformity position to maintain palmar width and breadth is critical to successful outcome.

Existing data demonstrate satisfactory results with either operative or nonoperative treatment for dorsal partial-thickness burns of the hand. Effective mobilization, proper splinting, edema control, and a carefully orchestrated hand therapy program are the determinants of a successful outcome.

To be successful, skin grafting of the burned hand should be carried out in accordance with a number of established guidelines:

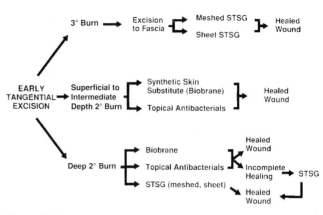

Figure 42-4.

- the recipient bed must be viable and devoid of eschar or infection;
- hemostasis must be complete;
- sheet grafts should be employed whenever possible;
- the maximum amount of skin should be provided by placing the hand in extreme positions, thereby accentuating the defect;
- immobilization and splinting must prevent mechanical disruption of the graft from the recipient bed; and
- darting or interposition of skin grafts with unburned skin should be carried out to diminish the likelihood of linear contractures or syndactyly.

Preservation of Motion

To preserve motion, splinting and positioning must be initiated as quickly as possible following injury. Elevation of the injured part to minimize edema formation is also important. Gentle active range of motion should be encouraged under the supervision of a hand therapist.

The hand should be splinted in the intrinsic-plus position with mild wrist extension, MP flexion, and IP extension. The thumb should be abducted and slightly circumducted into the palm. In the event of early excision and grafting, active range of motion exercises are initiated on the fifth postoperative day. Active assisted and passive range of motion is initiated in a graded fashion. Splints and continuous passive motion machines may be helpful in achieving full motion. In the event that early grafting is not done, attentive hand therapy is essential to achieving an optimal result. Range of motion should be documented and failure to progress should prompt reappraisal of the therapy program.

Achievement of Functional Rehabilitation

The return of optimal function is the primary goal in treating the burned patient as a whole and the burned hand in particular. This result may not be apparent immediately following wound closure, as complete wound healing and scar maturation require several months. During this period, close supervision, scar pressure exercise, massage, and edema control are critical. The degree of functional recovery must be based on objective measurement and the patient's ability to perform specific tasks. Work evaluation and functional capacity testing are frequently necessary to determine the degree and permanence of disability.

Reconstruction of the Burned Hand

Reconstruction of the burned hand is often a formidable challenge. The need for reconstruction is the result of several contributing factors acting independently or in various combinations. They include: severity of initial injury; specific areas of involvement; adequacy of initial care; prior management of the burn wound; postoperative management; quality of hand therapy; and motivation and reliability of the patient and/or caretakers. Frequently, reconstruction must address established deformities and their functional sequelae. The ultimate success or failure of reconstructive attempts hinges upon these factors as well.

The global goals of reconstructive surgery are the restoration of form and function. In the hand, this translates into power, delicacy, mobility, dexterity, and tactile sensibility. The hand must operate in concert with the more proximal regions of the upper extremity. Therefore, proximal deficits need to be addressed and successfully managed to optimize hand function.

The spectrum of deformities and problems requiring reconstruction is broad in array and severity. Some can be solved with straightforward methods, whereas others may defy satisfactory resolution. A thoughtful, stepwise delineation of the deformity, the involvement of tissues and structures, and a thorough assessment of function are the keystones of any reconstructive effort. Photography, radiographs, scans, and vascular studies may be required. A thorough and realistic discussion with patient, family, employer, or insurance carrier is necessary.

The wide array of problems and the multiple techniques described to treat them are beyond the scope of this chapter. However, a few basic rules apply:

- adhere to the reconstructive ladder, from simple to complex;
- choose the best reconstruction for the patient;
- plan alternatives and "lifeboats" in advance;
- review the options with the patient and let the patient participate in the process;
- do not allow pride to distort the objective; and
- amputation of a part may be a reasonable alternative.

Insufficiency or instability of skin mandates the provision of adequate stable skin coverage. The original defect must be recreated by removal of the entire scar. Skin grafts may be inadequate for coverage, necessitating the use of local, regional, or distant flaps. Fixed deformities of subcutaneous structures both soft and hard may require releases, bone fusions, amputations, transpositions, or grafts.

Peripheral compression neuropathies involving the median and ulnar nerves have been described in as many as 30% of burned patients. These problems often resolve with conservative treatment.

Electrical Injuries

High-voltage electricity produces devastating injuries to the hands. Injuries to the dominant hand predominate and frequently result in amputation (33% to 50%). Rarely is function sufficient to permit the individual to resume previous employment. Low-voltage injuries may produce small circumscribed burns, resulting in localized tissue necrosis, or occasionally, loss of a digit. At the site of entrance, and exit, high temperatures are generated, and thermal injury results. In addition, all intervening tissues may be affected to varying degrees by the flow of current.

The severity of an electrical injury depends upon a number of physical factors. These include voltage, amperage, resistance, type of current, duration of contact, and the pathway of the current through the body. Voltage is the amount of electromotive force, amperage is the current flow, and resistance is the quality of any material which resists the flow of electrons. The highest resistance is at the skin surface and is dependent on thickness, cleanliness, and moisture. The greatest heat is generated at the site of entry and exit from the body resulting in implosive and explosive injuries, respectively. Although a gradation in resistance among body tissues has been described, with nerve offering the least resistance and bone offering the greatest resistance, the flow of electrical current through the body is essentially uniform throughout all tissues once skin resistance has been overcome. In addition, cross-sectional area is a significant determinant of current density and, thus, the severity of injury. In the hand, wrist, and forearm, because of the small cross-sectional areas, there exist relatively high concentrations of current in the presence of high-voltage electrical injury and, a greater degree of tissue damage.

Electrical energy produces tissue injury by one of three mechanisms: (1) direct current effect at the point of contact and intervening body tissues; (2) arc burn; and (3) ignition of clothing and flame burn. The effect of high-voltage electrical injury has been likened to that seen with crush injury. A large volume of tissue is affected, in contradistinction to the pure surface injury characteristic of thermal burns.

The exact method by which deep tissues sustain damage has not been clearly defined. The most commonly accepted pathogenesis is the conversion of electrical injury to heat. However, recent data challenge this theory as the sole explanation for electrical injury. Experiments employing a computer model demonstrated that the heat generated is dependent upon whether the conducting layers are arranged in series or in parallel. If arranged in series, the layer with the greatest tissue resistance generates the most heat. If arranged in parallel, however, the layer with the highest conductivity (least resistance) generates the highest temperature. In addition, experimental data described the phenomenon of electroporation as a significant component in the pathogenesis of high-voltage electrical injury. Although many authors believe that the extent of tissue necrosis is determined at the time of the initial injury, other investigators demonstrated experimentally that some progression of injury may be the consequence of the release of potent vasoconstrictors such as thromboxane following high-voltage electrical injury.

Initial Management

The initial management of high-voltage electrical injury to the hand must be undertaken within the framework of total patient care. Adherence to the principles of resuscitation and the care of the multiply traumatized patient are imperative. Assessment for possible systemic injuries should be carried out. Adequate fluid replacement to maintain urine output in excess of 100 ml/hr with alkalinization of the urine is imperative. Mannitol, tetanus prophylaxis, and prophylactic antibiotics (including penicillin for clostridia) should be administered. Baseline evaluations of renal function, electrocardiograms, cardiac and liver enzymes, as well as electrolytes should be obtained and carefully followed. In addition, regular determinations of myoglobin and hemoglobin breakdown products are necessary. Once stabilization has been achieved and life-threatening problems have been managed, attention should be turned to the wound.

High-voltage electricity produces wounds of various sizes and the extent of injury may not be apparent during the initial examination. In most cases, the severity of the injury can be ascertained by the posture of the hand, the inability to passively extend the wrist or digits from their extremely flexed position, and the tenderness of forearm musculature. In addition, charring of skin, marked edema, or frank necrosis and tissue destruction may be apparent. The presence of large amounts of myoglobin or hemoglobin in the urine is an additional indicator of the severity of injury. Further evidence of severity may be obtained by careful examination of the neurovascular status of the hand and upper extremity.

Treatment

Injuries involving the hand and upper extremity should be treated as surgical emergencies, and the initial management requires prompt surgical decompression. Following stabilization, the patient should be taken to the operating room for fasciotomy of involved muscle compartments to release nerves at known sites of compression. This provides an opportunity for direct examination of the injured tissues to determine the extent and severity of injury and to provide both diagnostic and prognostic information, and therapeutic intervention in the early postinjury phase. Surgical decompression may, to varying degrees, preserve nutrient blood flow to nerves and muscle compartments. It should be undertaken after a thorough assessment of the patient's neurologic and circulatory status. Not all patients who have been exposed to electrical current require surgical management and decompression. Those who demonstrate signs of neurosensory deficits and circulatory embarrassment in the presence of obvious cutaneous or subcutaneous injury should undergo surgical decompression and exploration. In marginal cases, direct measurements of compartment pressures should be carried out. Following fasciotomy and initial debridement, the wound should be dressed with a topical antimicrobial. The topical antimicrobial of choice following high-voltage electrical injury is mafenide acetate cream (Sulfamylon), because it penetrates tissues to a greater degree than other topical antimicrobial agents and is effective against anaerobic species. In addition, because of its activity as a carbonic anhydrase inhibitor, it acts in concert with the alkalinizing agents to produce an alkaline urine that is desirable during this phase of treatment.

Following initial debridement and dressing, the hand should be splinted in the intrinsic plus position. In addition, more proximal areas of involvement should be similarly dressed and splinted to optimize positioning and the potential for restoration of function. The patient should be returned to the operating room until all devitalized tissue has been debrided. Because of the severity of these injuries, debridement frequently results in amputations. In situations where nerve, tendon, bone, or joint are exposed, and are in need of vascularized durable coverage, the use of biologic dressings may prevent desiccation and permit additional time for planning of the definitive reconstructive procedure. Following complete debridement of devitalized tissues, wound coverage is necessary. In many cases, exposure of important structures such as nerve, tendon, bone, joints, or blood vessels necessitates the use of flaps. Split-thickness skin grafts are often inadequate to achieve satisfactory closure and permanent coverage of these structures. In many instances, the use of local or regional flaps may not be possible due to extensive regional involvement. In the presence of small defects, local flaps provide ideal coverage for small and important structures such as flexor tendons and digital nerves. In the case of larger defects, several options may be available. Specific examples include the groin flap, the abdominal flap, the pectoralis major island flap, latissimus dorsi muscle and myocutaneous flap, or a variety of free-tissue transfers, and a wide array of fasciocutaneous, as well as muscle and myocutaneous flaps from distant donor sites throughout the body. Selection of these options requires thoughtful planning and must encompass the needs of the patient, the technical concerns inherent in the procedure, and functional considerations.

Amputation and Prosthetics

Amputation is rarely indicated at the initial treatment of the patient with the high-voltage electrical injury. However, amputations are frequent in the later stages of the patient's care to avoid sepsis or to address a nonviable, nonfunctional, and insensate extremity. Such decisions are difficult and may necessitate consultation with an experienced colleague in order to restore objectivity to this decision.

Chemical Burns

Chemical burns to the hands are generally localized but may require admission to the burn center and produce variable degrees of tissue necrosis. Chemical burns are different from thermal burns as the causative agent may remain in contact with the skin for a prolonged period, producing extensive and progressive tissue damage or destruction. The degree and extent of damage is dependent upon the chemical agent, quantity, concentration, contact time with the skin, and the type of chemical reaction that the agents produce. In general, acids cause coagulation necrosis, alkalis produce liquefaction, and vesicants result in ischemic and anoxic injury. Although most chemical agents produce a thermal burn as a result of an exothermic reaction, this is short lived and the vast majority of tissue damage from a chemical agent continues relentlessly until it is washed away from the skin, neutralized, or until its toxicity is spent by reaction with the tissues. Certain chemical agents may produce systemic toxicity by virtue of their absorption.

First Aid

Effective first-aid treatment is immediate and continuous irrigation with tap water. A continuous flow of water removes heat that may be produced. In addition, it dilutes, or totally removes the offending agent. Irrigation should continue until pain has subsided. Water irrigation is preferable to the use of specific neutralizing agents, for these agents may react with the offending chemical, producing an exothermic reaction and further thermal injury. The management of chemical injuries is very similar to that of thermal burns. Once wound cleansing has been accomplished, topical antimicrobial agents and debridement in wound closure are the mainstays of treatment.

Hydrofluoric Acid Burns

Burns caused by hydrofluoric acid mandate special atten-

tion. Hydrofluoric acid is a strong inorganic acid used in many industries as both a cleaning agent and a solvent. It is highly corrosive and penetrates tissue, producing cytotoxic injury at the cellular level. It produces liquefaction necrosis of the soft tissues and bony erosion. The severity and onset of symptoms are directly related to the area of skin exposure, the concentration of the acid, and duration of exposure. The clinical appearance is that of swelling, a yellowish-white area of necrosis, associated blistering, erythema, and severe pain. The treatment consists of immediate irrigation with copious amounts of water, followed by attempts to neutralize or eliminate the free fluoride ions that are responsible for tissue damage. When injuries involve the fingertips, 2.5% calcium gluconate gel may be applied topically and the hand placed in a rubber glove to achieve sufficient contact of the calcium gluconate and the hydrofluoric acid. Such a regimen is successful in relieving pain as the calcium combines with the fluoride ion and precipitates as an insoluble complex. When larger areas of the hand are involved, 10 cc of calcium gluconate and 40 cc of normal saline are infused via the radial or ulnar artery over a four-hour period. This method replaces previously recommended subcutaneous injections of 10% calcium gluconate. In the event that the forearm and hand are involved, 20 cc of 20% calcium gluconate and 80 cc of normal saline are infused via the brachial artery over a four-hour period.

Annotated Bibliography

American Burn Association, Guidelines for service standards and severity classifications in the treatment of burn injury. *American College of Surgeons Bulletin,* 69:10, 1984.

This document is a concise description of the standards for providing care to the burned patient.

Dimick AR: Experience with the use of proteolytic enzyme (Travase) in burn patients. *J Trauma,* 17:948-955, 1977.

This article describes a philosophy and practical application of enzymatic debridement in the management of the burned patient.

Edstrom L, Robson MC, Macchiaverna JR, Scala AD: Management of deep partial thickness dorsal hand burns. *Orthop Review,* 8:27-33, 1979.

A prospective randomized study that addresses the issue of spontaneous healing vs. delayed excision and grafting, which supports the notion that surgical and nonsurgical results are comparable when dealing with deep partial-thickness burn wounds of the hand.

Gant TD: The early enzymatic debridement and grafting to deep dermal burns to the hand. *Plast Reconstr Surg,* 66:185-189, 1980.

Describes a useful technique for enzymatic debridement and early grafting of deep dermal burns to the hands, which may be valuable in the management of selected patients.

Goodwin CW, Maguire MS, McManus WF, Pruitt BA: Prospective study of burn wound excision of the hands. *J Trauma,* 23:510-517, 1983.

A prospective evaluation of 164 burned hands, which seems to indicate that excision and grafting of hands with deep dermal burns, whether early or late, offers no distinct advantage over physical therapy and primary healing in maintaining hand function.

Heggers JP, Ko F, Robson MC, Heggers R, Craft KE: Evaluation of burn blister fluid. *Plast Reconstr Surg,* 65:798-803, 1980.

A concise description of the content of burn blister fluid and its protective effect against bacterial contamination.

Janzekovic Z: A new concept in the early excision and immediate grafting of burns. *J Trauma,* 10:1103-1107, 1970.

The landmark article describes early intradermal debridement and grafting of burn wounds and sets the stage for modern aggressive burn wound management.

Krizek TJ, Flagg SV, Wolfort FG, Jabaley ME: Delayed primary excision and skin grafting of the burned hand. *Plast Reconstr Surg,* 51:524-529, 1973.

The rationale for delayed primary excision and skin grafting of the hands is presented in this historical article.

Kurtzman LC, Stern PJ: Upper extremity burn contractures, *Hand Clin,* 6:261-279, 1990.

A concise and practical overview of the various upper extremity burn scar contractures and an approach to their management.

Lee RC, Gottlieb LJ, Krizek TJ: Pathophysiology and clinical manifestations of tissue injury in electrical trauma. *Advances Plast Reconstr Surg,* 8:1-29, 1992.

An interesting article which provides another theory on the pathogenesis of high-voltage electrical injury.

Pribaz JJ, Eriksson E, Smith DJ: Acute management of the burned hand. *Plast Reconstr Surg,* 209-225, 1989.

A broad overview of management of the acutely burned hand.

Robson MC, Smith DJ, VanderZee AJ, Roberts L: Making the burned hand functional. *Burn Rehab Reconstr,* 19:663-671, 1992.

Provides an overview and an algorithm for the management and treatment of the acutely burned hand.

Robson MC, Smith DJ: Plastic surgery, principles and practice, burned hand. 1:781-801, 1990.

A broad overview of management of the burned hand, not a detailed assessment.

Simpson RL, Flaherty ME: The burned small finger. *Burn Rehab Reconstr,* 19:673-682, 1992.

A detailed and useful analysis of problems associated with burns of the fifth finger and their pathogenesis and correction.

Smith DJ, McHugh TP, Philips LG, Robson MC, Heggers JP: Biosynthetic compound dressings–management of hand burns. *Burns,* 14:405-408, 1988.

A description of the clinical experience in 218 cases of burns managed with the biosynthetic dressing Biobrane, and the description of its advantages and cost effectiveness over standard wound management techniques.

Stern PJ, Neale HW, Graham TJ, Warden GD: Classification and treatment of postburn proximal interphalangeal joint flexion contractures in children, *J Hand Surg,* 12A:450-453, 1987.

A useful article which provides a classification system based on severity of burn contractures and an assessment of treatment results.

Terrill PJ, Kedwards SM, Lawrence JC: The use of GORE-TEX bags for hand burns. *Burns,* 17:161-165, 1991.

A description of both the clinical and laboratory assessment of water vapor permeable GORE-TEX bags and their application in the treatment of burned hands. An alternative method of treatment which may be useful in selected patients.

Upton J, Rogers C, Durham-Smith G, Swartz WM: Clinical applications of free temporoparietal flaps in hand reconstruction. *J Hand Surg,* 11A:475-483, 1986.

An anatomical and practical description of the applications of free temporoparietal flaps in reconstruction of a variety of hand defects.

43

Cumulative Trauma Disorders

Dean S. Louis, MD

Introduction

Cumulative trauma disorders: the epidemic of the 90s. CTDs are also called repetitive strain injuries, cervicobrachial syndromes, occupational overuse syndromes, and work-related disorders. Carpal tunnel syndrome, deQuervain's, various other forms of tenosynovitis, epicondylitis about the elbow, and proximal shoulder impairments in the work place are a major concern to large and small manufacturers, insurance carriers, health-care providers, and the federal government.

Epidemiology

Cumulative trauma disorders are largely due to repetitiveness and forcefulness of work and cause localized stresses in tissues, thus altering their homeostasis. The tissue changes that occur in CTDs may or may not be reversible, and they may or may not best be treated by surgical management. There are no simple solutions to these problems and no definitive algorithm to guide management.

Cumulative trauma disorders generally develop over periods of time, varying from weeks to years. Certain occupations have been the subject of reports regarding cumulative trauma disorders and include the poultry industry, the meat-packing industry, automotive assembly, electronic parts manufacturers, and video display terminal operations. In this latter regard, a recent law was passed in San Francisco mandating a rest period between periods of activity for video display terminal operators.

It would appear that much of modern work involves such intense repetitive activity and/or forceful use of the hands and upper extremities that the involved tissues are unable to recover satisfactorily. The daily repetition of these tasks may be additive, such that symptoms do not subside at the end of the working day and persist between work intervals. The exact nature of an individual's working tasks is important in delineating precipitating factors in the symptom complex. Included should be an assessment of the specific components of each task performed, the frequency with which it is performed, and the total motions or repetitions involved in the particular task. The forcefulness with which tasks are performed should also be assessed. For example, the heavy gripping that is necessary to operate air guns and power tools may be a significant factor in symptom production. The length of time a person has been on a particular job may also be related to symptom production, especially in older workers who are prone to certain degenerative processes. It is also important to evaluate a person's nonoccupational activities, i.e. sporting activities that may additionally aggravate the symptom complex.

Ergonomics

Ergonomic assessment involves the evaluation of how an employee performs work tasks. This requires an on-site evaluation of the way the individual performs the job. The factors mentioned in the preceding section regarding frequency, duration, and forcefulness of tasks are part of this assessment, but equally important are the positions of various parts of the upper extremity required to perform the tasks. Working overhead with the shoulders forward flexed or elevated is likely to produce upper extremity symptoms. The positions of extreme wrist flexion or extension are accompanied by increased pressures within the carpal tunnel, and may aggravate carpal tunnel symptoms. Modification of positions, repetitiveness, and forcefulness may require redesign or modification of the work place. Changing the position of the wrist at a keyboard, for example, by either raising or lowering the height of the chair, may effectively diminish symptoms. In addition, job rotation and periods of rest may compensate for periods of intense activity so that constant aggravation may be alleviated.

The Department of Labor and the Occupational Safety and Health Administration have recently been alarmed by the report from the Bureau of Labor Statistics, which stated that disorders associated with repeated trauma have more than tripled since 1984. DOL and OSHA are concerned with ergonomic disorders, particularly repetitive motions, forceful exertions, vibration, and sustained or awkward posturing involving the hand, wrist, arm, neck, and shoulder as significant ergonomic stressers. Specifically, OSHA is concerned with problems relating to carpal tunnel syndrome and various forms of tendon and muscle irritation, as well as lower back injuries. They have targeted changes in production processes and technologies, resulting in specialized tasks with increasing repetitions and higher assembly-line speed; and the failure of such changes to include ergonomic interventions.

Liberty Mutual, the largest underwriter of workers compensation coverage in the United States, has declared that since 1987, the cost of upper extremity cumulative trauma disorders as a percentage of all workers compensation costs has quadrupled. On July 31, 1991, the United Food and Com-mercial Workers Union, the AFL-CIO, and 29 other labor organizations petitioned OSHA to take immediate action to reduce the risk of employees from exposure to ergonomic hazards. These organizations requested that OSHA issue an emergency temporary standard on ergonomic hazards to protect workers from work-related musculoskeletal disorders (cumulative trauma disorders). Such a standard would set limits on repetitive and forceful work place activities. Some industries have been able to effectively control the incidence of problems by utilizing reasonable ergonomic measures. One suture manufacturer reduced its incidence of CTDs by incorporating rest and exercise programs into their work environment.

In certain settings, especially Australia, the incidence of CTDs (repetitive strain injuries) escalated during the early 80s. When it was understood that this was not a specific disease entity, but was the product of a sociopolitical-psychological mind-set, its incidence diminished dramatically. This brings into perspective the psychological aspects of these conditions. A worldwide debate continues regarding the casual relationship of work activities and clinical symptom complexes. The economic cost of cumulative trauma disorders continues to rise and is a matter of great national concern. To what degree surgical interventions are appropriate is still a matter of conjecture. It does appear that in the carpal tunnel syndrome, the tenosynovium becomes thickened without inflammation in response to repetitive and forceful mechanical stress. The nature of modern working tasks, i.e. manufacturing, keyboard use, computers, meat and poultry processing, seem so intense that the tissues cannot recover sufficiently, leading to persistent symptom states involving various different anatomic sites.

Cumulative Trauma Specific Conditions

The effect of vibration as a cause of cumulative trauma disorders has been documented. In one study, 43% of forestry workers had numbness in their hands, 50% had weakness of grip, and 27% had Raynaud's phenomenon. Another recent study showed that workers in the textile industry who were surveyed by questionnaire and examined confirmed that more physically demanding jobs resulted in more upper extremity symptoms ranging from carpal tunnel syndrome to epicondylitis. Another study noted that surgery was not a panacea for patients with de Quervain's tenosynovitis and suggested that women with this problem had other associated diagnoses and that complications of release were prevalent.

Disorders of Musicians

In one study it was shown, using a computer piano keyboard model to analyze finger motions in pianists, that the intrinsic mobility of the wrist and the hand was related to the production of symptoms. Another study revealed that musicians who use keyboards were more likely to develop symptoms than those who used strings, flutes, or plucked instruments. There are varying reports as to which type of instrument is most likely to result in problems. More studies in this regard are needed. The prolonged hours required for practice and performance in musicians leave them particularly susceptible to tendonitis, carpal tunnel syndrome, and other overuse syndromes. The only effective treatment for these individuals has been rest. The analogy between the musician, the athlete, and the worker is clear in that repetitive activities, the prolonged time of the activities, and the forcefulness involved seem to be common factors. In one study, of 71 piano majors responding to a questionnaire regarding upper extremity discomfort, 42% experienced discomfort that lasted more than one week, causing them to curtail practice. Fifty-eight percent, however, experienced little or no discomfort.

Athletes

There is perhaps no group, aside from musicians and industrial workers, who have such high performance requirements. The specific athletic task involved may engender precise upper extremity problems. This is particularly evident in baseball players, especially pitchers, and in gymnasts. In the former group, stresses on musculotendinous units and ligaments in a repetitive fashion may create cumulative stress at localized areas. In gymnasts, compressive forces such as those that are involved in vaulting are far less likely to cause symptoms than those which are distractive, such as in ring exercises. In one study of competitive gymnasts, 75% of the men and 32% of the women had wrist pain for at least four months.

Work Therapy and Rehabilitation

Work therapy, work hardening, and functional capacities evaluation are buzz words in the current milieu relating to the disorders that have been previously discussed. One study has shown that 75% of a surveyed population underwent work hardening and returned to work at their regular or modified jobs. Patients who were covered by workers compensation took much longer to return to the work place. Educational programs regarding modification of activities and utilizing ergonomic evaluations of the work place diminished symptoms in another group of patients.

Interestingly, blood flow after repetitive work tasks in both radial and ulnar arteries after 90 minutes of manual work improved with an exercise program as compared to a program of rest. One study showed that a trained occupational therapist could use functional capacities evaluation to predict a worker's ability to return to their usual occupation.

The status of work hardening programs and functional capacities assessments is currently unclear. The expense/benefit ratio has never been seriously challenged and is an area for further investigation.

Annotated Bibliography

Cumulative Trauma - General Including Epidemiology

Blair SJ, Armstrong TJ, Louis DS, Bear-Lehman J (eds): Occupational disorders of the upper extremity. *J Hand Surg,* 12A:821-970, 1987.

The history and development of occupational disorders of the upper extremity are reviewed; included are sections on epidemiology, prevention, biomechanics, cost effectiveness, work capacity evaluation, and rehabilitation.

Kasdan ML et al (ed): *Occupational Hand and Upper Extremity Injuries and Diseases.* Philadelphia: Hanley and Belfus, 1991.

This text details diagnosis and treatment of specific occupational injuries. All major areas of occupational involvement are covered. It also considers such areas as workers compensation, ergonomics, and return-to-work programs for the injured.
The authors validated the NIOSH surveillance case definition for work-related carpal tunnel syndrome. They used nerve conduction studies as the gold standard. The authors believe that improved diagnostic techniques are still needed.

Millender LH, Louis DS, Simmons BP (ed): *Occupational Disorders of the Upper Extremity.* New York: Churchill Livingstone, 1992.

This text is issue-oriented. It develops a format about the current industrial milieu that leads to an understanding of particular confounders in this complex area. Included are chapters related to legal and industrial perspectives, workers compensation, anatomical sites of involvement, an extensive chapter regarding musicians' afflictions, as well as chapters on impairment and disability evolution.

Ergonomics

Armstrong TJ, Fine LJ, Goldstein SA, Lifshitz YR, Silverstein BA: Ergonomic considerations in hand and wrist tendonitis. *J Hand Surg,* 12A:830-837, 1987.

Epidemiologic data suggest that the risk of hand and wrist tendonitis is 29 times greater in persons who perform forceful and repetitive tasks. This preliminary but unproven hypothesis has been the foundation of current thinking about these two factors in the causation of cumulative trauma disorders.

Department of Labor. Occupational Safety and Health Administration. *Ergonomic Safety and Health Management Federal Register,* Vol. 57, No. 149, pp 34192-34200, August 3, 1992.

The federal government's awareness of ergonomic problems in the work place and proposed new rules for management are outlined here.

Lutz G, Hansford T: Cumulative trauma disorder controls: the ergonomics program at Ethicon, Inc. *J Hand Surg,* 12A:863-866, 1987.

An ergonomics task force in an industrial setting succeeded in controlling cumulative trauma disorders.

Stock S: Work place ergonomic factors and the development of musculoskeletal disorders of the neck and upper limbs: a meta-analysis. *Am J Industr Med,* 19:87-107, 1991.

This rigorous analysis of 54 relevant studies revealed three met inclusion criteria. The author concludes that there is strong evidence of a causal relationship between repetitive, forceful work and the development of musculoskeletal disorders of the upper extremities. Workers with a combination of high force and high repetition were 32 times more likely to develop hand/wrist tendonitis and 15 times more likely to develop carpal tunnel syndrome than workers where these factors are not present.

Cumulative Trauma - Specific Conditions

Arons MS: De Quervain's release in working women: a report of failures, complications and associated diagnoses. *J Hand Surg,* 12A:540-544, 1987.

De Quervain's tenosynovitis does not occur as an isolated process. Sixteen women had 23 associated diagnoses and 14 surgical complications.

Ireland DCR: Psychological and physical effects of occupational arm pain. *J Hand Surg,* 13B:5-10, 1988.

This is a succinct analysis of the Australian experience with repetitive strain injuries. It presents strong arguments about the psychological genesis of these disorders.

Koskimmies K, Forkkela M, Pgykko I, et al: Carpal tunnel syndrome in vibration disease. *Br J Int Med,* 47:411-416, 1990.

Forty-three percent of forestry workers had numbness of their hands; 15% had weakness of grip; 27% had Raynaud's phenomenon.

McCormack RR Jr, Inman RD, Wells A, et al: Prevalence of tendonitis and related disorders of the upper extremity in a manufacturing work force. *J Rheumatology,* 17:958-964, 1990.

A large population of textile workers was surveyed and examined (2,047), confirming that more physically demanding jobs resulted in more upper extremity symptoms ranging from carpal tunnel syndrome to epicondylitis.

Schwind F, Ventura M, Posteck JL: Idiopathic carpal tunnel syndrome: Histologic study of flexor tendon synovium. *J Hand Surg,* 15A:497-503, 1990.

The flexor tenosynovium was characterized as showing fibrous hypertrophy believed to be the result of mechanical stresses.

Disorders of Musicians

Lee SH: Pianists hand ergonomics and touch central. *Med Probl Perform Art,* 5:72-78, 1990.

A computer piano keyboard was used to analyze finger motions in pianists. Wrist and hand mobility were related to the performance of specified piano exercises.

Lockwood AH: Medical problems of musicians. *N Engl J Med,* 320:221-226, 1989.

Almost half of performing musicians experience overuse syndromes, usually manifested by pain while playing. String players were most commonly affected and percussionists the least in this study. Repetitive movement, long hours of practice, and awkward body postures seem to play a part. Rest is the most important part of the treatment.

Revak JM: Incidence of upper extremity discomfort among piano students. *Am J Occup Ther,* 43:149-154, 1989.

Seventy-one piano majors responded to a questionnaire regarding upper extremity discomfort. Forty-two percent experienced discomfort that lasted more than one week; 58% experienced little or no discomfort. Those who experienced hand, wrist or forearm pain were improved after six months or less.

Disorders of Athletes

Mandelbaum BR, Bartolozzi AR, Davis CA, et al: Wrist pain syndrome in the gymnast: Pathogenetics, diagnostic, and therapeutic considerations. *Am J Sports Med,* 17:305-317, 1989.

Thirty-eight collegiate gymnasts were evaluated; 75% of men and 33% of women had wrist pain for at least four months. Pain appeared to be related to impaction maneuvers with compression, but not with distraction.

Strickland JW, Rettig AC, et al (eds): *Hand Injuries in Athletes.* Philadelphia: W. B. Saunders, Co., 1992.

This comprehensive text reviews all aspects of athletic injuries to the upper extremity. It contains thorough coverage of physiology, pathomechanics, epidemiology, treatment for specific injuries, and rehabilitation techniques.

Work Therapy and Rehabilitation

Ballard M, Baxter P, Bruening L, Fried S: Work therapy and return to work. *Hand Clin,* 2:247-258, 1986.

Seventy-five percent of a surveyed population doing a one-year period of work tolerance program (work hardening) returned to work at their regular or modified jobs. Patients who were covered under workers compensation took 63% longer to return to work than those who were covered by private insurance.

Dortch H, Trombly C: The effects of education on hand use with industrial workers in repetitive jobs. *Am J Occup Ther,* 44:777-782, 1990.

An educational program was used to help workers eliminate at risk movements known to cause cumulative trauma.

Hansford T, Blood H, Kent B, et al: Blood flow changes at the wrist in manual workers after preventive interventions. *J Hand Surg,* 11A:503-508, 1986.

Blood flow after repetitive work tasks diminished in both radial and ulnar arteries after 90 minutes of manual work. A five-minute exercise program resulted in greater blood flow than did a five-minute rest period.

Smith S, Cunningham S, Weinberg R: The predictive validity of functional capacities evaluation. *Am J Occup Ther,* 40:564-567, 1986.

An analysis of the predictive value of functional capacities evaluation was used in 52 subjects. The results suggest that a trained occupational therapist could use this data to predict a patient's ability to return to work.

44

Hand Rehabilitation

Roslyn B. Evans, OTR/L

Introduction

This chapter reviews recent contributions that have influenced the practice of hand rehabilitation in the areas of assessment, wound healing, and management of tendon and nerve tissues.

It is widely agreed among hand rehabilitation specialists that the most significant changes in the treatment of upper limb disorders during the past five years are related to the management of soft-tissue wounds during the first two stages of wound healing. This trend is not only a response to new basic science and clinical studies, which support early therapeutic intervention, but to medical/economic pressures. Long-term treatments required for tissues mismanaged in the first few critical weeks of healing, or tissues treated with excessive immobilization, are poorly received in today's medical economic climate.

Accurate assessment, physiologic approach to the management of healing tissues, and appreciation for therapy-induced problems define current clinical treatment provided by the hand rehabilitation specialist.

Assessment

The American Society for Surgery of the Hand and the American Society of Hand Therapists are currently rewriting guidelines for a common assessment language. These guidelines include recommendations for measurement of range of motion, strength, sensibility, volume, vascular status, and coordination. The validity and sensitivity of evaluation techniques and instrument control are key factors in establishing clinical reliability. Few assessment tools meet the criteria for being both reliable and valid.

Goniometric measurement is technically not a standardized assessment tool for joint range of motion; however, it does provide reliable and accurate information for which norms have been established. Intra-tester reliability is a recognized problem, especially with passive joint range of motion (PROM) measurements. Torque range of motion (TROM) is a precise and accurate method for measuring PROM in which the force applied to a joint at a given distance from the joint axis and the position of the proximal joints are controlled. Standard measurements and the use of TROM in the hand clinic have been described, providing the clinician and researcher with a reliable and reproducible method of measuring PROM (Fig. 44-1).

Twenty-nine uninjured healthy human subjects underwent proximal interphalangeal cast immobilization for periods of one to six weeks. Resultant curves were compared to baseline curves and to conventional measures of lost ROM. The primary finding was that torque angle curves were objective measures of quantity and quality of joint stiffness.

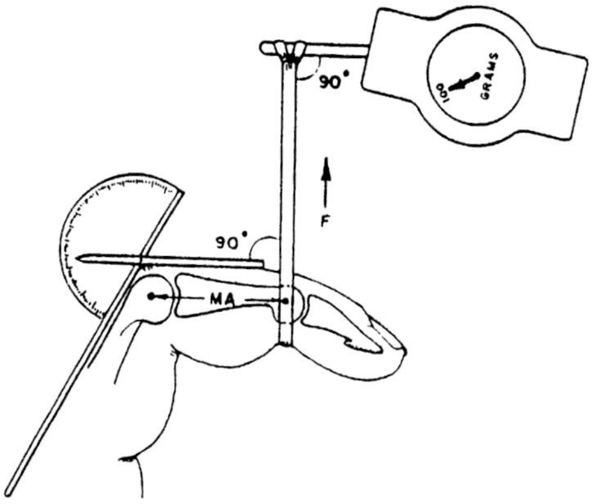

Figure 44-1. Torque is applied to extend the PIP joint at right angles in the middle segment of the finger. Torque = Force x Moment Arm. (Moment Arm: perpendicular distance from the joint axis.) Reproduced with permission from Breger-Lee D, Bell-Krotoski J, Brandsma JW: Torque range of motion in the hand clinic. *J Hand Ther,* 3:(1)7-13, 1990.

Sensibility function relying on neural continuity, impulse transmission, receptor activity, and cortical perception is evaluated by the ability to detect, discriminate, quantify, and recognize stimuli. Most currently used testing instruments for measuring tactile cutaneous sensation depend upon the application of a touch stimulus by the hand of the examiner. Hand-held instruments introduce variables in instrument application force from examiner to examiner, resulting in limited repeatability and limited reliability of the stimulus.

In a study describing the dynamic properties inherent in any hand-held touch stimuli, the measurement of variance in the force of instrument application and the measurement of the frequency produced by the instrument stimulus (force/time measurement) was recorded for the paperclip (two-point discrimination), the tuning fork (30 Hz and 256 Hz, a model for vibration), and the Semmes-Weinstein monofilaments to model touch-pressure threshold. This study demonstrates the consistency of force-application of the Semmes-Weinstein monofilaments and the inconsistency of the other tests. It addresses the fact that any hand-held instrument that does not have sufficient control over levels of force application produces variables that exceed the sensitivity needed by several orders of magnitude. Other caveats of this paper provide us with the concept that 30 Hz and perception of pain represent academic but not functional sensibility, whereas the Semmes-Weinstein monofilaments are a measurement of functional ability. This study also demonstrates that current instruments are too gross to differentiate between quickly and slowly adapting fibers (frequency spectrum test).

The Semmes-Weinstein monofilament kit as an evaluation tool for touch recognition threshold is reliable only if calibrated correctly. The physical characteristics, manufacturing problems, and test application for the monofilaments have recently been studied with equipment and material criteria established. The use of a 5-filament instead of a 20-filament kit with numbers 2.83, 3.61, 4.31, 4.56, and 6.65 has been proposed for clinical use as being less prone to inaccuracy and manufacturing problems.

The Automated Tactile Tester (ATT), a computer-controlled device designed to measure cutaneous perception of touch, vibration, temperature, and pain, may help to solve the problems of the hand-held instrument. The ATT provides repeatable and reliable measurements of sensory function in the skin and has potential application in the diagnosis and evaluation of compression and other peripheral neuropathies. Threshold values for skin indentation (touch), high- and low-frequency vibration, pin prick (sharpness), warmth, and 2PD were obtained from the fingers of 62 normal subjects to derive age-adjusted criteria for normal sensory function in the glabrous skin of human fingers. All tests with the ATT except pin prick showed a statistically significant increase in threshold with age. No difference was attributed to digit, hand, or sex. These results differ from those of Weinstein who found no change with age in his Semmes-Weinstein studies.

A companion study examined 61 patients with symptoms of median nerve compression at the wrist. A comparison was made of data obtained from five tests for threshold values on the ATT to values obtained in the same patients tested manually with the monofilaments, manual 2PD, and electrophysiologic nerve conduction studies. The ATT detected abnormal sensibility in 71% of the patients tested, nerve conduction velocity was abnormal in 44% of the cases, and the manual tests indicated abnormality in 42% of the hands. They found that the most indicative test for sensory abnormality in these patients was threshold to a 50 Hz vibration administered by the ATT. They concluded that the ATT is a sensitive tool for the evaluation and diagnosis of compressive peripheral neuropathy and may allow objective documentation in a higher percentage of patients than more traditional testing methods.

By comparison, a much earlier study demonstrated that 256 Hz applied with a hand-held instrument and the Semmes-Weinstein monofilaments were the best indicators of threshold sensibility. Other researchers in the field of sensibility testing point out that neurophysiologists do not agree that vibration as a separate nerve function even exists, and they propose that loss of vibratory sensation may not be the earliest symptom of nerve compression, but one of the last. Other problems exist concerning the use of vibration as an evaluation of nerve function. Some researchers feel that current evaluation instruments have not been controlled enough for testing and that sufficient research does not exist to correlate vibration detection

threshold to hand function.

The sequence of accepted sensory recovery has been challenged. A retrospective chart review of 20 nerve injury cases demonstrated that the orderly sequence of sensory recovery may vary from person to person and that clinical methods for evaluation of vibration may not be precise enough to prevent error. Nine median, three ulnar, and eight combined median/ulnar divided nerves were evaluated for sequence of recovery. Eleven of 20 patients recovered 30 Hz vibration prior to pain, nine recovered pain prior to 30 Hz. No patient demonstrated return of temperature or touch pressure modalities prior to pain or 30 Hz vibration. The authors point out that the classic study on the sequence of recovery was established in a very small sample. This earlier study on 12 patients (six with crush, six with nerve repair) predicts the sequence of recovery in this order: pin prick (pain), 30 Hz, moving touch, constant touch, and 256 Hz.

The fact that 30 Hz may be recovered before pain may be a moot point. They represent academic, not functional, sensibility and the clinician assumes that the nerve is recovering and adopts a "wait and see" attitude with either sign.

Other clinical diagnostic tests for evaluation of nerve compression or traction do not meet the criteria for reliability and validity but are a helpful adjunct to diagnosis. Recent findings demonstrate that a compressed nerve has a lower irritability threshold than a normal nerve to mechanical pressure. Pressure provocative tests demonstrate entrapment points along peripheral nerves. Gentle pressure over the nerve at the entrapment site in question produces a paresthesia in that nerve distribution. Nerve pressure tests are an adjunct to provocative positional tests in the assessment of single or multiple compression sites.

More attention is being directed to the problem of dynamic nerve compressions. Many hand therapists perform innervation density and threshold tests, not only with the patient at rest, but also following provocative pressure, positional tests, or simulated work activity.

Symptoms related to subclinical nerve entrapment may be reproduced by tension testing. The nervous system, while conducting its primary function of impulse conduction, must accommodate stresses imposed on that system during body movement. Complex anatomical adaptations which protect neurons and allow conduction in any desired posture are built into the healthy system. Changes that occur in the loose connective tissue framework of nerve from compression or injury which may result in neurodesis alter the nerve's ability to slide and adapt to anatomical joint changes.

Tension testing is a technique of clinical evaluation for intraneural pressure and tension of the nervous system. The joints of the limb being tested are manually placed in various anatomical positions to produce elongation or tension on the nerve being evaluated to determine the nerve's ability to glide and tolerate joint maneuvers.

Tests of neural tension proposed for the upper limb, Upper Limb Tension Tests (ULTTs), have been discussed in the literature, but recently have received more attention as therapists look more proximal for the answers to the problems of cumulative trauma disorders, multiple- or double-crush syndromes and myofascial pain. ULTTs are recommended as an evaluation tool for patients whose complaints suggest impaired nervous system mechanics. One author recommends four basic tension tests for the upper extremity as a means of defining and treating nerve irritability. Clinically, it appears that tension testing is a sensitive evaluation technique for identifying subclinical or subtle nerve injury. ULTTs are important to evaluation of the upper limb nervous system and treatment by mobilization.

The volumeter, an instrument for measuring composite hand mass, is based on Archimedes' principle of water displacement. A commercial hand volumeter has been found to be accurate within 10 ml when used according to manufacturer's specifications. Instrument reliability has been established to within 1% for intra-examiner measurements. This tool is invaluable in the hand therapy clinic as a means of assessing the effect of modalities and exercise on hand edema and in affirming or negating the patient's perception of the effect of activity on hand edema. Volume measurements are usually taken before and after physical capacity evaluation testing to provide some objective measure of tissue tolerance to stress.

Functional capacity is defined as the ability to work and reflects the integration of all systems. It is measured in terms of grip, pinch, coordination, and dexterity. A high instrument reliability has been established for the Jamar Dynamometer, an instrument used for measuring grip strength, when calibrated. A minimum tolerance criterion of +.9994 has been established as well as the need and method for calibrating both new and used Jamars. Sixty-five percent of all instruments tested in this study, new and used, needed to be recalibrated.

This instrument is helpful in evaluating submaximal effort. One study concluded that if maximal performance is not achieved in the static grip test, then the rapid exchange grip test demonstrates a significant increase in grip strength on the affected side. In the same study, more patients claiming workers compensation had positive rapid grip exchange grips than patients not claiming workers compensation.

In a study of 123 patients with chronic wrist pain, grip strength was assessed on five settings of the Jamar Dynamometer with both static and rapid grip exchange. The results demonstrated a significant decrease of grip strength in patients with a positive bone scan or confirmed wrist pathology as compared to those with negative bone scans ($P < 0.01$). The conclusion of this study was that detection of weakness of grip is a simple indicator of true pathology in "obscure" wrist pain.

The 10% rule states that the dominant hand possesses a 10% greater grip strength than the nondominant hand. Three hundred and ten normal subjects were studied with a factory-calibrated Jamar Dynamometer. Results showed that an overall 10.74% grip strength difference between dominant and nondominant hands verified the 10% rule. However, when the data were separated into left-handed and right-handed subjects, a 12.72% difference for right-handed subjects and a -0.08% difference for left-handed subjects was found. This study showed that the 10% rule is valid for right-handed persons only; for left-handed persons, grip strength should be considered equivalent in both hands.

The validity and reliability of the Baltimore Therapeutic Equipment Simulator, a widely used computerized exercise and evaluation tool, has recently been studied; its validity and reliability as an assessment tool had been questioned. The static mode with each BTE was found to be accurate but there was a statistically significant variation from simulator to simulator which means that normative data cannot be used. In the dynamic mode, unexplained mechanical fluctuations were noted dependent on the time of day testing was performed and statistical differences between real or applied torque were recorded. The author of that study recommends the BTE as an exercise but not as an assessment tool.

In summary, recent studies have found the volumeter, torque range of motion, the Jamar Dynamometer, the Semmes-Weinstein monofilaments, and the Automated Tactile Tester to be reliable and valid assessment tools for the upper extremity. Previously established standardized tests (currently recognized by hand therapists as reliable and valid) for assessing manual dexterity and coordination include the Jebson Hand Function Test, the Minnesota Rate of Manipulation Test, the Purdue Pegboard Test, and the Crawford Small Parts Test.

Wound Management

While the management of complex wounds has not been the focus of much research in hand surgery literature, scientific contributions from other disciplines have influenced wound treatment in the hand therapy clinic.

In an effort to simplify wound evaluation and treatment for the hand therapist, the American Society of Hand Therapists has recommended a universal classification system for open wounds, introduced by Marion Laboratories, in its second edition of Clinical Assessment Recommendations. This classification system simplifies wound description as it relates to each phase of wound healing for the open wound, and correlates wound description to wound treatment. This approach uses color to describe wound status. Wounds are described as either red, yellow, black, or a combination of two or three colors. Wound evaluation and treatment based on the Three Color Concept™ with guidelines for debridement, cleansing, disinfecting and dressing are summarized in Table 44-1.

Treatments in hand therapy for cleansing, disinfecting, and dressing wounds has been altered by new research which emphasizes (1) the importance of wound fluids and a moist wound environment for facilitating a positive cellular response, and (2) the cytotoxic effects of antiseptic agents. It has been demonstrated that incised and sutured wounds may be washed with mild soap and water as early as 24 hours postoperatively.

Hexachlorophene and povidone-iodine or Betadine scrubs, two commercially available wound-cleansing solutions, instantaneously lyse white blood cells that are critical for wound defense, and in the case of povidone-iodine,

Table 44-1.   Simplifying Clinical Decision Making for the Open Wound.

	Black Wound	Yellow Wound	Red Wound
Description	covered with thick, necrotic tissue or eschar	generating exudate, looks creamy, will contain pus, debris and viscous surface exudate	uninfected, properly healing with definite borders, may be pink or beefy red, granulated tissue and neovascularization
Cellular Activity	1. autolysis, collagenase activity, 2. defense, phagocytosis; 3. macrophage cell	1. immune response, defense 2. phagocytosis; 3. macrophage cell	1. endothelial cells - angiogensis 2. fibroblast cells - collagen and ground substance 3. myofibroblast - wound contraction 4. epidermal cells - migration and mitosis of epithelium
Debridement	1. surgical, preferred 2. mechanical, whirlpool, dressings 3. chemical, enzymatic digestion	separate wound debris with aggressive scrubs, irrigation, or whirlpool	N.A. – avoid any tissue trauma or stripping of new cells
Cleansing	1. whirlpool 2. irrigation 3. soap and water scrubs	1. use no antiseptics 2. soap and water 3. surfactant soaked sponge 4. polaxmer 188, Pluronic F-68	1. no antiseptics 2. ringers lactate 3. sterile saline, sterile water
Topical TX	topical antimicrobials with low WBC or cellulitis	1. topical antimicrobials to control bacterial contamination 2. silver sulfadiazine, bactroban, neomycin, polymixin B, neosporin	1. N/A for simple wounds 2. vitamin A for patients on steroids 3. antimicrobials for immuno-suppressed
Dressing	1. wet to dry for necrotic tissue 2. proteolytic enzyme to debride 3. synthetic dressing, autolysis 4. dress to soften eschar	1. wet to dry – wide mesh to absorb drainage 2. wet to wet – saturated with medicants 3. hydrocolloid or semipermeable foam dressings, hydrogels	1. occlusive or semi-occlusive dressings; semipermeable films 2. protect wound fluids and prevent desiccation
Desired Goal	1. remove debris and mechanical obstruction to allow epithelialization, collagen deposition to proceed 2. evolve to clean, red wound	1. light debridement without disrupting new cells 2. exudate absorption 3. bacterial control 4. evolve to red wound	1. protect new cells 2. keep wound moist and clean to speed healing 3. promote epithelialization, granulation tissue formation, angiogenesis, wound contraction

Reproduced with permission from Evans RB: An update on wound management. *Hand Clin,* 7:(3), 409-432, 1991.

damage red blood cells as well as result in considerable hemolysis. Wound epithelization and early tensile strength are affected by 1% povidone-iodine solution. This solution must be diluted to 0.001% concentration to be nontoxic to the cultured human fibroblast. The use of povidone-iodine solution on gauze dressings or in whirlpools is not recommended because of proven negative cellular effects. Cleansing solutions, such as Hibiclens™ are recommended only for periwound areas. Most cleansing solutions damage the wound's defense system and invite infection.

Hydrogen peroxide is perhaps misused as much as povidone-iodine. It has little bactericidal action and should be used only to cleanse periwound skin or to loosen dried exudate on the wound surface. Hydrogen peroxide should not be used after crust separation, on new granulation tissue, or on closed wounds. Topical antibiotics are the only antimicrobial agents recommended by wound specialists for wound care.

The new microenvironmental dressings, which function to modify and not just protect the wound environment, sequester wound fluids and prevent wound desiccation. Experimental studies have demonstrated that 90% more macrophages and 50% fewer neutrophils are present in moist wounds as compared to dry wounds, suggesting that the inflammatory phase of repair in moist wounds is accelerated. Fibroblasts and endothelial cell activity increase more rapidly in moist wounds.

Substantial differences exist in the various environmental dressings, but they share as a common characteristic their ability to utilize wound fluids to aid in healing by maintaining a moist environment. Some absorb exudate, and some permit exchange of gases. Preliminary studies indicate that the development of breaking strength may be delayed in an occluded wound, and that occlusion may affect collagen cross linking. Oxygen permeable dressings demonstrate increased epithelization whereas the use of gas impermeable dressings has been found to stimulate angiogenesis and to suppress epithelialization.

The discipline of physical therapy continues to contribute to our knowledge of the effects of electrical stimulation on the migration, proliferation, and functional capacity of cells involved in the healing process. Isolated epidermal cells, cell clusters, and cell sheets demonstrate galvanotaxis in migrating toward the cathode in *in vitro* studies. Macrophages migrate toward the anode, whereas neutrophils have been observed to migrate toward both anode and cathode.

Growth factors, which play an important part in wound healing, may be stimulated by electrical current. It has been demonstrated that dermal fibroblasts in culture, stimulated with pulsed current at 100 pulses per second and 100 v, had increases in the expression of receptors for transforming growth factor-B that were six times greater than those of control fibroblasts.

A recent clinical study has indicated that pulsed electrical stimulation has a beneficial effect on healing Stage II, III, and IV chronic dermal ulcers. The results of this multicenter study support other research in that treatment time to enhance tissue healing does not need to exceed 60 minutes per day, five to seven days per week. This study indicates that 3.7 to 7 hours per week of electrical stimulation is beneficial and sufficient. This treatment time is in contrast to the 20 to 42 hours of electrical stimulation treatment per week recommended in earlier studies.

Ultrasound as a means of facilitating tendon healing continues to be a controversial issue with regard to timing, duration, and intensity of application. Its clinical efficiency in the human model for healing flexor or extensor tendons has not been determined.

The effect of low-intensity ultrasound was studied on the healing strength of 24 repaired rabbit Achilles tendons. The tendons were excised after nine treatments and compared with non-ultrasound tendons for differences in tensile strength, tensile stress, and energy absorption capacity. The ultrasound group demonstrated a significant increase in tensile strength, tensile stress, and energy absorption capacity. The findings suggest that high-intensity ultrasound is not necessary to augment the healing strength of tendons, but low-intensity ultrasound may enhance the healing process of surgically repaired human Achilles tendons.

A study that describes the influence of ultrasound administered at different postoperative intervals on several aspects of healing of surgically repaired flexor tendons in Zone II in 76 white leg horn chickens has indicated that use during the early stages of wound healing increases ROM, decreases scar formation, and shows no adverse affect on strength.

Some researchers emphasize that because each stage of healing entails a different set of ultrastructural events, therapeutic interventions must be modified to address specific events. Timing appears to be a critical variable. Positive effects have been reported in those studies that limit sonication to the earliest stages of healing; negative results were obtained when sonication was not limited but continued for several weeks.

The effect of ultrasound on the healing human tendon has not been established.

Scar Management

Scar management by pressure garments, serial casting, and elastomers has been used for some time. Topical silicone gel sheeting (SGS) is a relatively new technique used to prevent, control, and reduce hypertrophic scar formation. The mechanism of action of the SGS is unknown. Pressure exerted by the SGS applied with paper tape is negligible

($< 3mm$ Hg). Temperature and differences in oxygen transmission have been excluded. The gel is occlusive with a water vapor rate lower than that of skin (4.5 vs. 8.5 g/m_2 per hour). However, other occlusive dressings such as polyurethane film do not have the same effect on hypertrophic scar. It is postulated that since the scar surface does not become wet or macerated with prolonged wear, the SGS may promote hydration of the scar, but changes in scar water content have not been directly measured. There is no histological or scanning electron microscopic evidence of silicone absorption, but a chemical effect has not been excluded. A number of clinical studies have demonstrated the efficacy of SGS in minimizing hypertrophic scar in surgical incisions, burn scar, and keloid scars with at least 12 hours of treatment daily over periods of up to six months. Recently SGS has been found to prevent development of these scars. In a controlled analysis of fresh surgical incisions, SGS was found to significantly inhibit the formation of hypertrophic scar when used at least 12 hours daily for two months.

Tendon

Therapeutic management concepts for the repaired tendon are reviewed in terms of timing, stress application, duration of exercise, excursion, splint geometry, and force application. The goal of all tendon rehabilitation is to reestablish functional tendon glide.

Timing

Preliminary experimental studies indicate that timing in relation to stress during the early inflammatory stage is critical. A study on chicken flexor tendons demonstrated that tendons treated with controlled passive motion significantly improved strength by five days after repair compared to immobilized digits. The difference in strength between the two groups increased with time. The authors concluded that immediate constrained digital motion following repair allows progressive tendon healing without an intervening phase of tendon softening.

In another study of early tensile properties of healing chicken flexor tendons, early controlled motion was found to improve efficiency. Controlled passive motion tendons demonstrated greater values for rupture load, stress, and energy absorbed when studied at intervals during the 30 days following repair.

Fibronectin, which appears to be an important component of the early tendon repair process, has been localized in a clinically relevant tendon repair model. Fibroblast chemotaxis and adherence to the substrate in the days after injury and repair appear to be directly related to fibronectin concentration.

Early passive motion correlated to an increased fibronectin concentration in an experimental study of 20 adult dog flexor tendons (the clinically relevant tendon repair model of the previous study). Fibronectin was elevated by the third day after injury in both early passive motion and immobilized tendons, but by seven days after surgery controlled motion flexor tendon had a fibronectin concentration two times that of immobilized tendon.

These studies offer documentation that increased cellular activity and strengthening occur with early motion during the immediate post-repair period, and emphasizes the critical relationship between stress application and timing.

Duration of Exercise

A prospective multicenter clinical study of 51 patients with flexor tendon repair determined that greater durations of daily passive motion following flexor tendon repair result in increased active interphalangeal joint motion. Two groups of patients treated with continuous passive motion and traditional EPM techniques were compared in terms of interphalangeal motion. The authors conclude that the duration of daily controlled motion interval is a significant variable in post-repair flexor tendon function.

Excursion

Studies of flexor and extensor tendon excursion have altered clinical application of stress. The importance of PIP joint motion with Zone II flexor tendon repair has been documented experimentally and clinically in several recent works (Fig. 44-2). These studies support postoperative flexor tendon splinting with a pulley in the palm and emphasize the importance of PIP extension to 0° during exercise. The question of actual tendon excursion with passive motion programs has been raised, and poor tendon excursion with low tendon tension has been reported. Therapeutic treatments to increase excursion include alterations in splint geometry, wrist tenodesis, changes in exercise position, and the application of minimal active tension as an adjunct to passive motion for both flexor and extensor systems.

In a study examining excursion between the flexor digitorum profundus (FDP) and tendon sheath in both human and canine digits, the amount of tendon excursion was found to be small in regions distal to the joint in motion (0.1 mm per 10° of joint rotation). Tendon excursion relative to the tendon sheath was the largest in Zone II during PIP joint motion (1.7 mm per 10° of joint rotation).

An *in vivo* study in which intratendinous metal markers were used to study FDP excursions during early controlled motion with dynamic flexion traction found that the size of excursions reported at the proximal phalangeal level had a significant effect on IP motion results. Distal interphalangeal joint motion mobilized the FDP (36% efficiency) and PIP motion (90% efficiency).

Comparative flexor tendon excursions after passive mobilization have been investigated in two *in vitro* studies. The first study evaluated tendon excursions due to passive joint motion and various loading conditions. In the second study, the efficacy of a new technique that uses synergistic wrist motion (S-splint) was compared to traditional dorsal splinting methods (the Kleinert Splint {K-Splint} and the Brooke Army Hospital/Walter Reed Modified Kleinert Splint with a palmar bar {P-Splint}) (Fig. 44-3). The first study demonstrated that the measured tendon excursion under a condition of low tendon tension was almost half that of theoretically predicted values and that actual tendon

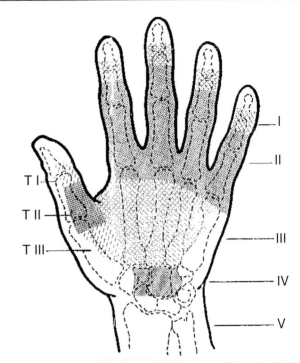

Figure 44-2. Flexor tendon zones defined by the Committee on Tendon Injuries for the International Federation of Societies for Surgery of the Hand. Reproduced with permission from Kleinert HE, Schepel S, Gill T: Flexor tendon injuries. *Surg Clin North Am*, 61:267-286, 1981.

excursion is equal to the predicted tendon excursion of earlier studies only when greater than 300 g of tension is applied. Excursion of the FDP at zero load was 5 ± 1 mm (mean $\pm$ SD); after muscle tendon load was increased to 330 g, excursion increased to 13 ± 2 mm. Passive PIP joint motion produced only 3 mm of differential excursion between the FDP and the flexor digitorum superficialis; with an increase in load, differential excursion increased from 3.5 mm to 9.5 mm.

In the second study, the magnitude of excursion introduced by the three mobilization methods was in descending order: S-Splint, P-Splint, K-Splint ($p < 0.05$) See Table 44-2. Differential excursions between the FDP and FDS were similar with all three methods. Simulated postoperative passive mobilization with a dorsal splint was found to produce crimping of the tendon beneath the annular pulleys as well as in the palm. These authors and others found that the most effective means of providing increased amplitude of tendon gliding in Zone II is PIP joint motion, and that passive DIP motion did not increase excursion in Zone II as much as previously predicted.

Increased excursions with early mobilization programs may produce gaping or rupture at the repair site. Earlier studies, which concluded that gaps greater than a few millimeters have a negative effect in terms of adhesion forma-

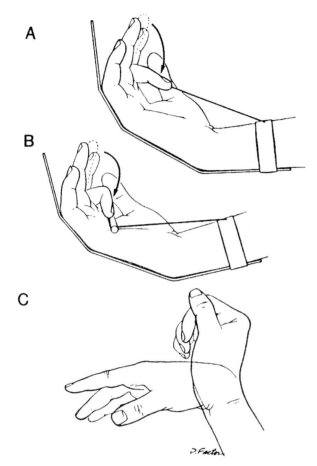

Figure 44-3. Finger and wrist positions under the three methods. **(A)** The Kleinert Splint (K-Splint). Dorsal extension block splint with rubber band traction to the fingertip. **(B)** The Kleinert Splint with a palmar bar (P-Splint). The direction of traction is changed by a palmar bar. **(C)** The synergistic wrist motion. The splint could be designed to control this motion (S-Splint). Reproduced with permission from Horii E, Lin G-T, Cooney WP, Linscheid RL, An KN: Comparative flexor tendon excursions after passive mobilization: an *in vitro* study. *J Hand Surg,* 17A:561, 1992.

tion and functional results, have been challenged by a recent *in vivo* study that demonstrates that gaps up to 10 mm in FDP repairs are compatible with good function. The results of this study support greater excursions in postoperative flexor tendon management and indicate that controlled motion, is effective in restricting the formation of adhesions associated with gap formation during postoperative immobilization.

Extensor tendon injuries in Zones V, VI, and VII have been managed for the past decade with controlled passive motion, allowing short arc motion at the MP joint with the wrist immobilized in 30° to 40° of extension to produce some passive tendon excursion at the repair site (Fig. 44-4). Tendon buckling with passive mobilization programs is a concern for extensor repairs as well as for flexor repairs, and clinical techniques to improve postoperative excursions, including controlled wrist tenodesis, immediate active place and hold exercise, increased range of motion for the digits with repairs in Zones V, VI, and VII, and early active short arc motion for the Zone III tendon are being utilized in the hand therapy clinic.

The importance of wrist position and its effect on extensor tendon excursion was studied in eight fresh cadaver limbs to measure extensor tendon gliding in Zones III to VIII when active grip and passive extension were simulated at different wrist positions. This study demonstrated that if the wrist were extended more than 21° that the extensor tendons glide with little or no tension in Zones V and VI throughout full simulated grip to full passive extension.

In a recent clinical study of 52 patients with extensor repairs from the midportion of the proximal phalanx to the wrist level treated with full digital flexion (within the confines of a static wrist extension splint and dynamic digital traction) two to five days after repair, all patients recovered complete digital flexion with no ruptures.

Results of 112 complex (tendon injury with associated fracture or crush) extensor injuries in Zones V, VI, VII, T IV, and T V report excellent results with more limited digital motions. This study followed a protocol for controlled passive motion defined in 1986 which limited MP joint rotation to one-half radian to produce 5 mm of excursions

Table 44-2.   Tendon Excursion Associated With Three Different Splinting Techniques.

Zone	Methods	FDP	FDS	FDP-FDS
II	K-splint	8 ± 2[c]	5 ± 2[b]	3 ± 1
	P-splint	14 ± 3[b]	11 ± 2[a]	3 ± 1
	S-splint	16 ± 3[a]	13 ± 3[a]	3 ± 2
III	K-splint	11 ± 2[b]	9 ± 2[b]	3 ± 1
	P-splint	13 ± 3[b]	10 ± 2[b]	4 ± 2
	S-splint	31 ± 4[a]	30 ± 3[a]	2 ± 1
V	K-splint	5 ± 3	5 ± 2	2 ± 1
	P-splint	6 ± 2	5 ± 2	2 ± 1
	S-splint	5 ± 3	3 ± 3	3 ± 1

Tendon excursions in three different passive mobilizations are compared (mean ± 1 SD, in millimeters). Any two values in the vertical columns with superscript letters in common are not significantly different from each other *(p > 0.05),* whereas those with a different letter are significantly different (Duncan's multiple range test, *p > 0.05).* Reproduced with permission from Horii E, Lin G-T, Cooney WP, Linscheid RL, An KN: Comparative flexor tendon excursions after passive mobilization: an *in vitro* study. *J Hand Surg,* 17A:561, 1992.

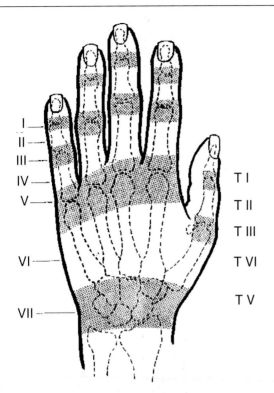

Figure 44-4. Extensor tendon zones as defined by the Committee on Tendon Injuries for the International Federation of Societies for Surgery of the Hand. Reproduced with permission from Kleinert HE, Schepel S, Gill T: Flexor tendon injuries. *Surg Clin North Am*, 61:267-286, 1981.

in Zones V, VI, and VII. This study reported a total active motion of 240° for the digits, and 116° for the thumb with complex injury by four to six weeks after surgery with a program of more limited excursion.

The electrophysiologic basis of dynamic extensor splinting has been studied in normal volunteers. Only 16% had quiescent extensor digitorum muscle activity within the dynamic extensor splints typically used for extensor tendon rehabilitation which rests the MP joint at 0°. MP joints splinted at 15° flexion were found to exhibit no extensor activity. This study demonstrates that patients move their digits actively in extension as well as flexion in their dynamic extension splints.

Excursion for the central slip has been calculated by the radian concept to be 3.75 mm with PIP joint motion of approximately 30° (one-half radian) in a newly defined protocol for early active short arc motion for the repaired central slip.

Force Application

Early passive motion protocols may not provide predicted excursions. Many clinicians feel that active muscle/tendon tension is required to glide a tendon repair site in a proximal direction to maintain functional glide. While the ideal tendon repair, capable of withstanding immediate active

flexion without the controls of splinting and specific exercise regimens, has not been created, we do have techniques of force application that apply physiologic stress application that is less than the tensile strengths of presently available suture materials and repair techniques.

A study designed to evaluate the influence of wrist position on the "minimal active tension" (minimal tension required to overcome the viscoelastic force of the antagonistic tendons) in flexor tendons demonstrated that the position of wrist extension and metacarpophalangeal flexion is associated with the least flexor force. The study concludes that this position should be utilized for postoperative protection of flexor tendon repair in which active mobilization is utilized.

Through the application of low-profile force transducers placed within the carpal tunnel under local anesthesia, forces were recorded within flexor tendons during passive and active motion as well as during pinch and grip. This study demonstrated that forces in the range of 0.1 to 0.6 kilograms of force (kgf) can be expected at the level of suture during passive mobilization of the wrist, and in the range of 0.1 to 0.9 kgf during passive mobilization of the fingers. Therefore, given the currently reported breaking forces of tendon repair, passive motion of either wrist or fingers should not have a deleterious effect on tendon healing or gap formation. Forces up to 0.4 kgf might be expected during unrestricted active mobilization of the wrist, and up to 3.5 kgf during unrestricted active mobilization of the fingers. The amount of flexor tendon forces during active motion of the fingers is greater than the current strength of common flexor tendon repairs.

The effect of different methods of early controlled mobilization on excursion and dehiscence of the FDP was examined during the treatment of 20 tendons in 18 patients with radiographic stereophotogrammetric analysis. Excursions were found to be dependent on the type of mobilization and level of injury within Zone II. The use of a mobilization technique that includes a component of controlled active motion was suggested for A_3 and A_4 levels. At the A_3 level, the active-hold technique was found to be superior. The Kleinert technique utilizing four fingers was found to be superior to the technique utilizing one finger. At the A_4 level, the Kleinert technique utilizing both one and four fingers was ineffective.

Postoperative management by immobilization, passive motion, and active motion remains a controversial subject, but the trend in experimental and clinical research is moving toward some degree of active muscle tendon tension as a part of postoperative rehabilitation. The concept of "active motion" with postoperative tendon rehabilitation needs to be redefined as "minimal active tension" in prescribed anatomical positions.

The increased angular rotation of both PIP and DIP joints with the addition of a palmar pulley to the original Kleinert splint has been studied not only in terms of tendon excursion but in terms of the force required to extend the PIP joint against the rubber band traction.

The flexion moment of the PIP joint with three commonly used postoperative flexor tendon techniques of elastic band mobilization was studied to identify which factors contribute to the development of PIP joint flexion contractures. The authors demonstrate that the line of force should be kept close to the axis of the PIP joint to reduce the flexion moment, which they identify as a major contributing factor to PIP joint flexion contracture. Flexion moments were found to be lower with splinting techniques that hold the distal phalanx into the distal palmar crease independent of MP joint motion, or with conventional forearm attachment when the MP is flexed to only 20°.

One group of clinicians reported 76.1% excellent and 23.9% good results with a new postoperative flexor tendon (PFT) brace that lessens resistance to finger extension and increases the arc of motion through full passive flexion of the injured fingers (Fig. 44-5). The forces exerted on the tip of the finger as it moved from flexion through extension measured 65 g to 85 g with the PFT brace, but much greater (65 g to 210 g) with the traditional Kleinert splint.

A study of 28 flexor tendons treated with a palmar pulley demonstrated less PIP flexion contracture when compared to 78 tendons (Zone II) anchored at the wrist. The authors found that by adding a palmar pulley with the vectors of forces redirected to the palm, that full DIP flexion was obtained. This splint design held the wrist at 50° to 60° flexion, MPs at 20°, and dynamic traction that included a palmar pulley and spring wire with elastic band traction.

A new concept in early application of resistive force to adherent flexor tendons treated with immobilization has been proposed. In a clinical study of 25 digits in 20 patients with flexor tendon injuries in Zones I through III treated with an average of 24 days of immobilization, resistance was applied to scarred tendons when the difference between active and passive IP motion exceeded 50° at three-and one-half weeks postoperatively. The authors report good results with the application of resistance that they describe as "vigorous blocking by three-and one-half weeks and squeezing a light grade of putty by four-and one-half weeks" with adherent flexor tendon.

The application of force to extensor tendons in the healing phase has not received much attention. While there are numerous studies on the biomechanical strengths of flexor tendon repairs, there is only one study published on extensor tendon repairs. The biomechanical characteristics of the extensor tendon suture techniques with measurements at 2 mm gapping and at failure were reported as follows: the mattress suture gapped at 2 mm at 488 g, failed at 840 g; figure-of-eight gapped at 587 g, failed at 696 g; Kessler gapped at 1,353 g, failed at 1,830 g; Bunnell gapped at 1,435 g, failed at 1,985 g. All techniques studied shortened the tendon and produced significant losses of flexion at the MP and PIP joints. In addition, repairs achieved with suture techniques were weaker than those achieved when comparable techniques were used for flexor tendons.

Resistance to the extensor digitorum has been measured by a mathematical formula at 300 g of force for the central slip with active extension of the PIP joint from 30° flexion to 0° extension in a protocol for early short arc motion for the repaired central slip. Resistance to the EDC in Zone V has been measured with active extension from 30° to 0° at 300 g of force in an unpublished, associated study.

The working equation between force application and ten-

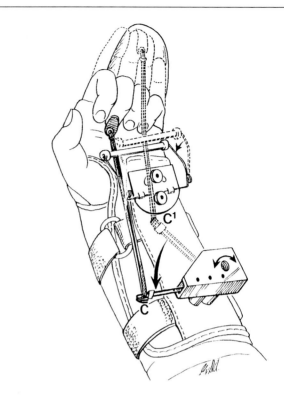

Figure 44-5. The postoperative flexor tendon traction brace. A housing over the distal forearm contains a coil lever that attaches to the rubber band; the hole in the palmar surface of the housing allows the tension of the coiled lever to be adjusted when more than one finger has been injured (double arrow). The rubber band runs from the coiled lever, under the springloaded roller bar at the distal palmar crease, to the tip of the injured finger. When the finger extends (dotted lines), the roller bar moves out from the palm and the lever arm rotates distally from C to C1. This enables the rubber band to stay significantly closer to its resting length and minimizes the force exerted on the finger. Reproduced with permission from Werntz JR, Chesher SP, Breidenbach BC, et al: A new dynamic splint for postoperative treatment of flexor tendon injuries. *J Hand Surg*, 14A:561, 1989.

sile strength of the repair is the main concern when applying physiologic stress to the healing tendon. The author utilizes the concept of minimal active tension immediately after tenorrhaphy in the management of both flexor and extensor tendons in all zones except extensors in Zone I with improved clinical results.

New Techniques for Clinical Management

The Zone I isolated flexor tendon injury was studied in 99 FDP injuries in 89 patients. Traditional treatment was compared to a postoperative management technique that addresses the problem of gap formation and active gliding of the uninjured FDS. The protocol uses a dorsal protective splint which holds the wrist at 30° flexion, MPs at 30° to 40°, PIPs at 0°, and maintains 40° to 45° flexion of the DIP joint in a dorsal digital one-joint splint the first three-and-one-half weeks postoperatively. Traction is not used. Wrist tenodesis, active place and hold for the FDS, and passive motion for the DIP from 40° to 70° ensure tendon glide while preventing gap formation. Average improvement of DIP motion was 23.9° to 41.2°, and percentage of normal range from 56.6% to 74% when the two groups were compared. The author suggests this technique when quality of the repair is questionable.

A retrospective study of 20 patients with Zone I tendon-to-tendon repair noted a complication rate of 35% (loss of the ability to flex the DIP and PIP flexion contracture). These authors advocate treating Zone I tendon injuries differently from Zone II injuries, but recommend complete passive DIP motion with the PIP held manually in a flexed position.

Other researchers have not found gap formation, rupture, or adhesion formation to be more of a problem with mobilization techniques that employ a larger range of excursion with the Zone I profundus injury.

A review of 60 fingers with complete laceration of FDP and FDS in Zone II treated with a modified Kleinert splint with a palmar pulley produced excellent results (52 excellent, four good, one fair, three poor) with a technique that rested the fingers in composite flexion between exercise sessions and at night. Other researchers believe that the PIP should rest in extension when not being exercised.

In a comparison of three methods of treatment for Zone II flexor tendon repair, TAM was significantly improved both at six weeks and at one year in a protocol that emphasized PIP extension and facilitated some active muscle tendon tension by utilizing four-finger traction. The daytime splint was cut away at the PIP joint to ensure extension to 0°. The concept of four-finger traction is favored as it facilitates a stronger EDC contraction for extension and a larger component of involuntary active flexion.

In the past decade, a number of clinical studies on extensor tendon repair treated with early passive motion protocols demonstrated improved results when compared to those treated with immobilization. The techniques vary in the amount of digital motion recommended. Recently, early passive motion protocols for extensor tendon injuries in Zones III and IV have been recommended; however, protocols for timing, splinting, exercise, and case selection vary from study to study.

An analysis of the factors that support early active short arc motion for the repaired central slip and a companion clinical study defined a protocol for early motion in this zone which has produced superior results in terms of PIP extension lag, composite IP flexion, and treatment time when compared to similar injuries treated with immobilization. This protocol recommends splinting only the PIP and DIP joints with a volar static extension splint between exercises. The exercise position of 30° wrist flexion, MP at 0° and active flexion-extension of the PIP joint to 30° applies 300 g of force to the tendon repair site and excursion of 3.75 mm to the tendon in Zone III and IV, preventing tendon to bone adherence in the broad tendon bone interface of Zone IV. This active motion is performed in the prescribed anatomic position without dynamic splint assis-

tance. A study of anatomy supports this technique as do the clinical results.

Nerve

Therapeutic management of nerve tissue has been altered by a new appreciation for the biomechanics and continuum of the nervous system. The complex patterns of multiple neuropathies from overuse, improper posturing, imbalance of function, and fibrous fixation of nerve tissue that limits mechanical gliding, have been addressed with job modification, myofascial treatment, and nerve gliding techniques.

Nerve symptoms are evaluated both statically and dynamically and treated by manual techniques which mobilize the entire upper quarter. While there are a number of publications available that describe treatment by mobilization, nerve gliding, and job modification, controlled clinical studies supporting specific therapeutic techniques are not available. This concept of early nerve gliding is integrated by many hand therapists into early intervention programs following decompression surgeries or injury to adjacent tissues to prevent the problems associated with neurodesis. Nerve gliding is performed by placing the cervical, shoulder, elbow, and wrist joints through maneuvers to facilitate nerve excursion. These practices, however, lack scientific documentation.

A national survey of hand therapists indicated that sensory re-education as part of a nerve recovery program is often not prescribed or is prescribed as an afterthought. Experimental work in adult monkeys has demonstrated cortical sensory plasticity after nerve injury providing a rationale for the efficacy of sensory re-education.

The effectiveness of sensory re-education on recovering nerve has been demonstrated in two clinical studies. In a study of 46 adult patients with median nerve laceration at the wrist level, repaired primarily with microsurgical grouped fascicular technique, 22 patients treated with a normal sensory re-education program demonstrated better (lower) recovery of cutaneous pressure threshold as measured by the Semmes-Weinstein monofilaments, than the 24 patients who received no structured sensory re-education program. Lower threshold readings were obtained regardless of age in the experimental group; however, patients who were less than 30 years of age had even better recovery.

Normal thresholds were not recovered in any patient. This study further demonstrated that the Semmes-Weinstein pressure anesthesiometer accurately describes quantitative improvement at the earlier, more critical stages of sensory recovery.

A later report by the same authors with presumably the same 46 patients reported that sensory re-education significantly diminished (p<0.01) the severity of postoperative paresthesias. It also gave significantly better improvement in moving two-point discrimination than in static two-point discrimination within the time frame evaluated (p<0.002), and demonstrated significantly better (p<0.005) object identification.

Annotated Bibliography

Assessment

Bell-Krotoski J, Buford WL: The force/time relationship of clinically used sensory testing instruments. *J Hand Ther,* 1:76-85, 1988.

The problems of hand-held instruments used to assess touch stimuli are defined. The consistency of force application of the Semmes-Weinstein monofilaments and inconsistency of 2PD and the tuning fork (30 Hz and 256 Hz) are demonstrated.

Breger-Lee D, Bell-Krotoski J, Brandsma JW: Torque range of motion in the hand clinic. *J Hand Ther,* 3:(1)7-13, 1990.

A method of controlled torque and joint position that has been used experimentally and clinically as a tool for objective assessment of passive range of motion is presented.

Fess EE: A method for checking Jamar Dynamometer calibration. *J Hand Ther,* 1:28-32, 1987.

High-instrument reliability is established for the Jamar Dynamometer when calibrated. A minimum tolerance criterion of .9994 is established.

Horch K, Hardy M, Jimenez S, Jabaley M: An Automated Tactile Tester for evaluation of cutaneous sensibility. *J Hand Surg,* 17A:829-37, 1992.

The Automated Tactile Tester, a computer-controlled device designed to measure a patient's cutaneous perception of touch, vibration, temperature, and pain, has been shown to provide repeatable and reliable measurements of sensory functions in the skin and may have application in the diagnosis of compression and other peripheral neuropathies.

Wound Healing

Enwemeka CS, Rodriguez O, Mendosa S: The biomechanical effects of low intensity ultrasound on healing. *Ultrasound in Med Biol,* 16:807-810; 1990.

The effect of low-intensity ultrasound studied on the healing strength of 24 repaired rabbit Achilles tendons indicates that the ultrasound group showed a significant increase in tensile strength, tensile stress, and energy absorption capacity when compared to a nonultrasound group. The findings suggest that low-intensity ultrasound may enhance the healing process of surgically repaired human Achilles tendons.

Evans RB: An update on wound management. *Hand Clin,* 7:(3) 409-432, 1991.

This chapter provides an extensive review of current experimental and clinical studies on wound healing that defines wound management techniques. Guidelines for cleansing, disinfecting, and for use of the new microenvironmental dressings and modalities are presented in terms of positive or negative cellular response. Wound evaluation by the Three Color Concept™ by Marion Laboratories is described.

Freedar JA, Kloth LC, GentzKow G-D: Chronic dermal ulcer healing enhanced with monophasic pulsed electrical stimulation. *Phys Ther,* 71:639-649, 1991.

This is a randomized, double-blind multicenter clinical study that demonstrates significantly improved healing rates in healing Stage II, III, and IV chronic dermal ulcers treated with pulsed electrical stimulation. Treatment time with electrical stimulation does not need to exceed 60 minutes per day, five to seven days per week to satisfactorily enhance tissue healing.

Huys S, Gan BS, Sherebrin MV, Scilley CG: The effects of ultrasound treatment on flexor tendon healing in the chicken limb. Submitted *J Hand Surg.*

The use of ultrasound during the early stages of wound healing increases ROM, decreases scar formation, and shows no adverse effects of decreased strength in an experimental study of surgically repaired flexor tendons in Zone II in the white leghorn chicken animal model.

Kloth LC, Mc Culloch JM, Freedar JA: *Wound healing: alternatives in management.* FA Davis Co., Philadelphia, 1990.

This work provides a comprehensive review of current experimental and clinical research studies that define the use of electrical stimulation, ultrasound, light, hyperbaric oxygen, and microenvironmental dressings that influence wound healing.

Tendon

Amiel D, Gelberman R, Harwood F, Siegel D: Fibronectin in healing flexor tendons subjected to immobilization or early controlled passive motion. *Matrix,* Vol II, (3):184-189, 1991.

Fibronectin concentrations (found to be higher in injured tissue than in control tissues) were found to be approximately twice as high in the controlled passive motion tissues as in the immobilized tissues by seven days after injury/repair. It was concluded that early immobilization depresses the accumulation of tissue fibronectin during the early stages of healing following injury.

Burge PD, Brown M: Elastic band mobilization after flexor tendon repair: Splint design and risk of flexion contracture. *J Hand Surg,* 15B:4433-4488, 1990.

The mechanics of three types of elastic band mobilization were analyzed from lateral video recordings of finger movement and the flexion moment at the PIP was derived every 10° of flexion. MP joint flexion of 45° or more will increase the risk of PIP flexion contraction unless a palmar pulley or dorsal elastic band (both decrease the flexor moment at the end range of PIP extension) is used.

Collins DC, Schwarze L : Early progressive resistance following immobilization of flexor tendon repairs. *J Hand Ther,* Vol 4(3) 111-116, 1991.

The problem of adherent flexor tendons treated with immobilization for an average of 24 days is treated by applying early resistance by three-and one-half to four-and one-half weeks postoperative when the discrepancy between active and passive TAM exceeds 50.

Evans RB: A study of the Zone I flexor tendon injury and implications for treatment. *J Hand Ther,* 133-148, 1990.

This study demonstrates significantly improved results with Zone I FDP tendon repairs as compared to tendons in this zone treated with the traditional Kleinert or Duran method when treated with a new postoperative management technique. The technique does not allow DIP extension beyond 40° the first three-and one-half weeks and promotes active muscle tendon tension in both FDP and FDS tendon systems.

Evans RB, Thompson DE: An analysis of factors that support early active short arc motion for the repaired central slip. *J Hand Ther,* Vol 5, No 4, 187-201, 1992.

Safe parameters for excursion, force application, and anatomical position during controlled active exercise are defined for a new postoperative management technique that proposes immediate constrained active motion for the Zone III extensor tendons.

Gelberman RH, Nunley JA, Osterman AL, Breen TF, Dimick MP, Woo SL-Y: Influences of the protected passive mobilization interval on flexor tendon healing: a prospective randomized clinical study. *Clin Orthop Rel Res,* 264:189-196, 1991.

This prospective multicenter study demonstrates that by increasing the duration of daily passive motion in the early stages of Zone II flexor tendon healing, increased interphalangeal motion is achieved as a final result.

Hagberg L, Selvik G: Tendon excursion and dehiscence during early controlled mobilization after flexor tendon repair in zone II: An x-ray stereophotogrammetric analysis. *J Hand Surg,* 16A: 669-680, 1991.

Considerable differences of tendon excursion were found between the various methods of mobilization and were dependent on the level of injury within Zone II. A component of active flexion is suggested for injuries at the A_3 and A_4 levels.

Horii E, Lin GT, Cooney WP, Linscheid RL, An KN: Comparative flexor tendon excursions after passive mobilization: an *in vitro* study. *J Hand Surg,* 17A:559-566, 1992.

Two experimental studies conducted to investigate flexor tendon excursions demonstrate that (1) measured tendon tension under a condition of low tendon tension is almost half that of theoretically predicted values; and that (2) of the three mobilization methods studied, excursions introduced were the greatest with a new splinting technique that uses synergistic wrist motion, and least with the original Kleinert splint.

May EJ, Silfverskiold KL, Sollerman CJ : Controlled mobilization after flexor tendon repair in Zone II. A prospective comparison of three methods. *J Hand Surg,* 17A:942-952, 1992.

Interphalangeal motion is improved at six weeks and one year with a postoperative management technique that incorporates four-digit traction with a dorsal splint that ends at the level of the PIP joint, and night splinting that rests the PIP joints at absolute 0° with dynamic extension assists.

Minamikawa Y, Peimer CA, Yamaguchi T, Banasiak NA, Kambe K, Sherwin FS : Wrist position and extensor tendon amplitude following repair. *J Hand Surg,* 17A:268-271, 1992.

Extensor tendon excursions measured in eight fresh cadaver hands in Verdan's Zones III to VIII indicate that if the wrist is extended more than 21° the extensor tendon glides with little or no tension in Zones V and VI throughout full simulated grip to full passive extension.

Newport ML, Shukla A: Electrophysiologic basis of dynamic extensor splinting. *J Hand Surg,* 17A:272-277, 1992.

This study demonstrates that the extensor digitorum communis (EDC) is not quiescent within dynamic extension splints that rest the MP joint at 0°, but that by resting the MP at 15° the EDC demonstrates no extensor activity. Dynamic extension splints used in postoperative extensor tendon repair programs appear to facilitate controlled active motion.

Schuind F, Garcia-Elias M, Cooney WP, An KN: Flexor tendon forces : *In vivo* measurements. *J Hand Surg,* 17A:291-298, 1992.

In vivo force measurements were studied with S-shaped force transducers along intact flexor tendons during surgery on five patients being operated on for treatment of carpal tunnel syndrome. Tendon forces up to 0.9 kgf were present during passive mobilization of the fingers, and in the range of 0.1 to 0.6 kgf during passive mobilization of the wrist. Tendon forces up to 3.5 kgf were present during active unrestricted finger motion.

Silfverskiold KL, May EJ, Tornvall AH: Flexor digitorum profundus tendon excursions during controlled motion after flexor tendon repair in Zone II: a prospective clinical study. *J Hand Surg,* 17A:122-131, 1992.

An *in vivo* study of FDP excursions during early controlled motion with dynamic flexion traction demonstrates that controlled motion of the DIP mobilized the FDP with 36% efficiency, and that PIP joint motion mobilized the FDP with 90% efficiency.

Nerve

Butler DS : *Mobilization of the nervous system.* Churchill Livingstone, New York, 1991.

This text describes the neurophysiological sequelae of adverse tension in the nervous system, evaluation by tension testing, and treatment by mobilization of the nervous system.

Imai H, Tajima T, Natsum Y: Successful re-education of functional sensibility after median nerve repair at the wrist. *J Hand Surg,* 16A:60-65, 1991.

The results of this clinical comparison study of adults with median nerve repair at the wrist indicate that sensory re-education after median nerve repair at the wrist minimizes discomfort and improves sensibility in the postoperative period.

Mackinnon SE: Double and multiple "crush" syndromes. *Hand Clin,* Vol 8(2), 369-390, 1992.

This chapter defines the physiology of the double-crush hypothesis of nerve compression and recommends maximum job modification before surgical intervention. Pressure provocative and positional provocative testing for upper extremity nerve compression are outlined.

45

Amputation and Prosthetics

James M. Kleinert, MD

Amputation

The most common reason for surgical amputation in the upper extremity today is traumatic injury that renders part of the limb unsalvageable. Less commonly, vascular insufficiency, infectious disorders, nerve problems, and tumors of the upper extremity make surgical amputation necessary. Approximately 43% of amputations occur in the workplace, especially in the manufacturing industry. In a high percentage of these injuries, surgical amputation of a digit, hand, or extremity plays a significant role.

The time to decide whether to amputate or to reconstruct is the day of the injury. Once begun, a course of treatment is not easy to alter until enough time has elapsed to determine its final outcome. Patients with severely mutilated digits or hands may be best served by early amputation, which allows them a shorter period of recovery and an earlier return of function and interaction with society.

Digital Amputation

While clean-cut injuries at the level of the distal phalanx can be microsurgically reconstructed, crushing or mutilating injuries often are best treated by revision amputation at the distal interphalangeal level. Proximal injuries may also require amputation if they entail severe joint destruction, tendon loss, soft-tissue loss, and nonreconstructible nerve deficit. Patients with associated complex fractures and other soft-tissue injury to the index finger who had surgical amputation of that digit demonstrated an improved outcome compared to those who had prolonged reconstructive procedures. A finger cleanly amputated through the proximal interphalangeal joint could be replanted with the joint fused in a functional position. Silicone implants have also been utilized selectively in lieu of fusion to maintain at least some motion.

Ray Amputation

Ray amputation may be indicated if the injury includes the metacarpophalangeal joint. If the metacarpophalangeal joint and a portion of the proximal phalanx are relatively intact, preservation of these structures may improve the hand's balance and grip strength. Many patients prefer to retain their proximal phalanx rather than have a ray amputation. Ray amputation can be performed later as an elective procedure if the patient wishes. Patients with severe injuries to the border digits, however, often choose to undergo ray amputation because such a hand is less conspicuous than one with an amputated digit.

Hand Amputation

Injuries necessitating amputation of the entire hand are rare.

In severe injuries where a large portion of the hand cannot be salvaged, amputation is often necessary. When such an injury occurs, preservation of portions of the thumb and hand (including the thumb metacarpal to maintain opposition) allows later reconstruction with possible toe transfer. Another priority is preservation of the carpus. If the wrist joint is also destroyed, the amputation is done so as to preserve maximum forearm length. The longer the forearm, the greater the potential for pronation and supination. With forearm and arm level amputations, myoplasty is performed, ie, the flexor and extensor muscles are sutured together over the bone end.

Elective amputation of the hand is sometimes done as a result of severe tissue loss, chronic pain, poor appearance, or infection, or to better meet a patient's functional requirements. Psychological and economic factors and body image may also contribute to this decision. After elective amputation of the hand, most patients are able to use a prosthesis successfully and believe they actually gain function.

Patients with replanted thumbs with return of sensibility perform better in tasks requiring fine dexterity or the holding of certain tools than those with revision amputation. Patients with isolated thumb revision amputations have stronger pinch strength than those with replanted thumbs. Thus a surgical amputation is not a failure but a reconstructive procedure that allows the patient to heal in the most beneficial way.

Psychological Impact

One must never lose sight of the important role the hand plays in body image. Patients undergo a natural grieving process when suffering the loss of a body part. As Gordan Grant commented, "Loss or mutilation of the hand especially deals a blow to the person's inner image that reverberates through their entire psyche." Patients may need help dealing with their loss whether it be of a portion of a digit, a hand, or an entire upper extremity.

The team approach for patients who have suffered traumatic amputation includes the physician, nurse, prosthetist, physical therapist, and a psychologist for selected patients. The goals for patient recovery include early acceptance of the injury; early acceptance of a new self-image, which involves the less-than-perfect appearance of a part; early restoration of function; and return to independence. A significant component of each of these goals is psychological. While hand therapists are instrumental in helping patients realize these goals, a psychologist may also play a role in reestablishing a patient's healthy self-image.

A traumatic amputation can lead to serious emotional disorders such as depression, anxiety, posttraumatic stress syndrome, and other personality adjustment disorders. Most patients suffering from depression and anxiety following an amputation respond to a combination of medication and psychotherapy. Murray noted that "the hand is one of the so called emotionally charged areas of the body and there is a propensity for a patient to develop emotional and psychiatric complications when it is disabled."

Techniques of Amputation

The basic principles of revision amputation of a digit are as follows: (1) The bone is contoured to make the stump look more natural and prevent a bulbous appearance. (2) If the amputation occurs at the level of a joint, the condyles are usually removed. The remaining bony edges are smoothed with a rasp. (3) Soft-tissue coverage is necessary for padding. (4) The digital nerves are identified at the level of the amputation and resected a centimeter or more. (5) The extensor tendons are not sutured to the flexor tendons. If the amputation occurs at the level of the distal phalanx, the profundus tendon may be sutured near the A4 pulley to prevent proximal migration and later lumbrical plus deformity.

Some patients suffer amputation of both hands in blast injuries and are simultaneously blinded. These patients can be treated successfully with the Krukenberg procedure; however, it produces significant anatomical change in the upper extremity and is considered unsightly, albeit functional. Another procedure of value for blind patients, reported by Vilkki, is toe-to-stump transplantation after wrist amputation (Fig. 45-1). This technically demanding microsurgical procedure involves transfer of a second toe with web space skin from the great toe to the remaining portion of the distal forearm stump and allows the patient return of functional pinch. A major advantage for the blind patient is that this procedure permits some return of sensibility.

Patients with transmetacarpal amputations of all digits may also lose their thumbs. In carefully selected and motivated patients, the thumb can be restored through a toe transfer, and the digit through a transfer of the ring finger from the opposite hand. The procedure is technically demanding in terms of microsurgical skill, but it restores useful pinch and grasp and at least some sensation.

Transplantation of severed digits to the forearm stump for restoration of partial hand function (Figs. 45-2 and 45-3) enables a small group of patients to preserve some digital function even though most of the wrist and hand has been destroyed. Patient acceptance prior to this procedure is critical because the hand anatomy is greatly altered.

These procedures represent viable alternatives to prosthetic fitting or reconstruction in select groups of patients.

Length

Restoration of length following amputation is important for regaining function. One patient with an amputated thumb had the stump of the small finger from the opposite hand microsurgically transferred to reconstruct his thumb and thus regained useful function without sacrificing significant function in the opposite hand. Microsurgical free-tissue

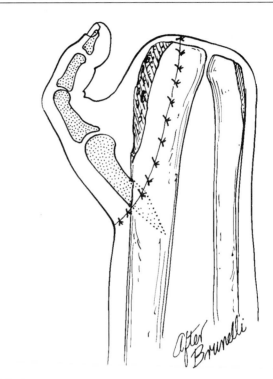

Figure 45-1.   Vilkki procedure of toe-to-stump transplantation after distal forearm level amputation used primarily as an alternative to the Krukenberg procedure in patients who are blind.

transfer can provide soft-tissue coverage of a degloved stump which traditionally would be amputated to achieve primary wound closure. Using this means to preserve the elbow joint, for example, allows a more functional extremity. Both salvageable tissue from an unreplantable amputated part (a microvascular volar forearm flap) and distant free-tissue transfers, such as the latissimus dorsi muscle or gracilis muscle, can be utilized to increase stump length and preserve functional joints. This improved soft-tissue coverage also provides more durable skin coverage for later prosthetic fitting.

Treatment of Painful Neuromas

Most patients require simple resection of the nerve proximal to the level of amputation. Thus, the nerve end is not in direct contact with the end of the stump, the prosthesis, or the external environment during use of the extremity. Techniques also recommended are suture ligation of the nerve end and bipolar cauterization of the distal nerve end after resection. Should a painful neuroma occur, it can be placed within a bed of a muscle or in the bone. Proximally, the nerve should be free, not tethered, so that motion of the joint produces no traction upon it.

Some patients with amputation at the forearm level have significant pain at the neuroma site. Should the patient develop a painful neuroma, the author typically resects 3 cm to 4 cm of the nerve 5 cm proximal to the amputation stump. The amputation stump itself is not violated.

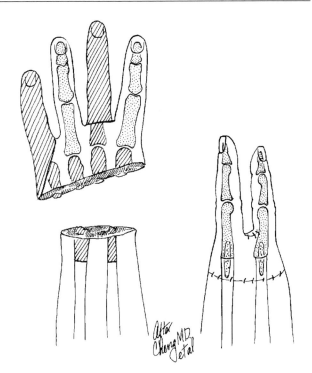

Figure 45-2.   Preservation of pinch by utilizing two digits from an amputed hand. Few patients would be candidates for this type of reconstruction.

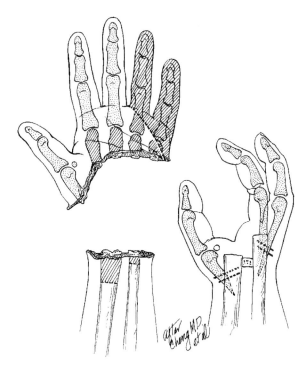

Figure 45-3.   Palm and wrist destruction prevented hand replantation. The thumb and two digits were replanted to the distal forearm to provide small and large object pinch. Few patients would be candidates for this type of reconstruction.

Following are descriptions of techniques for treating painful neuromas that do not respond to simple resection, including coaptation of the ends of the median and ulnar nerves after forearm amputation; the use of a vascularized island transfer; and the use of epineurial tube closure. Coaptation of the ends of the median and ulnar nerves underneath the pronator muscle has resulted in significant but not complete reduction of pain.

Painful neuromas in the stump of an amputated digit may be treated with a vascularized island transfer from a less important digit. The neuroma is excised and the remaining nerve end is coapted to a nerve in a neurovascular flap from the donor digit. A normal regeneration process occurs in the nerve stump by allowing regenerating axons to reach uninjured sensory receptors. At this time, it is not known how often patients develop symptomatic neuromas in the donor site.

Another technique for treating intractable neuromas entails epineurial tube closure using a synthetic tissue adhesive (histoacryl, presently not available in the U.S.) with fascicular shortening. This technique is based on the premise that a water-tight closure of the epineurium can prevent neuroma formation. The nerve is identified under the microscope and the fascicles are shortened within the epineurial tube (Fig. 45-4). The end of the epineurial tube is sealed with tissue glue. Applying tissue glue to the nerve end without resecting the fascicles is not sufficient to elim-

inate pain. Most patients who have this procedure were either improved or cured, and none were made worse. These patients had pain of long duration and had undergone multiple conservative treatments and surgical procedures, including resection of the nerve, ligation, and silicone capping.

Prosthetics

The ideal prosthesis would provide durability as well as a pleasing appearance. A patient's desires, needs, recreational and extracurricular activities, and occupation are all significant factors in determining the best prosthesis for the individual. Approximately 90% of upper extremity amputees with prostheses utilize the body-powered type. This type of prothesis is relatively inexpensive, functional, and reliable, and provides some sensory proprioceptive feedback from the shoulder harness and cable control system.

Cosmetic Prostheses

The first objective of the aesthetic prosthesis is psychological. Pillet described the problem: "There is little relation between the degree of actual physical loss and the psychological weight each individual patient will give to it and the degree [to which] it will influence performance. The man

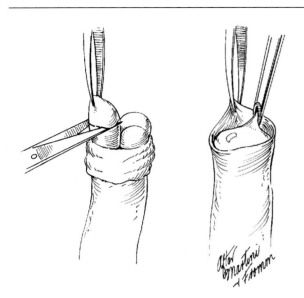

Figure 45-4. Preparation of the nerve end. Fascicles are shortened within the epineurial tube, which is then sealed with tissue glue.

who finds himself unable to take his hand from his pocket, even though it is very 'functional,' may be as handicapped as if it were lost. Thus, in a global sense of function, the aesthetic prosthesis may be beneficial even if it at times introduces some restriction of the prehensile capability of remaining parts. In allowing use of a stump that the amputee considers too repulsive to expose and use, overall function may well be improved."

Cosmetic or static prostheses are currently made of polyvinyl chloride or silicone (dimethyl siloxane polymer). Silicone prostheses, static or cosmetic, are more durable and more expensive. Overall, silicone prostheses are preferred. The cosmetic prosthesis gives some prehensile assistance, providing opposition of the part for the remaining digits or thumb. The most common part replaced by a cosmetic prosthesis is the digit. The cosmetic hand prosthesis must be of high quality technically, especially the digits because they are viewed alongside normal fingers. Silicone prostheses have excellent finger and nail detail and can be pigmented to correspond to the patient's skin color. In areas where seasonal climate varies significantly, two prostheses may be necessary to accommodate for seasonal pigmentation changes. Improvements prevent silicone prostheses from being stained by newsprint; this remains a problem with polyvinyl chloride prostheses.

The cosmetic hand prosthesis works best for a unilateral amputee who is well adjusted and has realistic expectations of what it can and cannot do. Approximately 36% of patients discontinue use of digital prostheses after three years. Reasons include inhibition of function, poor color match, and improved self-confidence regarding the amputation deformity.

Body-powered Prostheses

In body-powered prostheses, previously the gold standard

for the upper limb amputee, a cable control system is utilized to guide the terminal device. The cable obtains its energy from joint motion proximal to the level of amputation. A harness is used across the chest or shoulder region with the cable system.

The two basic types of mechanisms for the external device are voluntary opening and voluntary closing.

In the voluntary opening system, the hook remains closed by a built-in spring or elastic resistance system. Shoulder or elbow motion operates the cable to provide the force required to open the hook. This system provides constant tension that enables the patient to hold an object without concentrated effort. The amount of force applied is predetermined by the spring system, not by the patient. In any voluntary closing device, contrastingly, the tension used to hold the object can be controlled by the patient, and, as such, only the exact force required need be used. The appropriate choice depends on the patient's needs and preferences.

Today, the most commonly used body-powered terminal device is the voluntary opening split-hook (Fig. 45-5). Besides the basic split-hook, many other types of external devices are available, including tool holders, tweezers, functional hands, and a variety of split-hooks (Fig. 45-6). Passive devices can also be utilized as a terminal device, including knife, fork, spoon, plain hooks, an assortment of tools, typewriter key punch, automobile steering-wheel appliance, kitchen appliances, nail brush holder, garden tool holder, and fishing rod holder. Generally, patients with a prosthesis prefer not to interchange a multitude of terminal devices but rather to have a functional, stable, durable device that they can use in their everyday work.

Since the early 80s several new designs have been developed, such as those offered by Therapeutic Recreation Systems of Boulder, Colorado (Fig. 45-7). In these systems terminal devices for infants and small children and a sport series for all ages have been developed. The latter are flexible passive devices that absorb shock, store and release energy, and can be utilized for sports and other activities.

Wrist components are available, allowing attachment of various terminal devices and positioning of the terminal device prior to operation. Designs include the constant-friction wrist unit, quick-change unit, and rotational wrist unit. The latter is a cable-controlled, positive-locking mechanism providing greater resistance to rotation than a friction wrist unit. Also available are flexion wrist units that allow manual positioning of the hook.

The figure-of-eight ring-type harness is the most popular body-powered harness for below-elbow amputees. When a patient engages in heavier work, a chest strap or a shoulder-saddle harness may be required instead of the figure-of-eight ring-type harness.

The above-the-elbow amputee utilizing a body-powered prosthesis usually needs a locking elbow joint for efficient operation. Here, the most popular harness is the figure-of-eight dual control design. The terminal control device is attached to a lever on the forearm so that tension in the cable produces elbow flexion when the elbow is unlocked. When the elbow is locked, the cable controls the terminal device.

The long-term advantages of the body-powered prosthesis are its relatively low maintenance requirements, patient

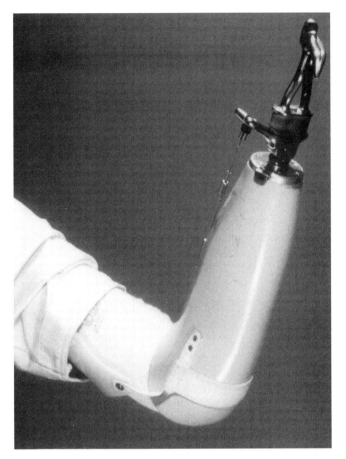

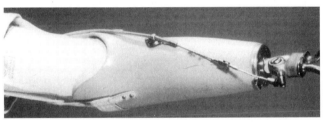

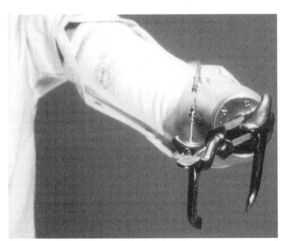

Figure 45-5. Below-elbow amputee with voluntary opening split-hook, elbow flexed **(Top)** and extended **(Center). (Bottom)** Hook in open position.

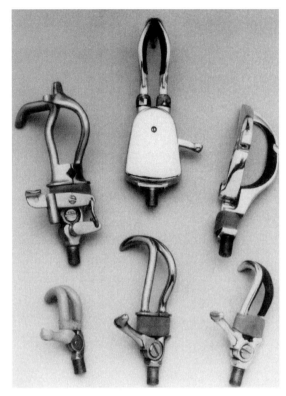

Figure 45-6. Various Hosmer Dorrance prosthetic device hooks, including pediatric sizes. (Photograph courtesy of Hosmer Dorrance Corporation).

acceptance, and functional capabilities. Many below-elbow amputees may return to work using a body-powered prosthesis with a terminal hook device. Unfortunately, many patients find the functional hook unacceptable in social situations and use a cosmetic hand even though it is less functional. Several new designs are being evaluated for use as prosthetic prehensors (Fig. 45-8).

External-powered Prostheses

Initially, external-powered prostheses were pneumatic "gas powered" prostheses. However, due to their size and mechanical problems, they were never popular. With the development of the electric-powered (myoelectric) prosthesis, external-powered prostheses became more acceptable. Their advantages are noteworthy. Overall appearance is better. An external-powered prosthesis usually has no external cable hardware; its harness is either simple or absent; a hand-shaped terminal device is common; it has a modern, high-tech appeal for patients; and its modular components are easily serviced. Now that external-powered myoelectric prostheses have interchangeable terminal devices, the patient can use one hand for lighter activities and a durable terminal device known as a Greifer for heavier activities (Fig. 45-9). These external-powered prostheses thus combine the advantages of a cosmetic prosthesis with those of the body-powered functional hook.

Handlike electric-powered prehensors are available from

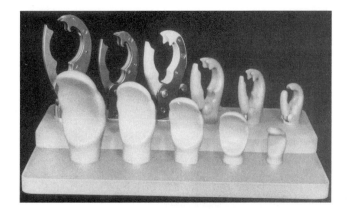

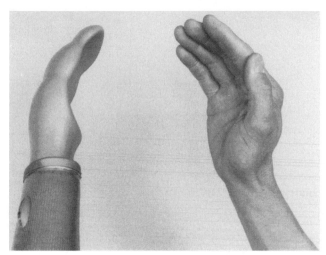

Figure 45-7. **(Top)** Therapeutic Recreation System. Back row: various terminal devices. Front row: corresponding passive flexible devices for sports. (Photograph courtesy of TRS, Inc.). **(Bottom)** Passive flexible terminal device with opposite normal hand in position to hold a large ball. (Photograph courtesy of TRS.).

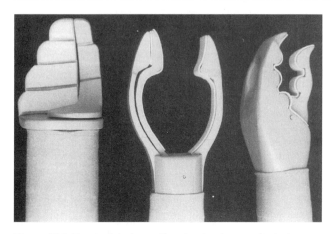

Figure 45-8. Terminal devices still under development for body-powered prostheses. (Photograph courtesy of Maunce LeBlanc, MSME,CP).

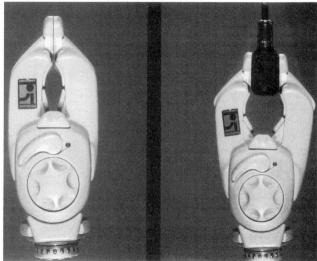

Figure 45-9. Greifer (Otto-Bock) which is interchangeable with the myoelectric hand (Otto-Bock). The Greifer is durable and suited for heavy manual work.

Otto-Bock and Steeper. Electric-powered prehensors without a handlike appearance include the Greifer, Hosmer NU-VA synergetic prehensor, and the Steeper powered gripper. Presently, electric-powered shoulder components are not commercially available.

The most common on-off switch presently utilized is the Myoswitch (the Otto-Bock system), a simpler system than that associated with true myoelectric control. Here the patient must generate a sufficiently strong signal to cross a threshold and trigger an electronic switch. Unfortunately, the Myoswitch does not allow proportional control. Hosmer-Dorrance Corp. and Motion Control both offer proportional myoelectric controls. With proportional control a mild myoelectric impulse will produce slow, gentle hand movement, and a stronger impulse produces more rapid, powerful movement. Overall, this approach is more physiologic in nature. A third control system, Switch Control (Otto-Bock), is the least expensive and least bulky and is used in juvenile below-elbow designs. Its switch controls include a cable pull switch, harness pull switch, and rocker switch.

External-powered Prostheses and Level of Amputation

The use and choice of prostheses varies with the level of amputation. The amount prostheses are used is approximately 80% for below-elbow amputees compared to 69% for above-elbow amputees and 70% for high-level amputees. Above-elbow and high-level amputees prefer electrically powered prostheses to cable-operated prostheses, possibly because they provide superior pinch force and require less energy expenditure than body-powered prostheses.

Some patients with above-elbow amputation use a body-powered prosthesis to control the elbow and a myoelectric unit to control the hand. Body-powered elbows can be controlled by a motorized lock (Steeper Electric Elbow Lock). Other patients with above-elbow amputation have a myoelectric hand with an electric elbow of the Utah, Boston, or NY-Hosmer type. These have different mechanical configurations, drive mechanisms, and control options. The active lifting capacity for these electric elbows is between 0.65 kg and 1.55 kg. The passive lifting capacity (elbow locked) is between 8 kg and 23 kg. Some above-elbow amputees use a body-powered cable-controlled terminal device with a myoelectric elbow. Presently, elbow controllers determine the velocity of motion but not position.

The myoelectric prosthesis is the most common device utilized in a below-elbow amputee (Fig. 45-10). A self-contained unit is usually powered by a six-volt battery placed on the volar aspect of the prosthesis. An articulated hand is utilized with a three-prong pincer-type grip. The grip varies from 1 kg to 10 kg with a digit opening of from 6 cm to 10 cm.

Comparison of Body-powered and Electrically Powered Prostheses

Several studies have compared body-powered and electrically powered prostheses. In one series, upper extremity amputees with myoelectric prostheses used the prosthesis 9.5 hours a day compared to 14 hours a day for patients with conventional cable-control hook prostheses. Patients using conventional prostheses took 2.5 times as long to complete tasks as persons with a normal hand, but those using myoelectric prostheses took five times longer. Nonetheless, more than 60% of below-elbow amputees preferred the myoelectric prosthesis to the conventional one with which they had previously been fitted.

In a series of patients followed for 15 years, 83% of patients using an electrically powered prosthesis did so successfully compared to 68% of those using a cable-operated hook. A large number of patients used more than one prosthesis. In general, fitting patients with more than one type of prosthesis may be beneficial.

The main reasons that patients do not use a prosthesis are pain and limited function. Other reasons include harness and stump problems. Cable-operated hook-type prostheses are best suited to jobs requiring heavy lifting or handling of dirty, greasy materials and sharp objects. Under extreme weather conditions, the body-powered prosthesis proves more functional; cold weather can interfere with battery function and warm weather causes hyperhidrosis and loss of control in myoelectric protheses. (Recent advances in circuitry may eliminate this problem.) Patients who supervise in an office or interact with the general public usually prefer a myoelectric prosthesis. In summary, the advantages of the electrically powered prosthesis include
- increased patient comfort for below-elbow amputees because of elimination of harness suspension;
- better appearance;
- superior pinch force (15 to 25 lbs. for electric-powered prostheses vs. seven to eight pounds for the cable-operated hook);
- more natural control because movement of the hand and elbow units is independent of body position; and

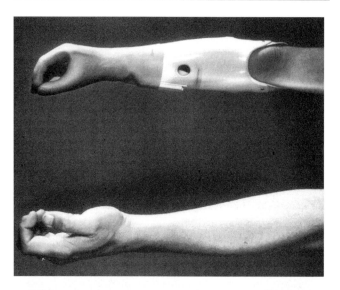

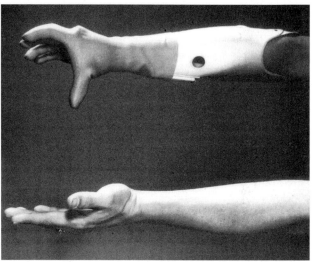

Figure 45-10.   (Top) Below-elbow myoelectric prosthesis with opposite normal hand. **(Bottom)** Myoelectric hand in maximum abduction and extension. Note full web space opening.

- reduced energy expenditure for the high-level amputee.
  The disadvantages of electrically powered prostheses are
- high cost;
- increased maintenance needs;
- less durability; and
- greater weight.

Electric-powered Prostheses in Children

In preschool children with congenital limb deficiency, training in the use of myoelectric prostheses was effective with either the parent or the therapist as primary trainer. The home program with the parent as trainer is much less costly.

In one study of children fitted with electric-powered prostheses, the acceptance of myoelectric prostheses by below-elbow amputees (90%) was comparable to that of conventional body-powered prostheses (87%). Children with above-elbow amputations preferred using myoelectric prostheses over conventional prostheses. Patients with the highest acceptance of myoelectric prostheses were congenital bilateral amputees. Approximately three-fourths of the upper-limb-deficient children felt that function was more important than appearance, but one-fifth rated appearance higher than function. Furthermore, two-thirds felt the myoelectric arm allowed better function, compared to one-third for the cable-operated hook.

The earlier myoelectric prosthetic training is begun, the greater the likelihood of long-term use by the amputee. Children with congenital and acquired upper-limb deficiency are more likely to continue to use a prosthesis if fitted before age two. Half of the children fitted after the age of two years abandon their prosthesis, while a quarter of patients fitted before the age of two years do the same. The highest drop-out rate occurs around age 13. This applies equally to patients with congenital and acquired deficiencies.

The level of amputation affects whether prosthesis use is continued. The more distal the level of the deficiency in the child, the more likely is discontinuation of the prosthetic use. In other words, a child with an amputation just below the elbow is likely to continue using a prothesis, while a child with a long forearm stump is likely to discontinue use. This is especially true if the child has a mobile carpal remnant, ie, a below-wrist deficiency.

A study of congenitally abrachial children found only a small percentage to be using the prosthesis after 25 years. Those using the prosthesis did so more during social than work activities. Congenitally abrachial children develop remarkable ability to carry out all necessary activities of daily life with their feet, and a prosthesis may be a burden.

In summary, fitting of children with congenital upper extremity deficiencies occurs ideally by two to three years of age. Between the age of six and 24 months, static prostheses are often utilized prior to fitting with a functional prothesis. Myoelectric prostheses in children with below-elbow amputations are as well accepted as body-powered prostheses. For children with above-elbow amputations, the myoelectric or external-powered prosthesis is superior in terms of acceptance and functional improvement. Nonetheless, patients have different needs and demands, so prosthetic selection, whether of myoelectric, body-powered, or hybrid, must vary accordingly.

Multifunctional Control Systems

In the future, myoelectric designs will include increasingly complex control techniques. A means of control called extended physiological proprioception has been demonstrated using an above-elbow prosthesis: an Intel 8751 microcomputer controls an electric-powered wrist and elbow joint allowing the motion of the intact shoulder to control the prosthesis. Grasp is regulated separately through EMG signals from the biceps and triceps. The principle of extended physiological proprioception allows the intact shoulder to provide both input to the prosthesis and proprioceptive feedback to the amputee. The amputee

associates the position of the shoulder with the position of the prosthesis. Preprogrammed linkages produce coordinated motions of the elbow and wrist. Preliminary investigation shows great promise for this myoelectric prosthesis, especially in higher level amputees.

Other potential improvements in myoelectric prostheses involve the use of multiple-state and myoelectric control units. Unfortunately, as the complexity of the control system increases, so does the needed concentration by the amputee. A level-sensitive, single-site, three-state control system has been available for some time. This allows one muscle unit to control two prosthetic movements, with different EMG levels executing different tasks. One Otto-Bock system utilizes a dual-site, five-state control system constructed from two single-site, three-state controllers. With a multiple-state control system, for instance, the patient could use flexor and extensor muscles to control prosthesis hand closing and opening and also forearm pronation and supination. For an above-elbow amputee, a dual system with multiple-state controls could cause elbow flexion and elbow extension, forearm rotation, and hand closing and opening.

A myoelectric prosthesis with fingertips that have touch, slip, and position sensors and a microprocessor-based controller is under development. If a prosthetically held object starts to fall, the controller automatically identifies the problem via the sensors and signals the motor to increase the grip power, allowing the amputee to hold the object without continuous conscious effort.

Orthotics

Hand neuroprostheses offer functional gains for quadriplegic patients by providing hand grasp through neuromuscular stimulation of paralyzed forearm and hand muscles. Percutaneous electrodes (controlled by contralateral shoulder movement) electronically stimulate hand and forearm muscles providing keygrip and three-finger pinch. Patients who performed various activities with and without the hand neuroprosthesis did significantly better with the prosthesis. Those patients benefiting most were the C5 and C6 quadriplegics, who were able to perform almost 90% of the activities of daily living with a neuroprosthesis as compared to less than half without. Some improvements were important: for example, five of 20 patients were unable to eat finger foods unless they used the neuroprosthesis.

Myoelectric hand orthoses have also been developed for patients with C5 and C6 quadriplegia. Presently, these patients are often fitted with a wrist-driven, flexor-hinge tenodesis orthosis. Patients with weak wrist extension, however, could gain the ability to grip by using the myoelectric orthosis. The myoelectric hand orthosis has been used in a few patients and it may enhance the rehabilitation and independence of a select group.

The integration of myoelectric components, including elbow, wrist, and hand devices, as well as interchangeable terminal devices combined with multistate control systems, will ensure continued future development in the field of upper limb prosthetics.

Annotated Bibliography

Indications for Amputation

Arnaud JP, Mallet T, Pecout C, et al: Isolated complex injuries to the index: the place of amputation. *J Chir*, (Paris) 123:321-325, 1986.

A study involving 20 male patients who sustained severe complex open fractures of the index finger was presented. Ten underwent initial amputation and the other 10 were treated with reconstruction. Overall results were better in those who underwent primary amputation. Cold intolerance and pain occurred in eight of the 10 patients whose digits were preserved. Complex trauma involving the extremity was felt to be best treated by amputation than by preservation of the digit.

Brown, PW: Sacrifice of the unsatisfactory hand. *J Hand Surg*, 4A:417-423, 1979.

Fifteen patients who had elective hand amputation were reviewed. The indications for amputation included severe tissue loss, pain, appearance, infection, functional requirements, sexual reasons, psychological makeup of the patients, economics, safety, the time elapsed since the injury, the patient's body image and desires, and the surgeon's opinion. Twelve of the 15 patients successfully used protheses.

Goldner RD, Howson MP, Nunley JA, et al: One hundred eleven thumb amputations: replantation vs. revision. *Microsurg*, 11:243-250, 1990.

Ninety percent of the amputations in subsequent replantations were performed between the metacarpophalangeal joint and the proximal third of the distal phalanx. Range of motion averaged 42% of the uninjured thumb. Lateral pinch was approximately 68% in the replanted group compared to the opposite normal side vs. 91% in the amputation group. Overall, a uniform superiority of replantation over revision amputation was not found. Patients who underwent replantation of the thumb did perform slightly better on the Jebsen test.

May JW Jr: Amputation stump closure: a reconstructive procedure, not a failure. *J Hand Surg*, 9A:828-829, 1984.

This report by May holds that microvascular replantation and prosthetic fitting as a combined approach achieve better results for patients with amputation than either approach separately.

Olson DK, Gerberich S: Traumatic amputations in the workplace. *J Occup Med*, 28:480-485, 1986.

In this study of 109 patients with amputation in the workplace over a one-year period in Minnesota, men were five times more frequently injured than women. Over 43% of the amputations occurred in manufacturing. The 109 patients had 135 amputations involving 126 digits of the hand. Only six involved digits of the foot, and only three amputations were at the hand or arm level.

Psychological Impact

Grant GH: The hand and the psyche. *J Hand Surg*, 5A:417-419, 1980.

This editorial reviews the psychological importance of the subjective image of the hand for patients with severe injuries.

Mendelson RL, Burech JG, Polack EP, et al: The psychological impact of traumatic amputations. A team approach: physician, therapist, and psychologist. *Hand Clin* 2:577-583, 1986.

The roles of the physician, hand therapist, and clinical psychologist are reviewed in terms of patients who had amputations involving the upper extremity. Neurotic depression, anxiety, posttraumatic stress syndrome, and other personality adjustment disorders can occur. A team approach for caring for these patients is described.

Murray JF: The patient with the injured hand. *J Hand Surg*, 7A:543-548, 1982.

The importance of caring for the whole patient with the injured hand is presented by Murray in his presidential address to the American Society for Surgery of the Hand, as are factors involved in rehabilitation.

New Techniques of Amputation

Cheng GL, Pan DD, Qu ZY: Transplantation of severed digits to forearm stump for restoration of partial hand function. *Ann Plast Surg*, 15:356-366, 1985.

Three patients with mutilating injuries to the distal end of the forearm, wrist, and palm with preservation of the digits were treated by transplantation or replantation of the severed digits to the forearm stump. This procedure allows for one-stage reconstruction providing pinch, grasp, and sensation and avoiding later sacrifice of the toes.

Kessler I: Cross transposition of short amputation stumps for reconstruction of the thumb. *J Hand Surg*, 10B:76-78, 1985.

A case report of a patient who suffered a previous amputation of the thumb and the long finger is presented. A remnant stump of the long finger is transposed to the thumb position to allow for reconstruction. The second digit was transposed to the third ray to complete the reconstruction in this case.

Vilkki SK: A technique for toe-to-stump transplantation after wrist amputation: a modern alternative to the Krukenberg operation. *Handchirurgie*, 17:92-97, 1985.

Three patients with a previous amputation at the wrist level underwent reconstruction utilizing an Allen flap from the big toe and the second toe. This modern alternative to the Krukenberg procedure is recommended for patients who are blind.

Morrison WA, O'Brien BM, MacLeon AM: Ring finger transfer in reconstruction of transmetacarpal amputations. *J Hand Surg*, 9A:4-11, 1984.

Four patients with previous transmetacarpal amputations had the ring finger from the normal hand transposed to the injured hand for reconstruction. The thumb was reconstructed by hallux transfer. The advantages of the ring finger transfer include length and mobility, strength, wider span, and appearance.

Moss ALH, Waterhouse N: One stage thumb reconstruction using a previously injured little finger from the contralateral hand. *J Hand Surg*, 10B:73-75, 1985.

A case report of a patient with a small finger previously amputated at the mid proximal phalanx level is presented. This patient also had amputation of the contralateral thumb. Using microvascular techniques, the fifth ray was transferred to the opposite thumb for reconstruction.

Preservation of Length

May JW Jr, Gordon L: Palm of hand free flap for forearm length preservation in nonreplantable forearm amputation: a case report. *J Hand Surg,* 5A:377-380, 1980.

A patient with a forearm level amputation could not have hand replantation. Preservation of forearm length to allow for a below-elbow prosthesis was achieved by replantation of palmar skin as a free flap on the remaining forearm stump.

Rees MJW, de Geus JJ: Immediate amputation stump coverage with forearm free flaps from the same limb. *J Hand Surg,* 13A:287-292, 1988.

Three patients with traumatic amputations of the upper extremity had forearm free flaps. This allowed for preservation of length and created a durable surface for later prosthetic fitting.

Treatment of Neuromas

Martini A, Fromm B: A new operation for the prevention and treatment of amputation neuromas. *J Bone Joint Surg,* 71B:379-382, 1989.

The technique involves excision of the fascicles for 5 mm, maintaining the length of epineurial sleeve, and sealing the end with a synthetic tissue adhesive. All 36 patients had been treated operatively or conservatively with success. Only three of the 36 patients with intractable neuroma pain continued to have pain after treatment with this technique.

Tada K, Nakashima H, Yoshida T, et al: A new treatment of painful amputation neuroma: a preliminary report. *J Hand Surg,* 12B:273-276, 1987.

Two patients with painful amputation neuromas were treated by a vascularized island transfer from a less important digit. The accompanying nerve was divided and its distal end sutured to the proximal end of the nerve in the recipient digit after excision of the neuroma. This treatment was utilized only after previous standard neuroma resection had failed.

Wood VE, Mudge MK: Treatment of neuromas about a major amputation stump. *J Hand Surg,* 12A:302-306, 1987.

Five patients with intractable pain secondary to neuromas after wrist and forearm amputation were successfully treated with resection of the neuromas and coaptation of the median and ulnar nerves under the pronator teres muscle. One patient also had anterior interosseous nerve coaptation to the superficial radial nerve below the muscles of the forearm.

Prosthetics

Bowker JH, Michael JW (eds): *Atlas of Limb Prosthetics: Surgical, Prosthetic, and Rehabilitation Principles,* Second ed, Mosby-Year Book, St. Louis, 1992.

This up-to-date reference is an indispensable guide to the entire field of limb prosthetics. Its sections range from surgical management of amputations to emerging trends in lower limb prosthetics.

Cosmetic Prostheses

Alison A, Mackinnon SE: Evaluation of digital prostheses. *J Hand Surg,* 17A:923-926, 1992.

Of 33 patients treated with 51 digital silicone-type prostheses, 36% discontinued the use of the prosthesis after three years. Forty-two percent felt better about their hands while wearing the prosthesis, and 51% felt their digits were less noticeable with the prosthetic digit. Overall, 80% of the patients felt that the cosmetic appearance of the prosthesis was acceptable, compared to 17% who felt it was not; 3% were undecided. Functional improvement was noted in 33%, compared to 21% who felt no functional improvement; 46% were undecided.

Pillet J: The aesthetic hand prosthesis. *Orthop Clin North Am,* 12:961-969, 1981.

This overview of the cosmetic hand prosthesis for treatment and management of upper limb amputations covers its functional potential, contraindications, and considerations according to the level of amputation.

Body-powered Prostheses

Atkins DJ, Meier RH III (eds): *Comprehensive Management of the Upper Limb Amputee.* Springer-Verlag, New York, 1989.

This text reviews the treatment of upper limb amputees, including amputation level and surgical techniques, pre- and postoperative therapy programs, evaluation and planning for upper limb amputee rehabilitation, surgical reconstruction of the amputated arm, body-powered upper limb components, adult upper limb prosthetic training, adult myoelectric upper limb prosthetic training, painful residual limb treatment strategies, evaluation of the pediatric amputee, electric pediatric and adult prosthetic components, and several centers' experience with various types of prostheses.

Law HT: Engineering of upper limb prostheses. *Orthop Clin North Am,* 12:929-951, 1981.

This overview of upper limb prostheses includes the passive prosthesis, body-powered prosthesis, and external-powered prosthesis.

LeBlanc M, Parker D, Nelson C: New designs for prosthetic prehensors. *Adv Extern Control Hum Extrem,* 9:475-481, 1987.

Three new prosthetic prehensors are described, including the Parker design, the LeBlanc design, and the Nelson design. These designs were developed to provide a terminal hook that is not only functional but aesthetically acceptable. Presently, these new designs are not utilized on a large scale and are still under development.

Wilson AB: *Limb Prosthetics,* Sixth ed, Demos Publications, New York, 1989.

This text is devoted to prosthetics and includes history, surgical options, treatment and early post-surgical period, as well as prostheses available for upper limb amputees.

External-powered Prostheses

Heger H, Millstein S, Hunter GA: Electrically powered prostheses for the adult with an upper limb amputation. *J Bone Joint Surg,* 67B:278-281, 1985.

This study evaluated 164 amputees fitted with an electrically powered prosthesis. Eighty percent of below-elbow amputees, 69% of above-elbow amputees, and 72% of high-level amputees utilized their prosthesis. Upper limb amputees, especially those with a high-level loss, had a more satisfactory result utilizing an electrically powered prosthesis than a cable-operated or body-powered prosthesis.

Kritter AE: Myoelectric prostheses. *J Bone Joint Surg,* 67A:654-657, 1985.

This article provides an overview of the myoelectric prosthesis and its utilization in children, in adults with below-elbow amputations, and in high-level amputees.

Michael JW: Upper limb powered components and controls: Current concepts. *Clinical Prosthetics and Orthotics,* 10:66-77, 1986.

Basic concepts, components, and controversies in the field of upper limb electrically powered prostheses is presented. Externally powered control options, as well as the commercially available powered components, are also detailed.

Millstein SG, Heger H, Hunter GA: Prosthetic use in adult upper limb amputees: a comparison of the body powered and electrically powered prostheses. *Prosthetics and Orthotics International* 10:27-34, 1986.

In this excellent article, a series of 314 adult upper-limb amputees was reviewed retrospectively.

Stein RB, Walley M: Functional comparison of upper extremity amputees using myoelectric and conventional prostheses. *Arch Phys Med Rehabil,* 64:243-248, 1983.

Function of upper extremity amputees was measured utilizing a standard series of tasks. A myoelectric prosthesis, a conventional prosthesis, and the normal hand were evaluated.

Prostheses in Children

Glynn MK, Galway HR, Hunter G, *et al:* Management of the upper-limb deficient child with a powered prosthetic device. *Clin Orthop,* 209:202-205, 1986.

This article reports on children with both congenital and traumatic upper limb deficiencies who were treated with electrically powered upper limb prosthetics over an 18-year period.

Hubbard S, Galway HR, Milner M: Myoelectric training methods for the preschool child with congenital below-elbow amputation. A comparison of two training programmes. *J Bone Joint Surg* 67B:273-277, 1985.

Home-based training for the preschool child utilizing a myoelectric prosthesis vs. a center-based technique with a therapist as the primary teacher was evaluated. Both training programs were felt to be equally effective.

Marquardt EG: A holistic approach to rehabilitation for the limb-deficient child. *Arch Phys Med Rehabil,* 64:237-242, 1983.

Seventy-four congenitally abrachial children were fitted with an externally powered prosthesis over a 25-year period. Only six were still utilizing their prosthesis. Recommendations for rehabilitation include physical medicine, orthopaedic surgery, occupational therapy, physical therapy, prosthetics and orthotics, education, psychology, and social work.

Scotland TR, Galway HR: A long-term review of children with congenital and acquired upper limb deficiency. *J Bone Joint Surg,* 65B:346-349, 1983.

In this series, 131 children fitted with an upper limb prosthesis were evaluated over a 10-year period, with follow-up care ranging from seven to 17 years. Children fitted after age two had a 50% likelihood of abandoning their prosthesis compared with 22% of those who had prosthetic fitting prior to age two. The dropout rate was similar for congenital and acquired amputees.

Multifunctional Control Systems

Chappell PH, Nightingale JM, Kyberd PJ, et al: Control of a single degree of freedom artificial hand. *J Biomed Eng,* 9:273-277, 1987.

The fingertips of this artificial hand were fitted with touch, slip, and position sensors using a microprocessor-based controller, which interprets signals from the sensors and then controls the response.

Charles D, James KB, Stein RB: Rehabilitation of musicians with upper limb amputations. *J Rehabil Res Dev,* 25:25-32, 1988.

Skin-conductivity touch control technique is utilized in three saxophone players with upper limb amputations.

Gibbons DT, O'Riain MD, Philippe-Auguste S: An above-elbow prosthesis employing programed linkages. *IEEE Trans Biomed Eng* BME34:493-498, 1987.

A prototype of a self-contained above-elbow prosthesis with electrically powered wrist and elbow controlled by a microcomputer is presented. The position of the above-elbow prosthesis is controlled by the motion of the intact shoulder, utilizing extended physiologic proprioception.

Philipson L, Sorbye R: Control accuracy and response time in multiple-state myoelectric control of upper-limb prostheses. Initial results in nondisabled volunteers. *Med Biol Eng Comput,* 25:289-293, 1987.

Control performance was evaluated in 49 nondisabled volunteers without previous prosthetic experience to determine their response time and control accuracy utilizing myoelectric control with complex control systems. Seven and nine control states were utilized successfully. This multifunctional control system would most likely be of value to the unilateral upper arm amputee.

Orthotics

Benjuya N, Kenney SB: Myoelectric hand orthosis. *Journal of Prosetics and Orthotics,* 2:149-154, 1989.

A myoelectric hand orthosis for utilization in two patients with C5 and C6 level spinal cord injury was presented. A flexible shaft on the forearm component is connected to the digits to allow for pinch with a force of six to seven pounds and an opening as much as 10 cm.

Wijman CAC, Stroh KC, Van Doren CL, et al: Functional evaluation of quadriplegic patients using a hand neuroprosthesis. *Arch Phys Med Rehabil,* 71:1053-1057, 1990.

A neuroprosthesis was utilized in 22 quadriplegic patients. Patients with C5 level injury had greater relative improvement with a neuroprosthesis as compared to those with C6 level injury.

Index